Hematological Complications in Obstetrics, Pregnancy, and Gynecology

There are many hematological complications associated with obstetrics, pregnancy, and gynecology and, unfortunately, they often lead to significant morbidity or mortality for both mother and child. As the first comprehensive reference on all aspects of hematological complications of obstetrics, pregnancy, and gynecology, this book will be a valuable resource to hematologists, obstetricians, gynecologists, reproductive medicine specialists, internists, anesthesiologists and others. The chapters are written by acknowledged experts in the field and, for each condition covered, the etiology, pathophysiology, clinical and laboratory diagnosis and management are discussed where appropriate.

Rodger Bick is Clinical Professor of Medicine and Pathology at the University of Texas Southwestern Medical Center (Dallas, Texas, USA).

Eugene Frenkel is Professor of Medicine at the Harold C. Simmons Comprehensive Cancer Center, University of Texas Southwestern Medical Center (Dallas, Texas, USA).

William Baker is Professor of Medicine at the University of California (Los Angeles, California, USA).

Ravindra Sarode is at the Transfusion Medicine and Coagulation Laboratory, University of Texas Southwestern Medical Center (Dallas, Texas, USA).

Hematological Complications in Obstetrics, Pregnancy, and Gynecology

Edited by

Rodger L. Bick (*Editor in Chief*)
University of Texas Southwestern Medical Center, Dallas, Texas, USA

Eugene Frenkel (*Editor*)
Harold C. Simmons Comprehensive Cancer Center, Dallas, Texas, USA

William Baker (*Editor*)
Thrombosis Center, Bakersfield, California, USA

and

Ravindra Sarode (*Editor*)
University of Texas Southwestern Medical Center, Dallas, Texas, USA

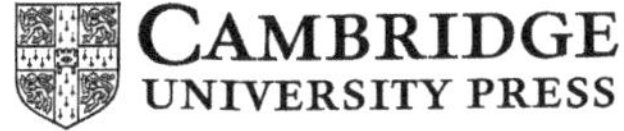

CAMBRIDGE UNIVERSITY PRESS
Cambridge, New York, Melbourne, Madrid, Cape Town, Singapore, São Paulo, Delhi

Cambridge University Press
The Edinburgh Building, Cambridge CB2 8RU, UK

Published in the United States of America by Cambridge University Press, New York

www.cambridge.org
Information on this title: www.cambridge.org/9780521108690

First published 2006
Reprinted 2007
This digitally printed version 2009

A catalogue record for this publication is available from the British Library

ISBN 978-0-521-83953-2 hardback
ISBN 978-0-521-10869-0 paperback

This textbook is dedicated to the important women in my life:

To my daughters, *Shauna Nicole Bick* and *Michelle Leanne Gage*

To the memory of my late wife, *Marcella Ann Bick*

And to:

All the hundreds of women with complications of pregnancy and their subsequent children whom I have had the privilege of caring for – this experience has been the most gratifying of my entire medical career.

Contents

Contributors

Adeboye H. Adewoye
Assistant Professor of Medicine, Department of Medicine, Section of Hematology-Oncology and the Center of Excellence in Sickle Cell Disease, Boston Medical Center, Boston, MA 02118, USA
adeboye.adewoye@bmc.org

William F. Baker Jr.
Center for Health Sciences, David Geffen School of Medicine at University of California-Los Angeles, Los Angeles, CA, USA

Rodger L. Bick
Department of Medicine, University of Texas Southwestern Medical Center, Dallas Thrombosis Hemostasis Clinical Center, 10455 North Central Expressway, Suite 109, PMB 320, Dallas, TX 75231, USA
rbick@thrombosis.com

Katharine Downes
Assistant Professor, Department of Pathology, University Hospitals of Cleveland, Cleveland, OH, USA

Jawed Fareed
Professor of Pathology and Pharmacology, Loyola University Chicago, Maywood, Illinois, USA

Arthur Fontaine
Chairman of Radiology, Mercy Hospital, 2215 Truxtun Ave., Bakersfield, CA 93301, USA

Eugene P. Frenkel
Professor of Medicine and Radiology, Harold C. Simmons Comprehensive Cancer Center, University of Texas Southwestern Medical School, 2201 Inwood Road, Dallas, TX 75235-8852, USA
eugene.frenkel@utsouthwestern.edu

Franklin Fuda
Fellow, Department of Pathology, UT Southwestern Medical Center, 5323 Harry Hines Blvd., Dallas, TX 75390-9073, USA

Barbara B. Haley
Professor of Medicine, Sherry Wigley Crow Cancer Research Endowed Chair in Honor of Robert Lewis Kirby, M.D., University of Texas Southwestern Medical School, 5323 Harry Hines Blvd., Dallas, TX 75390-8852, USA

Lothar Heilmann
Department of Obstetrics and Gynecology, City Hospital, August-Bebel-Str. 59, 65428 Russelsheim, Germany
dr_lothar_heilmann@yahoo.de

Karen Heller
Faculty Associate, Department of Pathology, University of Texas Southwestern Medical Center, Dallas, Texas, USA

Debra A. Hoppensteadt
Department of Pathology, Loyola University Medical Center, 2160 S. First Ave., Maywood, Illinois, USA
dhoppen@lumc.edu

Robyn Horsager
Associate Professor, Division of Maternal Fetal Medicine, Department of Obstetrics and Gynecology, University of Texas Southwestern Medical Center, Dallas, TX, USA

Omer Iqbal
Research Assistant Professor, Department of Pathology, Loyola University Chicago, Maywood, Illinois, USA

Ray Lee
Associate Professor of Internal Medicine University of Texas Southwestern School of Medicine, 5323 Harry Hines Blvd., Dallas, TX 75390-8889, USA
ray.lee@utsouthwestern.edu

Joseph Mansour
Associate Professor, Department of Obstetrics and Gynecology, Kern Medical Center, 1830 Flower St., Bakersfield, CA 93305, USA

Harry L. Messmore
Professor Emeritus, Department of Medicine, Loyola University Chicago, Maywood, Illinois, USA

Albert J. Phillips
Clinical Professor of Obstetrics and Gynecology, University of Southern California, School of Medicine, 1301 20th Street, Suite 270, Santa Monica, CA 90404, USA
ajphillips@pol.net

Werner Rath
Department of Obstetrics and Gynecology, University of Aachen, 52057 Aachen, Germany

Raymond W. Redline
Department of Pathology, University Hospitals of Cleveland, 11100 Euclid Avenue, Cleveland, OH 44106, USA

Ravindra Sarode
Professor, Department of Pathology, UT Southwestern Medical Center, 5323 Harry Hines Blvd., CS3.114, Dallas, TX 75390-9073, USA

Martin H. Steinberg
Professor of Medicine, Pediatrics, Pathology and Laboratory Medicine, Department of Medicine, Section of Hematology-Oncology and the Center of Excellence in Sickle Cell Disease, Boston Medical Center, Boston, MA 02118, USA

Georg-Friedrich von Tempelhoff
GP Rüsselsheim, Department of Obstetrics and Gynecology, August Bebel Strasse 59 65428 Rüsselsheim, Germany
G-F.von.Tempelhoff@gmx.de

William Wehrmacher
Professor Emeritus, Department of Physiology, Loyola University Chicago, Maywood, Illinois, USA

Preface

Hematological complications of obstetrics, pregnancy and gynecology are many, and, unfortunately, often lead to significant morbidity or mortality for both mother and child, for example disseminated intravascular coagulation, amniotic fluid embolism or postoperative deep vein thrombosis/pulmonary embolus, not only in obstetrical patients but also common in postoperative gynecological patients – particularly those having surgery for a malignancy. These complications range from hemorrhagic complications, thrombotic complications, combinations (such as disseminated intravascular coagulation), various anemias, hemoglobinopathies and others. A textbook on this topic was last written in the 1970s, and for the past several decades, hematologists, obstetricians, gynecologists, reproductive medicine specialists, internists, anesthesiologists and others have had to rely upon research reports, small clinical trials, opinion, rare review articles and very brief chapters in obstetrical and gynecological textbooks. An additional problem is that busy specialists in the aforementioned areas have a difficult time keeping up with a logarithmic increase in medical information relative to their particular areas. Thus, we have compiled a textbook, written by experienced experts in the various aspects of hematological complications of obstetrics, pregnancy and gynecology to serve as a ready reference for practicing physicians in these specialties to quickly find information relative to these problems. In each instance, where appropriate, the etiology, pathophysiology, clinical and laboratory diagnosis and management are discussed. It is hoped this text will help the practicing specialists caring for women with these hematological complications of pregnancy and the end result will be improved understanding, improved diagnosis, improved principles of management, and enhanced morbidity and mortality for these too often catastrophic problems.

1

Disseminated intravascular coagulation in obstetrics, pregnancy, and gynecology: Criteria for diagnosis and management

Rodger L. Bick, M.D., Ph.D., F.A.C.P.[1] and
Deborah Hoppensteadt, Ph.D., D.I.C.[2]

[1]Clinical Professor of Medicine and Pathology, University of Texas Southwestern Medical Center, Director: Dallas Thrombosis Hemostasis and Vascular Medicine Clinical Center, Dallas, Texas, USA
[2]Associate Professor of Pathology, Loyola University Medical Center, Maywood, Illinois, USA

Syndromes of disseminated intravascular coagulation in obstetrics, pregnancy and gynecology Objective criteria for diagnosis and management

Introduction

Disseminated intravascular coagulation is a confusing syndrome, regarding diagnostic and therapeutic modalities. Confusion and controversy stem from (1) the fact that many unrelated clinical scenario may induce DIC (2) a lack of uniformity in clinical manifestations (3) confusion regarding appropriate laboratory diagnosis and (4) unclear guidelines for management with respect to specific therapeutic modalities potentially available. Recommendations for and evaluation of management becomes even more difficult because: (1) the morbidity and survival is often dependent on the specific cause of DIC and (2) few of the generally used specific modes of therapy, heparin, antithrombin concentrate, protein C concentrate, and others, have been subjected to objective prospective randomized trials, except antithrombin concentrates.

This chapter provides specific and objective guidelines and criteria for (1) the clinical diagnosis, (2) laboratory diagnosis, and (3) to provide objective systems to assess efficacy of any given specific therapeutic modality, independent of influences of the underlying (inducing) disease causing the DIC in obstetrical, pregnancy or gynecological patients.[1,2] This approach allows for objective decisions regarding diagnosis and management in particular obstetric and gynecological settings and in

Hematological Complications in Obstetrics, Pregnancy, and Gynecology, ed. R. L. Bick *et al.* Published by Cambridge University Press.

individual patients. A general review of the etiology, pathophysiology, clinical and laboratory diagnosis, and management modalities suggested for DIC in obstetrics and gynecology is provided.

Disseminated intravascular coagulation (DIC) is an intermediary mechanism of disease usually seen in association with well-defined clinical disorders.[3,4,5,6] In obstetrics, pregnancy and gynecology, those disorders include amniotic fluid embolism, placental abruption, missed abortion, retained fetus syndrome, placenta previa (occasionally), preeclampsia/eclampsia, HELLP syndrome, ovarian cancer, uterine cancer and breast cancer. Of course, as will be discussed, the obstetric and gynecologic patient may also develop DIC secondary to other medical and surgical complications not specifically unique to obstetrics, pregnancy and gynecology, for example inflammation, infection, sepsis, etc.

The pathophysiology of DIC serves as an intermediary mechanism in many disease processes, which sometimes remain organ specific. This catastrophic syndrome spans all areas of medicine and presents a broad clinical spectrum that is confusing to many. DIC was called "consumptive coagulopathy" in early literature;[7,8] this is no longer an adequate description as very little is consumed in DIC; most factors and plasma constituents are plasmin biodegraded. Terminology following this phrase was "defibrination syndrome". The modern term is disseminated intravascular coagulation; this is a beneficial descriptive pathophysiological term if one accepts the concept that "coagulation" is expressed as both hemorrhage and thrombosis.[1,3,4,5,6] Most physicians consider DIC to be a systemic hemorrhagic syndrome however, this is only because hemorrhage is obvious and often impressive. Less commonly appreciated is the formidable microvascular thrombosis and sometimes, large vessel thrombosis occurring. The hemorrhage is often simple to contend with in patients with fulminant DIC but it is the small and large vessel thrombosis, with impairment of blood flow, ischemia, and associated end-organ damage that usually leads to irreversible morbidity and mortality. Throughout this review, fulminant DIC versus "low-grade" compensated DIC and the attendant

Table 1.1 Definition of disseminated intravascular coagulation (minimal acceptable criteria).

A systemic thrombohemorrhagic disorder seen in association with well-defined clinical situations
and
Laboratory evidence of
(1) Procoagulant activation
(2) Fibrinolytic activation
(3) Inhibitor consumption and
(4) Biochemical evidence of end-organ damage or failure

differences in clinical manifestations, laboratory findings, and treatment are discussed. However, these are often pure and theoretical, clinical spectrums of a disease continuum; patients may present anywhere in this continuum and may lapse from one end of the spectrum into another. A clear definition of DIC is outlined in Table 1.1.

Historical perspectives

The first description of disseminated intravascular coagulation comes from a lecture delivered by Dr. Walter H. Seegers titled "Factors in the Control of Bleeding".[9] Major clinical extensions of this early observation were shortly reported thereafter by Dr's. Ratnoff, Pritcher, and Colopy in an article entitled "Hemorrhagic States During Pregnancy."[10,11] In this two part article, many important observations were described including recognition that the hemorrhagic syndromes of pregnancy, now called DIC, included premature separation of the placenta, amniotic fluid embolism, the presence of a dead fetus in utero and severe pre-eclampsia or overt toxemia of pregnancy. Subsequently, more reports and descriptions of disseminated intravascular coagulation began to appear and in the mid-1960's, DIC became a clinically accepted and recognized syndrome. We owe our basic understanding and appreciation of this syndrome to the astute clinical and laboratory observations of Dr. Walter H. Seegers and Dr. Oscar D. Ratnoff and their co-workers.

Etiology

DIC is usually seen in association with well-defined clinical entities.[1,2,3,4,5,6,12,13] Those clinical disorders specific for obstetrics and gynecology are found in Table 1.2. The clinical disorders common to all medical specialties, and sometimes complicating the course of an obstetrical or gynecological patient and inducing to DIC are summarized in Table 1.3.

DIC syndromes unique to pregnancy and obstetrics

Obstetrical accidents are common events leading to disseminated intravascular coagulation. Amniotic fluid embolism with DIC is the most catastrophic and common of the life threatening obstetrical accidents.[1,2,4,5,6,7]

The syndrome of amniotic fluid embolism (AFE) is manifest by the acute onset of respiratory failure, circulatory collapse, shock and the serious thrombohemorrhagic syndrome of disseminated intravascular coagulation (DIC). The first careful description of this syndrome was by Steiner and Lushbaugh in 1941;[14] in

Table 1.2 Common causes of DIC syndromes in obstetrics and gynecology.

Obstetric accidents
Amniotic fluid embolism
Placental abruption
Placenta prevea
Prceclampsia
Eclampsia
HELLP syndrome
Retained fetus syndrome
Abortion
Gynecologic malignancy
Ovarian cancer
Uterine cancer
Breast cancer
Paraneoplastic syndromes

this landmark article, these authors describe the clinical histories of 8 obstetrical patients and demonstrated that these patients formed a distinct group with a unique pathophysiologic basis for the constellation of symptoms now associated with this syndrome. These authors were also able to duplicate this syndrome in animal models and demonstrated that amniotic fluid embolism is a relatively common cause of sudden death during labor or in the immediate post-labor period. These eight patients came from 4,000 consecutive autopsies performed over a period of 15 years, representing an incidence of 0.2% of deaths in this autopsy series. In this study, it was noted that these 8 cases were among a total of 24,200 deliveries, representing an incidence of 1 in 8,000 of their obstetrical cases. When analyzing their obstetrical deaths these authors were the first to show that amniotic fluid embolism was the most common cause of maternal death in the period during labor and within the first nine hours after labor.

Etiology of AFE

The common etiologic factor in the syndrome of amniotic fluid embolism is the entrance, by various proposed mechanisms and routes, of amniotic fluid, with or without meconium, into the systemic maternal circulation followed by embolization of amniotic fluid and it's contents to the lungs; subsequently, circulatory collapse and the development of disseminated intravascular

Table 1.3 Accepted disease entities generally associated with DIC.

Fulminant DIC	Low-grade DIC
Intravascular hemolysis	Cardiovascular diseases
Hemolytic transfusion reactions	Peripheral vascular diseases
Autoimmune diseases	Autoimmune disorders
Minor hemolysis	Renal vascular disorders
Massive transfusions	Hematologic disorders
	Inflammatory disorders
Septicemia	
Gram negative (endotoxin)	
Gram positive (mucopolysaccharides)	
Viremias	
HIV	
Hepatitis	
Varicella	
Cytomegalovirus	
Metastatic malignancy	
Leukemia	
Acute promyelocytic (M-3)	
Acute myelomonocytic (M-4)	
Many others	
Burns	
Crush injuries and tissue necrosis	
Trauma	
Acute liver disease	
Obstructive jaundice	
Acute hepatic failure	
Prosthetic devices	
Leveen or denver shunts	
Aortic balloon assist devices	
Vascular disorders	

coagulation occurs almost uniformly and instantaneously.[15] The incidence has been reported to be between 1 in 8,000 and 1 and 30,000 births.[16,17] The syndrome is commonly fatal for both the mother and child.[16] The mortality for the mother is generally 60%–80% and 50% of survivors have permanent neurological sequelae.[18,19] One recent series, however, reported a 26.4% mortality.[20] Of those surviving, thrombotic stroke is a major sequelae.[18,21,22] While the finding of amniotic fluid in maternal blood is not physiological there have been instances where

Table 1.4 Amniotic fluid embolism risk factors.

Older age
Multiparity
Physiologic intense uterine contractions
Drug-induced intense uterine contractions
Cesarean section
High cervical tear
Premature placental separation
Intra-uterine fetal death
Placental abruption
Trauma to abdomen
80% of cases develop during labor
20% may develop before or after labor

amniotic fluid may enter the systemic maternal circulation without any significant manifestations of this catastrophic syndrome.[15] In 1970, it was noted that the syndrome of amniotic fluid embolism represented 10% of all maternal deaths and a study in Sweden from 1965 to 1974 demonstrated that the syndrome of amniotic fluid embolism accounted for 22% of all maternal deaths.[15,23] Asner and co-workers have described amniotic fluid embolism to account for DIC in only 1 of 6 patients with clinically obvious disseminated intravascular coagulation and in none of 35 obstetrical patients with laboratory evidence of disseminated intravascular coagulation.[24] However, it has also been noted in a combined retrospective and prospective study of disseminated intravascular coagulation taken from the records of Massachusetts General Hospital, consisting of 60 prospectively studied patients and 15 retrospectively studied patients, that not one of these patients developed DIC in association with amniotic fluid embolism.[25] However, of these 75 DIC patients, 3 were associated with various other obstetrical accidents. Thus, when assessing the etiologic "triggers" of patients with DIC as a group, amniotic fluid embolism is quite rare. The risk factors associated with development of amniotic fluid embolism (Table 1.4) consist of older age, multiparity, marked exaggeration of uterine contraction following rupture of the uterine membranes, or markedly exaggerated uterine contraction due to the use of oxytocics or other uterine stimulatory agents, cesarean section, uterine rupture, high cervical laceration, premature separation of the placenta and intra-uterine fetal death.[17,26,27] Other factors have been spontaneous rupture of the fetal membranes and blunt trauma to the abdomen.[28,29] The syndrome can, on rare occasions, occur late in pregnancy but most commonly occurs during labor in 80% of patients; in only up to 20% of patients does the syndrome occur before labor

Table 1.5 Amniotic fluid embolism: General characteristics.

1 in 8,000 to 1 in 30,000 deliveries
10% of all maternal deaths in USA
22% of all maternal deaths in Sweden
80% overall mortality
25% will die within one hour
50% with fetal death or distress before maternal symptoms

begins and before rupture of the amniotic sac.[30,31] Twenty-five percent of women die within one hour of developing this syndrome and up to 80% will die within the first nine hours.[32,33] In 10% of women the syndrome develops without warning, usually during delivery, as amniotic fluid enters the systemic maternal circulation during an apparently normal labor and delivery unassociated with pre-delivery complications.

There is generally rapid onset of signs and symptoms of pulmonary failure and circulatory collapse; in at least 50% of patients this is followed by systemic bleeding. Fifty percent of fetuses die or develop intra-uterine asphyxia/distress before the sudden maternal onset of acute respiratory failure and circulatory collapse. In one series of 30,000 deliveries described by Graeff, there were six cases of amniotic fluid embolism; two patients died and four recovered.[15] The syndrome has also been described to occur immediately post-delivery but almost always occurs during delivery. Typically, the patient is in active delivery with the amnion intact and suddenly develops respiratory failure and circulatory collapse followed by a systemic thrombohemorrhagic disorder. The cause is only partially understood but the common etiologic event is entrance into the systemic maternal circulation of amniotic fluid which then causes extensive pulmonary micro-circulatory occlusion and local pulmonary activation of the procoagulant system; in addition, there is systemic activation of the procoagulant system.[34,35] This occurs in conjunction with intense induction of pulmonary fibrinolytic activity, presumably via release of pulmonary endothelial plasminogen activator activity in the lungs.[36,37]

Since this is a life threatening and not uncommon syndrome, all clinicians involved with obstetrics and care during delivery should be familiar with the potential of this syndrome when a patient presents with the risk factors depicted in Table 1.4, and when a patient immediately preceding, during, or immediately after delivery suddenly develops respiratory distress, shock and uncontrolled bleeding. The general characteristics of amniotic fluid embolism are presented in Table 1.5.

Pathophysiology of AFE

Amniotic fluid contains much cellular material including vernix caseosa, squamous epithelial cells and debris from the fetus.[17,38] The lipid content, cellular content, fetal debris, procoagulant activity and viscosity of amniotic fluid increase with duration of pregnancy and is at a maximum at time of delivery.[15,39,40] In most incidences, the actual mechanism(s) and site of entry of amniotic fluid into the uterine and subsequently, the systemic maternal circulation remain unclear. Indeed, several investigators examining pathologic specimens of patients with amniotic fluid embolism have, in most incidences, been unable to clearly define portals of entry.[41,42] Thus, the mechanism(s) by which amniotic fluid enters the maternal circulation in general often remains undefined. However, lacerations of the membrane and placenta may be portals of entry to the maternal venous sinuses in the uterus.[15] Entrance may be via a tear in the membranes at the placental margin with compression-injection of fluid into the maternal vessels or lacerated veins in the posterior vaginal wall or the entrance of amniotic fluid into the systemic maternal circulation may occur in the face of defect in the fetal membranes if this defect is in proximity to areas of maternal venous vessels.[15] In general, the site of entry is thought to be the area of the placental insertion or the area of the lower uterus or cervix.[15] It is possible that the cervical veins which open during labor permit entry of amniotic fluid after rupture of the membranes when the fetal head obstructs the intracervical canal, therefore blocking drainage and causing retrograde (upward) hydrostatic pressure thereby injecting amniotic fluid into open cervical veins and thus allowing entrance into the systemic returning circulation.[15] It is clear that amniotic fluid may enter the maternal circulation via a rupture of the uterus or through an abnormal placental placement site or as a part of the placental abruption syndrome. If meconium accompanies the amniotic fluid, the syndrome is accompanied by more intense DIC than occurs without meconium.[43] There appears to be many possible mechanisms by which amniotic fluid may enter the uterine and subsequently the systemic maternal circulation; however, these mechanisms are rarely documented on pathologic analysis.[41,42] Figure 1.1 demonstrates a fetal squamous cell in the maternal pulmonary microcirculation. It has recently been demonstrated that the monoclonal antibody THK-2 may be a specific pathological marker for amniotic fluid embolism.[44,45] Another suggestion is that finding fetal megakaryocytes and syncytiotrophoblastic cells in the maternal pulmonary circulation by monoclonal antibodies (CD-61 – GPIIIa, Beta-HCG and Factor VIII-vW hPL antibodies) may be diagnostic.[46]

On entering the systemic maternal circulation amniotic fluid simultaneously activates the procoagulant system leading to profound disseminated intravascular coagulation, and addition, causes intense and extensive pulmonary micro-embolization via

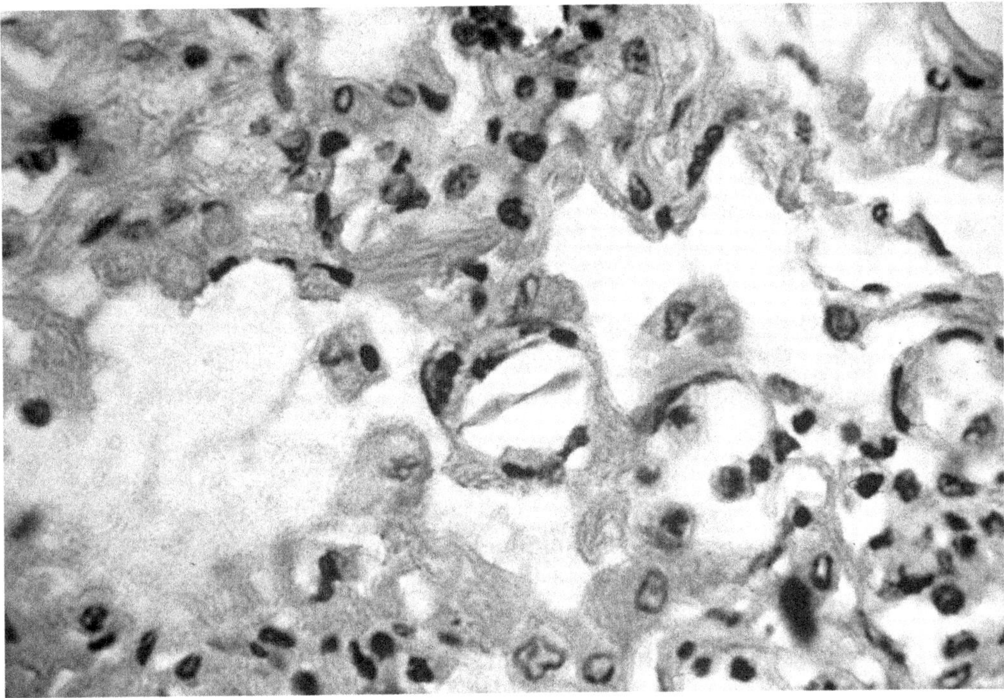

Figure 1.1 Fetal squamous cell in maternal pulmonary circulation.

not only activation of the coagulation system, but also due to hyperviscous amniotic fluid and amniotic fluid debris. As noted, this process appears more pronounced in the presence of meconium contamination.[43]

Pulmonary pathophysiology in AFE

The severity of the pulmonary manifestations are highly dependent upon the contents, amount and viscosity of amniotic fluid reaching the maternal pulmonary circulation. Of course, the higher the content of cellular elements the more viscous the material will be with cellular elements being vernix, caseosa and fetal squamous epithelial cells and complexes of squamous cellular material.[15,17] Amniotic fluid itself, as well as amniotic fluid content, will mechanically obstruct the pulmonary circulation occluding both large and small vessels with the subsequent usual manifestations of severe pulmonary embolization. This then leads to defective perfusion, defective diffusion capacity and intense vaso-constriction which, in turn, is accompanied by right heart failure and the findings of acute cor pulmonale, increased pulmonary artery pressure with subsequent decreased left ventricular filling, decreased cardiac output and resultant tissue hypoxia and ischemia, metabolic acidosis and finally, cardiogenic shock.

Hemostasis pathophysiology in AFE

Amniotic fluid contains a highly potent total thromboplastin-like activity; this procoagulant activity increases with time of gestation.[39,40] In addition, amniotic fluid contains a relatively strong anti-fibrinolytic activity and, as such, causes a non-specific inhibition of the fibrinolytic system; this activity of amniotic fluid also increases during gestation.[24] The fibrinolytic inhibition activity may predispose a patient to DIC and diffuse thrombotic phenomenon by inhibiting or dampering the usual secondary fibrinolytic response seen in DIC patients.[1,2,34] The secondary fibrinolytic response which usually occurs in DIC is responsible for hemorrhage due to plasmin digestion of numerous clotting factors; however, this secondary fibrinolytic response also serves to help keep the circulation free of thrombi.[47] It remains controversial if amniotic fluid itself has a direct effect on the vasculature or if this is a secondary effect of procoagulant/platelet activation.[48] However, Endothelin – 1, a potent vasoconstrictor and bronchoconstrictor, appears to be released, systemically, from circulating fetal squamous cells and may intensify the severe hemodynamic alterations noted in amniotic fluid embolism.[49]

The procoagulant activity of amniotic fluid correlates very well with the lecithin/sphingomyelin (LS) ratio during gestation.[50] Amniotic fluid, in vitro, will accelerate the prothrombin time, the activated partial thromboplastin time, the Russell's Viper Venom time and will accelerating the clotting of Factor VII deficient plasma.[51] Thus, amniotic fluid not only acts as a "total thromboplastin", but acts as a substitute for "tissue phase activation". The mechanism(s) by which amniotic fluid activates the procoagulant system is by the direct activation of Factor X, in the presence of calcium ions, to Factor Xa.[52] Factor Xa is one of the most thrombogenic substances known. Factor Xa, in the presence of Factor V and additional phospholipid (including amniotic fluid and platelet surfaces) will rapidly convert prothrombin to thrombin. Once thrombin is formed, fibrinogen is converted to fibrin.[53] Thus patients with amniotic fluid embolism may develop platelet-fibrin microthrombi throughout the systemic and pulmonary circulation. This disseminated intravascular coagulation syndrome is therefore associated with micro-circulatory thrombosis, thrombo-embolism, and hemorrhage. The pathophysiology of activation in AFE is depicted in Figure 1.2. The pathophysiology of disseminated intravascular coagulation, associated with hemorrhage and thrombosis throughout the circulation is depicted in Figure 1.3.

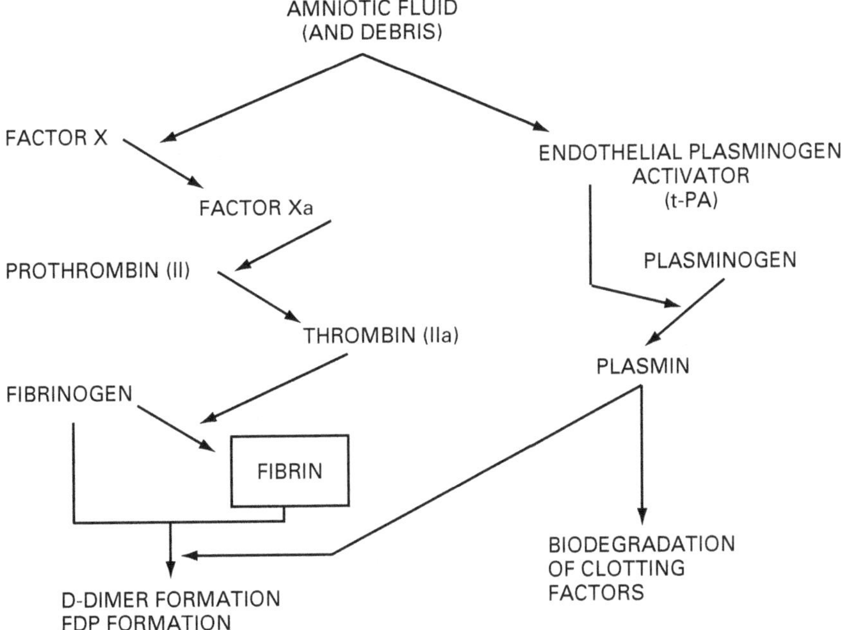

Figure 1.2 Pathophysiology of activation in AFE.

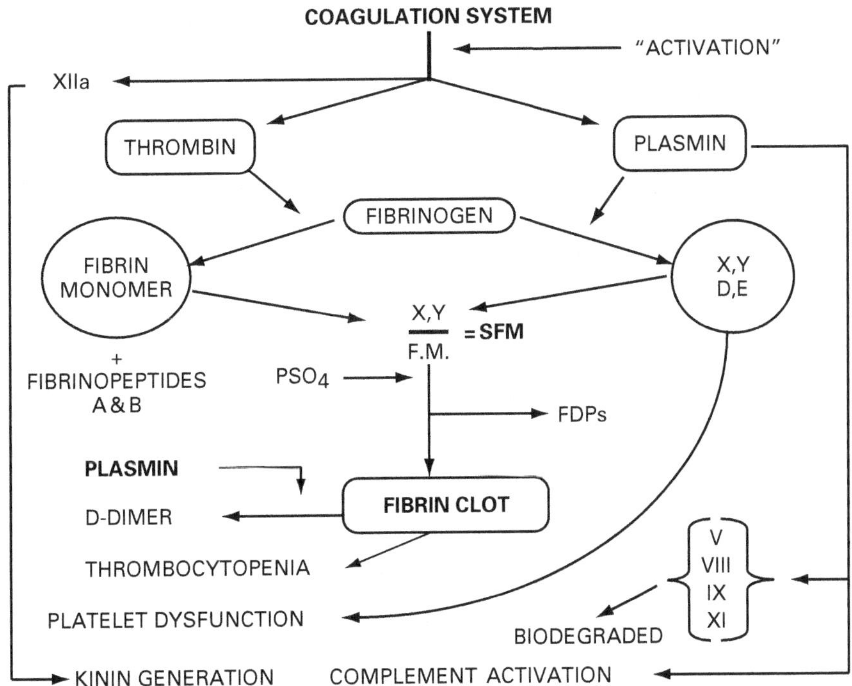

Figure 1.3 Pathophysiology of DIC.

Diagnosis of AFE

The diagnosis of amniotic fluid embolism should be strongly suspected when there is a sudden development of acute respiratory failure in an otherwise normal delivery. The acute respiratory failure occurs from occlusion of pulmonary vessels by amniotic fluid, intense vasoconstriction of pulmonary vessels and then further occlusion by platelet-fibrin thrombi. This initial event is usually followed by cardiogenic shock and systemic cardiovascular and pulmonary collapse. The usual clinical findings of acute pulmonary insufficiency are the sudden onset of tachypnea, dyspnea and peripheral cyanosis due to the abrupt development of abnormal perfusion and diffusion. These findings are usually accompanied by acute cor pulmonale with resultant right sided failure with subsequent decreased filling of the left ventricle and low output failure with subsequent peripheral end organ hypoxia, ischemia and metabolic acidosis. Arterial blood gases will reveal decreased PO_2 and PCO_2. Abnormal diffusion capacity, metabolic acidosis, and elevating central venous pressure will also be noted.

These events typically occur early in delivery and are usually without any clinical warning. Following the development of acute respiratory failure, cardiogenic shock, and peripheral circulatory collapse, there will usually be excessive uterine bleeding followed by systemic bleeding from multiple sites. As DIC develops, the sites of bleeding can be numerous and unpredictable; however, the most common bleeding sites noted will be oozing from IV puncture sites, hematuria, hemoptysis and, at times, intracranial bleeding.[1,2] In addition, the development of petechia and purpura usually are rapidly noted throughout the skin and mucosal membranes. As DIC progresses, there will be additional systemic microcirculatory occlusion by platelet-fibrin thrombi in multiple end organs, especially the renal, hepatic and central nervous system. This will further compromise adequate end-organ perfusion and thus lead to even more compromised end-organ hypoxia, ischemia and failure. The most reliable laboratory test to evaluate the development of DIC are the AT-III level, Fibrinopeptide A level, D-Dimer level, Prothrombin Fragment 1.2 (PF 1.2) and platelet count. More global tests, including the PT, PTT and fibrinogen level are helpful if abnormal; however, these tests may frequently be normal in DIC (discussed in detail in Laboratory Diagnosis of DIC section).

Management of AFE

The approach to management of acute respiratory failure is straightforward and consists of immediate establishment of an airway by use of an oropharyngeal tube, an endotracheal tube, or tracheostomy. Oxygen should be started immediately via nasal cannula or prongs, venturi mask, or a reservoir mask. A mechanical ventilator will probably be needed. Circulatory collapse must be managed immediately with the use of vaso-constrictive agents, usually dopamine. A central venous line should immediately be established and the central venous pressure carefully monitored. The patient should be digitalized if the central venous pressure is elevated. There should also be immediate institution of measures to induce uterine contraction and thus reduce bleeding from the placental site and uterus. Circulatory collapse is further managed by volume replacement. Those surviving amniotic fluid embolism have been treated with large amounts of blood and blood components.[54,55] One report suggests aerosolized prostacyclin may be highly effective.[56] Management of DIC should be via immediate consideration of heparinization or antithrombin concentrate to quickly stop the further deposition of platelet-fibrin thrombi and to stop the further generation of activated coagulation factors.[1,2,57] This author chooses to use antithrombin concentrate or subcutaneous unfractionated (UF) heparin at 100 units per kilogram, q 6 hours in this clinical setting or Low Molecular Weight (LMW) Heparin at 100–150 units/kg every 12–24 hours.[1,2] Following heparinization or antithrombin infusion, DIC should be further managed with the use of component therapy in the form of fresh frozen plasma and platelets depending upon the prothrombin time, PTT, and platelet count and sites and severity of hemorrhage. If there is enough time, and if available, antithrombin concentrates should be used to control DIC.[58,59,60,61] The neonate, if surviving birth, will usually require resuscitation and assessment for DIC.[61] The sequential management of amniotic fluid embolism is summarized in Table 1.6.

Placental abruption may induce DIC. In placental abruption with DIC, placental enzymes or tissues including procoagulants and thromboplastin-like material may be released into the uterine and next the systemic maternal circulation and lead to activation of the coagulation system. Rapid initiation of delivery will almost always cause cessation of DIC and only rarely are other treatment modalities needed.[1,2,3,4,5,6,12,13,62,63]

In the retained fetus syndrome, the incidence of DIC approaches 50% if the woman retains a dead fetus in-utero for greater than 5 weeks. The first findings are usually those of a low-grade compensated DIC which then progresses into a fulminant thrombohemorrhagic form. In this instance necrotic fetal tissue, including enzymes derived from necrotic fetal tissue, are released into the uterine and then the systemic maternal circulation and act at diverse sites to activate the procoagulant and fibrinolytic systems and trigger fulminant DIC.[1,2,3,4,5,6,7,12,13,62,63,64,65]

Toxemia of pregnancy is referred to as preeclampsia or eclampsia. Peeclampsia, usually occurring in the third trimester, is characterized by hypertension, edema, proteinuria, sodium retention, hyperreflexia and DIC. When frank convulsions

Table 1.6 Management of amniotic fluid embolism.

I. Treat respiratory failure
- Airway
- Mechanical ventilation

II. Treat shock and heart failure
- Vasopressors
- Digitalis preparations
- Fluids and electrolytes
- Establish central line

III. Treat hemorrhage and DIC
- Subcutaneous LMW heparin *or*
- Subcutaneous UF heparin
- Antithrombin concentrates
- Packed red blood cells as needed
- Platelets as needed
- Evacuate uterus
- Uterine contractions as needed
- Prostacyclins

LMW = low molecular weight
UF = unfractionated

occur in the face of preeclampsia, the term eclampsia is used to define the syndrome.[66] Preeclampsia, eclampsia and HELLP syndrome (discussed subsequently) appear to constitute a progressive spectrum of the same pathophysiological processes. Unfortunately, the pathophysiology remains elusive. It remains unclear if the process starts as one of endothelial damage which then activates procoagulant proteins and platelets or if the process starts as a procoagulant/platelet problem which then damages endothelium; most likely, the former is at play. If a woman develops eclampsia, the chances of developing isolated thrombocytopenia are about 18%, the chances of developing DIC are about 11% and the chances of developing HELLP syndrome are about 15%.[67,68] Also, in preeclampsia/eclampsia if a coagulation defect develops (thrombocytopenia, HELLP, and/or DIC) the maternal mortality is between 16%[159] to over 50%[68] and the perinatal mortality may be greater than 40%.[69] In addition, about 16% of patients with preeclampsia/eclampsia will develop placental abruption, thus enhancing probability of DIC and maternal/fetal demise.[68] In eclampsia DIC often remains low-grade and organ specific to the renal and placental microcirculation; however, in at least 10%–15% of women the process becomes systemic and fulminant.[1,2,70] Laboratory monitoring of hemostasis parameters has been found useful for assessing

Table 1.7 Features of preeclampsia/eclampsia.

1. Usually begins in third trimester
2. Usually occurs in primagravidas
3. Hypertension
4. Proteinuria
5. Edema
6. Oliguria +/−
7. Sodium retention
8. Hyperreflexia (preeclampsia)
9. Seizures (eclampsia)
10. Disseminated intravascular coagulation

potential progression from mild preeclampsia to more catastrophic syndromes of HELLP and DIC; these include the D-Dimer level, Thrombin-Antithrombin (TAT) complex, Prothrombin Fragment 1.2, plasminogen activator inhibitor Type-1 (PAI-1) and soluble fibrin monomer, all of which will progressively increase while fibrinogen, antithrombin, and plasminogen activator inhibitor Type 2 (PAI-2) will decrease.[71,72] Characteristics of eclampsia and complications are summarized in Table 1.7.

HELLP syndrome is generally thought to be a progression or complication of preeclampsia/eclampsia and comprises (1) microangiopathic *H*emolytic anemia (2) *E*levated *L*iver enzymes and (3) *L*ow *P*latelet count. HELLP syndrome occurs in about 0.5%–0.9% of all pregnancies[73,74,75] and between 15%–26% of preeclampsia/eclampsia patients.[67,76] The maternal mortality varies between 1.0% to 4%[77] and the perinatal mortality may be as high as 40%.[77,78] Some patients develop a prodrome of weakness and fatigue, nausea and vomiting, abdominal pain (particularly in the right upper quadrant), headache, visual changes and shoulder or neck pain.[78] In some women, the syndrome occurs post-partum.[74] The pathophysiology is poorly understood, but is thought due to initial inadequate placental vasculature with placental ischemia leading to systemic release of thromboxanes, angiotension, procoagulant prostaglandins, endothelin-1 and Tumor Necrosis Factor-alpha (TNF-α).[74,79] The subsequent DIC leads to micro and macrothrombi, with the placental, ovarian, renal, hepatic and cerebral vasculature being the most commonly involved. The thrombi then lead to endothelial damage and microangiopathic hemolytic anemia and, of course, varying degrees of end-organ failure in the organs involved with micro/macrothrombi. This includes not only hepatic failure, but also renal and pulmonary failure and cerebral edema and/or infarct.[80,81] Hepatic rupture is a catastrophic event in HELLP syndrome.[82,83] Laboratory monitoring for early DIC, as discussed above for preeclampsia, is recommended. Therapy is usually prompt delivery, control of hypertension and control of DIC; many have demonstrated efficacy of steroid therapy[84,85,86,87] and plasma exchange/plasmapheresis has been beneficial in some cases.[88,89] Maternal death is most commonly due to manifestations of uncontrolled DIC.[90]

Many patients enduring hypertonic saline-induced abortion develop a DIC-type process which, sometimes, becomes fulminant and at other times remains compensated until the abortion is completed.[91]

Obstetrical patients developing other complications not unique to obstetrics may also develop DIC; these conditions will be discussed subsequently.

DIC syndromes unique to gynecology

The most common setting for DIC in gynecological patients is malignancy; however, like obstetric patients, medical and surgical complications not limited to gynecology may also provide a triggering of DIC.

DIC is commonly seen with ovarian carcinoma, with or without complicating hemolytic anemia[2,92,93,94,95,96,97] and may be seen with metastatic uterine carcinoma.[98] Breast cancer may also be complicated by DIC.[92,93,94,96,97] Although thrombosis is more commonly the abnormality of hemostasis manifest with gynecological malignancies and hemorrhage is more commonly associated with acute leukemias, hemorrhage may be a significant clinical problem in patients with solid tumors as well.[96,97,99] Intravascular coagulation is present in many patients with malignancy and manifests varying clinical expressions, the most extreme form being acute fulminant disseminated intravascular coagulation with catastrophic hemorrhage and thrombosis.[62,96,97,100] DIC in cancer patients may be low-grade or fulminant. Patients with fulminant DIC will manifest oozing from intravenous sites or sites of other invasive procedures, such as intra-arterial lines, subclavian catheters, and hepatic artery catheters.[12,13,100,101,102,103,104] Although these are the most common bleeding manifestations, more life-threatening bleeding, such as intracranial and intrapulmonary hemorrhage with massive hemoptysis may also happen. Fulminant disseminated intravascular coagulation may be noted in association with carcinoma of the uterus, breast, and ovary. Initiation of chemotherapy has occasionally been associated with triggering or acceleration of disseminated intravascular coagulation.[97,105,106,107,108] Most patients with disseminated solid malignancy have some laboratory or clinical evidence of DIC; many patients with malignancy never develop clinical manifestations of DIC, but if one looks for laboratory findings of DIC, these are usually present. If present, molecular markers of activation should be monitored for evidence of progression to overt DIC and treatment instituted, when warranted. The patient with disseminated malignancy represents a special problem since DIC may be manifest as a fulminant, subacute, or low-grade form, and may, therefore be manifest as local thrombosis, diffuse thrombosis, thromboembolism, minor hemorrhage, diffuse hemorrhage, or any combination thereof.[12,13,97,102,103,104,109]

In patients with adenocarcinoma of gynecologic sites, the mechanism for disseminated intravascular coagulation may be multifaceted. However, the sialic acid moiety of secreted mucin from adenocarcinomatous tissue can invoke the non-enzymatic activation of Factor X to Factor Xa.[110,111] This can easily provide a trigger for systemic thrombin generation and a later course of fulminant or subacute disseminated intravascular coagulation.[12,109,112] Also, this sequence may lead to thrombosis alone.[12,100,102,113] It is probable that other less clearly defined mechanisms exist for initiating DIC in these malignancies. The systemic release of necrotic tumor tissue and/or enzymes with procoagulant or phospholipoprotein-like activity may activate the early phases of coagulation and/or platelet release. Also, many tumors undergo neovascularization; this process may produce abnormal endothelial cell lining which may either cause a platelet release or generation of Factor XIIa and XIa with subsequent procoagulant activation and the development of a fulminant, subacute, or low-grade DIC process. Another trigger for disseminated intravascular coagulation in the patient with malignancy is the use of LeVeen or Denver shunts for malignant ascites, commonly utilized in gynecological malignancies. Patients with malignant ascites must be carefully chosen for this procedure; if ascitic fluid is positive for malignant cells the placement of a LeVeen shunt is usually not successful,[114] does not lead to significant prolongation of quality life, and is commonly associated with the development of DIC.[1,12,13,115,116,117] DIC may be blunted or aborted by removal of ascitic fluid at the time of shunt placement.[118] Also, in this clinical setting a less common although significant complication of LeVeen shunting in the patient with malignant ascites is that of thromboembolism.[118]

DIC syndromes found in obstetrics, pregnancy, and gynecology complicated by or associated with other medical settings

Intravascular hemolysis of any etiology is a common cause of DIC. A frank hemolytic transfusion reaction is a triggering event for DIC; however, hemolysis of any etiology, even though minor, may trigger intravascular coagulation. During hemolysis the release of red cell ADP or red cell membrane phospholipoprotein activates the procoagulant system and a combination of these may account for DIC associated with major or minor hemolysis.[13,62,119,120,121,122]

Septicemia is often associated with DIC and certainly infection and septicemia is not uncommon in obstetrics and gynecology. An early organism to be associated with DIC was meningococcus.[123] Later, other gram-negative organisms were also associated with DIC.[124,125] The triggering mechanisms consist of the initiation of coagulation by endotoxin: bacterial coat lipopolysaccharide.[126,127,128] Endotoxin activates Factor XII to Factor XIIa, induces a platelet release reaction, causes endothelial sloughing with later activation of XII to XIIa or XI to XIa, and releases granulocyte procoagulant materials; any one of which might independently trigger DIC. What is most common is a clinical summation of several or all these activation events. Subsequently, many gram-positive organisms were also noted to be associated with DIC and the mechanisms have been aptly described.[3,5,13,62,129,130] Bacterial coat mucopolysaccharides induce DIC by the same mechanisms noted with endotoxin. However, as with gram-negative endotoxemia what is seen clinically is probably a summation of several or all these activation events.[3,5,13,62]

Many viremias seen in obstetric or gynecological patients, including Human Immunodeficiency Virus (HIV), are associated with DIC; the most common are varicella, hepatitis, or cytomegalovirus infections.[131,132] Many other acute viremias also induce DIC.[3,5,13,62] The triggering mechanisms are unclear but may represent antigen-antibody associated activation of Factor XII, a platelet release reaction, or endothelial sloughing with subsequent exposure of subendothelial collagen and basement membrane.[133]

Severe viral hepatitis and acute hepatic failure of any etiology, including drug, toxin or infectious can lead to DIC, which can be difficult to separate from the myriad of other coagulation abnormalities associated with severe hepatic dysfunction. Also, intrahepatic or extrahepatic cholestasis, especially when present for greater than five days, may be accompanied by DIC.[3,5,13,62]

Acidosis, and less commonly alkalosis, may also provide triggers for DIC.[3,5,13,62] In acidosis the triggering event is probably endothelial sloughing with the attendant activation of XII to XIIa and/or XI to XIa and/or platelet release with a later activation of the procoagulant system. However, the mechanisms in alkalosis are unclear. Vascular disorders may also be associated with DIC.[2,16]

Figure 1.4 illustrates the mechanisms by which a broad spectrum of unrelated pathophysiological insults found in obstetrics, gynecology or complications seen in these patients may give rise to the same common ultimate pathway, the syndrome of disseminated intravascular coagulation. There are many disorders associated with endothelial damage, circulating antigen-antibody complexes, endotoxemia, tissue damage, platelet damage or release, and red cell damage.[3,5,13,62,134] When one of these insults happens, there are many potential activation pathways by which systemically circulating plasmin and circulating thrombin may arise; when these two enzymes are circulating systemically, DIC is the usual result.[3,5,13,62,134] Conversely, both enzymes must be present for development of DIC. Frequently, the pathways leading from the first pathophysiological insult to the generation of systemic thrombin and plasmin are different; despite the differences in initiating the activation pathway, once triggered the resultant pathophysiology of DIC is the same.[3,5,13,62]

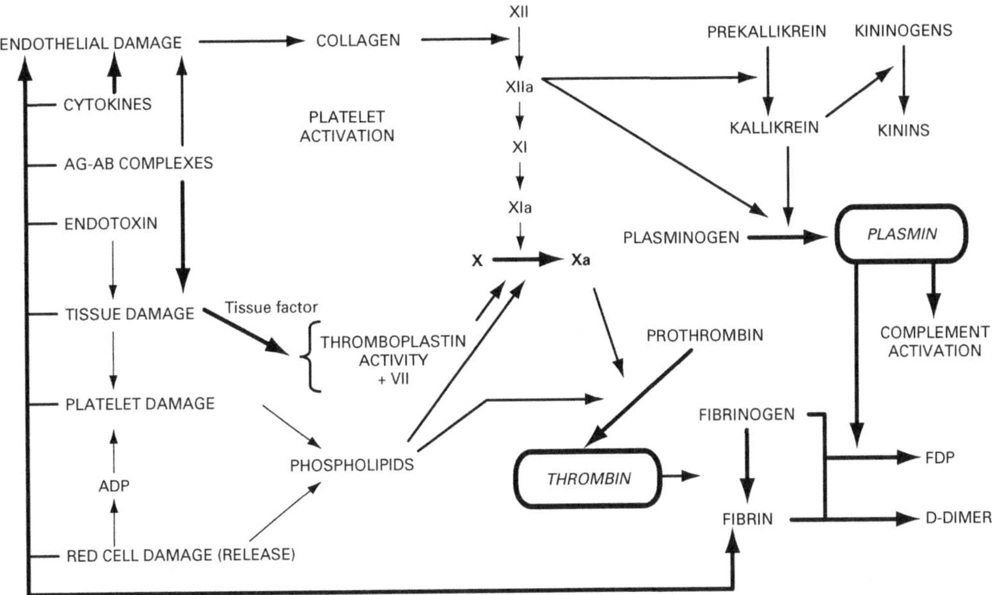

Figure 1.4 Triggering mechanisms for DIC.

Pathophysiological events

The pathophysiology of DIC, once a triggering event is provided, is summarized in Figure 1.3. After the coagulation system has been activated and both thrombin and plasmin circulate systemically, the pathophysiology of DIC is similar in all disorders. An exception may be the slight variant outlined for amniotic fluid embolism as depicted in Figure 1.2.

Consequences of systemic thrombin activity

When thrombin circulates systemically, fibrinopeptides A and B are cleaved from fibrinogen leaving behind fibrin monomer. Fibrin monomer polymerizes into fibrin (clot) in the circulation, leading to microvascular and macrovascular thrombosis and interference with blood flow, peripheral ischemia, and end-organ damage.[62,63,134,135] As fibrin is deposited in the microcirculation, platelets become trapped and thrombocytopenia follows.[4,62,63] On the other side of the "circle" depicted in Figure 1.3, plasmin also circulates systemically and cleaves the carboxy-terminal end of fibrinogen into fibrin(ogen) degradation products, creating the clinically recognized X, Y, D, and E fragments.[4,62,63,134,136,137,138] Plasmin also rapidly releases specific peptides, the B-beta 15–42 and related peptides, which may serve as diagnostic molecular markers. Fibrin(ogen) degradation products

(FDP) may combine with circulating fibrin monomer before polymerization and the fibrin monomer becomes "solubilized." This complex of FDPs and fibrin monomer is called soluble fibrin monomer; the presence of soluble fibrin monomer forms the basis of the "paracoagulation" reactions, the ethanol gelation and protamine sulfate tests.[139,140,141] When adding protamine sulfate or ethanol to a citrated tube of patient plasma containing soluble fibrin monomer, the ethanol or protamine sulfate will clear the fibrin(ogen) degradation products from fibrin monomer, fibrin monomer will complex and polymerize, hence, fibrin strands are formed in the test tube and this is interpreted as a positive protamine sulfate or ethanol gelation test.[5,12,140,142] Thus, systemically circulating fibrin(ogen) degradation products interfere with fibrin monomer polymerization; this further impairs hemostasis and leads to hemorrhage.[5,12,112] The later fragments (D and E) have a high affinity for platelet membranes and induce a profound platelet function defect.[5,12,143,144,145] Platelets remaining in the circulation are dysfunctional and may also lead to, or contribute to, clinically significant hemorrhage. FDP and D-Dimer, discussed later, induce synthesis and release of monocyte/macrophage-derived I. L.-1, I. L. 6 and plasminogen activator inhibitor-type (PAI-1); I. L.-1 and I. L.-6 induce additional vascular endothelial damage and disruption, thus more end-organ damage and elevated PAI-1 inhibits fibrinolysis, leading to accelerated thrombus formation.[146] Thrombin also induces monocyte release of Tumor Necrosis Factor (TNF), Interleukin-1 (I. L.-1), I. L.-6 and may induce endothelial release of soluble thrombomodulin and endothelin and selectin.[147,148] The endothelin release induced intense vasoconstriction, vasospasm and subsequent thrombus and vascular occlusion, leading to more end-organ damage and failure.[73] The selectin E (also known as ELAM-1) release binds to granulocytes and lymphocytes, monocytes/macrophages, inducing more cytokine release and release of Platelet Activating Factor (PAF), which may also be derived from damaged endothelium, mast cells, eosinophils, and platelets; PAF induces further thrombocytopenia.[73,148,149] Additionally, FDP are thought to induce monocyte release of monocyte-derived I. L.-1 and tissue factor (TF).[146] The release of I. L.-1 and tissue factor from monocytes both enhance thrombosis.[150] The release of I. L.-1 from monocytes by Thrombin appears to be further enhanced in the presence of lipopolysaccharide (usually derived from gram negative organisms).[151] The binding of granulocytes to endothelium, discussed above, also induces release of granulocyte cathepsins and elastases leading to direct end-organ damage, more cytokine release and these two compounds may also cause degradation of many procoagulant and profibrinolytic factors.[152]

Plasmin, unlike thrombin, is a global proteolytic enzyme and has equal affinity for fibrinogen and fibrin.[2,3,5,12] Plasmin also effectively biodegrades Factors V, VIII: C, IX, XI, and other plasma proteins including growth hormone, ACTH, insulin, and many more.[2,3,5,12,53,112,134,153,154,155] As plasmin degrades cross-linked fibrin, specific fibrin degradation products appear in the circulation; one of these is D-Dimer, discussed later. Also, as plasmin circulates systemically it may activate both C-1 and C-3 with the eventual activation of C-8,9 and subsequent red cell and platelet lysis.[5,12,53,112,134,156] Complement is also activated by TNF, via thrombin-mediated release of TNF from the monocyte/macrophage system.[147,157] Red cell lysis releases red cell ADP and red cell membrane phospholipids, supplying more procoagulant material. Also, complement-induced platelet lysis prompts further thrombocytopenia and provides more platelet procoagulant material. Of added clinical importance, activation of the complement system will increase vascular permeability leading to hypotension and shock.[2,3,5,12,53,100,112] Elevated levels of PAI-1 in DIC may blunt some of these activities and clearly leads to hypoactivity of overall fibrinolysis and fibrinogenolysis, thus enhancing fibrin precipitation.[158]

Activation of the kinin system is also an important pathophysiological event with serious clinical consequences in DIC. With generation of Factor XIIa in DIC, there is subsequent conversion of prekallikrein to kallikrein and later conversion of high molecular weight kininogen into circulating kinins.[53,159,160] This also leads to increased vascular permeability, hypotension, and shock.[1,2,3,5,62]

In summary, as thrombin circulates systemically the consequences are mainly thrombosis with deposition of fibrin monomer and polymerized (cross-linked) fibrin in the microcirculation and, occasionally, large vessels. Many of these consequences of thrombin are mediated by both the procoagulant system and consequences of other thrombin-activated systems and by thrombin-induced release of cytokines.[1,3,4,5] Many of these adverse actions in DIC are also mediated by subsequent endothelial damage/disruption, release of endothelial-derived products and cytokines and endothelial interactions with granolocytes, lymphocytes, and monocyte/macrophage cells.[1,3,4,5] Concomitantly, plasmin also circulates systemically and is primarily responsible for the hemorrhage seen in DIC because of the creation of fibrin(ogen) degradation products and the interference of FDP with fibrin monomer polymerization and platelet function. Plasmin-induced lysis of many aforementioned clotting factors also leads to hemorrhage. By appreciating this circular concept of pathophysiology, it is understandable why most patients with DIC are experiencing both hemorrhage and thrombosis. Clinicians are repeatedly misguided by appreciating only the hemorrhage evolving in DIC patients, as this is the most obvious physical finding observed during clinical assessment. However, of greater importance, is the substantial microvascular thrombosis and large vessel thrombosis that occurs, leading to irreversible end-organ damage. It is important to recognize that most patients with disseminated intravascular coagulation are not only experiencing significant hemorrhage but also significant and often diffuse thrombosis.[1,2,3,4,5,12,53,100,112,161,162] Understanding

Table 1.8 Laboratory criteria based upon DIC pathophysiology.

An understanding of the pathophysiology of DIC and the usual laboratory manifestations allows for clear development of criteria to meet the laboratory diagnosis of DIC, which are:
(1) Evidence of procoagulant activation
(2) Evidence of fibrinolytic activation
(3) Evidence of inhibitor consumption and
(4) Evidence of end-organ damage or failure
To meet these criteria, generally available laboratory tests are available

and appreciating the extraordinarily complex pathophysiology of DIC provides the dictum that DIC is always accompanied by (A) procoagulant system activation (B) fibrinolytic system activation (C) inhibitor consumption (D) cytokine release (E) cellular activation and resultant (F) end-organ damage, as summarized in Table 1.8. Findings of (1) procoagulant system activation (2) fibrinolytic system activation (3) inhibitor consumption and (4) end-organ damage must be present, and documented by appropriate laboratory parameters, for an objective diagnosis of DIC.[1,2,3,5]

Clinical diagnosis

The systemic signs and symptoms of DIC are variable and usually consist of fever, hypotension, acidosis, proteinuria, and hypoxia.[1,2,3,4,12] More specific signs found in patients with DIC that should immediately forewarn one to this possibility, in the appropriate clinical settings, are petechiae and purpura (found in most patients), hemorrhagic bullae, acral cyanosis and sometimes, frank gangrene.[1,2,3,12,163,164,165] Wound bleeding, especially oozing from a surgical or traumatic wound is common in patients who have undergone surgery or suffered trauma.[1,2,3,4,12,62] Oozing from venipuncture sites or intra-arterial lines is another common finding.[1,2,3,4,12,62] Large subcutaneous hematomas, and deep-tissue bleeding are also frequently seen.[21] The average patient with DIC usually bleeds from at least three unrelated sites and any combination may be seen.[1,2,3,4,12,62] A remarkable volume of microvascular and large vessel thrombosis may occur which is not clinically obvious unless and until looked for.[1,2,3,4,12,62] Those organ systems having a high chance of microvascular thrombosis associated with dysfunction include cardiac, pulmonary, renal, hepatic and central nervous system.[1,2,3,4,12,62,153] Thrombotic thrombocytopenic purpura (TTP) is commonly associated with CNS dysfunction however, it should be realized that this is observed just as commonly in DIC.[1,2,3,4,12,62]

Table 1.9 Minimal clinical findings required for a diagnosis of disseminated intravascular coagulation.

Understanding the usual clinical manifestations of DIC allow for minimal criteria required for the clinical component of a diagnosis of DIC:
(1) Clinical evidence of hemorrhage, thrombosis or both should be present

and

(2) Should be occurring in the appropriate clinical setting as defined in the text

Patients with low-grade DIC more commonly have subacute bleeding and diffuse thromboses instead of acute fulminant life-threatening hemorrhage.[1,2,3,4,12,62] These patients have been appropriately described as having a "compensated" DIC.[1,2,3,4,12,62,166] In this instance there is usually an increased turnover and decreased survival of many components of the hemostasis system including the platelets, fibrinogen, and Factors V, and VIII: C; because of this, most global coagulation laboratory tests are near normal or normal.[1,2,3,4,12,62,166] Patients with low-grade DIC, however, uniformly have elevated fibrin(ogen) degradation products, leading to impairment of fibrin monomer polymerization and a clinically significant platelet function defect resulting from the coating of platelet membranes by FDP. Also, molecular markers of hemostatic activation, subsequently discussed, are typically abnormal in low-grade DIC. Patients may also present with diffuse or singular thromboses that are quite taxing for clinical management.

The minimal clinical findings required for a diagnosis of fulminant or low-grade DIC are summarized in Table 1.9.

Morphological findings in DIC

Morphological findings in disseminated intravascular coagulation consist of characteristic peripheral smear findings and hemorrhage or thrombosis in any organ(s).[1,2,3,4,12,62,167] Early morphological findings are platelet rich microthrombi.[62,167,168] These are usually seen in association with intense vasoconstriction, resulting from compounds released from platelets including biogenic amines, adenine nucleotides, thromboxanes, and kinins.[1,2,3,4,12,62,169] These are later replaced by hyaline (fibrin)-rich microthrombi.[167,168] Another early finding is fibrin monomer deposition, occurring primarily in the reticuloendothelial system.[1,2,3,4,62,170] The precipitation of fibrin monomer may cause end-organ damage due both to primary parenchymal damage and to microvascular occlusion. Also, this may impair reticuloendothelial clearance of FDPs, activated clotting factors, and circulating soluble fibrin monomer. Later findings are the typical fibrin-rich hyaline microthrombi thought to replace earlier deposited platelet-rich microthrombi.[171] Patients with DIC may develop pulmonary hyaline membranes which account, in part, for significant pulmonary dysfunction and hypoxemia.[1,2,3,4,12,62] Schistocytes are red cell fragments seen in about 50% of individuals with DIC.[1,2,3,4,12,62,163,172,173] The mechanisms for the formation of schistocytes have been demonstrated by Bull and associates, who describe fibrin-red cell interactions.[174] Absence of schistocytes, however, does not rule out a diagnosis of DIC. Most patients with fulminant DIC will present with a mild reticulocytosis and a mild leukocytosis, usually associated with a mild to moderate shift to immature forms. Thrombocytopenia is usually present and often obvious by examination of the peripheral blood smear.[1,2,3,4,12,62] Also, large platelets are usually seen on the peripheral smear, representing an increased population of young platelets resulting from increased platelet turnover and decreased platelet survival, because of platelet entrapment in microthrombi.[1,2,3,4,12,62,163,175,176]

The platelet-rich microthrombi are later replaced by hyaline (fibrin) microthrombi.[1,2,3,4,168] Hyaline microthrombi account for significant end-organ damage; these are of three types. (1) Globular hyaline microthrombi may be seen on PAS-stained peripheral blood smears and are polymerized complexes of fibrinogen, fibrin, their degradation products and many intermediates.[1,2,3,4,12,62] (2) Intravascular hyaline microthrombi are typically seen by pathologists at postmortem examination in DIC patients. These intravascular hyaline microthrombi are homogeneous, compact, intravascular hyaline structures oriented parallel to the blood flow and occasionally contain platelets or white cell fragments. They are easily seen by PAS staining, trichrome staining, tryptophan staining, and fluorescein-labeled antifibrinogen antiserum staining and by electron microscopy.[177,178] (3) Pulmonary hyaline membranes are also a form of hyaline microthrombus and are highly polymerized complexes of fibrinogen, fibrin, their degradation products, and all types of intermediates.[179,180] They are usually seen to cover the alveolar epithelium with a preference for areas denuded of epithelial cells. Also, the interalveolar capillaries beneath these hyaline membranes typically exhibit abnormal vascular permeability with the circulation of endothelial cells, plasma protein precipitation between endothelial borders, and the formation of interstitial edema. Many patients with disseminated intravascular coagulation develop pulmonary hyaline membranes, leading to overt respiratory failure, abnormal arterial blood gases, or abnormal pulmonary function tests (especially altered diffusion capacity [DCO]).[1,2,3,4,62,163] Pure "adult shock-lung syndrome" shares similar pathophysiology with acute disseminated intravascular coagulation; in this instance, the pathophysiology frequently remains localized to the pulmonary microcirculation instead of becoming a systemic process.[1,2,3,4,12,62,181] The pulmonary hyaline membranes of adult shock-lung syndrome and those of pediatric respiratory distress syndrome are the same as those present in DIC.[62]

DIC is a process associated with hemorrhage and thrombosis, although thrombosis is less clinically evident and less commonly appreciated by the clinician until late in a course of DIC or until autopsy. Hemorrhage can often be successfully treated in patients with DIC while thrombosis in the microcirculation and macrocirculation often leads to end-organ damage with irreversible ischemic changes that lead to morbidity and death. Those parameters that accelerate or precipitate microthrombi and macrothrombi in patients with DIC are: (1) vasomotor reactions, including elevated catecholamines, acidosis, and progressive vasoconstriction accelerate the precipitation of thrombi in the circulation;[1,2,3,4,182,183] (2) use of exogenous glucocorticoids or endogenous ACTH elevation may contribute to the precipitation of microthrombi in DIC patients and cautious thought must accompany use of steroids in these patients; although frequently steroid use is desirable and warranted;[1,2,3,4,12,62,184] (3) impairment of reticuloendothelial clearance, resulting from fibrin monomer precipitation or use of steroids, of fibrin(ogen) degradation products, circulating soluble fibrin monomer, or activated coagulation factors may also enhance the precipitation of microthrombi.[1,2,3,4,12,62,163] These mechanisms and interplays between them lead to accelerated fibrin monomer precipitation in the circulation resulting in severe end-organ damage that may be irreversible and often associated with significant morbidity and mortality.[1,2,3,4,12,62,163]

Laboratory diagnosis

Because of the complex pathophysiology depicted earlier, many laboratory findings of DIC may be highly variable, complex, and difficult to interpret unless the pathophysiology is clearly understood and appropriate tests performed, but if ordered and interpreted appropriately, can provide objective criteria for diagnosis and monitoring.[1,2,3,4] The laboratory evaluation of patients with DIC, especially with respect to the significant tests useful for diagnosis, and monitoring efficacy of therapy, is complex. Fortunately, many newer modalities have become available to the routine clinical laboratory for easily assessing patients with DIC.[1,2,3,4,12,62,163,185,186,187] In this section, objective laboratory criteria required for a diagnosis of DIC, based upon knowledge of pathophysiology of DIC, are clearly defined.

Global coagulation tests in DIC

The prothrombin time should be abnormal in DIC for multiple reasons, but often is normal and is an unreliable test in this setting. The prothrombin time depends upon ultimate conversion of fibrinogen to fibrin and in DIC there is usually hypofibrinogenemia, and FDP and thrombin interference with fibrin monomer polymerization. Also, plasmin-induced lysis of Factors V and IX should prolong the prothrombin time. The prothrombin time is prolonged in about 50% to 75% of patients with DIC and in up to 50% of patients is normal or short. The reasons for normal or short times are: (1) the presence of circulating activated clotting factor(s) such as thrombin or Factor Xa, may accelerate the formation of fibrin and (2) early degradation products may be rapidly clottable by thrombin and quickly "gel" the test system giving a normal or fast prothrombin time.[1,2,3,4,5,12,62,163] The prothrombin time is generally unreliable and of minimal usefulness in evaluating DIC.[1,2,3,4,5,12,62,163]

The activated partial thromboplastin time (aPTT) should also be prolonged in fulminant disseminated intravascular coagulation for a variety of reasons, but is more unreliable than is the prothrombin time. There is plasmin-induced biodegradation of Factors V, VIII: C, IX, and XI which should prolong the aPTT. The aPTT, like the prothrombin time, is prolonged by fibrinogen levels less than 100 mg%. Also, the aPTT may be prolonged because of FDP inhibition of fibrin monomer polymerization. However, the activated PTT is prolonged in only 50–60% of patients with DIC and a normal PTT can certainly not be used to rule out the diagnosis. The reasons for a fast or normal PTT in 40–50% of patients are the same as for the prothrombin time.[1,2,3,4,5,12,62,163] Like the prothrombin time, the activated PTT is of minimal usefulness in DIC.[1,2,3,4,5,12,62,163]

A prolonged thrombin or reptilase time is expected in DIC. Both tests should be prolonged by the presence of circulating FDPs and interference with fibrin monomer polymerization and from the hypofibrinogenemia commonly present.[1,2,3,4,5,12,47,62,163] Both tests are often prolonged in DIC however, for reasons earlier mentioned they may sometimes be normal or fast. A "bonus test" of the thrombin or reptilase time is to observe the resultant clot for presence or absence of clot lysis.[1,2,3,4,5,12,47,62,163] This simple non-quantitative tool may provide significant clinical information; if the clot is not dissolving in 10 minutes, clinically significant fibrinolysis is unlikely to be present. However, if the clot begins to lyse within this period, a clinically significant amount of plasmin is probably present.[1,2,3,4,5,12,47,62,163]

Coagulation factor assays provide little, if any, meaningful information in patients with DIC.[1,2,3,4,5,12,47,62,163] In most patients with fulminant DIC, systemically circulating activated clotting factor(s), especially Factors Xa, IXa, and thrombin are present.[1,2,3,4,5,12,47,62,163] Coagulation factor assays done by the standard aPTT- or prothrombin time-derived laboratory techniques using deficient substrates will give uninterpretable and meaningless results in DIC patients. The reasons for this are obvious; for example, if a Factor VIII: C assay is attempted in the presence of circulating Factor Xa in a patient with DIC, a high level of Factor VIII: C is recorded since Factor Xa "bypasses" the necessity for Factor VIII: C in the test system [1,2,3,4,5,12,47,62,163] and a rapid conversion of fibrinogen to fibrin occurs; a rapid time will be recorded on the typical "standard curve" and this will be interpreted as a high Factor VIII: C level when there may be no Factor VIII: C present. Factor assays will give erroneous and meaningless results, are uninterpretable and add little or nothing to the diagnosis in DIC patients.[1,2,3,4,5,12,47,62,163]

Fibrin(ogen) degradation products are elevated in 85–100% of patients with DIC.[1,2,3,4,5,12,47,62,163,188,189] These degradation products are only "diagnostic" of plasmin biodegradation of fibrinogen or fibrin, and FDPs are, therefore, only indicative of the presence of plasmin.[1,2,3,4,5,12,47,62,163] The protamine sulfate or ethanol gelation tests for circulating soluble fibrin monomer are usually positive.[1,2,3,4,5,47,139,163,190,191] Like the FDP titer, however, these are not diagnostic as both elevated FDPs and circulating soluble fibrin monomer may occur in other clinical situations, including women using oral contraceptives, patients with pulmonary emboli, selected patients with myocardial infarction, patients with certain selected renal diseases, and patients with arterial or venous thrombotic or thromboembolic events.[1,2,3,4,5,143,163,192,193] Sometimes, the protamine sulfate test or ethanol gelation test may be negative. A quantitative assay for fibrin monomer, the FM-test by ELISA (Thrombin Precursor Protein) has been shown to be a sensitive marker in the management of DIC patients, however the data are preliminary.[194]

A newer test for DIC is the D-Dimer assay. D-Dimer is a neo-antigen formed when thrombin initiates the transition of fibrinogen to fibrin and activates Factor XIII to cross-link the fibrin formed; this neo-antigen is formed as a result of plasmin digestion of cross-linked fibrin.[195,196] The D-Dimer test is, therefore, specific for *fibrin* degradation products, whereas the formation of fibrinolytic degradation products (FDP), the X, Y, D and E fragments, discussed earlier, may be either fibrinogen or fibrin derived, following plasmin digestion. Recently, monoclonal antibodies have been harvested against the D-Dimer neo-antigen DD-3B6/22 that are specific for cross-linked fibrin derivatives containing the D-Dimer configuration.[197,198] Following the harvesting of monoclonal antibodies, a latex agglutination assay has been developed for the clinical laboratory. Of the common tests used in assessing DIC patients, the D-Dimer assay appears to be one of the most reliable test for the probability of being abnormal in patients with confirmed DIC.[1,102] Using our battery of DIC tests, in the appropriate clinical setting, the reliability of tests used, in descending order of reliability, are the D-Dimer and Prothrombin Fragment 1.2 assays (abnormal in over 90%) the anti-thrombin III level (abnormal in 89%) the fibrinopeptide A level (abnormal in 88%) and FDP titer (usually abnormal in 75% of patients).[5] Elms and co-workers have done D-Dimer assays in DIC patients and found elevated D-Dimer levels in

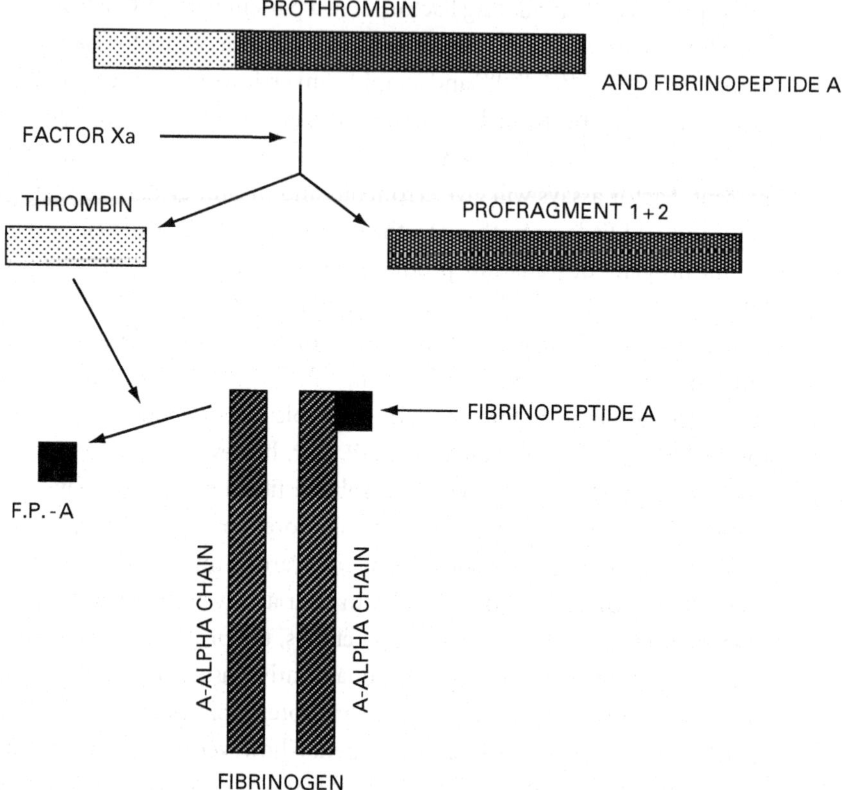

Figure 1.5 Formation of prothrombin fragment 1 + 2.

all patients with DIC.[199] Many of the newer D-Dimer assays commercially available do not use the DD-3B6/22 monoclonal antibody and have been found to be inadequate, as they are not specific for *fibrin* degradation products.[200] The formation of prothrombin fragment is depicted in Figure 1.5. In some instances, FDP titers and paracoagulation reactions may be negative in DIC. The available fibrin(ogen) degradation product determinations use latex particles that are "anti-fibrinogen" and since they are anti-fibrinogen, thrombin clot tubes are supplied to clot out fibrinogen so latex particles will not react with fibrinogen and erroneously measure fibrinogen instead of its degradation products.[1,2,3,4,5,47,163] However, fibrinogen and its degradation products have common antigenic determinants.[201] When these thrombin clot-tubes are used, not only is fibrinogen removed from the system but also Fragment X and Fragment Y. Currently available FDP methodologies measure Fragments D and E, and in some cases of DIC there may be minimal secondary fibrinolytic response and minimal plasmin circulating, thus there may

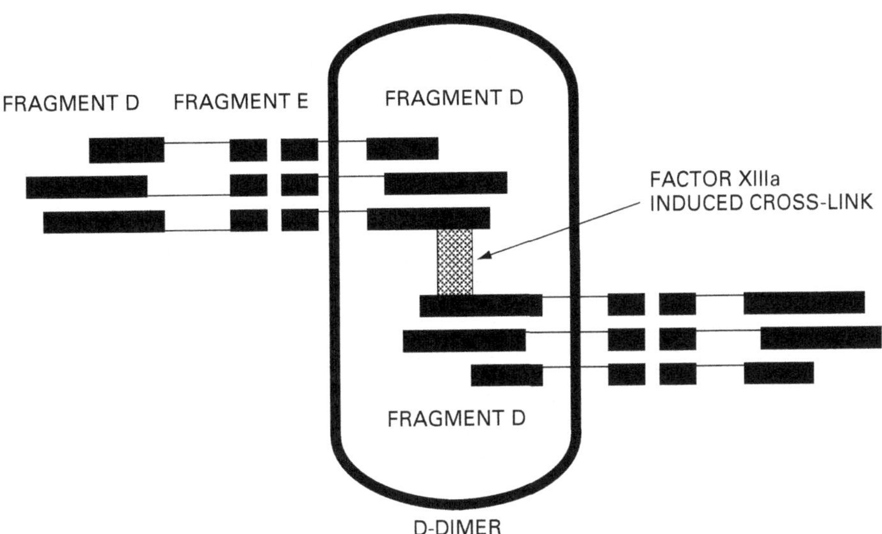

Figure 1.6 The formation of D-Dimer.

only be degradation to the X fragment stage or some intermediate between fibrin(ogen) and Fragment X. In this instance, there will be nothing for the test to measure since Fragment X and its intermediates will be removed from the test system by the thrombin clot-tubes used. Alternatively, in instances of acute DIC where there is a massive secondary fibrinolytic activation and overwhelming amounts of plasmin circulating, degradation past the D and E stage may happen. Fragments D and E are the last degradation products retaining antigenic determinants capable of being detected by the available commercial FDP titer kits. Another problem is that of overwhelming release of granulocyte enzymes, collagenases and elastases, which may also degrade all available D and E fragments and again, render false negative FDP titers in patients with acute disseminated intravascular coagulation.[1,2,3,4,5,12,163] Therefore, the presence of negative FDP titers does not rule out a diagnosis of DIC. Despite these difficulties, FDP titers are elevated in most DIC patients. However, with general availability of the D-Dimer assay, there is only limited use for the FDP titer, and no use for the protamine sulfate test in DIC patients. D-Dimer formation is shown in Figure 1.6.

Molecular markers for the diagnosis of DIC

The conversion of prothrombin to thrombin is a key event in the normal coagulation of blood; this activation results in the release of an inactive prothrombin fragment 1.2 (PF 1 + 2) from the amino terminus of the prothrombin molecule thus generating an intermediate species, prethrombin 2. The prethrombin 2 can be internally scissioned to yield thrombin; once produced this serine protease can

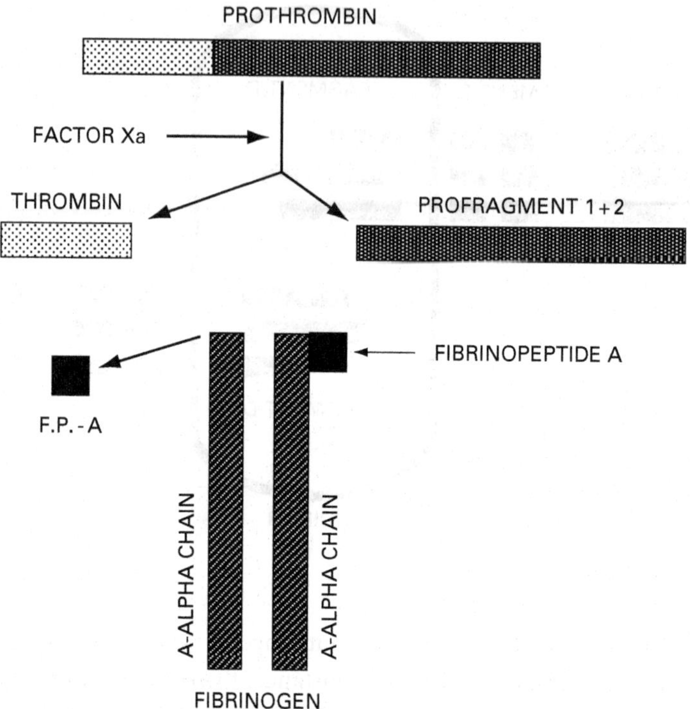

Figure 1.7 Formation of prothrombin fragment 1 + 2 and Fibrinopeptide A.

either proteolyze fibrinogen with the liberation of fibrinopeptide A (FPA) or combine with its major antagonist, antithrombin to form a stable inactive enzyme-inhibitor complex, the thrombin–antithrombin (TAT) complex.[202] Approved ELISA assays are now generally available to quantitate the levels of prothrombin fragment PF 1 + 2 and TAT within the circulation to provide evidence of excessive Factor Xa and thrombin generation.[203] The prothrombin fragment 1 + 2 assay is an easily performed reliable molecular marker for Factor Xa generation,[126,204,205,206,207,208] while the fibrinopeptide A assay, subsequently discussed, is an easily performed reliable marker for thrombin generation. These activation sequences are depicted in Figure 1.7.

The antithrombin determination is a key test for the diagnosis and monitoring of therapy in DIC.[1,2,3,4,5,12,112,163] During activation of DIC, there is irreversible complexing of thrombin and circulating activated clotting factors with antithrombin, leading to considerable decreases of functional antithrombin.[47,209] Several studies have compared the clinical applicability of various antithrombin methodologies and based upon these studies synthetic substrate assays are clearly the method of choice.[210,211] Immunological assays for antithrombin ignore biological function and may be low or normal in DIC; immunological assays for antithrombin in DIC patients should not be used.[1,2,3,4,5,12,143,163,212]

Fibrinopeptide A is usually elevated in patients with disseminated intravascular coagulation and provides an overall assessment of hemostasis activation, much like platelet factor 4 and beta-thromboglobulin levels provide for platelets. The presence of fibrinopeptide A is "diagnostic" of the presence of thrombin acting on fibrinogen. Also, fibrinopeptide A determinations may be of help in assessing efficacy of therapy in DIC.[1,2,3,4,5,12,143,163,213,214] The fibrinopeptide A level may be elevated in a wide variety of other micro- or macrovascular thrombotic events and also increases generally as a function of age.[215] The fibrinopeptide A level is available by ELISA assay.

To summarize, the prothrombin fragment 1 + 2 and Fibrinopeptide A elevation provide direct evidence of procoagulant activation, decreased antithrombin levels provide indirect evidence of both procoagulant activation and inhibitor consumption, and elevated TAT complex is direct evidence of procoagulant activation and inhibitor consumption.

Fibrinolytic system assays are now readily available in the clinical laboratory and provide useful information in DIC. Typically, plasminogen is decreased and circulating plasmin is present.[1,2,3,4,5,12,163] Intensity of the secondary fibrinolytic response is of clinical consequence for predicting potential microvascular thrombosis and resultant irreversible end-organ damage in patients with DIC. If there is impaired activation of the fibrinolytic system, morbidity and mortality resulting from end-organ damage may be even greater than expected. Fibrinolytic system activation can be assessed by measuring plasminogen and plasmin levels by currently available, simple, synthetic substrate techniques.[185,216,217] The euglobulin lysis time provides little or no clinically useful information for assessing the fibrinolytic system in clinical disorders, including DIC.[1,2,3,4,5,163,218,219] Direct measurement of plasmin in plasma can be difficult because it is rapidly inactivated by complexing with fast-acting alpha-2-antiplasmin[220,221] and slow acting alpha-2-macroglobulin.[222] Alpha-2-antiplasmin (A-2-AP) is also called alpha-2-plasmin inhibitor (alpha-2-PI). If these two fibrinolytic system inhibitors are markedly elevated, there may be an ineffective fibrinolytic response with resultant enhanced fibrin monomer precipitation, fibrin deposition, and vascular thrombosis. The plasmin-alpha-2-plasmin inhibitor (PAP) complex is measured by crossed immunoelectrophoresis, enzyme-linked immunoabsorbent assay (ELISA).[222,223,224] Alpha-2 macroglobulin-plasmin complexes can also be measured by ELISA.[225] The presence of these complexes is therefore a direct indicator of in vivo plasmin generation. The plasmin-alpha-2PI (PAP) complex has been shown to be markedly elevated in DIC at the time of presentation and changes in parallel with the course of DIC, with levels decreasing in clinical remission.[226] The PAP complex is useful in DIC because elevation documents (1) fibrinolytic system activation (plasmin) and (2) inhibitor (alpha-2-PI) consumption. Recently, assays for tissue (endothelial) plasminogen activator and tissue plasminogen activator inhibitor have become available; their potential role in DIC is unclear at present.

In summary, elevated plasmin and decreased plasminogen provide direct evidence of fibrinolytic activation, decreased alpha-2-PI provides indirect evidence of fibrinolytic activation and inhibitor consumption, and elevated PAP complex provides direct evidence of both fibrinolytic activation and inhibitor consumption.

The platelet count is typically decreased in DIC; however, the range may be variable, from as low as 2–3 $\times$ 10^9/l to greater than 100 $\times$ 10^9/l. In most patients with DIC, thrombocytopenia is obvious by examination of a peripheral blood smear and averages around 60 $\times$ 10^9/l.[1,2,3,4,5,12,163] Most tests of platelet function including the template bleeding time, platelet aggregation, and platelet lumi-aggregation are abnormal in patients with DIC.[175] This is caused by FDP coating of platelet membranes or partial release of platelet procoagulant materials. There is no reason for doing tests of platelet function in patients with fulminant DIC, as abnormal results are invariably found and add little to the diagnosis.[1,2,3,4,5,175] Increased platelet turnover and decreased platelet survival is usual in patients with DIC; Platelet factor 4 levels and beta-thromboglobulin levels are markers of general platelet reactivity and release and are usually elevated in DIC patients. Several reports have suggested that either of these may be worthwhile in DIC and for monitoring efficacy of therapy of the intravascular clotting process.[227,228] Both assays are readily available for the clinical laboratory and each has attendant advantages and disadvantages. Platelet factor 4 and beta-thromboglobulin are elevated in most DIC patients however, neither of these modalities are diagnostic of DIC, and may be elevated in pulmonary emboli, acute myocardial infarction, deep venous thrombosis, and in disorders associated with microvascular disease such as diabetes and autoimmunity. However, if elevated in DIC and then decrease after therapy, this suggests therapy has been successful in either blunting or stopping the intravascular clotting process.[1,2,3,4,5,12,163] Elevation of either platelet factor 4 or beta-thromboglobulin provides indirect evidence of procoagulant activation.

By understanding the pathophysiology of DIC, clearly hemostasis will be quite deranged and most common laboratory tests of hemostasis may be markedly abnormal.[1,2,3,4,5,12,134,163,229] It is therefore, useful to establish which tests are of practical significance for providing a high degree of reliability, specificity and availability in assessing patients with DIC. In this regard, hospital laboratories must be equipped to offer assays that will quickly and reliably allow assessment of DIC patients by objective means. If a hospital allows admission of patients with DIC or diseases associated with DIC, current standards of care require that the clinical laboratory can meet this need on a STAT basis.[1,2,3,4,5] Tests useful for aiding in a

Table 1.10 Clinical findings suggestive of DIC.

Disseminated intravascular coagulation
Petechiae
Purpura
Hemorrhagic bullae
Acral cyanosis
Gangrene
Surgical wound bleeding
Traumatic wound bleeding
Venipuncture site bleeding
Arterial line oozing/bleeding
Subcutaneous hematomas
Intracranial hemorrhage
Gastrointestinal hemorrhage
Intra-abdominal hemorrhage
Retroperitoneal hemorrhage
Genitourinary hemorrhage
Intrapulmonary hemorrhage
Clinical thrombosis/microvascular thrombosis

Table 1.11 Molecular markers useful for the differential diagnosis of DIC, primary lysis and thrombotic thrombocytopenic purpura.

Marker	DIC	Primary lysis	T. T. P.
Prothrombin Fragment 1 + 2	Elevated	Normal	Normal
D-Dimer	Elevated	Normal	Elevated
FDP	Elevated	Elevated	Elevated
Soluble fibrin monomer	Elevated	Normal	Normal
Fibrinopeptide A	Elevated	Normal	Normal
Fibrinopeptide B	Elevated	Normal	Normal
Platelet factor 4	Elevated	Normal	Elevated
Beta-thromboglobulin	Elevated	Normal	Elevated
Plasminogen activator	Elevated	Elevated	Decreased
Thromboxanes	Elevated	Normal	Elevated
6-keto-PGF-alpha	Normal	Normal	Decreased
Fibronectin	Decreased	Normal	Normal
B-beta 15–42 peptide	Elevated	Normal	Normal
B-beta 1–42 peptide	Elevated	Elevated	Normal
B-beta 15–118 peptide	Elevated	Elevated	Normal

Table 1.12 Laboratory diagnostic criteria.*

Tests currently suitable for evidence of procoagulant activation (*Group I tests*) are:
1. Elevated prothrombin fragment 1 + 2
2. Elevated fibrinopeptide A
3. Elevated thrombin-antithrombin complex (TAT)
4. Elevated D-Dimer**
5. Elevated soluble fibrin monomer (TPP) ELISA

Tests currently suitable as evidence for fibrinolytic activation (*Group II tests*) are:
1. Elevated D-Dimer
2. Elevated FDP
3. Elevated plasmin
4. Elevated plasmin-antiplasmin complex (PAP)
5. Elevated soluble fibrin monomer (TPP) ELISA

Tests currently suitable as evidence for inhibitor consumption (*Group III tests*) are:
1. Decreased AT-III
2. Decreased alpha-2-antiplasmin
3. Decreased heparin cofactor II
4. Decreased protein C or S
5. Elevated T. A. T. complex
6. Elevated P. A. P. complex

Tests currently suitable as evidence for end-organ damage or failure (*Group IV tests*) are:
1. Elevated LDH
2. Elevated creatinine
3. Decreased pH
4. Decreased pAO2

*Only one abnormality each is needed in group I, II, and III and at least two abnormalities are needed in group IV tests to satisfy criteria for a laboratory diagnosis of DIC.
**The D-Dimer is only reliable for this purpose if using the correct assay and monoclonal antibody, as discussed in the text.

diagnosis of DIC are depicted in Table 1.10.[1,2,3,4,5,12,47,163] Molecular marker profiling for DIC has become available and is performed in the laboratory by fully automated systems. These molecular markers are worthwhile for providing a differential diagnosis of DIC versus primary fibrinolysis or DIC versus TTP in particularly difficult situations. The differential diagnosis of DIC versus primary fibrinolysis versus TTP by molecular marker profiling is depicted in Table 1.11. In uncommon instances of a difficult differential diagnosis between DIC, TTP or primary fibrinolysis, use of these molecular markers may be quite helpful.[1,2,3,4,5,163,230]

In summary, the laboratory diagnosis of DIC requires documentation of (1) procoagulant system activation (Group I tests) (2) fibrinolytic system activation (Group II tests) (3) inhibitor consumption (Group III tests) and (4) end-organ damage (Group IV tests). The manner in which the above discussed tests are used to provide documentation of these four requirements is summarized in Table 1.12.

Management of disseminated intravascular coagulation

Fulminant disseminated intravascular coagulation

The treatment of disseminated intravascular coagulation is confusing and sometimes controversial.[1,2,3,4,5,12,62,231] Concomitant with controversy and confusion is the global perception that therapy is often futile and most patients succumb to the disease process. However, most published comments about therapy are based upon tradition instead of fact and emotion instead of clinical judgment.[1,2,3,4,5,12,62] The reasons for this are because very few objective series of DIC patients, for therapy given, morbidity, mortality, and survival, have been published. Difficulties in therapeutic clinical trials result because of the diverse etiologies and clinical manifestations associated with DIC; a given therapeutic approach may be proper for one particular etiology, but not necessarily another and one therapeutic approach may be appropriate for various types of hemorrhage, but not thrombosis. Thus, therapy must be highly individualized. If logical, aggressive, and sequential therapy is undertaken, morbidity and mortality rates are not as dismal as suspected.[1,2,3,4,5,12,62,163,231] Clinicians should exercise judgment with respect to therapy, formulated upon experience and published series of patients and documentation instead of dogma and mythology. Hopefully, the future will offer more guidelines than are available now with respect to successes and failures with various forms of potential therapy.

An acceptable approach to therapy in fulminant DIC is somewhat vigorous and is summarized in Table 1.13. Although this approach is aggressive, it is associated with a high survival rate and low morbidity in patients with classic, fulminant DIC.[1,2,3,4,5,12,62,163] As a guiding principle, therapy must be individualized for each patient depending on clinical findings and manifestations of the process.[1,2,3,4,5,12,62,112,163]

Therapy should be based upon etiology of the DIC, age, hemodynamic status, site and severity of hemorrhage, site and severity of thrombosis and other pertinent clinical factors. The essential therapeutic modality to be delivered to a patient with fulminant DIC is that of an aggressive but reasonable therapeutic approach to eliminate or treat the triggering disease process thought to be responsible for DIC.[1,2,3,4,5,12,62,112,163]

Table 1.13 Logical and sequential therapy for disseminated intravascular coagulation.

A. Individualize therapy
  - Site(s) and severity of hemorrhage
  - Site(s) and severity of thrombosis
  - Precipitating disease state
  - Hemodynamic status
  - Other clinical considerations

B. Treat or remove the triggering process
  - Evacuate/remove uterus
  - Antibiotics
  - Control shock
  - Volume replacement
  - Maintain blood pressure
  - Airway if needed
  - Antineoplastic therapy (GYN)
  - Other clinically indicated therapy

C. Stop intravascular clotting process
  - Subcutaneous LMW heparin
  - Subcutaneous UF heparin
  - Antithrombin concentrate
  - Intravenous heparin?
  - Investigational therapy
    - Concentrates?
    - Antiplatelet therapy?
    - Hirudin?

D. Replace missing blood components as indicated
  - Platelet concentrates
  - Packed red blood cells (washed/leuko-poor)
  - Antithrombin concentrate
  - Fresh frozen plasma
  - Cryoprecipitate?
  - Prothrombin complex concentrate

E. Inhibit residual fibrino(geno)lysis
  - *Aminocaproic acid*
  - Tranexamic acid

Treatments that remove or blunt the underlying disease process may in itself significantly blunt the intravascular clotting process. If however, control of the triggering event and pathophysiology is not achieved, later attempts at anticoagulant therapy, including heparin compounds, will rarely alleviate the disseminated intravascular clotting process.[1,2,3,4,5,12,62,112,163,231]

Sometimes, it is impossible, or unlikely that the underlying disease can be alleviated. However, frequently the removal of the triggering pathophysiology will stop the DIC process; the classical example of this is an obstetrical accident and another is septicemia. In cases of obstetrical accidents of any type (except amniotic fluid embolism), anticoagulant therapy, especially heparin, is rarely needed. Simply evacuating the uterus, or in rare instances uterine or hypogastric artery ligation or hysterectomy, will usually rapidly stop the intravascular clotting process.[1,2,3,4,5,12,62,112,163,232,233,234]

Although it is often difficult to pursuade the obstetrician/gynecologist to take a hemorrhaging thrombocytopenic, hypofibrinogenemic patient to the operating room, the results are usually immediate and dramatic.[1,2,3,4,5,12,62,112,163]

In septicemia, specific antibiotic therapy, alleviation of shock, volume replacement, possibly high-dose glucocorticoids, and other specific therapy to stabilize hemodynamics will often cause significant blunting of the intravascular clotting process and sometimes may stop the DIC process altogether.[1,2,3,4,5,12,62,112,163]

Each case must be evaluated on its own merits depending on the clinical situation and the clinician's assessment of the dominant triggering event. The crucial point is that an attempt to treat the triggering event is the essential therapeutic modality that must be administered to the patient with disseminated intravascular coagulation. Concomitant with therapy for the triggering or underlying event, indicated supportive therapy must be aggressively started. The particular supportive therapy needed will depend upon the clinical situation of the individual patient.

The second principle is to treat the intravascular clotting process, recalling that thrombosis, usually of small vessels, is the process which most impacts on morbidity and mortality in patients – not hemorrhage! Most patients, except those suffering from DIC secondary to obstetrical accidents or massive liver failure, will next usually need antithrombotic therapy of some form to stop the intravascular clotting process. The use of subcutaneous low-dose heparin or LMW heparin appears to be highly effective in DIC.[1,2,3,4,5,12,62,112,163]

Antithrombotic therapy is indicated if the patient continues to bleed or clot significantly for about 4–6 hours after the initiation of supportive therapy and therapy to stop or blunt the triggering pathophysiological event. This time period is somewhat empirical and depends upon the sites and severity of bleeding and thrombosis, the thromboses usually manifest as progressive end-organ failure. When the patient continues to bleed in this situation, subcutaneous porcine heparin at 80–100 units/kg every 4–6 hours, or LMWH as discussed previously, as the clinical situation, site and severity of bleeding and thrombosis, and patient size dictate, is begun. Low-dose subcutaneous heparin or LMWH appears to be as effective or possibly more effective than larger doses of intravenous heparin in disseminated intravascular coagulation.[1,2,3,4,235] With this approach one often notes cessation of antithrombin consumption, lowering of FDP, and increases in fibrinogen levels and slow or rapid correction of other abnormal laboratory modalities of acute DIC in 3–4 hours, followed shortly by blunting or cessation of clinically significant hemorrhage and thrombosis. The use of subcutaneous low-dose heparin, instead of intravenous heparin, appears reasonable for several reasons: (1) if the patient does not respond, larger doses of heparin can always be administered if thought appropriate (2) unlike fears with larger intravenous doses of heparin, low-dose subcutaneous heparin therapy is associated with minimal chances of increasing the patients' risk of hemorrhage, and (3) most importantly, the use of low-dose subcutaneous heparin or LMWH has been as efficacious as large-dose heparin therapy and is associated with a high percentage of patient survival when used with other therapeutic modalities.[1,2,3,4,5,12,62,112,163]

Other anticoagulant modalities available, depending on the clinician's experience, are intravenous heparin, the use of combination antiplatelet agents, or the use of antithrombin concentrates. Those clinicians using intravenous heparin therapy for acute disseminated intravascular coagulation usually deliver between 20,000 and 30,000 units per 24 hours by constant infusion and this may be associated with significant blunting or cessation of the intravascular clotting process however, aggravation of hemorrhage is a potential risk. The contraindications of subcutaneous heparin, or heparin in any dose, would be in patients with fulminant DIC and central nervous system insults of any type, DIC associated with fulminant liver failure, and in most instances obstetrical accidents.[1,2,3,4,5,12,62,112,163]

Combination antiplatelet agents are far less effective, but on occasion may be called for as the specific clinical situation dictates.[1,2,3,4,5,12,62,112,163]

Fulminant disseminated intravascular coagulation has been successfully treated with antithrombin concentrates.[1,2,3,4,5,12,58,59,60,62,163,234,236] Several investigators have also used antithrombin concentrates in fatty liver of pregnancy, and preliminary experience would suggest these to be quite effective.[237,238] Antithrombin concentrates have become this author's treatment of choice for most patients with fulminant DIC. The dose required is calculated as follows: total units needed = (Desired Level – Initial Level) × 0.6 × total body weight (kg).[1,2,3,4,5,12,62,112,163] The desired level should always be 125% or greater, and the dose calculation should be performed and the derived antithrombin dose delivered every eight hours. This author finds antithrombin to be highly effective in fulminant DIC; antithrombin concentrate has been subjected to objective prospective clinical trials which clearly establish efficacy.[59,60] Another agent of potential therapeutic benefit for fulminant DIC is recombinant hirudin. Extensive clinical experience with recombinant hirudin in DIC is limited.

About 75 percent of patients will respond to the two earlier outlined sequential therapeutic steps.[1,2,3,4,5,12,62,112,163] If patients continue to bleed after beginning reasonable attempts to treat the triggering pathophysiology responsible for DIC and anticoagulant therapy has been initiated, the most probable cause of continued bleeding is component depletion.[1,2,3,4,5,12,62,112,163] In this instance, the precise components missing and thought to be contributing to hemorrhage should be defined and administered. The delivery of certain components is associated with potential hazards in patients with *ongoing* DIC and as a general guideline, only concentrates and components void of fibrinogen should be delivered to a patient with ongoing DIC, especially if manifested by a continued severe depression of the antithrombin level. If, however, the antithrombin level, or another specific monitoring modality that the clinician chooses to follow, is returning to normal and it can be assumed the intravascular clotting process has been controlled, then any component or concentrate thought necessary can safely be given. Generally, the only components considered safe in patients with active, uncontrolled, DIC are *washed* packed red cells, platelet concentrates, antithrombin concentrates, and non-clotting protein containing volume expanders such as plasma protein fraction, albumin, and hydroxyethyl starch. Components containing clotting factors and/or fibrinogen may be associated with enhanced hemorrhage and especially thrombosis in a patient with active DIC to whom these components are unwisely delivered.[1,2,3,4,5,12,62,112,163,239] As would be expected from an understanding of the pathophysiology of DIC when whole blood, fresh frozen plasma, or cryoprecipitate is given to a patient with ongoing DIC, plasmin will rapidly biodegrade most, if not all, of the coagulation factors supplied.[1,2,3,4,5,12,62,112,163,239] This may not be particularly harmful but is not helpful.[1,2,3,4,5] Of greater significance is that these components contain fibrinogen and are associated with a potential for the creation of even higher levels of fibrin(ogen) degradation products that will further impair hemostasis by interference with fibrin monomer polymerization, further decrease already compromised platelet function, and will lead to enhanced microvascular deposition of fibrin thrombi and subsequent thrombocytopenia.[1,2,3,4,5,12,62,112,163,239] A reasonable approach is to assess the patient after initiation of antithrombotic therapy. If bleeding continues and the antithrombin level, or other selected monitoring modality, has returned to normal or near normal, any component thought significantly depleted and likely to be contributing to continued hemorrhage is reasonable to replace. Alternatively, if the patient continues to bleed after antithrombotic therapy has been delivered and the antithrombin level and other modalities used to monitor the patient remains abnormal and progressive end-organ damage (thrombosis) or deterioration in hemodynamic status is noted, it is highly likely in this situation that the intravascular clotting process has not been controlled. In this instance, the component(s) should be restricted to washed packed red cells, platelets, volume expanders, and if available, antithrombin concentrate.[1,2,3,4,5,12,62,112,163] By adhering to the above three sequential aggressive steps, most patients will stop hemorrhaging if they are going to survive.

In those rare instances where bleeding continues after the aforementioned three sequential steps are instituted, in conjunction with aggressive supportive therapy, the fourth step in the therapy of fulminant DIC is to consider inhibition of the fibrinolytic system. This is rarely needed and is only necessary in about 3% of patients. There are rare instances of DIC not associated with APL when the intravascular coagulation process and fibrin deposition has been alleviated and the patient continues to bleed because, for unexplained reasons, secondary fibrinolysis has continued with the concomitant biodegradation of the usual plasma protein targets of plasmin. In this rare instance, antifibrinolytic therapy may be indicated and should be considered as the clinical situation dictates. Antifibrinolytic therapy should not be routinely delivered to patients with ongoing DIC, as these patients need the fibrinolytic system to render the microcirculation clear of microthrombi.[1,2,3,4,5,12,62,112,163] Antifibrinolytic therapy is not delivered unless the first three sequential steps delineated above have been initiated and it has been established from the clinical and laboratory standpoint that the intravascular coagulation process has been eliminated by noting correction of biological antithrombin levels or other modalities used by the clinician to monitor the event. Also, antifibrinolytic therapy should never be used unless significant amounts of circulating plasmin have been documented by laboratory modalities such as a decrease in functional plasminogen or alpha-2-plasmin inhibitor and an increase in plasmin. In those rare instances where antifibrinolytic therapy is indicated, epsilon aminocaproic acid is given as an initial 5–10 grams slow intravenous push followed by 2–4 grams per hour for 24 hours or until bleeding stops. This agent may cause ventricular arrhythmias, severe hypotension, and severe hypokalemia.[240,241,242] Another antifibrinolytic is tranexamic acid, usually delivered as 1 to 2 grams, intravenously every eight to twelve hours; this agent is more potent and may be associated with fewer undesirable side effects.[112] If a fibrinolytic inhibitor is used in a patient with *ongoing* DIC, it may cause enhanced precipitation of fibrin in the microcirculation and macrocirculation and lead to fatal disseminated thrombosis.[1,2,3,4,5,12,62,112,163]

"Low-grade" DIC

Therapy of low-grade disseminated intravascular coagulation is often approached differently than for fulminant DIC. Many patients with compensated DIC do not suffer life-threatening hemorrhage but have bothersome bleeding and local or diffuse superficial or deep venous thrombosis and thromboembolus.[1,2,3,4,5,12,62,112,163,166,243] Essential therapy for low-grade DIC is treatment of the underlying disease process; frequently, this will produce cessation of the intravascular clotting process and alleviation of hemorrhage or thrombosis. As with fulminant DIC, indicated supportive therapy must be given. If this first step is accomplished and hemorrhage and/or thrombosis and/or thromboembolus continues, then anticoagulant therapy is indicated to stop the intravascular clotting process. However, since low-grade DIC patients usually do not suffer life-threatening hemorrhage, anticoagulant/antithrombotic therapy need not necessarily be vigorous. Aggressive antithrombotic therapy, particularly warfarin or heparin may be contraindicated in selected instances of malignancy, especially those with intracranial metastases.[1,2,3,4,5,12,62,97,112,163] Combination antiplatelet therapy is frequently successful in stopping a compensated DIC process after attempts to treat the triggering pathophysiology have also been started. Commonly, a combination of acetylsalicylic acid plus other agents, such as clopidogrel, will stop a low-grade intravascular coagulation process within 24 to 30 hours, as manifest by correction of coagulation laboratory parameters and cessation of bleeding or thrombosis. Low-dose subcutaneous heparin or LMW heparin therapy should be considered in patients with low-grade DIC who appear to be evolving into a fulminant process or who are developing significant thrombotic or thromboembolic problems. Replacement therapy is rarely indicated in compensated DIC. Also, inhibition of the fibrinolytic system is rarely, if ever, indicated in low-grade DIC.

Summary

Current concepts of the etiology, pathophysiology, clinical and laboratory diagnosis and management of fulminant and low-grade DIC as they apply to obstetrical, pregnant and gynecological patients have been presented. In addition, general medical complications leading to DIC, which may often be seen in obstetrics, pregnancy and gynecology are discussed. Considerable attention has been devoted to interrelationships within the hemostasis system. Only by clearly understanding these pathophysiological interrelationships can the Obstetrician/Gynecologist appreciate the divergent and wide spectrum of often confusing clinical and laboratory findings in patients with DIC. In this discussion, objective clinical and laboratory criteria for a diagnosis of DIC have been delineated, thus eliminating unnecessary confusion and empirical decisions regarding the diagnosis. Particularly in the obstetrical patient, if a condition exists noted to be associated with DIC or if any suspicion of DIC arises on either clinical or laboratory findings, it is imperative to carefully monitor these women with clinical and laboratory tools to assess potential progression to a catastrophic event. In most instances of DIC in obstetrics, the disease can easily be ameliorated at early stages. Many therapeutic decisions are straightforward, particularly in obstetrics and gynecology; for more serious and complicated cases of DIC in this patient population, however, efficacy and choices of therapy remain unclear and will remain so until more is published regarding response rates and survival patterns. Also, therapy must be highly individualized depending on the nature of DIC, age, etiology of DIC, site and severity of hemorrhage or thrombosis and hemodynamic and other clinical parameters. Finally, it should be appreciated that many syndromes which are often partitioned into organ specific disorders but either share common pathophysiology with disseminated intravascular coagulation or are simply a form of DIC are sometimes identified as an independent disease entity, such as amniotic fluid embolism syndrome, HELLP syndrome, adult shock lung syndrome, eclampsia, and many other isolated "organ-specific" disorders. All of these, however, represent DIC in its varied modes of clinical expression and serve to illustrate the very diverse clinical and anatomical manifestations of this fascinating syndrome.

REFERENCES

1 Bick, R. L. Disseminated intravascular coagulation: objective criteria for diagnosis and management. *Medical Clinics North America*, **78**: 511, 1994.

2 Bick, R. L. Disseminated intravascular coagulation syndromes in obstetrics, pregnancy and gynecology. In Bick, R. L., ed. *Hematology Oncology Clinics North America*, W. B. Saunders, Philadelphia, **10**: 999, 2000.

3 Bick, R. L. Disseminated intravascular coagulation: etiology, pathophysiology, diagnosis and management: guidelines for care. *Clinical Applied Thrombosis Hemostasis*, **8**: 1, 2002.

4 Bick, R. L. Disseminated intravascular coagulation: pathophysiological mechanisms and manifestations. *Sem. Thromb. Hemostas.*, **24**: 3, 1998.

5 Bick, R. L. Disseminated intravascular coagulation: objective laboratory diagnostic criteria and guidelines for management. *Clinics in Laboratory Medicine*, **14**: 729, 1994.

6 Bick, R. L. and Baker, W. F. Disseminated intavascular coagulation. *Hematologic Pathology*, **6**: 1, 1992.

7 Lasch, H. G. and Henne, D. L., Huth, K. and Sandritter, W. Pathophysiology, clinical manifestations, and therapy of consumptive coagulopathy. *Am. J. Cardiol.*, **20**: 381, 1967.

8 Rodriquez-Erdman, F. Bleeding due to increased intravascular blood coagulation: hemorrhagic syndromes caused by consumption of blood-clotting factors (consumption coagulopathies). *N. Eng. J. Med.*, **273**: 1370, 1965.

9 Seegers, W. H. Factors in the control of bleeding. *Cincinnati J. Med.*, **31**: 395, 1950.

10 Ratnoff, O. D., Pritchard, J. A., Colopy, J. A. Hemorrhagic states during pregnancy. I. *N. Engl. J. Med.*, **253**: 63, 1955.

11 Ratnoff, O. D., Pritchard, J. A., Colopy, J. A. Hemorrhagic states during pregnancy. II. *N. Engl. J. Med.*, **253**: 97, 1955.

12 Bick, R. L. Disseminated intravascular coagulation: objective criteria for clinical and laboratory diagnosis and assessment of therapeutic response. *Clin. Appl. Thrombosis Hemostasis*, **1**: 3, 1995.

13 Bick, R. L. Syndromes of disseminated intravascular coagulation. Chapter 2. In *Disseminated Intravascular Coagulation and Related Syndromes.* CRC Press, Boca Raton, FL, 1982.

14 Steiner, P. E. and Lushbough, C. C. Maternal pulmonary embolism by amniotic fluid as a cause of shock and unexplained deaths in obstetrics. *JAMA*, **117**: 1245, 1941.

15 Graeff, N. and Kuhn, W. The Amniotic Infection Syndrome In *Coagulation Disorders in Obstetrics.* W. B. Saunders, Philadelphia, 1980. pp. 91–5.

16 Sperry, K. Amniotic fluid embolism: to understand an enigma. *JAMA*, **255**: 2183, 1986.

17 Fiana, S. Maternal mortality in Sweden: 1955–1974. *Acta Obstet. Gynecol. Scand.*, **57**: 129, 1978.

18 Locksmith, G. J. Amniotic fluid embolism. *Obstetrics & Gynecology Clinics of North America*, **26**: 435, 1999.

19 Nadesan, K. and Jayalakshmi, P. Sudden maternal deaths from amniotic fluid embolism. *Ceylon Medical Journal*, **42**: 185, 1997.

20 Gilbert, W. M. and Danielsen, B. Amniotic fluid embolism: decreased mortality in a population-based study. *Obstetrics & Gynecology*, **93**: 973, 1999.

21 Lamy, C., Sharshar, T. and Mas, J. L. Cerebrovascular diseases in pregnancy and puerperium. *Revue Neurologique*, **152**: 422, 1996.

22 Mas, J. L. and Lamy, C. Stroke in pregnancy and the puerperium. [Review] [89 refs.] *Journal of Neurology*, **245**: 305, 1998.

23 Peterson, E. P. and Taylor, H. B. Amniotic fluid embolism: an analysis of 40 cases. *Obstet. Gynecol.*, **35**: 787, 1970.

24 Aznar, J., Gilabert, J., Estelles, A., *et al.* Evaluation of the soluble fibrin monomer complexes and other coagulation parameters in obstetric patients. *Thromb. Research*, **27**: 691, 1982.

25 Minna, J. D., Robboy, S. J. and Coleman, R. W. Disseminated intravascular coagulation in man. Charles C. Thomas, Springfield, IL, 1974, pp. 12–15 and pp. 156–7.

26 Aguillon, A., Andrus, T., Grayson, A., *et al.* Amniotic fluid embolism: a review. *Obstet. Gynecol. Survey*, **17**: 619, 1962.

27 Cortney, L. D. Amniotic fluid embolism. *Obstet. Gynecol. Survey*, **29**: 169, 1974.

28 D'Addato, F., Repinto, A. and Angeli, G. Amniotic fluid embolism in trial of labor. A case report. *Minerva Ginecologica*, **49**: 217, 1997.

29 Judich, A., Kuriansky, J., Engelberg, I., *et al.* Amniotic fluid embolism following blunt abdominal trauma in pregnancy. *Injury*, **29**: 475, 1998.

30 Morgan, M. Amniotic fluid embolism. *Anesthesia*, **34**: 20, 1979.

31 Price, T., Baker, V. V. and Cefalo, R. L. Amniotic fluid embolism: three case reports with a review of the literature. *Obstet. Gynecol. Survey*, **40**: 462, 1985.

32 Albrechtsen, O. K. Hemorrhagic disorders following amniotic fluid embolism. *Clinical Obstet. Gynecol.*, **7**: 361, 1964.

33 Russell, W. S. and Jones, W. H. Amniotic fluid embolism: a review of the syndrome with a report of 4 Cases. *Obstet. Gynecol.*, **26**: 476, 1965.

34 Gross, P. and Benz, E. J. Pulmonary embolism by amniotic fluid: report of three cases with a new diagnostic procedure. *Surg. Gynecol. Obstet.*, **85**: 315, 1947.

35 Reid, D. E., Weiner, A. E. and Roby, C. L. Intravascular clotting and afibrinogenemia, the presumptive lethal factors in the syndrome of amniotic fluid embolism. *Am. Journal Obstet. Gynecol.*, **66**: 466, 1953.

36 Aznar, J., Gilabert, J., Estelles, A., *et al.* Evaluation of plasminogen and other fibrinolytic parameters in the amniotic fluid (letter) *Thromb. Haemostas.*, **43**: 182, 1980.

37 Beller, F. K., Douglas, A. W., Debrovnet, C. H., *et al.* The fibrinolytic system in amniotic fluid embolism. *Am. Journal Obstet. Gynecol.*, **87**: 48, 1963.

38 Atwood, H. D. The histological diagnosis of amniotic fluid embolism. *Journal Path. Bacterial*, **76**: 211, 1958.

39 Yaffe, H., Eldor, A., Hornshtein, E., *et al.* Thromboplastic activity in amniotic fluid during pregnancy. *Obstet. Gynecol.*, **50**: 454, 1977.

40 Yaffe, H., Hay-am, E. and Sadovsky, E. Thromboplastic activity of amniotic fluid in term and postmature Gestations. *Obstet. Gynecol.*, **57**: 490, 1981.

41 Liban, E. and Raz, S. A clinicopathologic study of fourteen cases of amniotic fluid embolism. *Am. Journal Clinical Pathol.*, **51**: 477, 1969.

42 Sparr, R. A. and Prichard, J. A. Studies to detect the escape of amniotic fluid into the maternal circulation during parturition. *Surg. Gynecol. Obstet.*, **107**: 560, 1958.

43 Petroianu, G. A., Altmannsberger, S. H., Maleck, W. H., *et al.* Meconium and amniotic fluid embolism: effects on coagulation in pregnant mini-pigs. *Critical Care Medicine*, **27**: 348, 1999.

44 Kobayashi, H., Ooi, H., Hayakawa, H., *et al.* Histological diagnosis of amniotic fluid embolism by monoclonal antibody TKH-2 that recognizes NeuAc alpha 2–6GalNAc epitope. *Human Pathology*, **28**: 428, 1997.

45 Oi, H., Kobayashi, H., Hirashima, Y., *et al.* Serological and immunohistochemical diagnosis of amniotic fluid embolism. *Seminars in Thrombosis & Hemostasis*, **24**: 479, 1998.

46 Lunetta, P. and Penttila, A. Immunohistochemical identification of syncytiotrophoblastic cells and megakaryocytes in pulmonary vessels in a fatal case of amniotic fluid embolism. *International Journal of Legal Medicine*, **108**: 210, 1996.

47 Bick, R. L., Dukes, M. L., Wilson, W. L., *et al.* Antithrombin III (AT-III) as a diagnostic aid in disseminated intravascular coagulation. *Thromb. Res.*, **10**: 721, 1977.

48 Vedernikov, Y. P., Saade, G. R., Zlatnik, M., *et al.* The effect of amniotic fluid on the human omental artery in vitro. *Am. J. Obstet. Gynecol.*, **180**: 454, 1999.

49 Khong, T. Y. Expression of endothelin-1 in amniotic fluid embolism and possible pathophysiological mechanism. *Brit. J. Obstet. Gynaecol.*, **105**: 802, 1998.

50 English, C. J., Poller, L. and Burslem, R. W. A study of the procoagulant properties of amniotic fluid and their correlation with the lecithin/sphingomyelin ratio. *Brit. J. Obstet. Gynaecol.*, **88**: 133, 1981.

51 Pusey, M. L. and Mende, T. J. Studies on the procoagulant activity of human amniotic fluid I. Stability and coagulation factor requirements. *Throb. Res.*, **39**: 355, 1985.

52 Pusey, M. L. and Mende, T. J. Studies on the procoagulant activity of human amniotic Fluid II. The role of Factor VII. *Thromb. Res.*, **39**: 571, 1985.

53 Bick, R. L. and Murano, G. Physiology of hemostasis (Chapter 1) In *Disorders of Thrombosis & Hemostasis: Clinical & Laboratory Practice*, Lippincott Williams & Wilkins, Philadelphia, 2002, p. 1.

54 Bussen, S., Schwarzmann, G. and Steck, T. Clinical aspects and therapy of amniotic fluid embolism. Illustration based on a case report. *Zeitschrift fur Geburtshilfe und Neonatologie*, **201**: 95, 1997.

55 Davies, S. Amniotic fluid embolism and isolated disseminated intravascular coagulation. *Canadian Journal of Anaesthesia*, **46**: 456, 1999.

56 Van Heerden, P. V., Webb, S. A., Hee, G., *et al.* Inhaled aerosolized prostacyclin as a selective pulmonary vasodilator for the treatment of severe hypoxaemia. *Anaesthesia & Intensive Care*, **24**: 87, 1996.

57 Strickland, M. A., Bates, A. W., Whitworth, H. S., *et al.* Amniotic fluid embolism: prophylaxis with heparin and aspirin. *South. Med. Journal*, **78**: 377, 1985.

58 Bick, R. L., Fekete, L. F. and Wilson, W. L. Treatment of disseminated intravascular coagulation with antithrombin III. *Trans. Am. Soc. Hematol.*, 1976, p. 167.

59 Vinazzer, H. Antithrombin III in shock and disseminated intravascular coagulation. *Clin. Appl. Thromb. Hemost.*, **1**: 62, 1995.

60 Vinazzer, H. Hereditary and acquired antithrombin deficiency. *Seminars Thrombosis Hemostasis*, **25**: 257, 1999.

61 Suzuki, S. and Morishita, S. Hypercoagulability and DIC in high-risk infants. *Seminars in Thrombosis & Hemostasis*, **24**: 463, 1998.

62 Bick, R. L., Arun, B. and Frenkel, E. P. Disseminated intravascular coagulation: clinical and pathophysiological mechanisms and manifestations. *Haemostasis*, **29**: 111, 1999.

63 Bick, R. L. Disseminated intravascular coagulation: objective clinical and laboratory diagnosis, treatment and assessment of therapeutic response. *Seminars Thrombosis Hemostasis*, **22**: 69, 1996.

64 Hafter, R. and Graeff, H. Molecular aspects of defibrination in a reptilase-treated case of "dead-fetus syndrome". *Thromb. Res.*, **7**: 391, 1975.

65 Steichele, D. F. Consumptive coagulopathy in obstetrics and gynecology. *Thromb. Diath. Haemorrh. (Suppl.)*, **36**: 177, 1969.

66 Brenner, B. M. Vascular injury to the kidney (Chapter 277). In Fauci, A. S., Braunwald, E., Isselbacher, K. J., *et al.* eds. *Principles of internal Medicine*, Edn 14. McGraw-Hill, St. Louis, MO. 1998, p. 1558.

67 Mjahed, K., Hammamouchi, B., Hammoudi, D., *et al.* Critical analysis of hemostasis disorders in the course of eclampsia. Report of 106 cases. *Journal de Gynecologie, Obstetrique et Biologie de la Reproduction*, **27**: 607, 1998.

68 Porozhanova, V., Bozhinova, S. and Khristova, V. The perinatal outcome in adolescents with eclampsia and the HELLP syndrome. *Akusherstvo i Ginekologiia*, **35**: 14, 1996.

69 Yao, T., Yao, H. and Wang, H. Diagnosis and treatment of nephrotic syndrome during pregnancy. *Chinese Medical Journal*, **109**: 471, 1996.

70 Bonnar, J., McNicol, G. P. and Douglas, A. S. Coagulation and fibrinolytic systems in pre-eclampsia and eclampsia. *Br. Med. J.*, **1**: 12, 1971.

71 Schjetlein, R., Haugen, G. and Wisloff, F. Markers of intravascular coagulation and fibrinolysis in preeclampsia: association with intrauterine growth retardation. *Acta Obstetricia et Gynecologica Scandinavica*, **76**: 541, 1997.

72 Verduzco Rodriguez, L., Gonzalez Puebla, E., Manffrini Madrid, F., *et al.* D-dimer in different stages of pregnancy toxemia. A pilot study. *Ginecologia y Obstetricia de Mexico*, **66**: 77, 1998.

73 Ishibashi, M., Ito, N., Fujita, M., *et al.* Endothelin-1 as an aggravating factor of disseminated intravascular coagulation associated with malignant neoplasms. *Cancer*, **73**: 191, 1994.

74 Jones, S. L. HELLP: A cry for laboratory assistance – a comprehensive review of the HELLP syndrome highlighting the role of the laboratory. *Hematopathology & Molecular Hematology*, **11**: 147, 1998.

75 Carpani, G., Bozzo, M., Ferrazzi, E., *et al.* The evaluation of maternal parameters at diagnosis may predict HELLP syndrome severity. *J. Maternal Fetal Neonatal Medicine*, **13**: 147, 2003.

76 Cincotta, R. and Ross, A. A review of eclampsia in Melbourne: 1978–1992. *Australian & New Zealand Journal of Obstetrics & Gynaecology*, **36**: 264, 1996.

77 D'Anna, R. The HELLP syndrome. Notes on its pathogenesis and treatment. *Minerva Ginecologica*, **48**: 147, 1996.

78 Portis, R., Jacobs, M. A., Skerman, J. H., *et al.* HELLP syndrome (hemolysis, elevated liver enzymes, and low platelets) pathophysiology and anesthetic considerations. *AANA Journal*, **65**: 37, 1997.

79 Stone, J. H. HELLP Syndrome: hemolysis, elevated liver enzymes, and low platelets. *JAMA*, **280**: 559, 1998.

80 Debette, M., Samuel, D., Ichai, P., *et al.* Labor complications of the HELLP syndrome without any predictive factors. *Gastroenterologie Clinique et Biologique*, **23**: 264, 1999.

81 Paternoster, D. M., Rodi, J., Santarossa, C., *et al.* Acute pancreatitis and deep vein thrombosis associated with the HELLP syndrome. *Minerva Ginecologica*, **51**: 31, 1999.

82 Sheikh, R. A., Yasmeen, S., Pauly, M. P., *et al.* Spontaneous intrahepatic hemorrhage and hepatic rupture in the HELLP syndrome: four cases and a review. *Journal of Clinical Gastroenterology*, **28**: 323, 1999.

83 Weemhoff, R. A., van Loon, A. J. and Aarnoudse, J. G. Liver rupture in pregnancy: a life-threatening complication of the HELLP syndrome. *Nederlands Tijdschrift voor Geneeskunde*, **140**: 2140, 1996.

84 Magann, E. F. and Martin, J. N. Twelve steps to optimal managment of HELLP Syndrome. *Clinical Obstet. Gynecol.*, **42**: 532, 1999.

85 O'Boyle, J. D., Magann, E. F., Waxman, E., *et al.* Dexamethasone-facilitated postponement of delivery of an extremely preterm pregnancy complicated by the syndrome of hemolysis, elevated liver enzymes, and low platelets. *Military Medicine*, **164**: 316, 1999.

86 Vigil-De Gracia, P. and Garcia-Caceres, E. Dexamethasone in the post-partum treatment of HELLP syndrome. *International Journal of Gynaecology & Obstetrics*, **59**: 217, 1997.

87 Yalcin, O. T., Sener, T., Hassa, H., *et al.* Effects of postpartum corticosteroids in patients with HELLP syndrome. *International Journal of Gynaecology & Obstetrics*, **61**: 141, 1998.

88 Hamada, S., Takishita, Y., Tamura, T., *et al.* Plasma exchange in a patient with postpartum HELLP syndrome. *Journal of Obstetrics and Gynaecology Research*, **22**: 371, 1996.

89 Owen, C. A., Bowie, E. J. W. and Cooper, H. A. Turnover of fibrinogen and platelets in dogs undergoing induced intravascular coagulation. *Thromb. Res.*, **2**: 251, 1973.

90 Rath, W. Aggressive versus conservative management of HELLP syndrome – a status assessment. *Geburtshilfe und Frauenheilkunde*, **56**: 265, 1996.

91 Spivack, J. L., Sprangler, D. B. and Bell, W. R. Defibrination after intra-amniotic injection of hypertonic saline. *N. Engl. J. Med.*, **287**: 321, 1972.

92 Frenkel, E. and Bick, R. L. Thrombohemorrhagic defects associated with malignancy (Ch. 12) In *Disorders of Thrombosis & Hemostasis: Clinical & Laboratory Practice*, Lippincott Williams & Wilkins, Philadelphia, 2002, p. 265.

93 Bick, R. L. Alterations of hemostasis associated with malignancy (Ch. 11). In Murano, G., Bick, R. L., eds. *Basic Concepts of Hemostasis and Thrombosis*, CRC Press, Boca Raton, FL, 1980, p. 213.

94 Bick, R. L. Alterations of hemostasis in malignancy (Ch. 12) In *Disorders of Thrombosis and Hemostasis: Clinical and Laboratory Practice*, ASCP Press, Chicago, 1992, p. 239.

95 Bick, R. L., Strauss, J. F. and Rutherford, C. J., *et al.* Thrombosis and hemorrhage in oncology patients. *Hematology Oncology Clinics North America*, **10**: 875, 1996.

96 Cafagna, D. and Ponte, E. Pulmonary embolism of paraneoplastic origin. *Minerva Medica*, **88**: 523, 1997.

97 Frenkel, U. P. and Bick, R. L. Issues of thrombosis and hemorrhagic events in patients with cancer. *Anticancer Research*, **18**: 1, 1998.

98 Weltermann, A., Mitterbauer, G. J., Mittebauer, M., *et al.* Disseminated intravascular coagulation (DIC) with massive hyperfibrinolysis in metastatic uterine cancer: observations on the effects on the coagulopathy of various treatments. *Weiner Klinische Wochenschrift*, **110**: 53, 1998.

99 Bick, R. L. Coagulation abnormalities in malignancy. *Seminars Thrombosis Hemostasis*, **18**: 353, 1992.

100 Bick, R. L. Disseminated intravascular coagulation: section 6. *Conn's Current Therapy.* W. B. Saunders, Philadelphia, 2003, p. 442.

101 Bick, R. L. Disseminated intravascular coagulation: a clinical review. *Sem. Thromb. Hemostas.*, **14**: 299, 1988.

102 Bick, R. L. and Kunkel, L. Disseminated intravascular coagulation. *Int. J. Hematology*, **55**: 1, 1992.

103 Bick, R. L. and Scates, S. Disseminated intravascular coagulation. *Laboratory Medicine*, **23**: 161, 1992.

104 Bick, R. L. Disseminated intravascular coagulation and related syndromes. A review. *Am. J. Hematol.*, **5**: 265, 1978.

105 Davis, R. B., Theologides, A. and Kennedy, B. J. Comparative studies of blood coagulation and platelet aggregation in patients with cancer and non-malignant disease. *Ann. Intern. Med.*, **71**: 67, 1969.

106 Goodnight, S. H. Bleeding and intravascular clotting in malignancy: a review. *Ann. NY Acad. Sci.*, **230**: 271, 1974.

107 Gralnick, H. R. and Tan, H. K. Acute promyelocytic leukemia. A model for understanding the role of the malignant cells in hemostasis. *Human Path*, **5**: 661, 1974.

108 Leavy, R. A. Kahn, S. B. and Brodsky, I. Disseminated intravascular coagulation: a complication of chemotherapy in acute promyelocytic leukemia. *Cancer*, **26**: 142, 1970.

109 Bick, R. L. Disseminated intravascular coagulation: current concepts of etiology, pathophysiology, diagnosis and management. (Ch. 8) In *Hematology Oncology Clinics North America*, **17**: 149, 2003.

110 Pineo, G. F., Brain, M. C. and Gallus, A. S. Tumors, mucus production, and hypercoagulability. *Ann. NY Acad. Sci.*, **230**: 262, 1974.

111 Pineo, G. F., Regorczi, F., Hatton, M. W. C. The activation of coagulation by extracts of mucin: a possible pathway of intravascular coagulation accompanying adenocarcinomas. *J. Lab. Clin. Med.*, **82**: 255, 1973.

112 Harpel, P. C. Alpha-2-plasmin inhibitor and alpha-2-macroglobulin-plasmin complexes in plasma. *J. Clin. Invest.*, **68**: 46, 1981.

113 Bick, R. L. Basic mechanisms of hemostasis pertaining to DIC (Ch. 1). In *Disseminated Intravascular Coagulation and Related Syndromes.* CRC Press, Boca Raton, FL, 1983, p. 1.

114 Bick, R. L. Disseminated intravascular coagulation and related syndromes (Ch. 7). *In Disorders of Thrombosis and Hemostasis: Clinical and Laboratory Practice.* ASCP Press, Chicago, 1992, p. 137.

115 Cheung, D. K., Raaf, J. H. Selection of patients with malignant ascites for a peritoneovenous shunt. *Cancer*, **50**: 1204, 1982.

116 Harmon, D. C., Demirjian, Z. and Ellman, L. Disseminated intravascular coagulation with the peritoneovenous shunt. *Ann. Int. Med.*, **90**: 714, 1979.

117 Lerner, R. G., Nelson, J. C., Corines, P., *et al.* Disseminated intravascular coagulation: complication of LeVeen peritoneovenous shunts. *JAMA*, **240**: 2064, 1984.

118 Stein, S. F., Fulenwider, J. T. and Ansley, J. D. Accelerated fibrinogen and platelet destruction after peritoneovenous shunting. *Arch. Int. Med.*, **141**: 1149, 1981.

119 Bick, R. L. and Tse, N. Hemostasis abnormalities associated with prosthetic devices and organ transplantation. *Laboratory Medicine*, **23**: 462, 1992.

120 Egeberg, O. Blood coagulation and intravascular hemolysis. *Scand. J. Clin. Lab. Invest.*, **14**: 217, 1962.

121 Krevins, J. R., Jackson, D. P., Cowley, C. L., *et al.* The nature of the hemorrhagic disorder accompanying hemolytic transfusion reactions in man. *Blood*, **12**: 834, 1957.

122 Langdell, R. D. and Hedgpeth, E. M. A study of the role of hemolysis in the hemostatic defect of transfusion reactions. *Thromb. Diath. Haemorrh.*, **3**: 566, 1959.

123 Surgenor, D. M. Erythrocytes and blood coagulation. *Thromb. Diath. Haemorrh.*, **32**: 247, 1974.

124 Abildgaard, C. F., Corrigan, J. J., Seeler, R. A., *et al.* Meningiococcemia associated with intravascular coagulation. *Pediatrics*, **40**: 78, 1967.

125 Corrigan, J. J. Changes in the blood coagulation system associated with septicemia. *N. Engl. J. Med.*, **279**: 851, 1968.

126 Yoshikawa, T., Tanaka, R., and Guze, L. B. Infection and disseminated intravascular coagulation. *Medicine (Baltimore)*, **50**: 237, 1971.

127 Ceriello, A., Giacomello, R., Colatutto, A., *et al.* Increased prothrombin fragment 1 + 2 in Type I diabetic patients. *Haemostasis*, **22**: 50, 1992.

128 Cline, M. J., Melmon, K. L., Davis, W. C., *et al.* Mechanism of endotoxin interaction with leukocytes. *Br. J. Haematol.*, **15**: 539, 1968.

129 McKay, D. G., and Shapiro, S. S. Alterations in the blood coagulation system induced by bacterial endotoxin I: in vitro (generalized Schwartzman reaction). *J. Exp. Med.*, **107**: 353, 1958.

130 Cronberg, S., Skansberg, P., Nivenios-Larsson, K. Disseminated intravascular coagulation in septicemia caused by beta-hemolytic streptococci. *Thromb. Res.*, **3**: 405, 1973.

131 Rubenberg, W. L., Baker, L. R., McBride, J. A., *et al.* Intravascular coagulation in a case of clostridium perfringens septicemia: treatment by exchange transfusion and heparin. *Br. Med. J.*, **3**: 271, 1967.

132 Gagel, C., Linder, M., Muller-Berghous, G., *et al.* Virus infection and blood coagulation. *Thromb. Diath. Haemorrh.*, **23**: 1, 1970.

133 McKay, D. G. and Margaretten, W. Disseminated intravascular coagulation in virus diseases. *Arch. Intern. Med.*, **120**: 129, 1967.

134 Salmon, S. J., Lambert, P. H., Louis, J. Pathogenesis of the intravascular coagulation syndrome induced by immunological reactions. *Thromb. Diath. Haemorrh.*, **45**: 161, 1971.

135 Muller-Berghaus, G. Pathophysiologic and biochemical events in disseminated intravascular coagulation: dysregulation of procoagulant and anticoagulant pathways. *Sem. Thromb. Hemostas.*, **15**: 58, 1989.

136 McKay, D. G., Margaretten, W. and Csavossy, I. An electron microscope study of the effects of bacterial endotoxin on the blood-vascular system. *Lab. Invest.*, **15**: 1815, 1966.

137 Latallo, Z. S. Products of fibrin(ogen) proteolysis. *Thromb. Diath. Haemorrh. (Suppl.)*, **24**: 145, 1973.

138 Marder, V. J., Shulman, H. R. and Carroll, W. R. High molecular weight derivatives of human fibrinogen produced by plasmin. I. Physico-chemical and immunological characterization. *J. Biol. Chem.*, **244**: 2111, 1969.

139 Marder, V. J., Budzynski, A. Z. and James, H. L. High molecular weight derivatives of human fibrinogen produced by plasmin. III. Their NH2-terminal amino acids and comparison of the "NH2-terminal amino disulfide knot". *J. Biol. Chem.*, **247**: 4775, 1972.

140 Bang, N. U. and Chang, M. Soluble fibrin complexes. *Seminar Thromb. Hemost.*, **1**: 91, 1974.

141 Breen, F. A. and Tullis, J. Z. Ethanol gelation, a rapid screening test for intravascular coagulation. *Ann. Intern. Med.*, **69**: 111, 1968.

142 Fletcher, A. P., Alkjaersig, N., Fisher, S., *et al.* The proteolysis of fibrinogen by plasmin: the identification of thrombin-clottable fibrinogen derivatives which polymerize abnormally. *J. Lab. Clin. Med.*, **68**: 780, 1966.

143 Gurewich, V. and Hutchinson, E. Detection of intravascular coagulation by protamine sulfate and ethanol gelation tests. *Thromb. Res.*, **2**: 539, 1973.

144 Bick, R. L. The clinical significance of fibrinogen degradation products. *Seminars Thromb. Hemost.*, **8**: 302, 1982.

145 Kopec, M., Wegrzynowiczy, Z., Budzynski, A., *et al.* Interaction of fibrinogen degradation products with platelets. *Exp. Biol. Med.*, **3**: 73, 1968.

146 Niewiarowski, S., Regoeczi, E., Stewart, G., *et al.* Platelet interaction with polymerizing fibrin. *J. Clin. Invest.*, **51**: 685, 1972.

147 Robson, S., Shephard, E. and Kirsch, R. Fibrin degradation product D-dimer induces the synthesis and release of biologically active IL-1 beta, IL-6 and plasminogen activator inhibitors from monocytes in vitro. *Br. J. Haematol.*, **86**: 322, 1994.

148 Gando, S., Kameue, T., Nanzaki, S., *et al.* Cytokines, soluble thrombomodulin and disseminated intravascular coagulation in patients with systemic inflammatory response syndrome. *Thrombosis Research*, **80**: 519, 1995.

149 Okajima, K., Uchiba, M., Murakami, K., *et al.* Plasma levels of soluble E-selectin in patients with disseminated intravascular coagulation. *Am. J. Hematol.*, **54**: 219, 1997.

150 Ono, S., Mochizuki, H. and Tamakuma, S. A clinical study on the significance of platelet-activating factor in the pathophysiology of septic disseminated intravascular coagulation in surgery. *Am. J. Surgery*, **171**: 409, 1996.

151 Elsayed, Y., Nakagawa, K., Ichikawa, K., *et al.* Expression of tissue factor and interleukin-1 beta in a novel rabbit model of disseminated intravascular coagulation induced by carrageenan and lipopolysaccharide. *Pathobiology*, **63**: 328, 1995.

152 Hoffman, M. and Cooper, S. T. Thrombin enhances monocyte secretion of tumor necrosis factor and interleukin-1 by two distinct mechanisms. *Blood Cells, Molecules and Diseases*, **21**: 156, 1995.

153 Okajima, K., Fujise, R., Motosato, Y., *et al.* Plasma levels of granulocyte elastase-alpha 1-proteinase inhibitor complex in patients with disseminated intravascular coagulation: pathophysiologic implications. *Am. J. Hematol.*, **47**: 82, 1994.

154 Muller-Berghous, G. Pathophysiology of generalized intravascular coagulation. *Seminars Thromb. Hemost.*, **3**: 209, 1977.

155 Nilsson, I. M. Local fibrinolysis as a mechanism for haemorrhage. *Thromb. Diath. Haemorh.*, **34**: 623, 1975.

156 Stormorken, H. Relation of the fibrinolytic to other biological systems. *Thromb. Diath. Haemorrh.*, **34**: 378, 1975.

157 Schreiber, A. D., Austen, K. F. Interrelationships of the fibrinolytic, coagulation, kinin generation, and complement systems. *Seminars Hematol.*, **6**: 593, 1973.

158 Collins, P., Noble, K., Reittie, J., *et al.* Induction of tumor factor expression in human monocyte/endothelium cocultures. *Br. J. Haematol.*, **91**: 963, 1995.

159 Gando, S., Nakanishi, Y. and Tedo, I. Cytokines and plasminogen activator inhibitor-1 in post-trauma disseminated intravascular coagulation: relationship to multiple organ dysfunction. *Critical Care Medicine*, **23**: 1835, 1995.

160 Kaplan, A., Meier, H. and Mandel, R. The Hageman factor dependent pathways of coagulation, fibrinolysis, and kinin generation. *Seminars Thromb. Hemost.*, **3**: 6, 1976.

161 van Iwaarden, F. and Bouma B. Role of high molecular weight kininogen in contact activation. *Seminars Thromb. Hemost.*, **13**: 15, 1987.

162 Beller, F. K., Theiss, W. Fibrin derivitives, plasma hemoglobin and glomerular fibrin deposition in experimental intra-vascular coagulation. *Thromb. Diath. Haemorrh.*, **29**: 363, 1973.

163 McKay, D. G., Linder, M. M. and Cruse, V. K. Mechanisms of thrombosis of the microcirculation. *Am. J. Pathol.*, **63**: 231, 1971.

164 Bick, R. L. Disseminated intravascular coagulation. *Hematology Oncology Clinics North America*, **6**: 1259, 1992.

165 Lerner, R. G. The defibrination syndrome. *Med. Clin. N. Am.*, **60**: 871, 1976.

166 Robboy, S. J., Coleman, R. W. and Minna, J. D. Pathology of disseminated intravascular coagulation (DIC). Analysis of 26 cases. *Human Pathol.*, **3**: 327, 1972.

167 Owen, C. A. and Bowie, E. J. W. Chronic intravascular syndromes. *Mayo Clinical Proc.*, **49**: 673, 1974.

168 Skjorten, F. Hyaline microthrombi in an autopsy material. A quantitative study with discussion of the relationship to small vessel thrombosis. *Acta Pathol. Microbiol. Scand.*, **76**: 361, 1969.

169 Bleyl, U. Morphologic diagnosis of disseminated intravascular coagulation: histologic, histochemical, and electron-microscopic studies. *Seminars Thromb. Hemost.*, **3**: 247, 1977.

170 Morris, J. A., Smith, R. W. and Assali, N. S. Hemodynamic action of vaso-pressor and vaso-depressor agents in endotoxin shock. *Am. J. Obstet. Gynecol.*, **91**: 491, 1965.

171 Bleyl, U., Kuhn, W. and Graeff, H. Reticulo-endotheliale clearance intravascaler. Fibrinmonere in der milz. *Thromb. Diath. Haemorrh.*, **22**: 87, 1969.

172 Boyd, J. F. Disseminated fibrin-thromboembolism among neonates dying within 48 hours of birth. *Arch. Dis. Child.*, **42**: 401, 1967.

173 Bull, B., Kuhn I. N. The production of schistocytes by fibrin strands (a scanning electron microscope study). *Blood*, **35**: 104, 1970.

174 Heyes, H., Kohle, W. and Slijerpcevic, B. The appearance of schistocytes in the peripheral blood in correlation to degree of disseminated intravascular coagulation. *Haemostasis*, **5**: 66, 1976.

175 Bull, B., Rubenberg, M., Dacie, J., *et al.* Microangiopathic hemolytic anemia: mechanisms of red-cell fragmentation. *Br. J. Haematol.*, **14**: 643, 1968.

176 Bick, R. L. Acquired platelet function defects. *Hematology Oncology Clinics North America*, **6**: 1203, 1992.

177 Karpatkin, S. Heterogeneity of human platelets. VI. Correlation of platelet function with platelet volume. *Blood*, **51**: 307, 1978.

178 Blaisdell, F. W. and Stallone, R. J. The mechanism of pulmonary damage following traumatic shock. *Surg. Gynecol. Obstet.*, **130**: 15, 1970.

179 van Breeman, V. L., Heustein, H. B. and Bruns, P. D. Pulmonary hyaline membranes studied with the electron microscope. *Am. J. Pathol.*, **33**: 769, 1957.

180 Martin, A. M., Soloway, H. B. and Simmons, R. L. Pathologic anatomy of the lungs following shock and trauma. *J. Trauma*, **8**: 687, 1968.

181 Soloway, H. B., Castillo, Y. and Martin, A. M. Adult hyaline membrane disease. *Ann. Surg.*, **168**: 937, 1968.

182 Hardaway, R. M. Acute respiratory distress syndrome and disseminated intravascular coagulation. *South Med. J.*, **71**: 596, 1978.

183 Hardaway R. M. *Syndromes of Disseminated Intravascular Coagulation with Special Reference to Shock and Hemorrhage.* Charles C. Thomas, Springfield, Ill, 1966.

184 Muller-Berghous and Mann, G. B. Precipitation of ancrod-induced soluble fibrin by aprotinin and norepinephrine. *Thromb. Res.*, **2**: 305, 1973.

185 Latour, J. G., Prejean, J. B. and Margaretten, W. Corticosteroids and the generalized Schwartzman reaction. Mechanisms of sensitization in the rabbit. *Am. J. Pathol.*, **65**: 189, 1971.

186 Bick, R. L. Clinical hemostasis practice: the major impact of laboratory automation. *Seminars Thromb. Hemost.*, **9**: 139, 1983.

187 Fareed, J., Bick, R. L., Hoppenstedt, D., *et al.* Molecular markers of hemostatic activation: implications in the diagnosis of thrombosis, vascular and cardiovascular disorders. *Clinics Laboratory Medicine*, **15**: 39, 1995.

188 Messmore, H. L. Automation in coagulation testing: clinical applications. *Seminars Thromb. Hemost.*, **9**: 335, 1983.

189 Marder, V. J., Matchett, M. O. and Sherry, S. Detection of serum fibrinogen and fibrin degradation products: comparison of six techniques using purified products and application in clinical studies. *Am. J. Med.*, **51**: 71, 1971.

190 Myers, A. R., Bloch, K. J. and Coleman, R. W. A comparative study of four methods for detecting fibrinogen degradation products in patients with various diseases. *N. Engl. J. Med.*, **283**: 663, 1970.

191 Gurewich, V., Lipinsky, B. and Lipinska, I. A comparative study of precipitation and paracoagulation by protamine sulfate and ethanol gelation tests. *Thromb. Res.*, **2**: 539, 1973.

192 Hedner, U. and Nilsson, I. M. Parallel determinations of FDP and fibrin monomers with various methods. *Thromb. Diath. Haemorrh.*, **28**: 268, 1972.

193 Slaastad, R. A. and Godal, N. C. Coagulation profile and ethanol gelation test with special reference to components consumed during coagulation. *Scand. J. Haematol.*, **16**: 25, 1976.

194 Sonnabend, D., Cooper, D. and Fiddes, P., *et al.* Fibrin degradation products in thromboembolic disease. *Pathology*, **4**: 47, 1972.

195 Stibbe, J., Gomes, M. and de Ouda, A. The value of the FM-test (KABI) and thrombin-antithrombin-III complexes (TAT) in the management of DIC in cancer. *Throm. Haemost.*, **65**: 1238, 1989.

196 Francis, C. W. and Marder, V. J. A molecular model of plasmic degradation of cross-linked fibrin. *Sem. Thromb. Hemostas.*, **8**: 25, 1982.

197 Plow, E. F. and Edgington, T. S. Surface markers of fibrinogen and its physiologic derivatives related by antibody probes. *Seminars Thromb. Hemost.*, **8**: 36, 1982.

198 Matsumoto, T., Nishijima, Y., Teramura, Y., *et al.* Monoclonal antibodies to fibrinogen-fibrin degradation products which contain D-Domain. *Thromb. Res.*, **38**: 279, 1985.

199 Rylatt, D. B., Blake, A. S., Cottis, L. E., *et al.* An immunoassay for human D-Dimer using monoclonal antibodies. *Thromb. Res.*, **31**: 767, 1983.

200 Elms, M. J., Bunce, I. H., Bundesen, P. G. Measurement of cross-linked fibrin degradation products – an immunoassay using monoclonal antibodies. *Thromb. Haemostas.*, **50**: 591, 1983.

201 Ellis, D. R., Eaton, A. S., Plank, M. C., *et al.* A comparative evaluation of ELISA's for D-Dimer and related fibrin(ogen) degradation products. *Blood Coagulation and Fibrinolysis*, **4**: 537, 1993.

202 Murano, G. The molecular structure of fibrinogen. *Seminars Thromb. Hemost.*, **1**: 1, 1974.

203 Rosenberg, J. S., Beeler, D. L. and Rosenberg, R. D. Activation of human prothrombin by highly purified human factors V and Xa in the presence of human antithrombin. *J. Biol. Chem.*, **250**: 1607, 1975.

204 Tietel, J. M., Bauer, K. A., Lau, H. K., *et al.* Studies of the prothrombin activation pathway utilizing radioimmunoassays for the F_2/F_{1+2} fragment and thrombin-antithrombin complex. *Blood*, **59**: 1086, 1982.

205 Boneu, B., Bes, G., Pelzer, H., *et al.* D-dimers, thrombin antithrombin complexes and prothrombin fragments 1 + 2: diagnostic value in clinically suspected deep vein thrombosis. *Thromb. Haemost.*, **65**: 28, 1991.

206 Bruhn, H. D., Conard, J., Mannucci, M., *et al.* Multicentric evaluation of a new assay for prothrombin fragment F 1 + 2 determination. *Thromb. Haemost.*, **68**: 413, 1992.
207 Okamoto, K., Takaki, A., Takeda, S., *et al.* Coagulopathy in disseminated intravascular coagulation due to abdominal sepsis: determination of prothrombin fragment 1 + 2 and other markers. *Haemostasis*, **22**: 17, 1992.
208 Pelzer, H., Schwarz, A. and Stuber, W. Determination of human prothrombin activation fragment 1 + 2 in plasma with an antibody against a synthetic peptide. *Thromb. Haemost.*, **65**: 153, 1991.
209 Sorensen, J. V., Jensen, H. P., Rahr, H. R., *et al.* F 1 + 2 and FPA in urine from patients with multiple trauma and healthy individuals: a pilot study. *Thromb. Res.*, **67**: 429, 1992.
210 Bick, R. L. and Murano, G. Physiology of hemostasis (Ch. 84) In Bick, R. L., Bennett, J. M., Brynes, R. K., eds., *Hematology: Clinical and Laboratory Practice*, Mosby, Saint Louis, MO, 1993, p. 1285.
211 Bick, R. L. and McClain, B. J. A clinical comparison of chromogenic, fluorometric, and natural (fibrinogen) substrates for determination of antithrombin-III. *Thromb. Haemost.*, **46**: 364, 1981.
212 Fareed, J., Messmore, H. L., Walenga, J. M., *et al.* Laboratory evaluation of antithrombin III: a critical overview of currently available methods for antithrombin III measurements. *Seminars Thromb. Hemost.*, **8**: 288, 1982.
213 Bick, R. L. Clinical relevance of antithrombin III. *Seminars Thromb. Hemost.*, **8**: 276, 1982.
214 Cronlund, M., Hardin, J., Burton, L., *et al.* Fibrinopeptide-A in plasma of normal subjects and patients with disseminated intravascular coagulation and systemic lupus erythematosis. *J. Clin. Invest.*, **58**: 142, 1976.
215 Douglas, J. T., Shah, M., Lowe, G. D. O., *et al.* Fibrinopeptide-A and Beta-thromboglobulin levels in pre-eclampsia and hypertensive pregnancy. *Thromb. Haemost.*, **46**: 8, 1981.
216 Bauer, K. A., Weiss, L. M., Sparrow, D., *et al.* Aging-associated changes in indices of thrombin generation and protein C activation in humans. Normative aging study. *J. Clin. Invest.*, **80**: 1527, 1987.
217 Clavin, S. A., Bobbitt, J. L., Shuman, R. T., *et al.* Use of peptidyl-4-methoxy-2-naphthylamides to assay plasmin. *Anal. Biochem.*, **80**: 355, 1977.
218 Triplett, D. A., Harms, C., Hermelin, L., *et al.* Clinical studies of the use of fluorogenic substrate assay method for the determination of plasminogen. *Thromb. Haemost.*, **42**: 50, 1979.
219 Kowalski, E., Kopec, M. and Niewiarowski, S. An evaluation of the euglobulin method for the determination of fibrinolysis. *J. Clin. Pathol.*, **12**: 215, 1959.
220 Menon, I. S. A study of the possible correlation of euglobulin lysis time and dilute blood clot lysis time in the determination of fibrinolytic activity. *Lab. Pract.*, **17**: 334, 1968.
221 Aoki, N., Moroi, M. and Matsuda, M. The behavior of alpha-2-plasmin inhibitor in fibrinolytic states. *J. Clin. Invest.*, **60**: 361, 1977.
222 Collen, P. Identification and some properties of a new fast-acting plasmin inhibitor in human plasma. *Eur. J. Biochem.*, **69**: 209, 1976.
223 Harpel, P. C., Mosesson, M. W., Cooper, N. R. Studies on the structure and function of alpha-2-macroglobulin and C1 inactivator. In Reich, E., Rifkin, D. B., Shaw, E. (eds.), *Proteases and Biological Control*, Cold Spring Harbor Symp., Cold Spring Harbor, NY, 1975, p. 387.

224 Takahashi, H., Koike, T., Yoshida, N., *et al.* Excessive fibrinolysis in suspected amyloidosis: demonstration of plasmin-alpha-2 plasmin inhibitor complex and von Willebrand factor fragment in plasma. *Am. J. Hematol.*, **23**: 153, 1986.

225 Wiman, B., Jacobsson, L., Andersson, M., *et al.* Determination of plasmin-alpha-2-plasmin inhibitor complex in plasma samples by means of a radioimmunoassay. *Scand. J. Clin. Lab. Invest.*, **43**: 27, 1983.

226 Harpel, P. C. Alpha-2-plasmin inhibitor and alpha-2-macroglobulin-plasmin complexes in plasma. *J. Clin. Invest.*, **68**: 46, 1981.

227 Takahashi, H., Hanano, M., Takizawa, S., *et al.* Plasmin-alpha-2-plasmin inhibitor complex in plasma of patients with disseminated intravascular coagulation. *Am. J. Hematol.*, **28**: 162, 1988.

228 Matsuda, T., Seki, T., Ogawara, M., *et al.* Comparison between plasma levels of B-thromboglobulin and platelet factor 4 in various diseases. *Thromb. Haemost.*, **42**: 288, 1979.

229 Zahavi, J. and Kakkar, V. V. B-thromboglobulin – a specific marker of in vivo platelet release reaction. *Thromb. Haemost.*, **44**: 23, 1980.

230 Kwaan, H. C. Disseminated intravascular coagulation. *Med. Clin. N. Am.*, **56**: 177, 1972.

231 Bick, R. L. Clinical implications of molecular markers in hemostasis and thrombosis. *Seminars Thromb. Hemostas.*, **10**: 252, 1984.

232 Feinstein, D. I. Treatment of disseminated intravascular coagulation. *Sem. Thromb. Hemostas.*, **14**: 351, 1988.

233 Kuhn, W., Graeft, H. *Gerinnungsstorungen in der Geburtshilfe.* Theime Verlag, Stuttgart, 1977, p. 90.

234 Minna, J. D., Robboy, S., Coleman, R. W. Clinical aproach to a patient with suspected DIC. In Minna, J. D., Robboy, S. and Coleman, R. W. (eds). *Disseminated Intravascular Coagulation.* Charles C. Thomas, Springfield, IL, 1974, p. 167.

235 Thaler, E., and Lechner, K. Antithrombin III deficiency and thromboembolism. *Clin. Haematol.*, **10**: 369, 1981.

236 Bentley, P. G., Kakkar, V. V., Scully, M. F., *et al.* An objectice study of alternative methods of heparin administration. *Thromb. Res.*, **18**: 177, 1980.

237 Kakkar, V. V. The clinical use of antithrombin III. *Thromb. Haemost.*, **42**: 265, 1979.

238 Hellgren, M., Hagnevik K. and Robbe, H. Severe acquired antithrombin III deficiency in relation to hepatic and renal insufficiency and intruterine fetal death in late pregnancy. *Gynecol. Obstet. Invest.*, **16**: 107, 1983.

239 McGehee, W. G., Paul, R. H. and Feinstein, D. I. Antithrombin III concentrate in the management of patients with acute fatty liver of pregnancy. *Blood*, **66**: 282a, 1985.

240 Bick, R. L., Schmalhorst, W. R. and Fekete, L. F. Disseminated intravascular coagulation and blood component therapy. *Transfusion (Philadelphia)*, **16**: 361, 1976.

241 Gralnick, H. R., Greipp, P. Thrombosis with epsilon-amino-caproic acid therapy. *Am. J. Clin. Pathol.*, **56**: 151, 1971.

242 McNicol, G. P. and Douglas, A. S. Thrombolytic therapy and fibrinolytic inhibitors. In *Human Blood Coagulation, Haemostasis, and Thrombosis.* Oxford Press, London, 1972, p. 393.

243 Ratnoff, O. D. Epsilon aminocaproic acid: a dangerous weapon. *N. Engl. J. Med.*, **280**: 1124, 1969.

244 Patterson, W. P. and Ringenberg, Q. S. The pathophysiology of thrombosis in cancer. *Seminars Oncol.*, **17**: 140, 1990.

2

Recurrent miscarriage syndrome and infertility caused by blood coagulation protein/platelet defects

Rodger L. Bick, M.D., Ph.D., F.A.C.P.

Clinical Professor of Medicine and Pathology, University of Texas Southwestern Medical Center; Director: Dallas Thrombosis Hemostasis and Vascular Medicine Clinical Center, Dallas, Texas, USA

Introduction

Recurrent miscarriage syndrome (RMS) is a common obstetrical problem, affecting over 500,000 women in the USA per year;[1] infertility although less well defined in the population is also a common clinical problem.

Recurrent miscarriage, based upon literature available and our experience is generally due to well defined defects as follows: about 7% are secondary to chromosomal abnormalities, about 10% are due to anatomical abnormalities, about 15% appear due to hormonal abnormalities (progesterone, estrogens, diabetes or thyroid disease), about 6% cannot be explained and the remainder, about 55 to 62%, are due to blood coagulation protein/platelet defects.[1] The approximate prevalence of causes of RMS/infertility are summarized in Figure 2.1.[1] This is in contrast to first time miscarriage, which in about 90% of cases, is due to a chromosomal defect and may effect up to 25 percent of first time pregnancies.[1]

Blood coagulation protein/platelet defects

Recurrent miscarriage syndrome (RMS) due to blood protein or platelet defects may come about through two mechanisms, those disorders associated with a hemorrhagic tendency or those defects associated with a thrombotic tendency. Hemorrhagic (bleeding) defects associated with RMS are very rare, while thrombotic or hypercoagulable/thrombophilic defects are extremely common.[1,2] The hemorrhagic defects associated with fetal wastage syndrome presumably lead to inadequate fibrin formation, thus precluding adequate implantation of the

Hematological Complications in Obstetrics, Pregnancy, and Gynecology, ed. R. L. Bick *et al.* Published by Cambridge University Press.

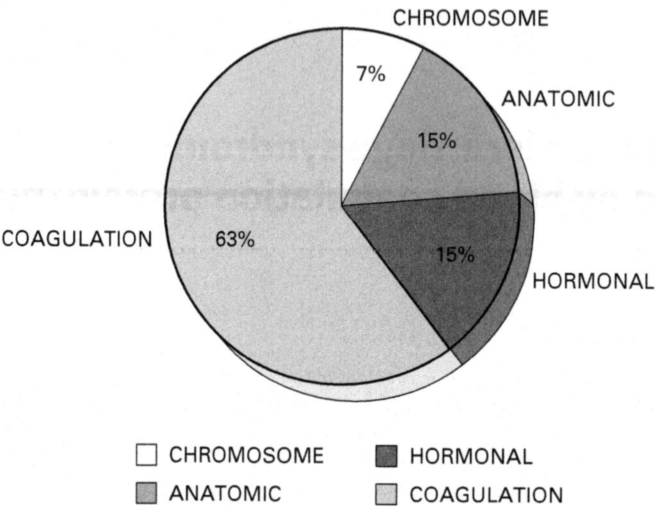

Figure 2.1 Defects causing recurrent miscarriage.

fertilized ovum into the uterus. The hemorrhagic defects associated with fetal wastage syndrome include Factor XIII deficiency,[3,4,5] Factor XII defects[6] Factor X deficiency,[7] Factor VII deficiency,[8] Factor V deficiency,[9] Factor II (prothrombin) deficiency[10] von Willebrand syndrome, carriers of Hemophilia and fibrinogen defects, including afibrinogenemia, those dysfibrinogenemias associated with hemorrhage and others.[11,12,13,14,15,16,17] Management of these patients is generally plasma substitution therapy or, in appropriate disorders DDAVP therapy.[1,2] Hemorrhagic/bleeding defects are rare causes of recurrent miscarriage as compared to thrombotic/thrombophilic disoders.[1,2]

The thrombotic defects associated with fetal wastage are thought to occur due to thrombosis of early placental vessels, with peak fetal wastage in the first trimester, but small peaks also occur in the second and third trimesters.[1,2] It appears the earlier the pregnancy, the smaller the placental and uterine vessels and, therefore, the greater the propensity to undergo partial or total occlusion by thrombus formation. Thrombotic occlusion of placental vessels, both venous and arterial, preclude adequate nutrition and, thus, viability of the fetus.[1,2]

The thrombotic hemostasis defects associated with RMS, include lupus anticoagulants and anticardiolipin antibodies (these two comprising the antiphospholipid syndromes associated with fetal wastage syndrome),[18,19,20] Factor XII deficiency,[21] dysfibrinogenemias associated with thrombosis,[22] Protein C defects,[23] Protein S defects, Antithrombin deficiency,[24] Heparin cofactor II deficiency,[25] and fibrinolytic defects associated with thrombosis, including plasminogen deficiency,[26] tissue plasminogen activator (t-PA) deficiency, elevated plasminogen

Table 2.1 Bleeding disorders associated with recurrent miscarriage syndrome (rare).

Factor XIII deficiency
Von Willebrand disease
Factor X deficiency
Factor VII deficiency
Factor V deficiency
Factor II deficiency
Hypofibrinogenemia
Dysfibrinogenemia
Hemophilia a carrier

Table 2.2 Thrombotic disorders associated with recurrent miscarriage syndrome (common).

Antiphospholipid syndrome
Sticky platelet syndrome
MTHFR mutations
Hyperhomocysteinemia
PAI-1 elevation/polymorphisms
Protein S deficiency
Factor V Leiden
Prothrombin G20210A
Protein C deficiency
Antithrombin deficiency
Heparin-Cofactor II deficiency
t-PA deficiency
Elevated lipoprotein (a)
Immune vasculitis

activator inhibitor Type 1 (PAI-1),[27] and PAI-1 polymorphism's.[28] Also, although sticky platelet syndrome has been known for over a decade and leads to a wide variety of arterial and venous events, only recently has it become apparent that this defect is a common cause of RMS[2] and, like other new defects, including Factor V Leiden, 5, 10-methyltetrahydrofolate reductase mutations (5,10-MTHFR) and prothrombin G20210 A gene mutation, should be added to the prothrombotic disorders associated with RMS.[2] It is anticipated that as new procoagulant factor mutations associated with hypercoagulability and thrombosis are discovered, they too will be found associated with placental thrombosis and RMS in many cases.

Table 2.1 summarizes the bleeding disorders which may give rise to RMS or infertility; it should be appreciated these are very rare causes as compared to prothrombotic disorders.

Table 2.2 summarizes the hypercoagulable, prothrombotic disorders leading to or potentially leading to RMS or infertility by inducing placental or uterine arterial or venous thrombosis; these defects are common causes of RMS and infertility.

Procoagulant defects

The antiphospholipid syndrome is clearly the most common thrombotic defect leading to fetal wastage syndrome/infertility and a variety of treatment programs have been advocated. One difficulty in evaluating these has been that some populations have addressed primarily patients with secondary antiphospholipid syndrome and fetal wastage, in particular those with underlying systemic lupus erythematosus or other autoimmune disorders, and only a few investigators have addressed populations with primary antiphospholipid syndrome, with no known underlying disease.

Antiphospholipid Syndrome (APLS) has long been recognized as a cause of miscarriage and infertility; it has long been recognized that treatment is often successful.[29] Many clinicians consider APLS to be the most common prothrombotic disorder among both hereditary and acquired defects and the most common thrombotic disorder causing recurrent miscarriage.[1,2,18,19,30,31,32,33,34] When assessing causes of infertility alone, APLS is thought to account for about 30% of infertility; however, in one series, abnormal CD 56+/CD 16 cell ratios were the single most common defect found (40%) in infertility patients.[35] In another recent series, only 21% of patients with RMS had APLS; however, when assessing women with APLS historically, 80% had suffered at least one miscarriage.[36] In a series reported by Granger, 384 unselected patients were assessed for APLS, of these 16% harbored APLS and of those with APLS 56% of APLS patients had a term delivery with low-dose ASA.[37] Borelli found that 60% of patients with "habitual" unexplained miscarriage harbored APLS.[38] Although the great majority of cases of APLS are clearly acquired,[32,33] familial APLS associated with RMS has been reported.[39] Clearly, however, screening for APLS is indicated in patients with RMS.[1,2,18,19,30,31,33,40] One recent study has suggested that monitoring miscarriage patients with APLS by use of prothrombin Fragment 1.2 may predict preclinical placental thrombi;[41] if this is confirmed, it may preclude the necessity of frequent sonograms, which is our current mode of careful following pregnant RMS patients on therapy. In addition since APLS is so common and since many of the hereditary thrombophilias, such as Factor V Leiden, are so prevalent in North America, it is not unexpected that some women with RMS will harbor APLS in combination with other procoagulant defects. Aznar has reported a case of RMS, complicated by DVT and thrombotic stroke in a patient with APLS, Factor V Leiden and congenital Protein S deficiency.[42] Many proposed mechanisms whereby APLS interfere with the hemostasis system and predispose to thrombosis have been proposed. These are summarized in appropriate references.[1,2,3,18,19,30,31,32,33,40] However, some investigators have proposed mechanisms specific for RMS. These proposed mechanisms have included the proposal the APLS induce acquired activated Protein C resistance (APC-R),[43] interference with prothrombin (Factor II), Protein C and Protein S, Tissue Factor and Factor XI[44] and the Tissue Factor/Tissue Factor Pathway Inhibitor (TF/TFPI) system.[45] Another study also found that patients with APLS also harbored antibodies to prothrombin, Protein C and Protein S.[46] Others have proposed these patients may also develop antibodies to "thromboplastin" and thrombin.[47] Another proposal is that antiphospholipid antibodies interfere with Annexin-V (also referred to as "Placental Anticoagulant Protein").[48] Two studies have shown Ig fractions of antiphospholipid antibody (APLA) or Beta-2-Glycoprotein-1 (APLA) decrease trophoblastic Annexin-V,[48,49,50] but several have shown this anti-Annexin-V activity to be limited to the antiphosphatidylserine subgroup antibody idiotype.[51,52] However, two carefully done studies have failed to demonstrate abnormalities of Annexin-V in miscarriage patients with APLS and concluded it plays no role in RMS.[53,54] In an additional study of lupus patients, anti-annexin antibodies were detected in only 19%; however, these were not miscarriage patients.[55] In an additional study in non-RMS lupus patients, only 3.8% harbored anti-Annexin-V antibodies.[44] In yet another study, patients with thrombosis and APLS were assessed; only 8% harbored Beta-2-Glycoprotein-1.[56] Testing for an antiphospholipid subgroup, in this case antiphosphatidylserine, was found useful in one study where RMS patients were negative for lupus anticoagulants and anticardiolipin antibodies; in this study it was thought useful to test for this subgroup.[57] In another study, however, the use of APL subgroup testing was not considered helpful.[58] It should be noted that on rare occasions antiphospholipid syndrome may be inherited (this author has seen three such families) and others have been reported,[39] suggesting that a positive maternal history may warrant evaluation at first pregnancy, as should a history of familial thrombosis.

Patients harboring other congenital or acquired thrombophilic states are also at high risk for placental thrombosis and RMS. In one study assessing a variety of these defects in 46 selected women (anatomic and hormone defects ruled out before hemostasis assessment) with RMS the following were found: 76% had anticardiolipin antibodies (void of lupus anticoagulants), 3% had a lupus anticoagulant (void of anticardiolipin antibodies), 11% had congenital protein S deficiency (three quantitative and one dysfunctional), 6.5% had "sticky platelet syndrome" (two with type I and one with type II), 3% had dysfibrinogenemia and 3% had congenital tPA deficiency.[2] In a study assessing prevalence of hereditary and acquired defects in RMS patients, 9% had isolated Factor XII deficiency, 7.4% had antiphospholipid syndrome, and fibrinolytic system defects, leading to hypofibrinolysis and hypercoagulability were found in 43% of patients.[59] This study concluded von Willebrand disease, fibrinogen deficiency, antithrombin deficiency, Protein C and Protein S deficiency, t-PA deficiency and PAI-1 defects played no role in RMS.[59] In a similar study assessing hereditary hemostasis defects in 125 RMS patients, quite different results were noted and Factor V Leiden mutation was found in 14%.[60] However, in another study of 50 RMS patients, it was concluded Factor V Leiden, Prothrombin G20210 A mutation and 5,10-methyltetrahydrofolate reductase mutations were not causes of RMS.[61] Factor V Leiden was discovered by Dahlback and associates in 1993[62], thus screening has only recently become common; for a summary of this inherited defect see reference 62.[62] As noted above, Kutteh failed to find an association between Factor V Leiden and recurrent miscarriage; however, in a recent study Factor V Leiden was found responsible for 48% of recurrent miscarriages.[63] In another study of pregnancy, it was found that although Factor V Leiden was responsible for a greater than 3-fold risk of DVT, there was no association with miscarriage.[64] In yet another study, however, Factor V Leiden was associated with a high incidence of second trimester miscarriages.[65] Also, two additional studies have clearly shown an association between Factor V Leiden mutation and recurrent miscarriages.[66,67] Thus, the preponderance of current evidence certainly strongly suggests that heterozygous Factor V Leiden mutation is a significant risk factor for recurrent miscarriage and increases the risk for miscarriage by at least 3.3 fold.[63] Another new common thrombophilic disorder, Prothrombin G20210A gene mutation, was described by Poort and associates in 1996.[68] Although Kutteh[61] found no association between this mutation and RMS, another study found an increased risk of recurrent miscarriage of 2.2-fold in women harboring this genetic procoagulant defect.[69] Another newly appreciated hereditary defect which leads to hypercoagulability and thrombosis is 5,10-methylenetetrahydrofolate reductase (MTHFR) C677 T mutation. One study found no association between this defect and recurrent miscarriage,[61] however another, more recent study, has shown a clear association between heterozygosity for this mutation and recurrent miscarriage with those harboring the mutation having a 2-fold enhanced risk.[69] Finally, although hypofibrinolysis, in general, has been shown to be associated with recurrent miscarriage,[27] only recently has the role of PAI-1 elevation and PAI-1 polymorphism(s) been shown as a cause of recurrent miscarriage syndrome.[28] Potential and proposed

Table 2.3 APL-T syndromes: proposed mechanisms of thrombosis.

1. Interference with endothelial phospholipids and thus, prostacyclin release
2. Inhibition of prekallikrein, thus inhibition of fibrinolysis
3. Inhibition of thrombomodulin, thus protein C/S activity
4. APC resistance (non-molecular)
5. Interaction with platelet membrane phospholipids
6. Inhibition of endothelial t-PA release
7. Direct inhibition of proteins
8. Inhibition of annexin V: a cell surface protein which inhibits tissue factor; also referred to as: "placental anticoagulant protein" (serine only!!)
9. Induce release of monocyte tissue factor

mechanism(s) of antiphospholipid antibody – induced thrombosis are summarized in Table 2.3

Dallas Thrombosis Hemostasis Clinical Center experience

Over the past five years we have carefully assessed 351 women referred for thrombosis and hemostasis evaluation after suffering recurrent miscariages. In the Dallas/Fort Worth Metroplex (DFW Metroplex), comprising a population of about 6 million, a flow protocol is followed to maximize success and keep costs of evaluation for etiology of RMS/infertility at a minimum, while providing the best chances for defining an etiology and, thus, providing ideal therapy for successful term pregnancy outcome.[1,2,3] This protocol is presented in Figure 2.2. In all instances, women with RMS/infertility are first seen by an obstetrician or reproductive specialist; at this stage anatomical defects and hormonal defects are assessed and, if found, the workup stops at this point and treatment is initiated (about 25% of all women). If no anatomical or hormonal defect is found, the patient is then seen by referral for hemostasis evaluation; the positive yield among this selected population is about 92%. If this evaluation is negative (about 8%), then if the patient desires, chromosomal evaluation is initiated (about a 7% yield). Most of the obstetricians/reproductive specialists in the DFW Metroplex refer after two or more miscarriages; however, some will refer after one miscarriage in the face of a positive family history for miscarriage and, occasionally, patients will request a work-up after only one miscarriage; our practice has been to accommodate the desires of the patient, after discussing the costs and other implications of evaluation. At the time of this writing, all 322 patients with a defect have been followed for at least 15 months, thus have been analyzed in detail and are presented below.

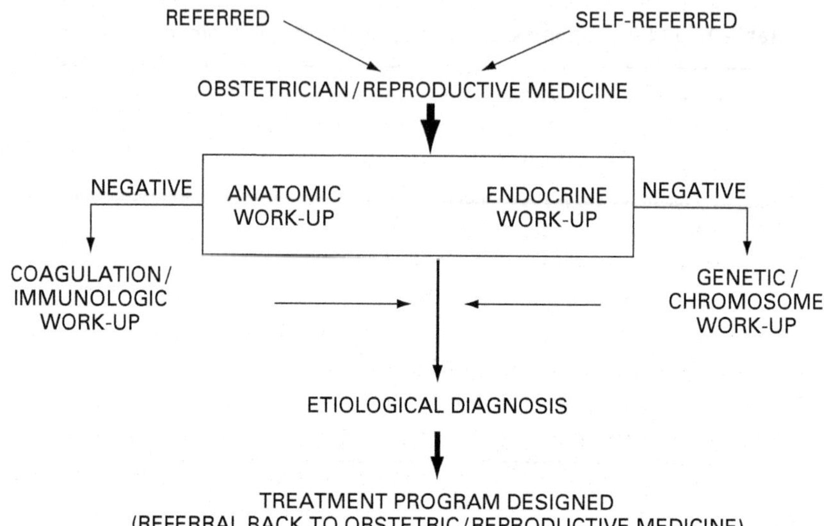

Figure 2.2 A suggested pathway for evaluation of the patient with recurrent miscarriage.

Characteristics of the first 351 women referred for hemostasis evaluation

The mean age of patients referred for a hemostasis evaluation is 33.3, the mean number of miscarriages before referral is 2.9 (range = 2–9) and the percent found with a hemostasis defect has been 92%. This information is provided in Table 2.4.

All patients underwent a thorough evaluation for thrombophilia and, when indicated, a hemorrhagic disorder. Of the 351 patients, 29 (8%) had no defect. Of the remaining 322 patients, 10 (2%) had a bleeding disorder: 3 with platelet dysfunction, 1 with Factor XIII deficiency, 3 with von Willebrands and 3 with Osler-Weber-Rendu. The remainder of the patients had a thrombophilia as follows: 195 (60%) had antiphospholipid syndrome, 64 (20%) had Sticky Platelet Syndrome, 38 (12%) had MTHFR mutation, 23 (7.1%) had PAI-1 polymorphism, 12 (3.7%) had Protein S deficiency, 12 (3.7%) had Factor V Leiden, 3 (1%), had AT deficiency, 3 (1%) had Heparin-Cofactor II deficiency, 3 (1%) had t-PA deficiency, and 6 (2%) had Protein C deficiency. There were a total of 364 defects found in the 312 patients harboring thrombophilia; thus, several harbored two and a few harbored three separate defects.

Like that found by most other investigators, discussed previously, the most common defect found has been antiphospholipid syndrome (APLS); however, unlike some groups, we assess for all phospholipid antibody subgroups including antiphosphatidylserine, antiphosphatidylethanolamine, antiphosphatidylglycerol,

Table 2.4 Patient demographics.

Patient characteristics: (All 351 patients)	Mean	S.D.	Max.	Min.
Age:	33.3	5.63	49	18
Number of miscarriages:	2.9	2.39	9	2
Percent with defect(s) = 322/351:	92%			

Table 2.5 Hemostasis (bleeding) disorders found in the population (7% of total seen).

Platelet dysfunction = 3
Von Willebrands = 3
Osler–Weber–Rendu = 3
Factor XIII deficiency = 1

antiphosphatidic acid, antiphosphatidylcholine, antiphosphatidylinositol, anti-annexin-V antibody, Beta-2-Glycoprotein-1, hexagonal phospholipid, and lupus anticoagulant (by dRVVT with correction by non-platelet derived phospholipid to avoid false positive results). We always assess all three idiotypes of anticardiolipin antibody (IgG, IgA and IgM), an incomplete evaluation continues to be made by many who evaluate these patients and leave out either IgA or IgM idiotypes. The most common defect we find is, again, antiphospholipid syndrome, followed by Sticky Platelet Syndrome SPS), followed by MTHFR mutations, PAI-1 defects – most commonly polymorphisms (4G/5G or 4G/4G), protein S deficiency, Factor V Leiden, antithrombin deficiency, heparin co-factor II deficiency, tissue plasminogen activator (tPA) defects, and protein C deficiency. It is of interest that by including all antiphospholipid subgroups, it is found that 29% of patients have a subgroup antiphospholipid antibody, but no anticardiolipin antibody or lupus anticoagulant; thus 29% of patients would remain undiagnosed if these subgroups are not performed. Interestingly, this is about the same finding recently noted in young age (<51) thrombotic stroke patients.[70] The hemostasis defects found in our population are summarized in Table 2.5. The particulars of the antiphospholipid patients, with demonstration of the idiotypes found, are summarized in Table 2.6.

All patients with a thrombophilic defect were treated with preconception aspirin at 81 mg/day and at documentation of conception were treated with the addition of subcutaneous unfractionated porcine mucosal heparin at 5,000 units every 12 hours

Table 2.6 APLS patients.

Antiphospholipid found	Percent of patients with APLS
ACLA-IgG only	32.6
ACLA-IgM only	23.4
ACLA-IgA only	7
ACLA-IgG + IgM	3
ACLA-IgG + IgA	1
ACLA IgA + IgM	0
Lupus anticoagulant only	2
ACLA + lupus anticoagulant	2
"subgroup" only*	
Antiphosphatidylserine	4
Antiphosphatidylinositol	2
Antiphosphatidylethanolamine	5
Antiphosphatidic acid	5
Antiphosphatidylcholine	7
Antiphosphatidylglycerol	1
Anti-annexin-V	5
Beta-2-Glycoprotein 1	0
Hexagonal phospholipid	0
Total:	
(9 Patients had ACLA + a "subgroup" antibody)	
Total with only a "subgroup" antibody:	29
Percent of APLS patients with only a "subgroup" antibody:	

*= No ACLA or LA present

by self-injection (first 120 patients) or subcutaneous low-molecular-weight (LMW) heparin dalterparin (Fragmin) at 5,000 units q 24 hours by self-injection (subsequent 192 patients). Both drugs (ASA + unfractionated heparin or LMW heparin) are used to term. All patients are instructed in heparin injections and are informed of all important side effects of heparin therapy and are extensively informed of the benefits and risks of heparin/LMW heparin therapy, including the fact that side effects, although rare, include heparin-induced thrombocytopenia (HIT) with and without paradoxical thrombosis/thromboembolism (HITT), osteoporosis, mild to moderate alopecia, skin and allergic reactions, including erythema and itching, at injection sites, eosinophilia (of little clinical consequence) and

Table 2.7 Protocol for fetal wastage syndrome associated with hypercoagulable blood protein/platelet defects.

Follow-up used by DFW Metroplex cooperative RMS group

Medications: All throughout pregnancy:

1. ASA: 81 mg/day, start preconception (time of diagnosis)
2. Porcine heparin: 5000 units subcutaneously Q 12 hours immediately post-conception (added to ASA – both to term) or Dalteparin: 5000 units subcutaneously Q 24 hours immediately post-conception (added to ASA – both to term)
3. Calcium: 500 mg, P. O. daily
4. Prenatal vitamins
5. Iron: 1 tablet P. O. daily
6. Folic acid: 1 mg, P. O. daily

Laboratory assessment:

1. CBC/platelet count and heparin level* weekly × 4 weeks, then
2. CBC/platelet count and heparin level monthly, to term
3. Sonogram initially, and frequently to term
4. Fetal activity chart daily starting at 28 weeks
5. Biophysical profile and color doppler flow of umbilical artery at 32, 34, 36, and 38 weeks
6. Delivery at the discretion of the obstetrician
7. At delivery (or loss) send placenta to pathology for analysis and search for placental vascular thrombosis

*By anti-Xa method.

potential bleeding. Patients are also informed that about 5%–10% of patients develop a transient transaminasemia during heparin/LMW heparin therapy, but this is without any known adverse clinical consequences. They are also instructed that the ideal injection sites are the anterior or lateral thighs, injection sites should be rotated with every injection and that each injection is likely to produce a bruise about 0.5 cm to 4.0 cm in diameter and pain of injection, if experienced, can usually be alleviated by applying a small piece of ice at the site for 20 seconds before and 20 seconds after the injection is given. All patients are instructed to return immediately if they note dark or black areas of the injection site, potentially indicative of skin necrosis. The methods of follow-up are summarized in Table 2.7.

Those clinicians considering the use of LMW heparin in pregnancy should be made aware of the US-FDA Medwatch Alert posted by the FDA in January of 2002 (see FDA website: LOVENOX (enoxaparin sodium) Injection [January 9, 2002:

Aventis]: *WARNINGS* FDA MedWatch 1/9/2002: http://www.fda.gov/medwatch/SAFETY/2002/jan02.htm#lovenox) regarding the use of enoxaparin (Lovenox) in pregnancy and women of child bearing age which is as follows:

[January 9, 2002: Aventis]

Warnings

Prosthetic Heart Valves: The use of Lovenox Injection is not recommended for thromboprophylaxis in patients with prosthetic heart valves. Cases of prosthetic heart valve thrombosis have been reported in patients with prosthetic valves who have received enoxaparin for thromboprophylaxis. Some of these cases were pregnant women in whom thrombosis led to maternal deaths and fetal deaths. Pregnant women with prosthetic heart valves may be at higher risk for thromboembolism (see PRECAUTIONS: Pregnancy).

Precautions

Pregnancy

Teratogenic effects

There have been reports of congenital anomalies in infants born to women who received enoxaparin during pregnancy including cerebral anomalies, limb anomalies, hypospadias, peripheral vascular malformation, fibrotic dysplasia, and cardiac defect. A cause and effect relationship has not been established nor has the incidence been shown to be higher than in the general population.

Non-teratogenic effects

There have been post-marketing reports of fetal death when pregnant women received Lovenox Injection. Causality for these cases has not been determined. Pregnant women receiving anti-coagulants, including enoxaparin, are at increased risk for bleeding. Hemorrhage can occur at any site and may lead to death of mother and/or fetus. Pregnant women receiving enoxaparin should be carefully monitored. Pregnant women and women of child-bearing potential should be apprised of the potential hazard to the fetus and the mother if enoxaparin is administered during pregnancy.

In a clinical study of pregnant women with prosthetic heart valves given enoxaparin (1 mg/kg bid) to reduce the risk of thromboembolism, 2 of 7 women developed clots resulting in blockage of the valve and leading to maternal and fetal death. There are postmarketing reports of prosthetic valve thrombosis in pregnant women with prosthetic heart valves while receiving enoxaparin for thromboprophylaxis. These events resulted in maternal death or surgical interventions. The use of Lovenox Injection is not recommended for thromboprophylaxis in pregnant women with prosthetic heart valves (see WARNINGS: Prosthetic Heart Valves).

Adverse Reactions

Ongoing Safety Surveillance: Since 1993, there have been over 80 reports of epidural or spinal hematoma formation with concurrent use of Lovenox Injection and spinal/epidural anesthesia or spinal puncture.

Outcomes

All of the 315 patients with a thrombophilic defect were treated with the aforementioned regimen of preconception low-dose ASA plus addition of postconception thromboprophylactic (low-dose) subcutaneous porcine heparin or thromboprophylactic doses of dalteparin. Patients with MTHFR mutations were also treated with folic acid at 5 mg/day plus pyridoxine at 50 mg/day. There were a total of four losses (= 2.6%); only two were treatment failures. One loss was during the second trimester and accompanied a cholycystectomy and one loss was during the first trimester in an individual with APLS and a fetal chromosomal defect; these were not considered treatment (ASA + heparin/LMW heparin) failures. However, two patients suffered loss, both first trimester, on ASA + heparin/LMW heparin and placental thrombi and infarcts were present; thus there were two losses which clearly represented treatment failure. The overall success in treating RMS patients with procoagulant/platelet defects in our program is, therefore, (312/315 =) 99% with respect to normal term delivery. All patients were followed for a minimum of 3 months post-delivery. No patient sustained a thrombotic episode during pregnancy, delivery or post-partum, except the two treatment failures, both of whom had placental vascular thrombi. In addition, no patient developed HIT/T, and none had a clinically significant hemorrhage. Almost all patients developed small ecchymoses at injection sites, but these were considered insignificant by both patient and physician. Ten percent of patients developed eosinophilia which had abated by 3 months post-partum and 7% developed mild to moderate elevations of hepatic transaminases; these also returned to normal by 3 months post-partum. As per obstetricians, reproductive medicine specialists and involved pediatricians, no neonatal or pediatric problems were associated with therapy. No patient sustained a fracture during or after treatment. Patients with a bleeding disorder (7) were untreated. No patient had a significant hemorrhage during pregnancy or delivery. None required any blood product therapy.

Treatment review

Because fetal loss associated with bleeding disorders is thought to come about due to interference with adequate fibrin formation for implantation of the fertilized ovum into the uterine lining, we chose to not use vigorous pre-conception antithrombotic therapy with those with thrombophilia and use low-dose ASA at 81 mg/day; this may be of theoretical concern only, in view of the recent report of Sher who used pre-conception low-dose heparin with a high success rate for in vitro fertilization techniques.[71] However, we remain concerned and continue to advocate low-dose ASA as the pre-conception antithrombotic therapy in most instances.[1,2,4] The regimen of post-conception addition of fixed low-dose porcine mucosal heparin at 5000 units every 12 hours is empirical, but higher doses seem to be associated with bleeding and a lower success rate.[48,72] However, it may be that even lower doses might suffice. We do not advocate using corticosteroid therapy in this population, based upon the negative experience of others in fetal wastage syndrome, and our own preliminary experience of using steroids, in conjunction with antithrombotics, in patients with antiphospholipid syndrome and other types of thrombosis, wherein the corticosteroid use could be shown to lower antiphospholipid antibody titers, but failed to abort thrombotic events.[1,2,18,19,31,32,33] In addition, it is thought steroid use in patients with APLS may be detrimental.[29]

A variety of treatment programs have been utilized for women with antiphospholipid (anticardiolipin antibodies or lupus anticoagulants) and fetal wastage syndrome; however many of these studies have studied only very small populations, or fail to distinguish between primary or secondary antiphospholipid syndrome in the information provided. Brown[73] reported a 90% failure rate (miscarriage) among untreated women, Perino[74] reports a 93% failure rate in untreated women and Many[75] reports a 93% failure rate in untreated patients. Lubbe,[76] in a small group of women noted a successful term pregnancy rate of 80% with use of prednisone and ASA and a similar success rate with this regimen was noted by Lin.[77] Cowchuck[78] noted a 75% success rate with prednisone alone or ASA alone, but also noted more undesirable effects in the prednisone treated population. Landy,[79] in a small population, reported a success rate of 90% with either ASA alone or prednisone alone. However, Many[75] only noted a 43% successful term pregnancy rate with ASA and prednisone and Semprini[80] noted only a 14% success rate with prednisone alone. Several studies have assessed the role of post-conception addition of heparin; however, most have used higher doses than used in our population. Rosove[72] reports a 93% success rate with dose-adjusted subcutaneous heparin, the mean heparin doses being about 25,000 units/day. Kutteh,[81] in a population of 25 patients treated with ASA plus dose-adjusted subcutaneous heparin noted a success rate of 76%; the mean heparin dose was 26,000 units/day. In Many's study,[75] patients treated with prednisone plus ASA plus heparin at 5000 units twice a day had a better outcome (69%) than did those treated with ASA plus prednisone (43%) or prednisone alone (7%). Based on our original and current results,[1,2] it appears that fixed low-dose porcine heparin is more effective than the high-dose, dose-adjusted regimens, with >98% of our RMS population with antiphospholipid syndrome or other prothrombotic propensity, having a normal term delivery. It may be that higher doses of heparin somehow contribute to adverse outcomes, such as small periplacental hemorrhages. Parke[82] reports on the combination of low-dose heparin used in conjunction with intravenous immunoglobulin (IVIG), her success rate, however, was only 27% suggesting that IVIG has little role in antiphospholipid fetal wastage syndrome.

Summary

Recurrent miscarriage syndrome and infertility are common problems in the USA with recurrent miscarriage effecting over 500,000 women annually. If properly screened through a cost-effective protocol as outlined above, the etiology will be found in almost all women. The most common singular defect in women with RMS is a hemostasis defect and the most common of these is APLS, if a thorough APLS evaluation is performed. Following APLS, other hereditary and acquired procoagulant defects are also commonly found if looked for. It is important to appropriately evaluate women with RMS as if an etiology is found, the majority will have positive outcomes with normal term delivery. Hemorrhagic defects are very rare hemostasis causes of RMS, but these also are treatable in many instances and should be looked for in appropriate women. Treatment of the common procoagulant defects consists of preconception low-dose ASA at 81 mg/day followed by addition of immediate postconception low-dose unfractionated porcine heparin or dalteparin. Based on our experience, low molecular weight heparin may be a suitable alternative.

REFERENCES

1 Bick, R. L., Recurrent miscarriage syndrome and infertility caused by blood coagulation protein or platelet defects. *Hematology Oncology Clin. North America*, **14**: 1117, 2000.

2 Bick, R. L., Laughlin, H. R., Cohen, B., *et al.* Fetal wastage syndrome due to blood protein/ platelet defects: results of prevalence studies and treatment outcome with low-dose heparin and low-dose aspirin. *Clin. Appl. Thrombosis Hemostasis*, **1**: 286, 1995.

3 Duckert, F. The fibrin stabilizing factor, Factor XIII. *Blut*, **26**: 177, 1973.

4 Dossenbach-Glaninger, A., van Trotsenburg, M., Dossenbach, Oberkanins, C., *et al.* Plasminogen activator inhibitor 1 4G/5G polymorphism and coagulation factor XIII Val34Leu polymorphism: impaired fibrinolysis and early pregnancy loss. *Clin. Chem.*, **49**: 1081, 2003.
5 Muszbek, I. A. Coagulation factor deficiencies and pregnancy loss. *Sem. Thromb. Hemost.*, **29**: 171, 2003.
6 Kumar, M. and Mehta, P. Congenital coagulopathies and pregnancy: report of four pregnancies in a Factor X-deficient woman. *Am. J. Hematol.*, **46**: 241, 1994.
7 Valnicek, S., Vacl, J., Mrazova, M., *et al.* Hemotherapeutic safeguarding of induced abortion in inborn proconvertin insufficiency (hemagglutination Factor VII) using exchange plasmapheresis. *Zentralblatt fur Gynakologie*, **94**: 931, 1972.
8 Nelson, D. B., Ness, R. B., Grisso, J. A. and Cushman, M. Influence of hemostatic factors on spontaneous abortion *Am. J. Perinatol.*, **4**: 195, 2001.
9 Slunsky, R. Personal experiences with the antifibrinolytic PAMBA in obstetrics and gynecology. *Zentralblatt für Gynakologie*, **92**: 364, 1970.
10 Owen, C. A., Henriksen, R. A., McDuffie, F. C., *et al.* Prothrombin quick: a newly identified dysprothrombinemia *Mayo Clinic Proceedings*, **53**: 29, 1978.
11 Pauer, H. U., Burfeind, P., Kostering, H., *et al.* Factor XII deficiency is strongly associated with primary recurrent abortions. *Fertil Steril. Sep.*, **80**: 590, 2003.
12 Jones, D. W., Gallimore, M. J. and Winter, M. Antibodies to factor XII: a possible predictive marker for recurrent foetal loss. *Immunobiology*, **207**: 43, 2003.
13 Sugi, T. and Makino, T. Antiphospholipid antibodies and kininogens in pathologic pregnancies: a review. *Am. J. Reprod. Immunol.*, **47**: 283, 2002.
14 Iinuma, Y., Sugiura-Ogasawara, M., Makino, A., *et al.* Coagulation factor XII activity, but not an associated common genetic polymorphism (46C/T), is linked to recurrent miscarriage. *Fertil. Steril.*, **77**: 353–6, 2002.
15 Yamada, H., Kato, E. H., Ebina, Y., *et al.* Factor XII deficiency in women with recurrent miscarriage. *Gynecol. Obstet. Invest.*, **49**: 80, 2000.
16 Evron, S., Anteby, S. O., Brzezinsky, A., *et al.* Congenital afibrinogenemia and recurrent early abortion. *European J. Obstet. Gynecol. Reproductive Biol.*, **19**: 307, 1985.
17 Mammen, E. F. Congenital abnormalities of the fibrinogen molecule. *Seminars Thrombosis Hemostasis*, **1**: 184, 1974.
18 Bick, R. L., Baker, W. F. Antiphospholipid syndrome and thrombosis. *Seminars Thrombosis Hemostasis*, **25**: 333, 1999.
19 Bick, R. L. The antiphospholipid thrombosis syndromes: a common mutlidisciplinary medical problem. *Clin. Appl. Thrombosis Hemostasis*, **3**: 270, 1997.
20 Scott, J. R., Rote, N. S. and Branch, D. W. Immunological aspects of recurrent abortion and fetal death. *Obstet. Gynecol.*, **70**: 645, 1987.
21 Schved, J. F., Gris, J. C., Neveu, S., *et al.* Factor XII congenital deficiency and early spontaneous abortion. *Fertility and Sterility*, **52**: 335, 1989.
22 Klein, M., Rosen, A., Kyrle, P., *et al.* Obstetrical management of dysfibrinogenemia with increased thrombophilia. *Geburtshilfe und Frauenheilkunde*, **52**: 442, 1992.
23 Barkagan, Z. S. and Belykh, S. I. Protein C deficiency and the multi-thrombotic syndrome associated with pregnancy and abortion. *Gematologia I Transfuziologiia*, **37**: 35, 1992.

24 Hellgren, M., Tengborn, L. and Abildgaard, U. Pregnancy in women with congenital antithrombin III deficiency: experience of treatment with heparin and antithrombin. *Gynecologic and Obstetric Investigation*, **14**: 127, 1982.

25 Simioni, P., Lazzaro, A. R., Coser, E., *et al.* Hereditary heparin cofactor II deficiency and thrombosis: report of six patients belonging to two separate cohorts. *Blood Coagulation and Fibrinolysis*, **1**: 351, 1990.

26 Satoh, A., Suzuki, K., Takayama, E., *et al.* Detection of anti-annexin IV and V antibodies in patients with antiphospholipid syndrome and systemic lupus erythematosus. *J. Rheum.*, **26**: 1715, 1999.

27 Gris, J., Neveu, S., Mares, P., *et al.* Plasma fibrinolytic activators and their inhibitors in women suffering from early recurrent abortion of unknown etiology. *J. Lab. Clin. Med.*, **125**: 606, 1993.

28 Glueck, C. J., Wang, P., Fontaine, R. N., *et al.* Plasminogen activator inhibitor activity: an independent risk factor for the high miscarriage rate during pregnancy in women with polycystic ovary syndrome. *Metabolism: Clinical & Experimental*, **48**: 1589, 1999.

29 Khamashta, M. A. Management of thrombosis and pregnancy loss in the antiphospholipid syndrome. *Lupus*, **7**(Suppl. 2): S162–5, 1998.

30 Amengual, O., Atsumi, T., Khamashta, M. A., *et al.* Advances in antiphospholipid (Hughes') syndrome. *Annals of the Academy of Medicine, Singapore*, **27**: 61, 1998.

31 Bick, R. L. Antiphospholipid thrombosis syndromes: etiology, pathophysiology, diagnosis and managment. *International J. Hematology*, **65**: 193, 1997.

32 Bick, R. L., Baker, W. F. The Antiphospholipid and Thrombosis Syndromes. *Medical Clinics North America*, **78**: 667, 1994.

33 Bick, R. L., Arun, B., Frenkel, E. P. Antiphospholipid thrombosis syndromes. *Haemostasis*, **29**: 100, 1999.

34 Festin, M. R., Limson, G. M., Maruo, T. Autoimmune causes of recurrent pregnancy loss. *Kobe Journal of Medical Sciences*, **43**: 143, 1997.

35 Roussev, R. G., Kaider, B. D., Price, D. E., *et al.* Laboratory evaluation of women experiencing reproductive failure. *Am. J. Reproductive Immunology (Copenhagen)*, **35**: 415, 1996.

36 Oshiro, B. T., Silver, R. M., Scott, J. R., *et al.* Antiphospholipid antibodies and fetal death. *Obstetrics & Gynecology*, **87**: 489, 1996.

37 Granger, K. A. and Farquharson, R. G. Obstetric outcome in antiphospholipid syndrome. *Lupus*, **6**: 509, 1997.

38 Borrelli, A. L., Brillante, M., Borzacchiello, C., *et al.* Hemocoagulative pathology and immunological recurrent abortion. *Clinical & Experimental Obstetrics & Gynecology*, **24**: 39, 1997.

39 Hellan, M., Kuhnel, E., Speiser, W., *et al.* Familial lupus anticoagulant: a case report and review of the literature. *Blood Coagulation & Fibrinolysis*, **9**: 195, 1998.

40 Ogasawara, M., Aoki, K., Matsuura, E., *et al.* Anti beta-2-glycoprotein I antibodies and lupus anticoagulant in patients with recurrent pregnancy loss: prevalence and clinical significance. *Lupus*, **5**: 587, 1996.

41 Zangari, M., Lockwood, C. J., Scher, J., *et al.* Prothrombin activation fragment (F1.2) is increased in pregnant patients with antiphospholipid antibodies. *Thromb. Res.*, **85**: 177, 1997.

42 Aznar, J. Factor V Leiden and antibodies against phospholipids and protein S in a young woman with recurrent thromboses and abortion. *Haematologica*, **84**: 80, 1999.

43 Aznar, J., Villa, P., Espana, F., *et al.* Activated protein C resistance phenotype in patients with antiphospholipid antibodies. *J. Lab. & Clin. Med.*, **130**: 202, 1997.

44 Schultz, D. R. Antiphospholipid antibodies: basic immunology and assays. *Seminars in Arthritis & Rheumatism*, **26**: 724, 1997.

45 Amengual, O., Atsumi, T., Khamashta, M. A., *et al.* The role of the tissue factor pathway in the hypercoagulable state in patients with the antiphospholipid syndrome. *Thrombosis & Haemostasis*, **79**: 276, 1998.

46 Martini, A. and Ravelli, A. The clinical significance of antiphospholipid antibodies. *Annals of Medicine*, **29**: 159, 1997.

47 Bussen, S. S. and Steck, T. Thyroid antibodies and their relation to antithrombin antibodies, anticardiolipin antibodies and lupus anticoagulant in women with recurrent spontaneous abortions (antithyroid, anticardiolipin and antithrombin autoantibodies and lupus anticoagulant in habitual aborters). *European J. Obs. Gyn. Repro. Biol.*, **74**: 139, 1997.

48 Rand, J. H. and Wu, X. X. Antibody-mediated disruption of the annexin-V antithrombotic shield: a new mechanism for thrombosis in the antiphospholipid syndrome. *Thrombosis & Haemostasis*, **82**: 649, 1999.

49 Rand, J. H., Wu, X. X., Andree, H. A., *et al.* Antiphospholipid antibodies accelerate plasma coagulation by inhibiting annexin-V binding to phospholipids: a "lupus procoagulant" phenomenon. *Blood*, **92**: 1652, 1998.

50 Rauch, J. Lupus anticoagulant antibodies: recognition of phospholipid-binding protein complexes. *Lupus*, **7**(Suppl. 2): S29, 1998.

51 Rote, N. S., Vogt, E., DeVere, G., *et al.* The role of placental trophoblast in the pathophysiology of the antiphospholipid antibody syndrome. *Am. J. Repro. Immunol. (Copenhagen)*, **39**: 125, 1998.

52 Vogt, E., Ng, A. K. and Rote, N. S. Antiphosphatidylserine antibody removes annexin-V and facilitates the binding of prothrombin at the surface of a choriocarcinoma model of trophoblast differentiation. *Am. J. Obs. Gyn.*, **177**: 964, 1997.

53 Lakasing, L., Campa, J. S., Poston, R., *et al.* Normal expression of tissue factor, thrombomodulin, and annexin V in placentas from women with antiphospholipid syndrome. *Am. J. Obs. Gyn.*, **181**: 180, 1999.

54 Siaka, C., Lambert, M., Caron, C., *et al.* Low prevalence of anti-annexin V antibodies in antiphospholipid syndrome with fetal loss. *Revue de Medecine Interne*, **20**: 762, 1999.

55 Kaburaki, J., Kuwana, M., Yamamoto, M., *et al.* Clinical significance of anti-annexin V antibodies in patients with systemic lupus erythematosus. *Am. J. Hematol.*, **54**: 209, 1997.

56 Eschwege, V., Peynaud-Debayle, E., Wolf, M., *et al.* Prevalence of antiphospholipid-related antibodies in unselected patients with history of venous thrombosis. *Blood Coagulation & Fibrinolysis*, **9**: 429, 1998.

57 Silver, R. M., Pierangeli, S. S., Edwin, S. S., *et al.* Pathogenic antibodies in women with obstetric features of antiphospholipid syndrome who have negative test results for lupus anticoagulant and anticardiolipin antibodies. *Am. J. Obs. Gyn.*, **176**: 628, 1997.

58 Branch, D. W., Silver, R., Pierangeli, S., *et al.* Antiphospholipid antibodies other than lupus anticoagulant and anticardiolipin antibodies in women with recurrent pregnancy loss, fertile controls, and antiphospholipid syndrome. *Obs. Gyn.*, **89**: 549, 1997.

59 Gris, J. C., Ripart-Neveu, S., Maugard, C., *et al.* Respective evaluation of the prevalence of haemostasis abnormalities in unexplained primary early recurrent miscarriages. The Nimes Obstetricians and Haematologists (NOHA) Study. *Thrombosis & Haemostasis*, **77**: 1096, 1997.

60 Tal, J., Schliamser, L. M., Leibovitz, Z., *et al.* A possible role for activated protein C resistance in patients with first and second trimester pregnancy failure. *Human Reproduction*, **14**: 1624, 1999.

61 Kutteh, W. H., Park, V. M. and Deitcher, S. R. Hypercoagulable state mutation analysis in white patients with early first-trimester recurrent pregnancy loss. *Fertility & Sterility.*, **71**: 1048, 1998.

62 Dhalback, B. Activated Protein C resistence and thrombosis: Molecular mechanisms of hypercoagulable state due to FVR506Q mutation. *Seminars Thrombosis Hemostasis*, **25**: 273, 1999.

63 Brenner, B., Mandel, H., Lanir, N., *et al.* Activated Protein C resistance can be associated with recurrent fetal loss. *Brit. J. Haematology*, **97**: 551, 1997.

64 Bokarewa, M. I., Bremme, K., Blomback, M. Arg 506-Gln mutation in factor V and risk of thrombosis during pregnancy. *Brit. J. Haematology*, **92**: 473, 1996.

65 Rai, R., Regan, L., Hadley, E., *et al.* Second-trimester pregnancy loss is associated with activated C resistance. *Brit. J. Haematology*, **92**: 489, 1996.

66 Grandone, E., Margaglione, M., Colaizzo, D., *et al.* Factor V Leiden mutation is associated with repeated and recurrent unexplained fetal losses. *Thromb. Haemostasis*, **77**: 822, 1997.

67 Ridker, P. M., Miletich, J. P., Buring, J. E., *et al.* Factor V Leiden mutation as a risk factor for recurrent pregnancy loss. *Ann. Internal Medicine*, **128**: 1000, 1998.

68 Poort, S., Rosendaal, F., Reitsma, P., *et al.* A common genetic variation in the 3′-untranslated region of the prothrombin gene is associated with elevated plasma prothrombin levels and an increase in venous thrombosis *Blood*, **88**: 3698, 1996.

69 Brenner, B., Sarig, G., Weiner, Z., *et al.* Thrombophilic polymorphisms are common in women with fetal loss without apparent cause. *Thrombosis & Haemostasis*, **82**: 6, 1999.

70 Toschi, V., Motta, A., Costelli, C., *et al.* High prevalence of antiphosphatidylinositol antibodies in young patients with cerebral ischemia of undetermined cause *Stroke*, **29**: 1759, 1998.

71 Sher, G., Feinman, M., Zouves, C., *et al.* High fecundity rates following in-vitro fertilization and embryo transfer in antiphospholipid antibody seropositive women treated with heparin and aspirin. *Human Reproduction*, **9**: 2278, 1994.

72 Rosove, M. H., Tabsh, K., Wasserstrum, N., *et al.* Heparin therapy for pregnant women with lupus anticoagulant or anticardiolipin antibodies. *Obstetrics Gynecology*, **75**: 630, 1990.

73 Brown, H. L. Antiphospholipid antibodies and recurrent pregnancy loss. *Clinical Obstetrics Gynecology*, **34**: 17, 1991.

74 Perino, A., Barba, G., Cimino, C., *et al.* Immunological problems in the recurrent abortion syndrome. *Acta Eurtopaea Fertilitatis*, **20**: 199, 1989.

75 Many, A., Pauzner, R., Carp, H., *et al.* Treatment of patients with antiphospholipid antibodies during pregnancy. *American J. Reproductive Immunology*, **28**: 216, 1992.

76 Lubbe, W. F. and Liggins, G. C. Role of lupus anticoagulant and autoimmunity in recurrent fetal loss. *Seminars Reproductive Endocrinology*, **6**: 181, 1988.

77 Lin, Q. Investigation of the association between autoantibodies and recurrent abortions. *Chinese J. Obstetrics Gynecology*, **28**: 674, 1993.

78 Cowchuck, F. S., Reece, E. A., Balaban, D., *et al.* Repeated fetal losses associated with antiphospholipid antibodies: a collaborative randomized trial comparing prednisone with low-dose heparin treatment. *American J. Obstetrics Gynecology*, **166**: 1318, 1992.

79 Landy, H. J., Kessler, C., Kelly, W. K., *et al.* Obstetric performance in patients with the lupus anticoagulant and/or anticardiolipin antibodies. *American J. Perinatology*, **9**: 146, 1992.

80 Semprini, A. E., Vucetich, A., Garbo, S., *et al.* Effect of prednisone and heparin treatment in 14 patients with poor reproductive efficiency related to lupus anticoagulant. *Fetal Therapy*, **4**(Suppl. 1): 73, 1989.

81 Kutteh, W. H. Heparin plus aspirin (Hep + ASA) is superior to aspirin alone (ASA) for the treatment of recurrent pregnancy loss (RPL) associated with antiphospholipid antibodies (APA). *Proceedings: American College Obstetricians & Gynecologists*, 1994 (abstract).

82 Parke, A. The role of IVIG in the management of patients with antiphospholipid antibodies and recurrent pregnancy losses. *IVIG Therapy Today*. Ballow, M., ed. Totowa, N. J., Humana Press, Inc., 1992, p. 105.

3

Von Willebrand disease and other bleeding disorders in obstetrics

Franklin Fuda, D.O.[1] and Ravindra Sarode, M.D.[2]

[1]Fellow: Hematopathology, Department of Pathology, University of Texas Southwestern Medical Center, Dallas, Texas, USA
[2]Professor of Pathology, University of Texas Southwestern Medical Center; Director: Transfusion Medicine and Hemostasis, Dallas, Texas, USA

Introduction

Bleeding disorders in the female population often present unique challenges to an obstetrician. The hormonal and physical changes that occur during the menstrual cycle, pregnancy, childbirth, and the post-partum period continually place strain upon the hemostatic system. Although severe bleeding disorders are usually easily recognized, mild bleeding disorders often go undiagnosed due to the "mild degree" of signs and symptoms (e.g. slightly abnormal menstruation). Unfortunately, even these mild bleeding disorders often lead to a decrease in the quality of life, variable degrees of morbidity, and even life-threatening hemorrhage.[1–3] Therefore, it is essential that the obstetrician be aware of the clinical clues, appropriate diagnostic tests, and treatment regimens for such disorders. This is particularly important for pregnant women, whose hemostatic system undergoes marked alterations in preparation for the unique challenge of delivery.

The hemostatic system

Basic knowledge of the hemostatic system assists in making clinical decisions regarding bleeding conditions in the obstetric population. Normal hemostasis is a highly regulated, physiologic process of clot formation and clot management that occurs in response to vascular injury. It involves 2 major systems: (i) primary hemostasis and (ii) secondary hemostasis. Although both systems are initiated at the same time and work together intricately to form stable platelet-fibrin clots, the influence that each system has upon clot formation in the arterial versus the venous systems is different. Primary hemostasis plays a major role in clot

Hematological Complications in Obstetrics, Pregnancy, and Gynecology, ed. R. L. Bick *et al.* Published by Cambridge University Press.

formation in areas of high blood flow velocity such as the arterial system, whereas secondary hemostasis predominates in areas of low blood flow velocity such as the venous system.

During primary hemostasis, platelets adhere to subendothelial collagen in areas of injury and secrete stimulating factors (e.g. ADP, thromboxane A2, etc.), and then aggregate to form a platelet plug. The process and the extent of platelet adhesion, secretion, and aggregation are tightly regulated by plasma and subendothelial von Willebrand factor (VWF), by the actions of neighboring endothelial cells, and perhaps by red blood cells, e.g. through release of ADP.[4–7] Figure 3.1 explains the scheme of primary hemostasis in more detail.

Secondary hemostasis begins concurrently with primary hemostasis through activation of the tissue factor (TF) pathway (a process known as initiation phase). TF, a molecule embedded in the plasma membranes of subendothelial fibroblasts and smooth muscle cells (as well as endothelium and monocytes/macrophages), interacts with activated plasma coagulation factor VII to initiate the coagulation cascade. This initial phase of coagulation ultimately leads to the formation of thrombin. Thrombin then initiates the intrinsic pathway by activating factor XI resulting in the propagation of coagulation. The end result of this coagulation process is the production of a cross-linked, polymerized fibrin clot at the site of injury. Termination of the coagulation cascade (involving the anticoagulation system) and restructure/dissolution of the fibrin clot (involving the fibrinolytic

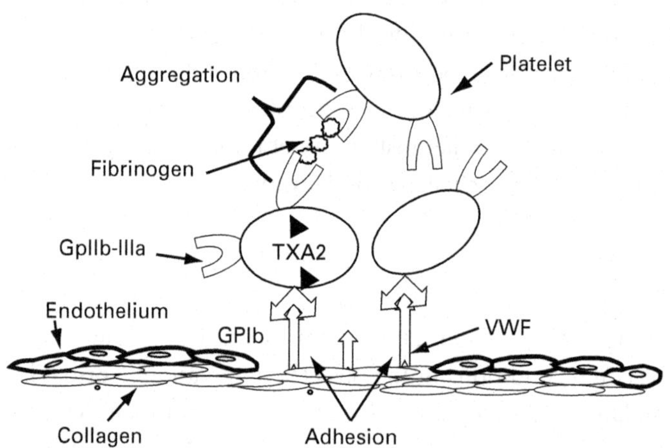

Figure 3.1 Primary hemostasis: Disruption of endothelial cells exposes subendothelial collagen and large multimers of VWF, which interact with GPIb receptors on platelets causing adhesion of platelets at the site of injury. This is followed by secretion of agonists (ADP) from platelet granules and thromboxane A2. This process results in a conformational change in GPIIb/IIIa, allowing bridging of adjacent platelets by fibrinogen, known as aggregation.

system) are directed by many soluble modulators from the plasma, by the neighboring endothelial cells, and by the platelets. The major components of the natural anticoagulant system include protein C, its cofactor protein S, and antithrombin. The major components of the fibrinolytic system include plasminogen/plasmin and tissue plasminogen activator (tPA). The dynamic interactions of the procoagulants, the anticoagulants, and the fibrinolytic system involved in secondary hemostasis are discussed in more detail in Figure 3.2(a)–(d).

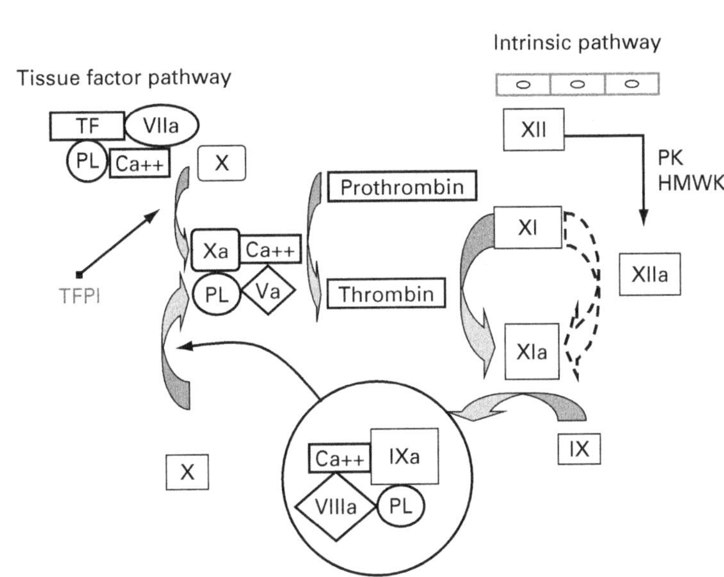

Figure 3.2a Coagulation cascade: Coagulation cascade begins with exposure of subendothelial tissue factor (TF) following disruption of the vascular endothelial lining. TF complexes with circulating activated FVII (FVIIa) and cleaves factor X to its active form (FXa), which then complexes with circulating activated factor V, calcium, and phospholipid to form the prothrombinase complex (Xa-Va-Ca^{2+}-PL). The prothrombinase complex cleaves prothrombin to produce thrombin. This initial phase or "tissue factor pathway" is quickly terminated by TF pathway inhibitor (TFPI); it does, however, generate enough thrombin to propagate coagulation by initiating the intrinsic pathway. Thrombin cleaves factor XI (i.e. in vivo initiation of the classic "intrinsic pathway") into its active form (FXIa), which in turn activates factor IX. FIXa complexes with FVIIIa, Ca++ and phospholipid to form the Tenase complex (IXa-VIIIa-Ca^{2+}-PL). As the name suggests, the Tenase complex produces FXa, which then assembles into a prothrombinase complex to produce more thrombin. In vitro, contact factors (FXII, prekallikrein (PK) and high molecular weight kininogen (HMWK) also activate FXI.

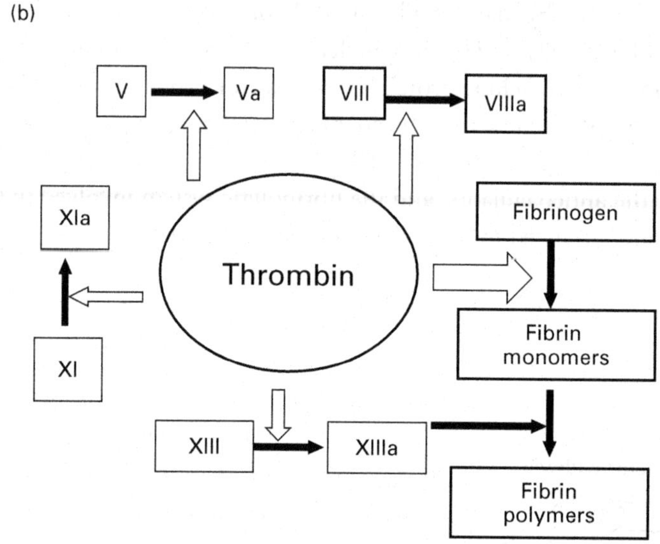

(b)

V
Va
VIII
VIIIa
XIa
Thrombin
Fibrinogen
XI
Fibrin monomers
XIII
XIIIa
Fibrin polymers

Figure 3.2b Thrombin: Thrombin converts fibrinogen to fibrin; in addition, however, it propagates coagulation by cleaving factors XI, V, and VIII into their activated forms. The fibrin monomers are then crossed linked by FXIIIa (also activated by thrombin) to form fibrin polymers (i.e. a stable red clot).

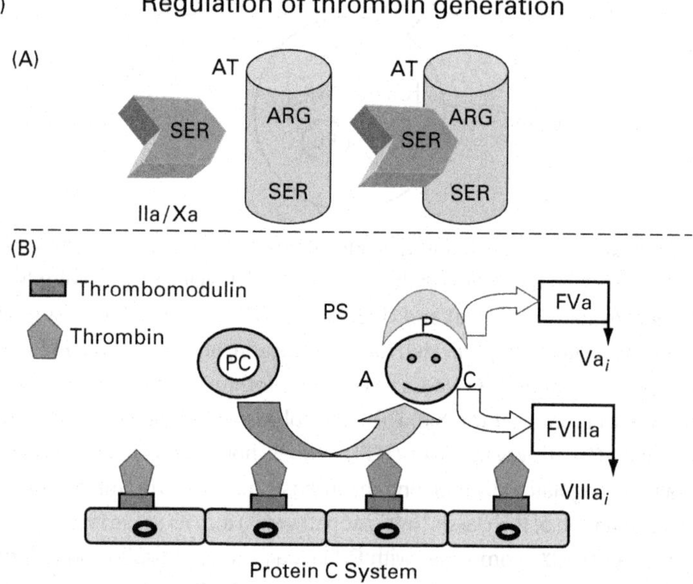

Figure 3.2c Anticoagulant system: (A) Antithrombin (AT) neutralizes predominantly thrombin and FXa, thus regulating fibrin formation. (B) The protein C system regulates thrombin generation. In this process thrombin forms a complex with thrombomodulin to activate protein C. Activated protein C assembles with protein S to inactivate both FVa and FVIIIa, thereby shutting down both prothrombinase and Tenase complexes.

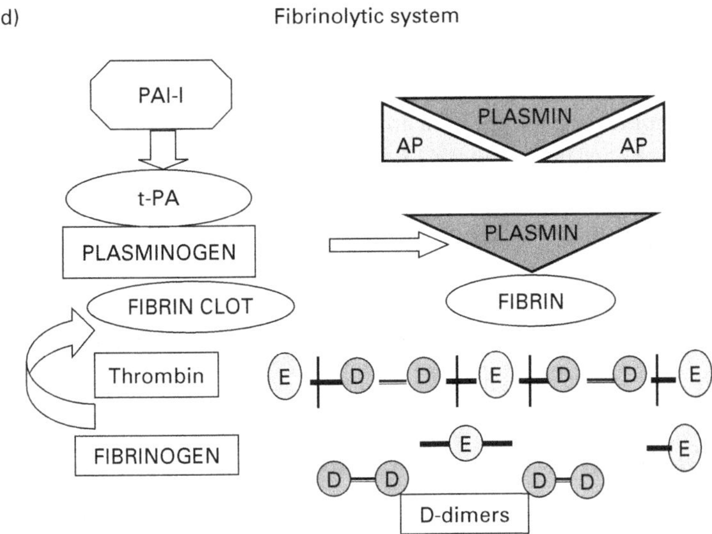

Figure 3.2d The fibrinolytic system dissolves the cross-linked fibrin clot. Plasminogen binds to the fibrin clot and undergoes a conformational change allowing tissue plasminogen activator (tPA) to bind to it; tPA cleaves plasminogen to plasmin, which cleaves the fibrin clot and results in the formation of D-dimers. This process is tightly regulated by plasminogen activator inhibitor-1 (PAI-1) and alpha 2-antiplasmin (AP), both of which function to inhibit fibrinolysis.

The clotting system during gestation

During pregnancy the body prepares itself for an extraordinary challenge to the hemostatic system. Many incompletely understood physiologic changes occur that increase the tendency of the hemostasis system toward clot formation. This propensity is believed to be largely due to changes in concentrations of procoagulant, anticoagulant, and anti-fibrinolytic factors. During the second half of gestation, two procoagulant factors that rise steadily during pregnancy are factor VIII and VWF (highest mean FVIII of 206% and VWF of 376%).[8–13] Other factors that are elevated include FVII, FX, and fibrinogen.[11,14] The remaining coagulation factor levels do not appear to change significantly.[14–17] In addition to the increase in procoagulant factors, there is a concurrent decrease in the anticoagulants protein S[18–21] and antithrombin[10,12] as well as a decrease in the activity of the fibrinolytic system, most likely due to an increase in plasminogen activator inhibitors.[22–24]

Evaluation of the patient with a history of a bleeding disorder

A complete history and physical exam (H&P) is essential for the evaluation of bleeding disorders in all obstetric patients. The history should include some form of objective criteria, since a patient's perception of abnormal bleeding does not always correlate with the actual presence or absence of a disorder.[25] For instance, when inquiring about menorrhagia, it is helpful to quantify the bleeding (e.g. how many tampons or pads are used and how saturated they become). Such questioning has obvious flaws (personal hygiene practices introduce variation in how often pads are changed) but when used as a component of a complete H&P does increase sensitivity for detecting abnormal bleeding.[26,27] The physical examination should include inspection of the skin, mucosal membranes, and the musculoskeletal system for signs of a bleeding disorder. Such signs may be subtle (e.g. the joint laxity seen in connective tissue diseases) but may also be the only clues when a patient is a poor historian.

Laboratory evaluation of the hemostatic system

The type of bleeding should guide the plan of the laboratory evaluation. In general, mucocutaneous type bleeding typically results from dysfunction of primary hemostasis (i.e. platelet or VWD), whereas deep tissue, retroperitoneal, or intra-articular types of bleeding typically arise as a result of secondary hemostatic dysfunction (i.e. coagulation factor deficiency). Laboratory evaluation, therefore, should begin with screening tests chosen to detect most hemostatic defects, i.e. platelet count, PT, PTT, fibrinogen level, or PFA-100™. Once further clues to the type of disorder are elicited, testing is then tailored to evaluate specific disorders. Currently, routine testing for bleeding disorders focuses upon isolating different segments of the hemostatic system for evaluation. All current tests, with exception of the now-mostly-obsolete bleeding time test, are performed *in vitro*.

Evaluation of the primary hemostatic system includes the following laboratory tests:

(a) *Platelet Count*: The platelet count is performed on an automatic blood counter. Typical normal ranges are approximately 150,000–450,000 × 10^9/l.

(b) *Platelet Function Analyzer-100 (PFA-100™ ®)*: The PFA-100™ ® evaluates components involved in primary hemostasis. The test cartridge simulates *in vivo* conditions that would promote primary hemostasis, i.e. an injured blood vessel wall. It accomplishes this by using a membrane with an aperture to simulate the lumen of a blood vessel. The membrane itself is coated with collagen and a platelet activator (either ADP or epinephrine) to simulate the milieu that promotes platelet aggregation. Whole blood passes through the aperture at a standardized, high velocity (simulating capillary/arterial blood flow). The time that it takes for the blood to stop flowing is designated as the closure time (CT). CT is dependent upon the concentration and functionality of platelets and VWF, and upon the hematocrit. It is recorded in seconds and represents the amount of time it takes for a primary clot to develop. Prolongation of the CT can result from von Willebrand disease (VWD), thrombocytopenia (below 100,000/dl), a qualitative platelet disorder, anti-platelet therapy, or a low hematocrit (below 20%). There are two different cartridges; the collagen-epinephrine (CEPI) cartridge and the collagen-ADP (CAPD) cartridge. Both cartridges detect primary hemostatic defects, but only the CEPI cartridge detects defects due to aspirin. Used in conjunction, therefore, these cartridges can differentiate between platelet dysfunction due to aspirin versus those due to other causes. Although the PFA-100™ is not specific for a particular disorder, it is more sensitive and has more clinical utility than the antiquated and inaccurate bleeding time.[26,28–30]

(c) *Specific Testing for platelet dysfunction*: *Platelet Aggregation Studies*: These studies measure platelet aggregation and secretion in response to exposure to various platelet agonists (e.g. ADP, collagen, arachidonic acid, ristocetin). Two methods to measure aggregation are currently in use: (i) an optical method which uses platelet rich plasma and measures the increase in light transmission as platelet aggregation proceeds and (ii) an impedance method which uses whole blood and measures the decrease in electric current between two oppositely charged electrodes as platelets aggregate and coat each electrode. Platelet ATP secretion is measured using chemiluminescence techniques. Certain aggregation and secretion profiles correspond to different defects in primary hemostasis or to different anti-platelet drugs. These studies are, therefore, useful in categorizing primary hemostatic defects.

Evaluation of the secondary hemostatic system includes the following laboratory tests:

(a) *Prothrombin Time (PT)*: The PT measures the classic extrinsic coagulation pathway (TF pathway), which is based upon the amount of time that it takes for a fibrin clot to form once the patient's citrate anti-coagulated plasma is added to tissue thromboplastin reagent that also contains calcium. Prolongation of the PT is caused by deficiency of factor VII, by deficiencies of the common pathway factors (X, V, II, I) and rarely by inhibitors to these factors, or by lupus anticoagulants.

(b) *Activated Partial Thromboplastin Time (aPTT)*: The aPTT measures the classic intrinsic coagulation pathway. In this test the patient's citrate anti-coagulated plasma is added to a contact activator (e.g. silica or ellagic acid), calcium and phospholipid. This mixture results in activation of factor XII (and other contact activators like high molecular weight kininogen, prekallikrein), which initiates the classic intrinsic pathway. It is important to remember, however, that although factor XII is essential to this *in vitro* test, its deficiency does not lead to bleeding disorder. The aPTT, therefore, detects deficiencies of factors XII, XI, IX, VIII and the common pathway factors (X, V, II, I) as well as the presence of any inhibitors to these factors or the presence of lupus anticoagulant. The most common cause of a prolonged aPTT in the hospital setting is heparin therapy or heparin contamination from intravenous catheters.

(c) *Thrombin Time* (TT): The TT specifically measures the conversion of fibrinogen to fibrin by bovine thrombin. Prolongation of the thrombin time is caused by deficiencies of fibrinogen, dysfibrinogenemia, inhibitors of thrombin (i.e. heparin), fibrin degradation products, and paraproteins.

(d) *Individual Factor assays*: Multiple laboratory techniques exist for antigen testing (quantitative) and activity testing (functional) of specific coagulation factors.

Primary hemostatic defect

Patients with primary hemostatic defect present with mucocutaneous type bleeding. Investigation of such bleeding focuses upon platelets and von Willebrand factor (VWF). The more common defects should be investigated first.

Antiplatelet medications

The first consideration in the investigation of mucocutaneous ("platelet-type") bleeding is to determine whether or not the patient has recently taken any antiplatelet medication. Currently available platelet inhibitors that result in clinically significant hemostatic defects include aspirin and clopidogrel (Plavix).

Aspirin (ASA) blocks platelet production of thromboxane A_2 (TXA_2) through irreversible acetylation of cyclooxygenase (COX-1). Without TXA_2, platelet aggregation in response to collagen, epinephrine, thrombin, and adenosine diphosphate (ADP) is impaired. With regard to aggregation, all circulating platelets at the time of ASA ingestion are essentially rendered inactive for their entire life span (8–10 days). Since ten percent of circulating platelets are replaced by healthy, younger, more active platelets each day, ASA impairment of primary hemostasis is typically mild unless it is taken regularly. Administration during pregnancy, however, can lead to excessive hemorrhage at delivery for both the mother and the neonate.[31]

In addition to aspirin, several other nonsteroidal anti-inflammatory drugs (NSAIDS) impair platelet aggregation. Similarly to ASA, the mechanism of action for all of these is through acetylation of COX-1. Unlike ASA, however, the remaining NSAIDS acetylate in a reversible fashion leading to shorter, less effective platelet inhibition. The more commonly administered NSAIDs include indomethacin, diclofenac, ibuprofen, sulfinpyrozone, meclofenamic acid, phenylbutazone, naproxene, ketoprefen, tolmetin, piroxicam, and sulinac. The selective

COX-2 inhibitors celecoxib (Celebrex)[32] and rofecoxib (Vioxx)[33,34] do not affect platelet function. Acetominophen is not an NSAID and does not impair platelet function.

Clopidogrel (Plavix) is an inhibitor of ADP receptors and leads to decreased aggregation primarily in response to ADP.[31,35] Unlike aspirin, the degree of inhibition varies amongst individual circulating platelets. Typically, the anti-platelet effect is not observed until 2 to 3 days after the initial dose, peaks at 4 to 7 days, and persists for 7 to 10 days following cessation of therapy.[31,35]

Thrombocytopenia

Thrombocytopenia, as a cause of mucocutaneous bleeding, is easily detected through a complete blood count (CBC). A mild or relative decrease in the platelet count, however, is common and expected during pregnancy due to the physiologic expansion of plasma volume. Nevertheless, platelet counts below 100,000/μl warrant further work-up.[36–38] Thrombocytopenia and its etiologies are discussed in Chapter 15.

Von Willebrand disease

With a prevalence of 1% in the general population and a prevalence of 7 to 20% in women presenting with menorrhagia, VWD is the most commonly inherited bleeding disorder.[39,40] It arises secondary to quantitative and/or qualitative abnormalities of VWF, an essential regulator protein for normal hemostasis. Numerous variants of congenital VWD exist, each resulting from a different mutation of the VWF gene on chromosome 12. To date, not all mutations have been elicited. In addition to these congenital VWD, many other medical conditions are associated with an acquired von Willebrand syndrome (aVWS). These conditions have clinical and diagnostic features of a VWD but are not caused by an inherited VWF gene mutation. The risk of hemorrhage in each individual case of VWD or aVWS is determined by the particular biological activity of the VWF. Since treatment strategies are dependent upon the type of VWD, it is, therefore, essential to correctly diagnose each individual case.

Understanding the classification scheme and treatment modalities for VWD requires basic knowledge of the structure and function of VWF. It is produced by megakaryocytes in the bone marrow and by vascular endothelial cells. The initial VWF gene product is a monomer that undergoes extensive post-translational processing to create the spectrum of VWF multimers found in the plasma. Although each monomer contains all of the essential binding sites for interaction with the receptors and molecules required to achieve normal hemostasis, only the larger multimers can achieve the spatial orientations required for such a function. In general, the multimeric size determines its activity; larger multimers with greater numbers of binding sites have greater activity than smaller ones.[41]

By acting as bridging molecules for both platelet adhesion and aggregation, VWF is an essential mediator of primary hemostasis. As mentioned above, platelet adhesion is the initial event that occurs during primary hemostasis. After vascular injury, residential subendothelial VWF is exposed and interacts with platelets that are flowing by the site of injury. In the arterial system, the high velocity of blood flow "drags" the larger VWF multimers from their globular structure into elongated filaments, thereby exposing numerous binding sites for platelet membrane glycoprotein (GP) Ib receptors.[41,42] Once the initial platelets are tethered to the site of injury, more platelets are recruited to build a larger clot, a process designated as platelet aggregation. VWF once again plays an essential role in this process by bridging activated platelet GP IIb/IIIa membrane receptors on neighboring platelets. Although these VWF bridges are quickly replaced by more stable connections, i.e. fibrinogen binding to GP IIb/IIIa, platelet adhesion and aggregation cannot proceed until the VWF bridges are in place.[41,43–46] Without appropriate quantities of properly acting VWF, primary platelet clots cannot develop, and platelet-like hemorrhage ensues, i.e. mucocutaneous bleeding.

Prior to discussing the different forms of VWD, one last essential aspect regarding VWF must be briefly discussed: hormonal influence upon VWF levels. The two hormones that are clinically most significant to the obstetric population are estrogen and thyroid hormone, as the plasma concentration of each is directly proportional to that of VWF. The increase in estrogen associated with pregnancy often results in correction of mild VWF deficiency during states of increased estrogen production (e.g. 3rd trimester of pregnancy)[47] whereas hypothyroidism can lead to an acquired VWF deficiency.[48–50]

Classification of von Willebrand disease

In general, VWD does not alter fertility or the course of pregnancy relative to the normal population, but it does significantly increase the risk of bleeding at parturition[51] and during any surgical procedures. There are three types of VWD. Types 1 and 3 are quantitative defects, whereas type 2 is a qualitative defect. Type 2 VWD has several subtypes.

VWD Type 1 is characterized by a mild to moderate decrease in VWF; however, the distribution of multimers is normal. With a prevalence of 1 per 1000, it accounts for approximately 70–75% of all VWD. Family history is not always helpful, as the disease penetrance is only 60 percent.[52] Clinical manifestations depend upon the severity of the VWF deficiency but typically include mild to moderate mucocutaneous bleeding. Treatment regimens, in turn, depend upon the clinical severity. Since these patients have the capacity to produce VWF, the heightened estrogen levels during pregnancy characteristically result in increases of VWF to levels sufficient for protection against abnormal bleeding. In most cases no particular treatment is warranted. There are, however, several caveats regarding VWD type 1 in pregnancy:

(1) Case reports have demonstrated that not all VWD type 1 patients show correction of VWF levels during pregnancy. In these studies, patients who have a particular genetic abnormality (VWF mutation C1130F) experienced significant immediate post-partum bleeding, i.e. requiring blood transfusions, when no prophylactic treatment was administered.[53] In contrast, these same patients showed no bleeding in subsequent pregnancies after receiving prophylaxis. Although the genetic defect was eventually determined in these particular patients, the specific genetic defect is rarely determined in most patients with VWD. Furthermore, there is no certainty whether or not other variants of VWD type 1 will have adequate pregnancy-induced rises in VWF. Due to the possibility of hemorrhagic complications, all VWD type 1 patients should be monitored throughout pregnancy and treated when necessary.
(2) Although VWF levels generally begin to rise in the 2nd trimester of pregnancy, protective levels are often not reached until the 3rd trimester. Therefore, bleeding risks during the 1st and 2nd trimester should be considered the same as during non-pregnant states.[54,55]
(3) Following delivery, plasma VWF rapidly decreases to pre-pregnancy levels, and the risk period for postpartum hemorrhage may be prolonged for as long as a few weeks compared to normal patients.[9,54] Due to this prolongation of hemorrhagic risk, weekly contact with the patient and medical intervention with any signs of abnormal bleeding is advised during the puerperium.

The various subcategories of VWD type 2 should be thought of as distinct clinical and pathologic entities.
(a) VWD type 2A constitutes 10 percent of reported VWD cases and has a prevalence of 1–3 per 10,000.[52] Family history is very revealing, as this variant has a full penetrance pattern. Clinical bleeding is typically mild to moderate and results from an absence of large and medium sized VWF.[56] The lack of larger, more functional VWF can either be due to abnormal processing, which results in the production of only smaller forms, or due to increased metabolism of the larger forms by VWF cleaving protease.[56] Depending upon the individual pathophysiologic process, primary hemostasis may or may not normalize during pregnancy.[47]

(b) VWD type 2B accounts for approximately 5 percent of cases with a prevalence of less than 1 per 10,000.[52] Once again, the typical clinical manifestation is mild to moderate mucocutaneous bleeding resulting from a lack of larger VWF multimers. In this variant, however, the absence of large molecular weight VWF is secondary to an overactive GP Ib binding domain. The heightened affinity for platelet GP Ib receptors leads to increased binding to platelets and ultimately to removal from the plasma. Interestingly, this increase in interaction between VWF and platelets often leads to a mild thrombocytopenia as well.

(c) VWD type 2M is extremely rare and results from an under-active GP Ib binding domain. Bleeding among these patients is variable depending upon the level of decreased affinity for platelet GP Ib receptors. Here, multimeric analysis may appear normal, but VWF activity levels are significantly decreased (See Table 3.1).[57,58]

(d) VWD type 2N, another rare disorder, is unique among variants of VWD in its clinical presentation. There is impaired binding of the FVIII molecule to VWF due to a genetic mutation of the binding site on VWF. Once again, the pathophysiology involves a derangement in a major function of VWF, i.e. its role as a chaperone molecule for coagulation factor VIII. Normal VWF regulates the plasma concentration of FVIII by binding to and protecting it from enzymatic degradation. As the plasma concentration of VWF increases or decreases, so too does the plasma concentration of FVIII (but not vice versa). If the FVIII binding site on the VWF molecule is altered so that FVIII cannot bind, the plasma levels of FVIII will drop regardless of the amount of

Table 3.1 Laboratory diagnosis of VWD.

	Type 1	Type 2A	Type 2B	Type 2N	Type 2M	Type 3
PTT	N or ↑	N or ↑	N or ↑	↑	N or ↑	↑
PFA-100™	Abn	Abn	Abn	N	Abn	Abn
VWF:Ag	↓	↓or/N	N	N	N	Absent
RCoF	↓	↓↓	↓↓	N	↓↓	Absent
FVIII	↓	N or ↓	N or ↓	↓	↓	↓↓↓
RIPA Std	↓	↓↓	↑↑↑		↓↓	Absent
Low	Absent	Absent	**Present**	Absent	Absent	Absent
Multimer analysis	Normal distribution	Large and intermediate absent	Large absent	Normal	Normal	Absent

PTT = partial thromboplastin time, PFA-100 ™ = platelet function analyzer, Abn = abnormal, N = normal, VWF:Ag = von Willebrand antigen, RCoF = ristocetin cofactor activity, RIPA = ristocetin induced platelet agglutination.

VWF present. Therefore, type 2N VWF indirectly leads to defective secondary hemostasis. Depending upon the extent of FVIII deficiency, the patient will experience mild to moderate bleeding. Generally females presenting with low FVIII and mild bleeding tendency are classified as hemophilia carriers, however they may need further investigation to rule out VWF-type 2N.

VWD Type 3 is an autosomal recessive disease that has a prevalence of 1–5 per million[59,60] and presents clinically as severe bleeding akin to hemophilia. The type of bleeding can be mucocutaneous, deep tissue/intra-articular, or both. Mucocutaneous bleeding is usually more pronounced and more frequent.[51] It is characterized by undetectable amounts of VWF and, secondarily, very low levels of FVIII (usually between 2 and 10 IU/dl). Since these patients have little or no production of VWF, increased estrogen levels cannot lead to compensation of the deficiency. These patients generally require lifelong therapy and will definitely need therapy prior to parturition, as discussed below.

Acquired von Willebrand syndrome

An acquired von Willebrand syndrome (aVWS) might account for late onset mucocutaneous bleeding in a patient with no family history of VWD. Laboratory tests will be indistinguishable from certain patterns seen in VWD (see Table 3.1). Although many different pathologic processes can lead to aVWS, the underlying etiology is usually associated with a hematopoietic malignancy (plasma cell dyscrasia being the most common), connective tissue disease, or hypothyroidism (all patients with menorrhagia should have a thyroid screen). Treatment is directed toward correcting the instigating disorder but can also include therapy used in congenital VWD.

Diagnosis of von Willebrand disease

When the clinical history and physical examination strongly suggest a primary hemostatic disorder in a patient with no obvious reason for platelet dysfunction (e.g. aspirin ingestion), and the initial laboratory results reveal a normal or only slightly decreased platelet count, VWD should be suspected. Diagnosis of VWD begins with a triad of diagnostic laboratory tests:

(a) Factor VIII Activity (FVIII: C)
(b) Von Willebrand Factor Antigen
(c) Von Willebrand Factor Activity as Ristocetin cofactor assay (VWF:RCoF)

All three tests are needed because of the heterogeneity of VWD. For instance, a functional assay in a patient with VWD type 2M will exhibit a qualitative defect of VWF, whereas the quantitative assay for VWF antigen in this same patient will be normal. Typical test result profiles for the various types of VWD are listed in Table 3.1. When testing for VWD, it is important to recall that the luteal phase of the menstrual cycle is a high estrogen state associated with increases in VWF concentrations,[61,62] and testing performed during this period may not reveal a true VWF deficiency. Baseline VWF levels should be obtained during either the follicular or the menstrual phase, which is the apparent nadir,[63] to limit false negative results. Furthermore, if the clinical suspicion for VWD is high but the initial triad testing is borderline normal, the tests should be repeated, as there can be artifact in the collection or testing of the sample.[29,64] Depending upon the pattern of abnormal test results, further workup to subcategorize the VWD may be necessary. Such work ups may include a Ristocetin-induced platelet agglutination test (RIPA), which is a different assay from VWF:RCoF, VWF multimeric assay[65,66] or a factor VIII binding assay.

Management of von Willebrand disease during pregnancy

The management of VWD during pregnancy requires appropriate monitoring throughout gestation as well as medical intervention when needed. In known VWD patients, VWF and FVIII activity levels should be measured when pregnancy is confirmed to establish baseline levels. These tests should then be repeated prior to any surgical intervention and prior to delivery to ensure adequate levels for normal hemostasis.[67] The hemostatic challenge determines the therapeutic approach to raise low levels. Dosing regimens for the various therapies are set to raise FVIII activity and VWF/RCoF activity to greater than 50%, and higher goals (80–100%) are set for C-section delivery. Above these levels, there should be no increased risk of bleeding. The greatest risk of bleeding is in the postpartum period and during the puerperium, when levels of VWF are rapidly decreasing,[17] and, therefore, clinical and possibly laboratory monitoring should be continued for at least 1–2 weeks postpartum.

Only a few treatment options exist. Most of the therapeutic agents are aimed at increasing the plasma concentrations of functional VWF. The available therapies include VWF replacement (FVIII/VWF concentrates and cryoprecipitate), stimulants of VWF production/release (DDAVP and conjugated estrogens), hemostatic agents (recombinant factor VIIa), and antifibrinolytics (e.g. Amicar). Among these therapies, FVIII/VWF concentrates and DDAVP are routinely used during pregnancy and/or the puerperium. All others are either contraindicated for pregnant women or only used as adjunctive therapy during hemorrhagic crises.

A variety of virus-inactivated plasma concentrates exist, but only one (Humate-P, Aventis-Behring) is approved for use in the United States for treating VWD. Humate-P is an intermediate-purity factor VIII concentrate used in the treatment of VWD. It has a factor VIII activity of 1–5 U/mg protein and contains large amounts of high molecular weight VWF, i.e. ~2.5 U ristocetin cofactor activity per 1 U FVIII: C.[13,68] Upon infusion, plasma VWF and FVIII rise immediately.[39] The rise in factor VIII coagulant activity (FVIII: C recovery) is expected to be at least 2 U/dl for every 1 U/kg of factor VIII infused.[13,68] The rise in VWF activity (VWF:RCoF) is expected to be at least 1.5 U/dl for every 1 U/kg VWF.[13] The half life of FVIII cannot be accurately determined. The half-life of VWF:RCoF is approximately 12 hours.[13] Side effects include urticaria, fever, weakness, and nausea.

Cryoprecipitate (Cryo) also contains sufficient amount of VWF for use in the treatment of VWD. As with infusion of Humate-P, FVIII and VWF rise concurrently with infusion of cryo. Although the cost of cryo is much less than Humate-P, the risk of infectious disease transmission remains, since to date no method exists for viral inactivation of Cryo. It is advised that this be used as a last-resort when other feasible treatments, i.e. Humate-P or DDAVP, are not available. Each bag of Cryo contains approximately 100 U of FVIII (and VWF). Depending upon the baseline level of VWF and desired increase in its activity, 25–50 U of FVIII (VWF)/kg is infused. This amounts to approximately 15–30 bags of Cryo as a loading dose and then half as much as a maintenance dose every 12 hours.

DDAVP (1-deamino-8-D-arginine, desmopressin) is a synthetic analog of antidiuretic hormone that induces the release of VWF from storage sites. The result is a 3- to 5-fold increase in plasma VWF levels within 30 minutes of administration (IV dose of 0.3 μg/kg).[69,70] The elevated levels last for eight to ten hours;[70] however, tachyphylaxis is commonly experienced after 6 to 7 doses, thus making long-term use impractical. Since response to DDAVP varies from patient to patient, evaluation of the drug's efficacy at the time of initial diagnosis for each individual patient is indicated.[69] Many physicians are reluctant to use DDAVP in the antenatal period because of (i) theoretic risk of placental insufficiency due to vasoconstriction, (ii) theoretic risk of premature labor due to uterine contraction, and (iii) the risk of maternal and/or neonatal hyponatremia.[69,71] It should be noted that DDAVP activity is very specific to V_2 receptors, which are not significantly involved in uterine contraction or vasoconstriction.[72] While potential hyponatremia secondary to its antidiuretic effect is not common with appropriate regulation of fluid intake, serum sodium levels should still be monitored during therapy.[73] With these factors taken into consideration, DDAVP has been used successfully as prophylaxis for antenatal testing, e.g. chorionic villus sampling, and as treatment for pregnant patients with diabetes insipidus, platelet storage diseases and Ehlers-Danlos syndrome.[74–78] DDAVP is most efficacious in VWD type 1.[79] Experience with its use in type 2M is limited, but response is predicted to be poor, since it would lead to an increase of only dysfunctional VWF.[70] Likewise, the effect of DDAVP in type 2N patients is an increase in only dysfunctional VWD.[80,81]

Therefore, it is not indicated in this population. It is contraindicated in VWD type 2B due to release of overactive VWF that will interact with platelets resulting in potential thrombocytopenia.[82] Lastly, it has no role in the treatment of type 3 patients due to their inability to produce VWF.

Planning for antenatal procedures such as chorionic villus sampling or amniocentesis must include the measurement of FVIII and, possibly, VWF:RCoF activity levels within one week of the procedure. Therapy should be administered to reach and maintain activity levels greater than 50% prior to and for 3 to 4 days following the procedure. The goal may be reached with either Humate-P or DDAVP, although a comprehensive discussion should be held with the patient regarding the risks and benefits associated with each therapy.[47,70] Similar steps and procedures can be used to prepare for epidural anesthesia, if so desired.[47,83,84]

The decision to employ antenatal/intrapartum therapeutic intervention for VWD patients depends upon the activity levels of VWF and the presence of clinically significant bleeding. Careful monitoring may preclude the necessity to treat type 1 or type 2A patients in the antenatal period. They will only require prophylactic treatment for delivery or procedures if FVIII: C and VWF:RCoF levels are below 50%. Unlike most type 1 and 2A patients, VWD type 3 patients will require antenatal treatment (see below). Antenatal management for the remaining subtypes of type 2 patients may also require therapy with Humate-P.

Mechanical hemostasis and postpartum prophylaxis are indicated at the time of delivery in all types of VWD. Aggressive uterotonic therapy with a 20–40 IU/l bolus of oxytocin should be instituted at the time of placental delivery.[83] Other uterotonic agents, i.e. Methergine, Hemabate, or Prostin E, can be added as needed.[83] DDAVP is typically the prophylactic treatment of choice for type 1 patients and Humate-P for all other types.

Since very few clinical trials have assessed the appropriate dosing for factor replacement (Humate-P) in pregnancy, recommendations are generated from anecdotal reports. Generalization of dosing schedules are extrapolated from those used for surgery.[47,85] For any type of VWD that requires Humate-P, cesarean section delivery is considered equivalent to major surgery and vaginal delivery to minor surgery. For planned cesarean section delivery, a loading dose of 50 to 75 U/kg Humate-P given prior to surgery should be followed by subsequent doses of 40 to 60 U/kg every 8 to 12 hours.[68] The goal is to maintain activity levels well above 50% of normal (preferably between 80 to 100%). If emergent C-section is indicated, an infusion of 50 to 75 U/kg should be started immediately.[68] Following delivery, doses of 40 to 60 U/kg Humate-P every 8 to 12 hours should be continued to keep the VWF nadir at or above 50% for 8 to 10 days.[47,85] Uncomplicated vaginal delivery with possible episiotomy or low-degree tear can typically be treated with smaller subsequent dosing (20 to 30 IU/kg) at the same frequency to keep levels above 50% for 3 to 4 days postpartum. Rarely, it may be necessary to transfuse cryoprecipitate if Humate-P is not available and DDAVP is contra-indicated or not indicated, e.g. treatment of VWD type 3. In such cases, a loading dose of 15–30 units of Cryo should be administered followed by one half of the loading dose every 12 hours to keep VWF:RCoF at or above 50% (see Chapter 17).

Uremic bleeding

Mucocutaneous bleeding can be a serious complication in patients with chronic uremia. The definitive etiology of the bleeding remains elusive, but defective platelet aggregation due to either platelet or VWF dysfunction is the ultimate result. The abnormal VWF or platelet function is believed to be secondary to accumulation of "middle molecules" during times of severe renal impairment.[86–88] The uremia, in itself, does not alter blood coagulation or prolong coagulation tests, e.g. aPTT and PT. Vitamin K deficiency, however, is common in uremic patients and may lead to prolongation of the PT alone or both the PT and aPTT. Uremic patients are also commonly afflicted with anemia, which contributes to ineffective platelet-vessel wall interactions. The minimal work up of uremic patients, who are bleeding, therefore, should include a complete blood count, blood urea nitrogen (BUN), creatinine level, PT, and PTT. Treatment can include the following: (i) dialysis to remove "middle molecules", (ii) packed red blood cell transfusion or (iii) erythropoietin to correct anemia, and (iv) DDAVP, (v) cryo, or (vi) estrogen derivatives to increase the levels of normal functioning VWF. It is important to note that renal failure leads to an increased half-life for both heparin and, especially, low molecular weight heparin (LMWH). This must be taken into consideration when using heparin for either dialysis or for treating hypercoaguability in pregnancy.

Primary platelet disorders

If VWD, thrombocytopenia, antiplatelet drugs, and uremia are not the cause of mucocutaneous bleeding, then more esoteric hemostatic defects must be considered. Most of the remaining causes of primary hemostatic defect are congenital primary platelet disorders. These are typically categorized by the type of defect: (i) disorders of adhesion, (ii) disorders of secretion and signal transduction, and (iii) disorders of aggregation.

The most common primary platelet defect of adhesion is Bernard-Soulier syndrome (BSS).[89] BSS results from a variety of mutations (most of which are autosomal recessive) that lead to quantitative or qualitative abnormalities of platelet GPIb-GPIX-GPV receptor complexes (GPIb). Since GPIb is essential to the initial interaction between platelets and subendothelial VWF, i.e. the process of adhesion and to the activation of GPIIb/IIIa receptors involved in platelet aggregation, the clinical presentation and laboratory testing of BSS are very similar to VWD. Like VWD types 1 and 3, platelet aggregation studies reveal normal responses to ADP, epinephrine, and collagen, but decreased or absent response to ristocetin. In addition, BSS patients exhibit mild to moderate thrombocytopenia with abnormally large platelets on peripheral blood smear.

Primary platelet defects of secretion and signal transduction include a long list of disorders that are due to (i) abnormalities of platelet granules, (ii) signal transduction defects, (iii) arachidonic acid pathway and thromboxane synthesis defects, or (iv) cytoskeletal assembly defects. The common denominator for these disorders is impaired platelet function due to diminished granule contents or a derangement in the mechanisms that control the secretion of these contents.[89]

Primary platelet defects of aggregation are seen in Glanzmann's thrombasthenia (GT).[90] GT is another very rare autosomal recessive disorder. It results from quantitative (types 1 and 2) or qualitative (other types) defects of platelet GPIIb/IIIa receptors.[90] Platelet counts and morphology are normal. Aggregation studies reveal absence of response to ADP, collagen, epinephrine, and arachidonic acid but normal response to ristocetin. Due to the frequent need for platelet transfusion in these patients, antenatal management requires evaluation for risk of fetal alloimmune thrombocytopenia (see Chapter 16).

Since hemorrhage in primary platelet defects is very common and often severe enough to necessitate hysterectomy, prophylactic transfusion of platelets and/or administration of DDAVP may be warranted during active labor for vaginal delivery or immediately prior to incision for cesarean section.[83,91] Similarly to VWD, uterotonic agents should be aggressively utilized at the time of delivery.[83] In the postpartum period, hormone therapy or encouragement of breast feeding to delay menses may also be useful.[91] Recently, recombinant FVIIa has been used successfully in primary platelet dysfunction.[92–95]

Secondary hemostatic dysfunction

A history of deep tissue, intra-articular, retroperitoneal, and/or immediate post surgical bleeding is most consistent with deficiency of secondary hemostasis (coagulation factor dysfunction/deficiency). These types of deficiencies typically result in prolongation of the activated partial thromboplastin time and/or the prothrombin time, as discussed above. With the exception of FXI, the reactivity of the majority of coagulation factors must decrease to levels below 30% of normal to lead to dysfunctional hemostasis.

Coagulation factor deficiencies

With exception of factor XII, congenital deficiencies in any of the coagulation factors could lead theoretically to secondary hemostatic dysfunction. The clinical occurrence of these disorders, however, is very rare. Since Hemophilia A (congenital FVIII deficiency) and Hemophilia B (congenital FXI deficiency) are transmitted as X-linked recessive disorders, they almost exclusively effect the male population. Exceptions do exist, however, and include the following: (i) heterozygous women who carry a single FVIII or FIX gene mutation but have a high degree of lionization,[96] (ii) Turner syndrome patients with 46, XX/45X mosaicism or 46, XX structurally abnormal sex chromosomes, (iii) testicular feminization women with an XY karyotype, (iv) VWD type 2N patients (discussed above) and (v) the extraordinarily rare homozygous patients. Patients with these conditions will develop varying degrees of factor VIII or IX deficiencies, some of which will exhibit activity levels below 5%. Activity levels below 30% may lead to classical Hemophiliac-type bleeding. The respective factor activity levels should be monitored at regular intervals throughout pregnancy (at least once per trimester).[47]

Factor XI deficiency is an autosomal recessive bleeding disorder with a genetic prevalence of 4.3% in Ashkenazi Jews,[97] although it is not restricted to the Ashkenazi Jewish population.[98] Bleeding does not occur spontaneously with this defect, but rather only under conditions of hemostatic challenge, e.g. menstruation or surgery. This is the only factor deficiency in which the tendency to bleed does not correlate well with factor activity levels.[99–101] Normal levels range between 70 to 150%. Patients with homozygous defects typically exhibit levels below 15%, but even those who have no detectable activity levels may never experience abnormal bleeding.[99–101] The absence of bleeding in such patients is not fully understood but is believed to result from the ability to generate fibrin through other pathways (TF pathway and activation of FIX by TF-VIIa complex) and through a potential FXI-like activity of platelets. Determining whether or not a particular patient will experience hemorrhagic problems is further complicated by the fact that bleeding tendencies are not consistent within an individual. Regardless of the tendency to bleed, it is reasonable to assess levels in all FXI deficient patients prior to any procedures and delivery. The decision to prophylactically treat FXI deficient patients who lack a history of bleeding, however, is based upon individual experience. If therapy is required, the goal is to reach activity levels of approximately 40–50%. The only therapeutic agent approved for use in the Unites States is fresh frozen plasma, although a factor concentrate does exist for use outside of the USA. A loading dose of 10 to 15 ml FFP/kg (not to exceed 30 IU/kg) prior to the procedure/delivery should be followed by the same dose every 48 hours for 3 to 5 days postpartum.

Other factor deficiencies that may affect the obstetric population include those of prothrombin, fibrinogen, and factors V, VII, X, and XIII. Clinical experience for managing these conditions in the obstetric population is quite limited, as only 1 to 2 cases per million occur in the general population. Therapy regimens for pregnant women afflicted with any of these disorders are therefore extrapolated from experience in managing surgical interventions and hemorrhage in the non-pregnant population. Appropriate therapy for each of these is determined by the factor activity levels, the half-lives of these factors, and the currently available therapies. Fresh frozen plasma (FFP) remains the treatment of choice for patients with factor V, X, or prothrombin deficiencies. Cryo is administered to treat factor XIII deficiencies. Recombinant FVIIa is now available for factor VII deficiency. Additionally, Factor XIII and, rarely, afibrinogenemia are associated with spontaneous abortion and should always be considered in this situation.[102]

Inhibitors of coagulation

In addition to congenital deficiencies, patients may develop acquired coagulation factor deficiencies secondary to production of inhibitors. Like factor deficiencies, specific inhibitors cause prolongation of the aPTT and/or PT. Since nonspecific inhibitors, i.e. lupus anticoagulants, may also prolong screening tests, algorithms have been developed to differentiate between these different conditions. In assessing the clinical history in congenital disorders, certain clues, such as the presence of abnormal bleeding from early childhood, assist in tailoring the laboratory investigation. The most important initial clue in assessing prolongation of coagulation screening tests, i.e. aPTT and/or the PT, is the presence or absence of bleeding. If the patient is not bleeding or if the patient is abnormally clotting, the appropriate first step for laboratory investigation is the lupus anticoagulant test. If the patient is bleeding, the first step is to test for specific factor deficiencies using functional factor assays. The most common disorders are investigated first. After identifying a specific factor inhibitor, it should then be quantified for treatment purposes. The best example of a quantification method, the Bethesda assay for FVIII inhibitor, is discussed below.

Acquired hemophilia

The most common inhibitor associated with the pregnant population is against FVIII, a condition known as acquired hemophilia. It typically develops one to four months postpartum but can develop more than one year after delivery or during the antepartum period. The bleeding manifestations are slightly different than those seen in Hemophilia A. Although patients with the acquired and congenital forms can both develop prolonged post-operative and postpartum bleeding, acquired hemophiliacs do not typically experience intra-articular hemorrhage. Rather, they exhibit deep muscle or mucocutaneous-type bleeding.[103] The severity of bleeding in acquired hemophilia is typically greater than that seen in hemophilia A, with a mortality rate of up to 6% in postpartum women and up to 22% in the general public.[103–105] Clinical vigilance, therefore, is essential, and any postpartum evidence of new onset menometrorrhagia, development of soft tissue hematomas, bleeding from multiple sites, or bleeding that cannot be controlled by usual measures are all suspicious. Although the inhibitor antibodies usually disappear spontaneously after a few months, they can persist for years. The prognosis for subsequent pregnancy, however, is favorable in cases with complete remission.

Characteristic laboratory findings include a significantly prolonged PTT with normal PT, platelet count, and fibrinogen level. Specific testing for FVIII will reveal a deficiency with levels <10%. Factor VIII inhibitor is a time and temperature dependent neutralizing autoantibody and, therefore, can not be detected by routine mixing PTT study. It requires incubation of the patient's plasma with normal pooled plasma at 37 °C for an hour. Once laboratory testing confirms the diagnosis, the Bethesda assay is used to quantify the inhibitor which is reported as Bethesda Units (BU). For therapeutic purposes BUs below 5 are considered to be low titer, whereas BUs of 5 or greater are considered to be high titer. A modified Bethesda assay using porcine FVIII in place of normal pooled plasma (NPP) is used to assess the feasibility of porcine FVIII concentrates for therapy. However, because a better product is available (recombinant FVIIa) the porcine FVIII is seldom used in the USA.

Since the clinical presentation of acquired hemophilia is often acute and life threatening, immediate medical intervention is necessary. Consultation with Hemophiliac specialists and management at a Hemophiliac Comprehensive Care Clinic is preferable, but care should never be delayed when these resources are not available. There are many therapeutic options to control acute bleeding episodes. The choice of treatment and treatment protocol depends on inhibitor titers, the severity of bleeding, and the past medical history (see references,[106,107] for detailed therapeutic suggestions).

Patients with inhibitor titers <5 BU can be treated with agents that raise FVIII plasma levels high enough to both saturate the inhibitor and still provide sufficient activity for normal hemostasis. For serious bleeding, recombinant factor VIII (rFVIII) or FVIII concentrates are used. The recommended loading dose of FVIII is 100–200 U/kg; this should be followed by continuous infusion of 5 to 10 U/kg/hour in order to achieve and maintain factor levels >50%.[108,109]

Patients with titers of inhibitor ≥5 BU can not be treated with high dose FVIII concentrates and require treatment that bypasses the FVIII inhibitor. Bypass strategies involve stimulating fibrin production through routes that do not involve FVIII. Several preparations are available for this purpose and include Activated Prothrombin Complex Concentrates, which contain partially activated factors II, VII, IX, and X, and Factor Eight Inhibitor Bypass Activity (FEIBA), which contain more fully activated factors especially FX. Among these two options, FEIBA at a dosage of 50–75 U/kg every 8 to 12 hours is the recommended treatment for patients with serious bleeding. Due to an increased risk of thromboembolism, the total amount of FEIBA should not exceed 200 U/kg in a 24-hour period and should not be given for more than 3–5 days. Furthermore, D-dimer and fibrinogen levels should be monitored during therapy. The other available therapy to bypass FVIII inhibition is recombinant FVIIa (rFVIIa), administered as 90–120 μg/kg (or even higher) every 2–4 hours to control bleeding.[106] Due to the inability to measure the efficacy of these treatments in the laboratory, these patients must be monitored clinically.

Patients with acquired Hemophilia require immunosuppressive therapy. Corticosteroids are often used alone or in conjunction with cyclophosphamide or azathioprine to suppress the formation of antibodies.[107,110,111] Many different dosing schedules can be used (see references.[106,107] However, cyclophosphamide or azathioprine can only be used in the non-pregnant, non-lactating population, as these are contraindicated during pregnancy and lactation.[106] Intravenous administration of immune globulin (IVIg) at 2 g/dl in 2 or 5 daily fractions has also been shown to decrease inhibitors in a subset of patients.[107,112,113] Other adjunctive treatments such as topical hemostatic agents, e.g. fibrin glue, topical gelatin sponges, 10% topical aminocaproic acid solution, and antifibrinolytic drugs, e.g. tranexamic acid or aminocaproic acid, may also be helpful in appropriate clinical settings.[106]

Genetic counseling and prenatal testing

In addition to diagnosis and treatment, management of bleeding disorders in obstetrics also requires appropriate counseling and perhaps prenatal testing for congenital disorders. A family history of a congenital bleeding disorder should encourage investigation for a carrier or disease state in the patient. If an abnormality is identified, it is essential that the patient understands the condition thoroughly and has adequate support to be able to make educated decisions regarding the particular condition. Prenatal diagnosis in carriers of hemophilia, severe forms of VWD, and severe FXI deficiency allows for the possibility of different approaches in prenatal care.[11]

REFERENCES

1 Kadir, R. A., Sabin, C. A., Pollard, D., *et al.* Quality of life during menstruation in patients with inherited bleeding disorders. *Haemophilia*, 1998; **4**(6): 836–41.

2 Kouides, P. A., Phatak, P. D., Burkart, P., *et al.* Gynaecological and obstetrical morbidity in women with type I von Willebrand disease: results of a patient survey. *Haemophilia*, 2000; **6**(6): 643–8.

3 Rozeik, C. H. Gynecological disorders and psychological problems in 184 women with von Willebrand disease (vWD). *Haemophilia*, 1998; **4**(3): 293.

4 Kulkarni, S., Dopheide, S. M., Yap, C. L., *et al.* A revised model of platelet aggregation. *J. Clin. Invest.*, 2000; **105**(6): 783–91.

5 Shattil, S. J., Kashiwagi, H. and Pampori, N. Integrin signaling: the platelet paradigm. *Blood*, 1998; **91**(8): 2645–57.

6 Watson, S. P. and Gibbins, J. Collagen receptor signalling in platelets: extending the role of the ITAM. *Immunol. Today*, 1998; **19**(6): 260–4.

7 Wickstrom, K., Edelstam, G., Lowbeer, C. H., *et al.* Reference intervals for plasma levels of fibronectin, von Willebrand factor, free protein S and antithrombin during third-trimester pregnancy. *Scand. J. Clin. Lab. Invest.*, 2004; **64**(1): 31–40.

8 Kadir, R. A., Lee, C. A., Sabin, C. A., *et al.* Pregnancy in women with von Willebrand's disease or factor XI deficiency. *Br. J. Obstet. Gynaecol.*, 1998; **105**(3): 314–21.

9 Conti, M., Mari, D., Conti, E., *et al.* Pregnancy in women with different types of von Willebrand disease. *Obstet. Gynecol.*, 1986; **68**(2): 282–5.

10 Stirling, Y., Woolf, L., North, W. R., *et al.* Haemostasis in normal pregnancy. *Thromb. Haemost.*, 1984; **52**(2): 176–82.

11 Economides, D. L., Kadir, R. A. and Lee, C. A. Inherited bleeding disorders in obstetrics and gynaecology. *Br. J. Obstet. Gynaecol.*, 1999; **106**(1): 5–13.

12 Cerneca, F., Ricci, G., Simeone, R., *et al.* Coagulation and fibrinolysis changes in normal pregnancy. Increased levels of procoagulants and reduced levels of inhibitors during pregnancy induce a hypercoagulable state, combined with a reactive fibrinolysis. *Eur. J. Obstet. Gynecol. Reprod. Biol.*, 1997; **73**(1): 31–6.

13 Dobrkovska, A., Krzensk, U. and Chediak, J. R. Pharmacokinetics, efficacy and safety of Humate-P in von Willebrand disease. *Haemophilia*, 1998; **4**(Suppl 3): 33–9.

14 Condie, R. G. A serial study of coagulation factors XII, XI and X in plasma in normal pregnancy and in pregnancy complicated by pre-eclampsia. *Br. J. Obstet. Gynaecol.*, 1976; **83**(8): 636–9.

15 Phillips, L. L., Rosano, L. and Skrodelis, V. Changes in factor XI (plasma thromboplastin antecedent) levels during pregnancy. *Am. J. Obstet. Gynecol.*, 1973; **116**(8): 1114–6.

16 Beller, F. K. and Ebert, C. The coagulation and fibrinolytic enzyme system in pregnancy and in the puerperium. *Eur. J. Obstet. Gynecol. Reprod. Biol.*, 1982; **13**(3): 177–97.

17 Hilgartner, M. W. and Smith, C. H. Plasma thromboplastin antecedent (Factor Xi) in the neonate. *J. Pediatr.*, 1965; **66**: 747–52.

18 Fernandez, J. A., Estelles, A., Gilabert, J., *et al.* Functional and immunologic protein S in normal pregnant women and in full-term newborns. *Thromb. Haemost.*, 1989; **61**(3): 474–8.

19 Clark, P., Brennand, J., Conkie, J. A., *et al.* Activated protein C sensitivity, protein C, protein S and coagulation in normal pregnancy. *Thromb. Haemost.*, 1998; **79**(6): 1166–70.

20 Edelstam, G., Lowbeer, C., Kral, G., *et al.* New reference values for routine blood samples and human neutrophilic lipocalin during third-trimester pregnancy. *Scand. J. Clin. Lab. Invest.*, 2001; **61**(8): 583–92.

21 Kjellberg, U., Andersson, N. E., Rosen, S., *et al.* APC resistance and other haemostatic variables during pregnancy and puerperium. *Thromb. Haemost.*, 1999; **81**(4): 527–31.

22 Chabloz, P., Reber, G., Boehlen, F., *et al.* TAFI antigen and D-dimer levels during normal pregnancy and at delivery. *Br. J. Haematol.*, 2001; **115**(1): 150–2.

23 Cadroy, Y., Grandjean, H., Pichon, J., *et al.* Evaluation of six markers of haemostatic systems in normal pregnancy and pregnancy complicated by hypertension or pre-eclampsia. *Br. J. Obstet. Gynaecol.*, 1993; **100**(5): 416–20.

24 Koh, C. L., Viegas, O. A., Yuen, R., *et al.* Plasminogen activators and inhibitors in normal late pregnancy, postpartum and in the postnatal period. *Int. J. Gynaecol. Obstet.*, 1992; **38**(1): 9–18.

25 Wahlberg, T., Blomback, M., Hall, P., *et al.* Application of indicators, predictors and diagnostic indices in coagulation disorders. I. Evaluation of a self-administered questionnaire with binary questions. *Methods Inf. Med.*, 1980; **19**(4): 194–200.

26 Kouides, P. A. Menorrhagia from a haematologist's point of view. Part I: initial evaluation. *Haemophilia*, 2002; **8**(3): 330–8.

27 Siegel, J. E. and Kouides, P. A. Menorrhagia from a haematologist's point of view. Part II: management. *Haemophilia* 2002; **8**(3): 339–47.

28 Peterson, P., Hayes, T. E., Arkin, C. F., *et al.* The preoperative bleeding time test lacks clinical benefit: College of American Pathologists' and American Society of Clinical Pathologists' position article. *Arch. Surg.*, 1998; **133**(2): 134–9.

29 Favaloro, E. J. Utility of the PFA-100™ for assessing bleeding disorders and monitoring therapy: a review of analytical variables, benefits and limitations. *Haemophilia*, 2001; **7**(2): 170–9.

30 Wuillemin, W., Gasser, K., Zeerleder, S., *et al.* Evaluation of a Platelet Function Analyser (PFA-100™) in patients with a bleeding tendency. *Swiss Med. Wkly.*, 2002(**132**): 443–8.

31 Roa, A. Disorders of platelet function. In Kitchens, C. S. A. B., and Kessler, C. M., eds. *Consultative Hemostasis and Thrombosis.* 1st edn. Philadelphia: W. B. Saunders; 2002. pp. 133–48.

32 Wilner, K. D., Rushing, M., Walden, C., *et al.* Celecoxib does not affect the antiplatelet activity of aspirin in healthy volunteers. *J. Clin. Pharmacol.*, 2002; **42**(9): 1027–30.

33 Silverman, D. G., Halaszynski, T., Sinatra, R., *et al.* Rofecoxib does not compromise platelet aggregation during anesthesia and surgery. *Can. J. Anaesth.*, 2003; **50**(10): 1004–8.

34 Homoncik, M., Malec, M., Marsik, C., *et al.* Rofecoxib exerts no effect on platelet plug formation in healthy volunteers. *Clin. Exp. Rheumatol.*, 2003; **21**(2): 229–31.

35 Coukell, A. J. and Markham, A. Clopidogrel. *Drugs*, 1997; **54**(5): 745–50; discussion p. 751.

36 Pritchard, J. A., Weisman, R., Jr., Ratnoff, O. D., *et al.* Intravascular hemolysis, thrombocytopenia and other hematologic abnormalities associated with severe toxemia of pregnancy. *N. Engl. J. Med.*, 1954; **250**(3): 89–98.

37 Pitkin, R. M. and Witte, D. L. Platelet and leukocyte counts in pregnancy. *JAMA*, 1979; **242**(24): 2696–8.

38 Dilley, A., Drews, C., Miller, C., *et al.* Von Willebrand disease and other inherited bleeding disorders in women with diagnosed menorrhagia. *Obstet. Gynecol.*, 2001; **97**(4): 630–6.
39 Rodeghiero, F., Castaman, G. and Dini, E. Epidemiological investigation of the prevalence of von Willebrand's disease. *Blood*, 1987; **69**(2): 454–9.
40 Edlund, M., Blomback, M., von Schoultz B., *et al.* On the value of menorrhagia as a predictor for coagulation disorders. *Am. J. Hematol.*, 1996; **53**(4): 234–8.
41 Ruggeri, Z. M. Structure of von Willebrand factor and its function in platelet adhesion and thrombus formation. *Best Pract. Res. Clin. Haematol.*, 2001; **14**(2): 257–79.
42 Siediecki, C. Shear-dependant changes in the three-dimensional structure of human von Willebrand factor. *Blood*, 1996; **88**: 2939–50.
43 Ruggeri, Z. M., Dent, J. A. and Saldivar, E. Contribution of distinct adhesive interactions to platelet aggregation in flowing blood. *Blood*, 1999; **94**(1): 172–8.
44 Fujimoto, T. and Hawiger, J. Adenosine diphosphate induces binding of von Willebrand factor to human platelets. *Nature*, 1982; **297**(5862): 154–6.
45 Ni, H., Denis, C. V., Subbarao, S., *et al.* Persistence of platelet thrombus formation in arterioles of mice lacking both von Willebrand factor and fibrinogen. *J. Clin. Invest.*, 2000; **106**(3): 385–92.
46 Goto, S., Ikeda, Y., Saldivar, E., *et al.* Distinct mechanisms of platelet aggregation as a consequence of different shearing flow conditions. *J. Clin. Invest.*, 1998; **101**(2): 479–86.
47 Seremetis S. and Afshani, V. Management of bleeding disorders in pregnancy. In Kitchens, C. S. A. B., and Kessler, C. M., eds. *Consultative Hemostasis and Thrombosis.* 1st edn. Philadelphia: W. B. Saunders; 2002. pp. 437–48.
48 Hennessy, B. J., White, B., Byrne, M., *et al.* Acquired von Willebrand's disease. *Ir. J. Med. Sci.*, 1998; **167**(2): 81–5.
49 Nitu-Whalley, I. C. and Lee, C. A. Acquired von Willebrand syndrome – report of 10 cases and review of the literature. *Haemophilia*, 1999; **5**(5): 318–26.
50 Attivissimo, L. A., Lichtman, S. M. and Klein, I. Acquired von Willebrand's syndrome causing a hemorrhagic diathesis in a patient with hypothyroidism. *Thyroid*, 1995; **5**(5): 399–401.
51 Lak, M., Peyvandi, F. and Mannucci, P. M. Clinical manifestations and complications of childbirth and replacement therapy in 385 Iranian patients with type 3 von Willebrand disease. *Br. J. Haematol.*, 2000; **111**(4): 1236–9.
52 Kroll, M. *Manual of Coagulation Disorders.* 1st edn. Malden, MA: Blackwell Science; 2001.
53 Castaman, G., Eikenboom, J. C., Contri, A., *et al.* Pregnancy in women with type 1 von Willebrand disease caused by heterozygosity for von Willebrand factor mutation C1130F. *Thromb. Haemost.*, 2000; **84**(2): 351–2.
54 Kouides, P. A. Obstetric and gynaecological aspects of von Willebrand disease. *Best Pract. Res. Clin. Haematol.*, 2001; **14**(2): 381–99.
55 Sorosky, J., Klatsky, A., Nobert, G. F. Von Willebrand's disease complicating second-trimester abortion. *Obstet. Gynecol.*, 1980; **55**(2): 253–4.
56 Meyer, D., Fressinaud, E., Hilbert, L., *et al.* Type 2 von Willebrand disease causing defective von Willebrand factor-dependent platelet function. *Best. Pract. Res. Clin. Haematol.*, 2001; **14**(2): 349–64.
57 Ginsburg, D. and Sadler, J. E. Von Willebrand disease: a database of point mutations, insertions, and deletions. For the Consortium on von Willebrand Factor Mutations and

Polymorphisms, and the Subcommittee on von Willebrand Factor of the Scientific and Standardization Committee of the International Society on Thrombosis and Haemostasis. *Thromb. Haemost.*, 1993; **69**(2): 177–84.

58 Ruggeri, Z. M. and Zimmerman, T. S. Classification of variant von Willebrand's disease subtypes by analysis of functional characteristics and multimeric composition of factor VIII/von Willebrand factor. *Ann. NY. Acad. Sci.*, 1981; **370**: 205–9.

59 Weiss, H. J., Ball, A. P. and Mannucci, P. M. Incidence of severe von Willebrand's disease. *N. Engl. J. Med.*, 1982; **307**(2): 127.

60 Mannucci, P. M., Bloom, A. L., Larrieu, M. J., *et al.* Atherosclerosis and von Willebrand factor. I. Prevalence of severe von Willebrand's disease in western Europe and Israel. *Br. J. Haematol.*, 1984; **57**(1): 163–9.

61 Kadir, R. A., Economides, D. L., Sabin, C. A., *et al.* Variations in coagulation factors in women: effects of age, ethnicity, menstrual cycle and combined oral contraceptive. *Thromb. Haemost.*, 1999; **82**(5): 1456–61.

62 Miller, C., Dilley, A. B., Drews, C., *et al.* Changes in von Willebrand factor and Factor VIII during the menstrual cycle. *Thromb. Haemost.*, 2002; **87**(6): 1082–3.

63 Mandalaki, T., Louizou, C., Dimitriadou, C., *et al.* Variations in factor VIII during the menstrual cycle in normal women. *N. Engl. J. Med.*, 1980; **302**(19): 1093–4.

64 Blomback, M., Eneroth, P., Andersson, O., *et al.* On laboratory problems in diagnosing mild von Willebrand's disease. *Am. J. Hematol.*, 1992; **40**(2): 117–20.

65 Budde, U., Drewke, E., Mainusch, K., *et al.* Laboratory diagnosis of congenital von Willebrand disease. *Semin. Thromb. Hemost.*, 2002; **28**(2): 173–90.

66 Enayat, M. S. and Hill, F. G. Analysis of the complexity of the multimeric structure of factor VIII related antigen/von Willebrand protein using a modified electrophoretic technique. *J. Clin. Pathol.*, 1983; **36**(8): 915–9.

67 Walker, I. D., Walker, J. J., Colvin, B. T., *et al.* Investigation and management of haemorrhagic disorders in pregnancy. Haemostasis and Thrombosis Task Force. *J. Clin. Pathol.*, 1994; **47**(2): 100–8.

68 Eikenboom, J. C. Congenital von Willebrand disease type 3: clinical manifestations, pathophysiology and molecular biology. *Best Pract. Res. Clin. Haematol.*, 2001; **14**(2): 365–79.

69 Batlle, J., Noya, M. S., Giangrande, P., *et al.* Advances in the therapy of von Willebrand disease. *Haemophilia*, 2002; **8**(3): 301–7.

70 Mannucci, P. M. How I treat patients with von Willebrand disease. *Blood*, 2001; **97**(7): 1915–19.

71 Chediak, J. R., Alban, G. M. and Maxey, B. Von Willebrand's disease and pregnancy: management during delivery and outcome of offspring. *Am. J. Obstet. Gynecol.*, 1986; **155**(3): 618–24.

72 Mannucci, P. M. Desmopressin (DDAVP) in the treatment of bleeding disorders: the first 20 years. *Blood*, 1997; **90**(7): 2515–21.

73 Mannucci, P. M. Hemostatic drugs. *N. Engl. J. Med.*, 1998; **339**(4): 245–53.

74 Charles, K., Preston, F. and Makris, M. Successful use of desmopression (DDAVP) in pregnant women with inherited storage pool disease. *Haemophilia*, 2000; **6**: 241.

75 Burrow, G., Wassenaar, W. and Robertson, G. DDAVP treatment of diabetes insipidus during pregnancy and the post-partum period. *Acta Endocrinol.*, 1981; **97**: 23–5.

76 Rochelson, B., Caruso, R., Davenport, D., *et al.* The use of prophylactic desmopressin (DDAVP) in labor to prevent hemorrhage in a patient with Ehlers-Danlos syndrome. *NY State J. Med.*, 1991; **91**(6): 268–9.
77 Weinbaum, P. J., Cassidy, S. B., Campbell, W. A., *et al.* Pregnancy management and successful outcome of Ehlers-Danlos syndrome type IV. *Am. J. Perinatol.*, 1987; **4**(2): 134–7.
78 Ray, J. G. DDAVP use during pregnancy: an analysis of its safety for mother and child. *Obstet. Gynecol. Surv.*, 1998; **53**(7): 450–5.
79 Mannucci, P. M., Lombardi, R., Bader, R., *et al.* Heterogeneity of type I von Willebrand disease: evidence for a subgroup with an abnormal von Willebrand factor. *Blood*, 1985; **66**(4): 796–802.
80 Sadler, J. E., Mannucci, P. M., Berntorp, E., *et al.* Impact, diagnosis and treatment of von Willebrand disease. *Thromb. Haemost.*, 2000; **84**(2): 160–74.
81 Mazurier, C., Gaucher, C., Jorieux, S., *et al.* Biological effect of desmopressin in eight patients with type 2N ('Normandy') von Willebrand disease. Collaborative Group. *Br. J. Haematol.*, 1994; **88**(4): 849–54.
82 Holmberg, L., Nilsson, I. M., Borge, L., *et al.* Platelet aggregation induced by 1-desamino-8-D-arginine vasopressin (DDAVP) in Type II B von Willebrand's disease. *N. Engl. J. Med.*, 1983; **309**(14): 816–21.
83 Fausett, B. and Silver, R. M. Congenital disorders of platelet function. *Clin. Obstet. Gynecol.* 1999; **42**(2): 390–405.
84 Sage, D. J. Epidurals, spinals and bleeding disorders in pregnancy: a review. *Anaesth. Intensive Care*, 1990; **18**(3): 319–26.
85 Phillips, M. D. and Santhouse, A. von Willebrand disease: recent advances in pathophysiology and treatment. *Am. J. Med. Sci.*, 1998; **316**(2): 77–86.
86 Pales, J. L., Lopez, A., Asensio, A., *et al.* Inhibitory effect of peak 2–4 of uremic middle molecules on platelet aggregation. *Eur. J. Haematol.*, 1987; **39**(3): 197–202.
87 Bazilinski, N., Shaykh, M., Dunea, G., *et al.* Inhibition of platelet function by uremic middle molecules. *Nephron*, 1985; **40**(4): 423–8.
88 Moal, V., Brunet, P., Dou, L., *et al.* Impaired expression of glycoproteins on resting and stimulated platelets in uraemic patients. *Nephrol. Dial. Transplant*, 2003; **18**(9): 1834–41.
89 Kunicki T. J. Platelet immunology. In Colman, R. W., Hirsh, J., Marder, V. J., *et al.*, eds. *Hemostasis and Thrombosis: Basic Principles & Clinical Practice.* 4th edn. Philadelphia: Lippincott Williams & Wilkins; 2001, pp. 461–77.
90 Ramasamy, I. Inherited bleeding disorders: disorders of platelet adhesion and aggregation. *Crit. Rev. Oncol. Hematol.*, 2004; **49**(1): 1–35.
91 Khalil, A., Seoud, M., Tannous, R., *et al.* Bernard-Soulier syndrome in pregnancy: case report and review of the literature. *Clin. Lab. Haematol.*, 1998; **20**(2): 125–8.
92 Laurian, Y. Treatment of bleeding in patients with platelet disorders: is there a place for recombinant factor VIIa? *Pathophysiol. Haemost. Thromb.*, 2002; **32**(Suppl. 1): 37–40.
93 Caglar, K., Cetinkaya, A., Aytac, S., *et al.* Use of recombinant factor VIIa for bleeding in children with Glanzmann thrombasthenia. *Pediatr. Hematol. Oncol.*, 2003; **20**(6): 435–8.
94 Poon, M. C., d'Oiron, R., Hann, I., *et al.* Use of recombinant factor VIIa (NovoSeven) in patients with Glanzmann thrombasthenia. *Semin. Hematol.*, 2001; **38**(4 Suppl. 12): 21–5.

95 Almeida, A. M., Khair, K., Hann, I. The use of recombinant factor VIIa in children with inherited platelet function disorders. *Br. J. Haematol.*, 2003; **121**(3): 477–81.

96 Lusher, J. M. and McMillan, C. W. Severe factor VIII and factor IX deficiency in females. *Am. J. Med.*, 1978; **65**(4): 637–48.

97 Seligsohn, U. High gene frequency of factor XI (PTA) deficiency in Ashkenazi Jews. *Blood*, 1978; **51**(6): 1223–8.

98 Bauduer, F., Dupreuilh, F., Ducout, L., *et al.* Factor XI deficiency in the French Basque Country. *Haemophilia*, 1999; **5**(3): 187–90.

99 Kadir, R. A., Economides, D. L. and Lee, C. A. Factor XI deficiency in women. *Am. J. Hematol.*, 1999; **60**(1): 48–54.

100 Bolton-Maggs, P. H., Young Wan-Yin, B., McCraw, A. H., *et al.* Inheritance and bleeding in factor XI deficiency. *Br. J. Haematol.*, 1988; **69**(4): 521–8.

101 Bolton-Maggs, P. H., Colvin, B. T., Satchi, B. T., *et al.* Thrombogenic potential of factor XI concentrate. *Lancet*, 1994; **344**(8924): 748–9.

102 Roberts, H. and Escobar, M. Less common congenital disorders of hemostasis. In Kitchens, C. S. A. B., and Kessler, C. M., eds. *Consultative Hemostasis and Thrombosis.* Philadelphia: W. B. Saunders; 2002, pp. 57–73.

103 Green, D. and Lechner, K. A survey of 215 non-hemophilic patients with inhibitors to Factor VIII. *Thromb. Haemost.*, 1981; **45**(3): 200–3.

104 Hauser, I., Schneider, B. and Lechner, K. Post-partum factor VIII inhibitors. A review of the literature with special reference to the value of steroid and immunosuppressive treatment. *Thromb. Haemost.*, 1995; **73**(1): 1–5.

105 Delgado, J., Jimenez-Yuste, V., Hernandez-Navarro, F., Villar, A. *et al.* Acquired haemophilia: review and meta-analysis focused on therapy and prognostic factors. *Br. J. Haematol.*, 2003; **121**(1): 21–35.

106 Rubinger, M., Rivard, G. E., Teitel, J., *et al.* Suggestions for the management of factor VIII inhibitors. *Haemophilia*, 2000; **6**(Suppl. 1): 52–9.

107 Ewenstein B., Putnam K. and Bohn R. Nonhemophilic inhibitors of coagulation. In Kitchens, C. S., Alving, B. M. and Kessler, C. M., eds. *Consultative Hemostasis and Thrombosis.* Philadelphia: W. B. Saunders; 2002, pp. 75–90.

108 Rubinger, M., Houston, D. S., Schwetz, N., *et al.* Continuous infusion of porcine factor VIII in the management of patients with factor VIII inhibitors. *Am. J. Hematol.*, 1997; **56**(2): 112–8.

109 Shulman, N. R. and Hirschman, R. J. Acquired hemophilia. *Trans. Assoc. Am. Physicians*, 1969; **82**: 388–97.

110 Green, D. Suppression of an antibody to factor VIII by a combination of factor VIII and cyclophosphamide. *Blood*, 1971; **37**(4): 381–7.

111 Spero, J. A., Lewis, J. H. and Hasiba, U. Corticosteroid therapy for acquired F VIII: C inhibitors. *Br. J. Haematol.*, 1981; **48**(4): 635–42.

112 Schwartz, R. S., Gabriel, D. A., Aledort, L. M., *et al.* A prospective study of treatment of acquired (autoimmune) factor VIII inhibitors with high-dose intravenous gammaglobulin. *Blood*, 1995; **86**(2): 797–804.

113 Sultan, Y., Kazatchkine, M. D., Nydegger, U., *et al.* Intravenous immunoglobulin in the treatment of spontaneously acquired factor VIII: C inhibitors. *Am. J. Med.*, 1991; **91**(5A): 35–9(S).

4

Hemolytic disease of the fetus and newborn caused by ABO, Rhesus, and other blood group alloantibodies

Katharine A. Downes, M.D.[1] and Ravindra Sarode, M.D.[2]

[1]Assistant Professor, Department of Pathology, University Hospitals of Cleveland, Cleveland, Ohio, USA
[2]Professor of Pathology, University of Texas Southwestern Medical Center; Director: Transfusion Medicine and Hemostasis, Dallas, Texas, USA

Introduction

This chapter presents an overview of immune mediated hemolytic disease of the fetus and newborn (HDFN) due to ABO, Rh(D) and other red cell alloantibodies. Section I reviews the pathophysiology of immune mediated HDFN. Section II describes HDFN due to different antigen incompatibilities (ABO, Rh, and other antigens). Section III focuses on the management of the non-sensitized Rh(D) negative female, the alloimmunized mother, the fetus, and the neonate.

Section I: Pathophysiology of hemolytic disease of the fetus and neonate (HDFN)

The cause of hemolytic disease of the fetus and neonate (HDFN) is immune mediated destruction of fetal and/or newborn erythrocytes by maternal antibodies directed against fetal erythrocyte antigens inherited from the father. HDFN occurs as the result of five distinct events:

(1) Fetal inheritance of a paternal erythrocyte antigen

The gene for red cell antigen is inherited from the father. If the father is homozygous for the gene that the mother lacks, 100% of his offspring carry that gene and will be at the greatest risk for HDFN. The offspring of a heterozygous father will have 50% chance of carrying that gene and therefore will be at a lesser risk.

Hematological Complications in Obstetrics, Pregnancy, and Gynecology, ed. R. L. Bick *et al.* Published by Cambridge University Press.

(2) Passage of fetal erythrocytes into the maternal circulation exposes the pregnant female to the "foreign" paternal erythrocyte antigen

Any clinical situation that introduces the possibility of fetomaternal hemorrhage (FMH)[1] may introduce fetal RBCs into maternal circulation and, thus, the possibility of maternal alloimmunization.[2,3] Repeated episodes of FMH may lead to increased maternal antibody titers, in turn leading to increased severity of HDFN. Invasive obstetrical procedures/interventions such as amniocentesis,[4] fetal blood sampling, abdominal trauma[5] intrauterine transfusion (IUT)[6] and delivery are all associated with FMH and the consequent possibility of maternal alloimmunization. While in most cases a small volume hemorrhage occurs, as little as 1 cm^3 of fetal cells may immunize the mother.[7] Additionally, another source of alloimmunization may come from exposure to foreign erythrocyte antigens by transfusion therapy or missed abortions and miscarriages.[8]

(3) Production of maternal IgG alloantibodies

The mother's ability to produce antibody varies, depending on complex genetic factors.[9] Destruction of fetal red cells by maternal anti-A or anti-B antibodies results in the clearance of fetal red cells before they have a chance to stimulate the maternal immune system to make antibody against non-ABO antigens. Thus, ABO incompatibility provides some protection against other red cell antigen alloimmunization, as will be described later.

(4) Passage of maternal IgG into the fetal circulation

Only immunoglobulin G class antibodies (IgG) are transported from the maternal circulation across the placental barrier and into the neonatal circulation,[10] leading to HDFN.[11] Antibody transport results from interactions between immunoglobulin and syncytiotrophoblast Fc receptors; only IgG_1 and IgG_3 are transportable and can bind macrophage Fc receptors.[12] Active transport of IgG starts in the second trimester and is continued until birth. The IgG subclass can affect the severity of HDFN; of the four IgG subclasses, IgG_1 and IgG_3 are more efficient in promoting RBC hemolysis than IgG_2 or IgG_4.

(5) Binding of maternal IgG to fetal erythrocytes leads to hemolysis

The erythrocyte antigen must be well developed and expressed on the cell surface for HDFN to occur. The blood group antigens A and B, and Rh antigens are well developed during fetal life. Similarly the blood group systems Duffy, Kell, and Kidd are well developed *in utero* and will allow antigen binding resulting in HDFN.[13] In such instances maternal IgG binds to and coats specific fetal erythrocyte antigens. Splenic macrophages target the antibody-coated RBCs and remove them from the circulation. The erythrocyte destruction rate depends on the antibody titer, the number of antigenic sites on the RBCs, and the antibody's specificity; if the titer is low enough, the maternal IgG will bind the fetal red cells but hemolysis will not be apparent. RBC antigens such as Lewis and Cartwright are not well developed at birth; consequently, the antigen is not available to bind with the maternal antibody.[14]

Effects on the fetus

RBC hemolysis results in anemia that stimulates rapid erythrocytopoiesis in the fetal bone marrow and extramedullary sites like the spleen and liver, thus resulting in hepatosplenomegaly. There is an ensuing release of erythroblasts into the fetal circulation; the term used to describe this phenomenon is *erythroblastosis fetalis.*[15] Erythrocyte destruction releases hemoglobin, which is metabolized to indirect bilirubin. This indirect bilirubin is transported across the placenta and conjugated in the maternal liver to direct bilirubin, which is then excreted by the mother. While bilirubin levels may be increased in the amniotic fluid, these do not cause disease in the fetus. However, the newborn liver is unable to conjugate bilirubin effectively, especially in the premature infant. Unconjugated or indirect bilirubin may reach levels that are dangerous to the infant's brain, and, if left untreated, such levels may cause *kernicterus*[16–18] or permanent brain damage and death.

Hydrops fetalis

Hepatosplenomegaly results in portal hypertension and hepatocellular damage. Decreased hepatic production of plasma proteins results in high-output cardiac failure, generalized edema, effusions, and ascites, i.e. generalized anasarca or *hydrops fetalis.* Hydrops fetalis[19] has been described in severe cases at 18–20 weeks' gestation and previously was uniformly fatal. Currently, most fetuses can be treated successfully. Maternal IgG persists for a variable period in the neonatal circulation depending upon the titer of antibody. With a half-life of 21 days, IgG can be detected for up to 3 months in the neonate and thus may cause some ongoing hemolysis.

Section II: Erythrocyte antigens implicated in HDFN

Up to 64 different specificities of antibodies have been implicated as causative agents in HDFN (Table 4.1).[20] This section focuses on the most common causes of HDFN – namely the ABO and Rh(D) antigens. Other alloantibodies are briefly discussed.

HDFN caused by ABO incompatibility

Overview of the ABO blood group system

The ABO blood group system was the first erythrocyte blood group system identified and consists of different carbohydrate antigens expressed on erythrocytes. The

Table 4.1 Alloantibodies identified in maternal prenatal specimens.

Common	Rare	Never
Anti-D	anti-Fy^a	anti-Le^a
Anti-D + C	anti-s	anti-Le^b
Anti-D + E	anti-M	anti-I
Anti-C	anti-N	anti-IH
Anti-E	anti-S	anti-P1
Anti-c	JKA	
Anti-e		
Anti-Kell		

ABO blood group is the most clinically significant blood group system because individuals have naturally occurring circulating antibodies (anti-A, anti-B, and/or anti-A, B – an antibody that reacts with both A and B antigens) against the A or B antigens that they lack. In the absence of transfusion or pregnancy, these antibodies are produced as a response to exposure to A or B antigen-like carbohydrates present in food and other substances in the environment.[21] These antibodies are predominantly IgM in nature and may therefore fix complement and cause intravascular hemolysis of incompatible RBCs. However, variable amounts of IgG antibodies are also present in the plasma.

ABO antigen expression is determined by the presence and/or absence of antigen determining sugars. Genes for ABO (chromosome 9),[22] Hh and *Sese* (chromosome 19) are located at 3 separate loci and control expression of ABO antigens.[23] Each A, B and H gene encodes a glycosyltransferase, which places a different sugar on the polypeptide or lipid to produce the unique antigen.[24] The A and B genes encode glycosyltransferases that produce the A and B antigens respectively. The O gene does not encode a functional enzyme. The ABH antigens are widely distributed throughout the different tissues of the body[25] and are part of endothelial and epithelial membranes.[26] They also occur in a soluble form in the plasma and other body fluids depending upon their secretory status that is determined by *Sese* gene.[27]

To determine a patient's ABO blood group, a front type and a reverse type are performed. In the front type, the patient's RBCs are reacted with anti-A and with anti-B reagent sera to determine what antigen(s) are expressed on the patient's RBCs. In a reverse type, the patient's plasma is reacted with A and B reagent cells to determine the presence or absence of anti-A, anti-B, and anti-A, B in the patient's plasma. Each individual's erythrocytes either lack or express one or both of the A and B antigen(s), and the plasma contains naturally occurring antibody against

Table 4.2 Comparison of ABO versus Rh(D) HDFN.

Feature	ABO	Rh(D)
First pregnancy	Yes	No
Titer predict disease severity	No	Yes
Antibody IgG	Yes	Yes
Bilirubin at birth	Normal	Elevated
Anemia at birth	No	Yes
Phototherapy	Yes	Yes
Spherocytes	Yes	Rare
Exchange transfusion	Rare	Common
Intrauterine transfusion	None	Sometimes

A or B antigens that are absent from the RBC. The frequency of these blood types varies among populations.[28,29]

Prevalence of ABO-HDFN

As HDFN due to anti-D has declined, ABO incompatibility has become the most common cause of HDFN.[30,31] A type O person carries a significantly higher amount of IgG component as compared to group A or B persons. ABO-HDFN typically occurs in A or B infants whose mothers are Group O with potent-high titer anti-A, anti-B or anti-A, B IgG.[32,33] ABO incompatibility associated HDFN can occur in the first pregnancy, whereas Rh(D) or other red cell antigens induced HDFN generally occurs in second or subsequent pregnancies unless the patient has been transfused with red cells in the past (Table 4.2).

Clinical presentation

AB antigens are poorly developed and simple in configuration on fetal RBCs. In adults these antigens are well developed with high density and complexity.[34] A and B antigens are also expressed on tissues (endothelium and epithelium) and are present in the fetal secretions/plasma where they absorb/neutralize most of the maternal antibodies crossing the placenta.[35] The clinical presentation is therefore generally subtle with mild postpartum hyperbilirubinemia and jaundice occurring within 48 hours of birth. Rarely, there can be a severe presentation with moderate to severe hyperbilirubinemia and anemia with risk of kernicterus.[36] Increasing bilirubin levels may be treated with phototherapy;[37] severe cases are rare and may require exchange transfusion[38,39] (see below).

Diagnosis

The laboratory diagnosis of ABO incompatibility induced HDFN is generally straightforward.[40] The neonate has increasing hyperbilirubinemia in the first 24–48 hours after birth. There is also a disproportionate decrease in hemoglobin values with respect to the expected decrease in the first few days. At this stage a work-up on cord blood is indicated that includes performing a Coomb's or direct antiglobulin test (DAT). Red cells coated with IgG, e.g., fetal red cells coated by maternal IgG, cannot agglutinate themselves in the test tube because IgG molecules are small; hence, they cannot bring red cells together. In the DAT, rabbit–human anti-IgG is added to the patient's red cells, which binds to the IgG molecules on the red cells causing agglutination. The DAT is weakly positive in A or B neonates born to O mothers; however, a positive DAT does not automatically indicate hemolysis because positivity may simply indicate that red cells are coated with IgG. Therefore, without evidence of hyperbilirubinemia or moderate to severe anemia, there is no HDN. Performing a DAT may be useful for diagnosis,[41] but it is not always positive in all cases of ABO-HDFN.[12]

If the DAT is positive then an elution technique is performed which pulls off IgG molecules from red cells by various means (e.g., acid or heat treatment);[42] these free IgG molecules in suspension are then tested against A and B reagent cells to confirm the specificity of the antibody causing positive DAT.[43] Since a positive DAT is not indicative of HDFN, performing routine DATs on the cord blood of all newborns or of those born to O mothers is not indicated unless there is clinical evidence of HDFN.

In a study of 80 ABO-incompatible newborn infants and their mothers, the hemolyzing effect of maternal IgG anti-A or anti-B antibodies by an antibody-dependent cell-mediated cytotoxicity (ADCC) assay was better correlated with clinical severity of HDFN.[44] Similarly, assay of A or B antigen density determination was demonstrated to be a more specific test.[45] In 230 primigravid mothers of ABO-HDFN-affected offspring, subsequent pregnancies had a recurrence rate of 88% in those infants with the same blood type as their index sibling with 62% of the affected infants requiring therapy.[46]

Rhesus (D)

Overview and history of the Rhesus system

The second most clinically significant RBC antigen system is the Rhesus (Rh) system,[47,48] and in particular the D antigen. The Rh(D) antigen is highly immunogenic; about 80% of Rh(D)-negative individuals who are transfused with 1 unit of Rh(D)-positive RBCs form anti-D. However, in the absence of RhIg prophylaxis, the risk of immunization for an Rh(D) negative mother with an Rh-positive fetus is only about 10% (described later).

In 1939 Levine and Stetson[49] first described the role of anti-D in HDFN when they reported the case of a woman who delivered an infant with HDFN and had a severe transfusion reaction after receiving a blood transfusion from her husband. This led to the hypothesis that the antibody that had caused the severe hemolytic transfusion reaction had also crossed the placental barrier and destroyed fetal RBCs. Later the antibody was identified as anti-D. To date, the incidence of anti-D alloimmunization has markedly decreased due to administration of anti-D (see below).[50]

Because Rh(D) is the most antigenic of all non-A and B-RBC antigens,[51] all Rh(D) negative women of childbearing age receive Rh(D) negative blood. Anti-D may cause serious clinical effects such as HDFN and transfusion reactions. The genetics of the Rh system are detailed by Bloy *et al.*[52]

Partial D

Rarely, HDFN occurs in women with genetic variants of the D antigen.[53–57] A partial D variant might be suspected when D antigen typing has a weak agglutination reaction. Historically, patients with a weak D phenotype have not been considered candidates for Rh immune globulin prophylaxis. However, there is a recent case of a gravida 2, para 1 woman with A-positive blood type, whose infant died of severe HDFN 6 days after birth.[58] Anti-D levels, which were undetectable at the first prenatal visit, were subsequently identified at delivery (titer 1:64). Further investigation revealed that the mother's RBCs were partial D (VI) phenotype.

Rh(D)-HDFN severity of hemolysis

Clinical presentation

Unlike ABO-HDFN, HDFN caused by the Rh(D) antigen is severe because the D antigen is well developed on fetal RBCs, and Rh(D) antibodies are primarily IgG, which readily cross the placental barrier.[59] Typically, an Rh(D) negative female's first child is not affected by HDFN. The mother has not yet been immunized unless she has been transfused with Rh(D) positive blood or has a past history of abortion or miscarriage that was not covered with RhIg. Whatever the method of exposure, once the woman has been exposed to the Rh(D) antigen and produces a high titer (>16–32) anti-D, subsequent offspring carrying the D antigen will be affected.

Rh(D)-HDFN is clinically moderate to severe in presentation and requires aggressive management. The neonate will have increasing hyperbilirubinemia with a decrease in hemoglobin within the first 48 hours. A DAT should be performed on the cord blood, and if positive, an elution may be performed to confirm the nature of the antibody causing hemolysis.[60] The other alternative would be to test the mother's serum for the causative antibody.

Maternal–fetal ABO-incompatibility is protective for other HDFN

As previously mentioned, the incidence of anti-D formation in the Rh(D) negative mother carrying an Rh(D) positive fetus is only 10% in the absence of RhIg prophylaxis as opposed to 80% when transfused with a unit of blood. This is dose-dependent, and as the amount of Rh(D) positive cell exposure increases, so does the chance of anti-D production.

However, the incompatibility between an ABO mother and her group A or B fetus may confer protection against Rh immunization. This occurs presumably by hemolysis or clearance of A or B Rh-positive fetal RBCs by anti-A or anti-B present in the mother's plasma before the Rh antigen (or other red cell antigens) is recognized by the mother's immune system.

Non-Rh antibodies

Apart from ABO and Rh group antigens, there are other red cell antigens that are also rarely associated with HDFN.[61]

Anti-Kell

Anti-Kell is the most potent of the non-Rh antibodies in causing HDFN.[62–64] The Kell blood group system is complex and contains over 20 different antigens. K1 (K, Kell), which is present in 9 percent of the population, is antithetical to the high-prevalence K2 (k) antigen. K1 is strongly immunogenic. Antibodies directed against K1 may cause severe transfusion reactions, if incompatible blood is transfused, and may cause HDFN in sensitized mothers.[65,66] The molecular basis of the K1/K2 polymorphism has been determined,[67] and it has been demonstrated that a C to T base substitution in exon 6 creates a Bsm I restriction enzyme site. This base change identifies the K1/K1 genotype. This test differentiates genotypes K1/K1, K2/K2, and the K1/K2 heterozygote and may be used in the prenatal diagnosis of K1-related HDFN.

Diagnosis

Molecular diagnostic techniques are now employed in pregnant women sensitized to the Rh(D) and Kell-1 antigens. Paternal genotypes may be determined using DNA amplification of Rh(D) specific sequences obtained from sperm cells, and paternal Kell phenotypes may be determined by serologic assays on peripheral blood.[68] Fetal Rh(D) and/or Kell type may be determined using polymerase chain reaction with amniotic cells.

Other antibodies (see Table 4.1): C,[69] E,[70,71] and c[72,73] are also potent immunogens, though less potent than D. These antigens are associated with less frequent and less severe HDFN.

Section III: Management of the Rh(D)-negative, unsensitized female, the alloimmunized pregnant female, the fetus and the neonate

Prevention of HDFN (anti-D) in the Rh(D) negative, unsensitized female

RhoGam (RhIG)

Administration of anti-D in the form of Rh immunoglobulin (RhIG) was developed to prevent Rh_0D-negative mothers from forming anti-D following pregnancy with an Rh_0D-positive fetus, thereby preventing Rh_0D HDFN.[74,75] RhIg is a preparation of hyper-immune gamma globulin from pooled human donor plasma collected from Rh(D)-negative sensitized donors with high levels of anti-D antibody.[76] Rh(D) negative women *with a negative antibody screen* receive RhIg during pregnancy to prevent the occurrence of HDFN. In the United States the standard of care is to give 300 μg of RhIg to all Rh(D) negative, non-sensitized women at 28 weeks gestation.[77] The drug was originally made from the plasma of women whose previous pregnancies were affected by Rh alloimmunization. As the incidence of the disease has declined[78–80] the drug is made from donors whose antibody levels are maintained by vaccination. RhIg may be stored in and issued by the hospital pharmacy or the blood bank. Since transfusion of as little as 0.1 cm^3 of red cells has been associated with anti-D production, prevention of alloimmunization of the mother during this period is critical. The current recommendations for the use of RhIg to prevent RBC alloimmunization are listed below:

All Rh(D) negative non-immunized females should receive:[81]

(1) A single intramuscular dose of 300 μg of RhIg at 28 weeks gestation.
(2) A second dose of 300 μg of RhIg within 72 hours of the birth of an Rh(D) positive infant.
(3) A 300 μg dose of RhIg in the first half of pregnancy (>12 weeks) for threatened abortion, spontaneous abortion, ectopic pregnancy, or any vaginal bleeding of uterine origin.
(4) Prophylaxis therapy (300 μg) for any procedures that carry the risk of feto-maternal hemorrhage (i.e. chorionic villus sampling, amniocentesis, cordocentesis, placental biopsy, percutaneous or open fetal surgery, external cephalic version).
(5) A maternal Kleihauer-Betke test for all cases in which FMH is suspected during either pregnancy or delivery. The Kleihauer-Betke[82] test is performed to quantify

how much fetal blood is in the maternal circulation.[8,83] If more than 30 ml of fetal whole blood (15 ml of fetal red cells) is detected, a corresponding increase in the dose of RhIg is given to prevent immunization. For example, if the calculated amount of fetal red cells is 45 cm^3, based on one vial of RhIg of 300 μg/15 cm^3 of RBCs, the patient should receive 3 vials plus one additional vial to account for any miscalculation. Thus, a total of 4 vials should be given to this patient. Other laboratory methods to detect FMH such as flow cytometry,[84] fluorescence microscopy,[85] and automated Kleihauer Betke[86] are being investigated and used but have not been adopted at this time in the majority of laboratories in the United States.[87–89] To optimize patient care, obstetricians and the transfusion medicine service should work closely to develop a process for identifying potential RhIg-eligible candidates as well as a system for delivering it to them.

Management of the alloimmunized female during pregnancy

Once an immune anti-D has been identified during pregnancy, RhIG is not necessary. The management of the alloimmunized female should include assessment of the previous pregnancy history, serial titers of maternal antibody, serial ultrasound measurements,[81,90–95] serial amniocentesis, fetal blood sampling and intrauterine transfusion when indicated (see below).[96]

History of a previously affected pregnancy is very helpful in predicting the outcome of the current pregnancy.[97] Generally, the severity of HDFN in subsequent pregnancies is either similar or worse than the previous pregnancy; however, in 5–10% of cases, it may be less severe. Thus, with a history of hydrops, there is a 90% chance of hydrops in the next pregnancy. The initial titer should be performed in the first trimester. Thereafter, it should be performed at 16 weeks and every 4 weeks until 28 weeks and, thereafter, every 2 weeks. The titer is reported as the inverse of the greatest tube dilution in which an agglutination reaction is observed. Thus, a titer of 32 represents a dilution of 1:32. Titer results may differ between laboratories depending on the methods employed, but should not vary by more than one dilution within the laboratory. While performing antibody titers in the blood bank, the current sample is tested along with the previous sample during that pregnancy. The titer level associated with risk for *fetal hydrops* is a critical titer value and may vary by institution based on the method of testing and clinical correlation. In most institutions a critical value for anti-D ranges between 16 and 64, depending on the method used.[95]

Management of the fetus with HDFN

Amniocentesis and Liley curves

In 1961 Liley first reported a correlation between elevated amniotic fluid OD450 (indicative of the bilirubin level) with the severity of HDFN and fetal anemia in women with Rh(D) alloimmunization.[98] Based on gestational age and the amount of bilirubin present in amniotic fluid as assessed by OD450, Liley developed a 3-zoned graph: Values in zone one showed slightly increased bilirubin and mild anemia, whereas values in zone three reflected severe disease with severe HDFN and anemia requiring immediate intervention – either intrauterine transfusion or induction of delivery. Some centers use a modification of the Liley curve.[99] Liley also introduced intraperitoneal transfusion for the treatment of the severely affected fetus.[100] However, red cell absorption from the peritoneal lymphatics is slow, and the increase in fetal hemoglobin may take up to 8–10 days. Currently, the correction of fetal anemia is accomplished by fetal intravascular transfusion where the correction of anemia is immediate.[101]

Intrauterine transfusion (IUT)

For a discussion of this topic, see chapter on blood component therapy (Chapter 17).

Indications: A pregnancy complicated by immune-mediated maternal isoimmunization to RBC in HDFN may result in a certain degree of fetal anemia, which can only be corrected by intrauterine transfusion of compatible RBCs.[102,103] IUT of RBC is usually recommended when the fetal hematocrit is less than 30 percent; the procedure is performed after 20 weeks' gestation. A variety of methods may be employed to determine the fetal hematocrit; the reader is referred to the following references.[92,104,105]

Red blood cells: RBCs must be ABO compatible with the maternal serum. Therefore, a crossmatch is performed with the mother's serum and donor cells. Group O Rh(D) negative fresh allogeneic RBCs (less than 7 days old) should be transfused. RBCs should be irradiated to inactivate lymphocytes, in order to prevent graft-versus-host disease, as fetuses have a poorly developed immune system. Irradiation should be performed just prior to transfusion because irradiated stored RBCs leak potassium, which may be detrimental.

Premature neonates have an especially immature immune system and are therefore at a greater risk for CMV infection. Therefore, RBCs should be derived either from a donor who has tested negative for CMV or should be leukocyte-reduced to remove lymphocytes containing CMV.[106–109] Fresher units maximize RBC survival *in vivo*. The hematocrit of the RBC unit should be about 80–90 percent to prevent volume overload. This high hematocrit is achieved by centrifugation of the unit and removal of supernatant plasma and anticoagulant. Normal saline is added to obtain a hematocrit of 80–90 percent. RBCs should be negative for the sickle cell trait. Using a direct intravascular fetal transfusion technique, the mean volume of transfusion is

50 ml/kg of estimated non-hydropic fetal weight and may be transfused in 10 ml aliquots over 1–2 minutes.[110] The frequency of IUT generally depends on the severity of anemia and the gestational stage. Generally, red cells will survive for 3–4 weeks. Therefore, some pregnancies may require several IUTs, whereas other pregnancies may need only one.

Management of the neonate with HDFN

The consequences of hyperbilirubinemia in HDFN are restricted to the neonate because bilirubin is processed *in utero* by transplacental passage to maternal circulation. Neonates have a decreased ability to produce glucuronyl transferase, leading to a diminished capacity to conjugate bilirubin. Additionally, the immature blood-brain barrier is more permeable to unconjugated bilirubin, and there is increased risk of kernicterus with rapidly increasing unconjugated bilirubin. Since the passive alloantibody from the mother will continue to cause hemolysis of neonatal red cells carrying the implicated antigen, it is very important to monitor HDFN neonates carefully.

Newborns with the maternal alloantibody should be monitored by frequent bilirubin testing because that is the best available clinical decision-making parameter. In the blood bank, the DAT should be performed on cord blood. Whenever a neonate suffering from HDFN presents to a hospital with no known previous antenatal care, the nature of the antibody will be unknown; in this case an elution of antibody from fetal red cells should be performed to identify the antibody. If available, maternal blood should also be used to identify the antibody, and the mother's serum may also be used for cross-matching.

Hyperbilirubinemia – exchange transfusion

Rh(D)-HDFN may be severe presenting with hyperbilirubinemia[111,112] and require aggressive treatment.[113] If an exchange transfusion is required,[114,115] a CBC, bilirubin, and DAT on cord blood should be performed. When performing an exchange transfusion, RBCs are selected that are negative for the antigen against which the antibody is directed. RBCs are Group O and Rh(D) negative, negative for the implicated antigen, fresh (<7 days old), pre-storage leukocyte reduced[116] and/or CMV seronegative[117–119] and irradiated for the prevention of graft-versus-host disease.[120,121] The hematocrit of the RBC unit is adjusted to ~50% by removing the supernatant anticoagulant and plasma and replacing it with AB plasma. Plasma is added to prevent coagulopathy in a neonate with immature liver and also to prevent potential hemolysis due to anti-A or anti-B present in O RBCs. Generally, a two blood volume exchange transfusion is performed manually. The infant should be monitored closely during the exchange.[122–125]

REFERENCES

1 Bowman, J. M., Pollock, J. M. and Penston, L. E. Fetomaternal transplacental hemorrhage during pregnancy and after delivery. *Vox Sang*, 1986; **51**(2): 117–21.

2 Biankin, S. A., Arbuckle, S. M. and Graf, N. S. Autopsy findings in a series of five cases of fetomaternal haemorrhages. *Pathology*, 2003; **35**(4): 319–24.

3 Pourbabak, S., Rund, C. R. and Crookston, K. P. Three cases of massive fetomaternal hemorrhage presenting without clinical suspicion. *Arch. Pathol. Lab. Med.*, 2004; **128**(4): 463–5.

4 Lele, A. S., Carmody, P. J., Hurd, M. E., *et al.* Fetomaternal bleeding following diagnostic amniocentesis. *Obstet. Gynecol.*, 1982; **60**(1): 60–4.

5 Shah, A. J. and Kilcline, B. A. Trauma in pregnancy. *Emerg. Med. Clin. North Am.*, 2003; **21**(3): 615–29.

6 Nicolini, U., Kochenour, N. K., Greco, P., *et al.* Consequences of fetomaternal haemorrhage after intrauterine transfusion. *BMJ*, 1988; **297**(6660): 1379–81.

7 Zipursky, A. and Israels, L. G. The pathogenesis and prevention of Rh immunization. *Can. Med. Assoc. J.*, 1967; **97**(21): 1245–57.

8 Banerjee, K., Kriplani, A., Kumar, V., *et al.* Detecting fetomaternal hemorrhage after first-trimester abortion with the Kleihauer-Betke test and rise in maternal serum alpha-fetoprotein. *J. Reprod. Med.*, 2004; **49**(3): 205–9.

9 Hadley, A. G. Laboratory assays for predicting the severity of haemolytic disease of the fetus and newborn. *Transpl. Immunol.*, 2002; **10**(2–3): 191–8.

10 Pollock, J. M. and Bowman, J. M. Placental transfer of Rh antibody (anti-D IgG) during pregnancy. *Vox Sang*, 1982; **43**(6): 327–34.

11 Lubenko, A., Contreras, M., Rodeck, C. H., *et al.* Transplacental IgG subclass concentrations in pregnancies at risk of haemolytic disease of the newborn. *Vox Sang*, 1994; **67**(3): 291–8.

12 Ukita, M., Takahashi, A., Nunotani, T., *et al.* IgG subclasses of anti-A and anti-B antibodies bound to the cord red cells in ABO incompatible pregnancies. *Vox Sang*, 1989; **56**(3): 181–6.

13 Toivanen, P. and Hirvonen, T. Antigens Duffy, Kell, Kidd, Lutheran and Xg a on fetal red cells. *Vox Sang*, 1973; **24**(4): 372–6.

14 Abhyankar, S., Silfen, S., Rao, S. P., *et al.* Positive cord blood "DAT" due to anti-Le(a): absence of hemolytic disease of the newborn. *Am. J. Pediatr. Hematol. Oncol.*, 1989; **11**(2): 184–5.

15 Bowman, J. M. and Pollock, J. M. Amniotic fluid spectrophotometry and early delivery in the management of erythroblastosis fetalis. *Pediatrics*, 1965; **35**: 815–35.

16 Stevenson, D. K., Wong, R. J., Vreman, H. J., *et al.* NICHD Conference on kernicterus: Research on prevention of bilirubin-induced brain injury and kernicterus – bench-to-bedside diagnostic methods and prevention and treatment strategies. *J. Perinatol.*, 2004; **24**(8): 521–5.

17 Bhutani, V. K. and Johnson, L. H. Urgent clinical need for accurate and precise bilirubin measurements in the United States to prevent kernicterus. *Clin. Chem.*, 2004; **50**(3): 477–80.

18 Ross, G. Hyperbilirubinemia in the 2000s: what should we do next? *Am. J. Perinatol.*, 2003; **20**(8): 415–24.

19 Diamond, L., Blackfan, K. and Baty, J. Erythroblastosis fetalis and its association with universal edema of the fetus, icterus gravis neonatorum and anemia of the newborn. *J. Pediatr.*, 1932; **1**: 269.

20 Vengelen-Tyler, V. The serological investigation of hemolytic disease of the newborn caused by antibodies other than anti-D. In Garratty, G., ed. *Hemolytic Disease of the Newborn*, Arlington, VA: American Association of Blood Banks; 1984. p. 145.

21 Springer, G. F. and Horton, R. E. Blood-group isoantibody stimulation in man by feeding blood-group-active bacteria. *J. Clin. Invest.*, 1969; **48**(7): 1280–91.

22 Ferguson-Smith, M. A., Aitken, D. A., Turleau, C., *et al.* Localisation of the human ABO: Np-1: AK-1 linkage group by regional assignment of AK-1 to 9q34. *Hum. Genet.*, 1976; **34**(1): 35–43.

23 Yamamoto, F., Clausen, H., White, T., *et al.* Molecular genetic basis of the histo-blood group ABO system. *Nature*, 1990; **345**(6272): 229–33.

24 Yamamoto, F. and Hakomori, S. Sugar-nucleotide donor specificity of histo-blood group A and B transferases is based on amino acid substitutions. *J. Biol. Chem.*, 1990; **265**(31): 19257–62.

25 Curtis, B. R., Edwards, J. T., Hessner, M. J., *et al.* Blood group A and B antigens are strongly expressed on platelets of some individuals. *Blood*, 2000; **96**(4): 1574–81.

26 Ravn, V. and Dabelsteen, E. Tissue distribution of histo-blood group antigens. *APMIS*, 2000; **108**(1): 1–28.

27 Kelly, R. J., Rouquier, S., Giorgi, D., *et al.* Sequence and expression of a candidate for the human Secretor blood group alpha(1,2)fucosyltransferase gene (FUT2). Homozygosity for an enzyme-inactivating nonsense mutation commonly correlates with the non-secretor phenotype. *J. Biol. Chem.*, 1995; **270**(9): 4640–9.

28 Bucher, K. A., Patterson, A. M., Jr., Elston, R. C., *et al.* Racial difference in incidence of ABO hemolytic disease. *Am. J. Public Health*, 1976; **66**(9): 854–8.

29 Levine, D. H. and Meyer, H. B. Newborn screening for ABO hemolytic disease. *Clin. Pediatr. (Phila)*, 1985; **24**(7): 391–4.

30 Shanwell, A., Sallander, S., Bremme, K., *et al.* Clinical evaluation of a solid-phase test for red cell antibody screening of pregnant women. *Transfusion*, 1999; **39**(1): 26–31.

31 Peevy, K. J. and Wiseman, H. J. ABO hemolytic disease of the newborn: evaluation of management and identification of racial and antigenic factors. *Pediatrics*, 1978; **61**(3): 475–8.

32 Cariani, L., Romano, E. L., Martinez, N., *et al.* ABO-haemolytic disease of the newborn (ABO-HDN): factors influencing its severity and incidence in Venezuela. *J. Trop. Pediatr.*, 1995; **41**(1): 14–21.

33 Desjardins, L., Blajchman, M. A., Chintu, C., *et al.* The spectrum of ABO hemolytic disease of the newborn infant. *J. Pediatr.*, 1979; **95**(3): 447–9.

34 Grundbacher, F. J. The etiology of ABO hemolytic disease of the newborn. *Transfusion*, 1980; **20**(5): 563–8.

35 Waldron, P. and de Alarcon, P. ABO hemolytic disease of the newborn: a unique constellation of findings in siblings and review of protective mechanisms in the fetal-maternal system. *Am. J. Perinatol.*, 1999; **16**(8): 391–8.

36 Dufour, D. R. and Monoghan, W. P. ABO hemolytic disease of the newborn. A retrospective analysis of 254 cases. *Am. J. Clin. Pathol.*, 1980; **73**(3): 369–73.

37 Sivan, Y., Merlob, P., Nutman, J., *et al.* Direct hyperbilirubinemia complicating ABO hemolytic disease of the newborn. *Clin. Pediatr. (Phila)*, 1983; **22**(8): 537–8.

38 Goraya, J., Basu, S., Sodhi, P., *et al.* Unusually severe ABO hemolytic disease of newborn. *Indian J. Pediatr.*, 2001; **68**(3): 285–6.

39 McDonnell, M., Hannam, S. and Devane, S. P. Hydrops fetalis due to ABO incompatibility. *Arch. Dis. Child Fetal Neonatal Ed.*, 1998; **78**(3): F220–1.

40 Contreras, M. Antenatal tests in the diagnosis and assessment of severity of haemolytic disease (Hd) of the fetus and newborn (hdn). *Vox Sang*, 1994; **67** (Suppl 3): 207–10.

41 Chuansumrit, A., Siripoonya, P., Nathalang, O., *et al.* The benefit of the direct antiglobulin test using gel technique in ABO hemolytic disease of the newborn. *Southeast Asian J. Trop. Med. Public Health*, 1997; **28**(2): 428–31.

42 Feng, C. S., Kirkley, K. C., Eicher, C. A., *et al.* The Lui elution technique. A simple and efficient method for eluting ABO antibodies. *Transfusion*, 1985; **25**(5): 433–4.

43 Haberman, S., Krafft, C. J., Luecke, P. E., Jr. *et al.* ABO isoimmunization: the use of the specific Coombs and heat elution tests in the detection of hemolytic disease. *J. Pediatr.*, 1960; **56**: 471–7.

44 Brouwers, H. A., Overbeeke, M. A., Ouwehand, W. H., *et al.* Maternal antibodies against fetal blood group antigens A or B: lytic activity of IgG subclasses in monocyte-driven cytotoxicity and correlation with ABO haemolytic disease of the newborn. *Br. J. Haematol.*, 1988; **70**(4): 465–9.

45 Brouwers, H. A., Overbeeke, M. A., van Ertbruggen, I., *et al.* What is the best predictor of the severity of ABO-haemolytic disease of the newborn? *Lancet*, 1988; **2**(8612): 641–4.

46 Katz, M. A., Kanto, W. P., Jr. and Korotkin, J. H. Recurrence rate of ABO hemolytic disease of the newborn. *Obstet. Gynecol.*, 1982; **59**(5): 611–14.

47 Avent, N. D. Molecular biology of the Rh blood group system. *J. Pediatr. Hematol. Oncol.*, 2001; **23**(6): 394–402.

48 Avent, N. D. and Reid, M. E. The Rh blood group system: a review. *Blood*, 2000; **95**(2): 375–87.

49 Levine, P. and Stetson, R. An unusual case of intragroup agglutination. *JAMA*, 1939; **113**: 126.

50 Chavez, G. F., Mulinare, J. and Edmonds, L. D. Epidemiology of Rh hemolytic disease of the newborn in the United States. *JAMA*, 1991; **265**(24): 3270–4.

51 Howard, H., Martlew, V., McFadyen, I., *et al.* Consequences for fetus and neonate of maternal red cell allo-immunisation. *Arch. Dis. Child Fetal Neonatal Ed.*, 1998; **78**(1): F62–6.

52 Bloy, C., Blanchard, D., Dahr, W., *et al.* Determination of the N-terminal sequence of human red cell Rh(D) polypeptide and demonstration that the Rh(D), (C), and (E) antigens are carried by distinct polypeptide chains. *Blood*, 1988; **72**(2): 661–6.

53 Wagner, F. F., Eicher, N. I., Jorgensen, J. R., *et al.* DNB: a partial D with anti-D frequent in Central Europe. *Blood*, 2002; **100**(6): 2253–6.

54 Lacey, P. A., Caskey, C. R., Werner, D. J., *et al.* Fatal hemolytic disease of a newborn due to anti-D in an Rh-positive Du variant mother. *Transfusion*, 1983; **23**(2): 91–4.

55 White, C. A., Stedman, C. M. and Frank, S. Anti-D antibodies in D- and Du-positive women: a cause of hemolytic disease of the newborn. *Am. J. Obstet. Gynecol.*, 1983; **145**(8): 1069–75.

56 Mayne, K. M., Allen, D. L. and Bowell, P. J. 'Partial D' women with anti-D alloimmunization in pregnancy. *Clin. Lab. Haematol.*, 1991; **13**(3): 239–44.

57 Mayne, K., Bowell, P., Woodward, T., *et al.* Rh immunization by the partial D antigen of category DVa. *Br. J. Haematol.*, 1990; **76**(4): 537–9.

58 Cannon, M., Pierce, R., Taber, E. B., *et al.* Fatal hydrops fetalis caused by anti-D in a mother with partial D. *Obstet. Gynecol.*, 2003; **102**(5 Pt 2): 1143–5.

59 Hadley, A. G. and Kumpel, B. M. The role of Rh antibodies in haemolytic disease of the newborn. *Baillieres Clin. Haematol.*, 1993; **6**(2): 423–44.

60 Nakamura, Y., Sada, I., Tanaka, S., *et al.* Significance of positive direct anti-globulin test for cord blood in administration of anti-d immunoglobulin for postpartum immunoprophylaxis. *Nippon Sanka Fujinka Gakkai Zasshi*, 1984; **36**(4): 623–5.

61 Geifman-Holtzman, O., Wojtowycz, M., Kosmas, E., *et al.* Female alloimmunization with antibodies known to cause hemolytic disease. *Obstet. Gynecol.*, 1997; **89**(2): 272–5.

62 Weiner, C. P. and Widness, J. A. Decreased fetal erythropoiesis and hemolysis in Kell hemolytic anemia. *Am. J. Obstet. Gynecol.*, 1996; **174**(2): 547–51.

63 Mayne, K. M., Bowell, P. J. and Pratt, G. A. The significance of anti-Kell sensitization in pregnancy. *Clin. Lab. Haematol.*, 1990; **12**(4): 379–85.

64 McKenna, D. S., Nagaraja, H. N. and O'Shaughnessy, R. Management of pregnancies complicated by anti-Kell isoimmunization. *Obstet. Gynecol.*, 1999; **93**(5 Pt 1): 667–73.

65 Moise, K. J., Jr. Non-anti-D antibodies in red-cell alloimmunization. *Eur. J. Obstet. Gynecol. Reprod. Biol.*, 2000; **92**(1): 75–81.

66 Babinszki, A., Lapinski, R. H. and Berkowitz, R. L. Prognostic factors and management in pregnancies complicated with severe kell alloimmunization: experiences of the last 13 years. *Am. J. Perinatol.*, 1998; **15**(12): 695–701.

67 Lee, S., Wu, X., Reid, M., *et al.* Molecular basis of the K:6,-7 [Js(a + b−)] phenotype in the Kell blood group system. *Transfusion*, 1995; **35**(10): 822–5.

68 Lipitz, S., Many, A., Mitrani-Rosenbaum, S., *et al.* Obstetric outcome after RhD and Kell testing. *Hum. Reprod.*, 1998; **13**(6): 1472–5.

69 Malde, R., Stanworth, S., Patel, S., *et al.* Haemolytic disease of the newborn due to anti-Ce. *Transfus. Med.*, 2000; **10**(4): 305–6.

70 To, W. W., Ho, S. N. and Mok, K. M. Anti-E alloimmunization in pregnancy: management dilemmas. *J. Obstet. Gynaecol. Res.*, 2003; **29**(1): 45–8.

71 Lee, C. K., Ma, E. S., Tang, M., *et al.* Prevalence and specificity of clinically significant red cell alloantibodies in Chinese women during pregnancy – a review of cases from 1997 to 2001. *Transfus. Med.*, 2003; **13**(4): 227–31.

72 Wu, K. H., Chu, S. L., Chang, J. G., *et al.* Haemolytic disease of the newborn due to maternal irregular antibodies in the Chinese population in Taiwan. *Transfus. Med.*, 2003; **13**(5): 311–14.

73 Hackney, D. N., Knudtson, E. J., Rossi, K. Q., *et al.* Management of pregnancies complicated by anti-c isoimmunization. *Obstet. Gynecol.*, 2004; **103**(1): 24–30.

74 Moise, K. J., Jr. and Brecher, M. E. Package insert for rhesus immune globulin. *Obstet. Gynecol.*, 2004; **103**(5): 998–9.

75 Bowman, J. M. Antenatal suppression of Rh alloimmunization. *Clin. Obstet. Gynecol.*, 1991; **34**(2): 296–303.

76 Greenough, A. The role of immunoglobulins in neonatal Rhesus haemolytic disease. *BioDrugs*, 2001; **15**(8): 533–41.

77 Ghosh, S. and Murphy, W. Implementation of the Rhesus prevention programme: A prospective study. *Obstet. Gynecol. Surv.*, 1995; **50**: 432–3.

78 Tovey, L. A. Haemolytic disease of the newborn – the changing scene. *Br. J. Obstet. Gynaecol.*, 1986; **93**(9): 960–6.

79 Moncharmont, P., Juron, Dupraz F., Vignal, M., *et al.* Haemolytic disease of the newborn infant. Long term efficiency of the screening and the prevention of alloimmunization in the mother: thirty years of experience. *Arch. Gynecol. Obstet.*, 1991; **248**(4): 175–80.

80 Narang, A. and Jain, N. Haemolytic disease of newborn. *Indian J. Pediatr.*, 2001; **68**(2): 167–72.

81 ACOG practice bulletin. Prevention of Rh D alloimmunization. Number 4, May 1999 (replaces educational bulletin Number 147, October 1990). Clinical management guidelines for obstetrician-gynecologists. American College of Obstetrics and Gynecology. *Int. J. Gynaecol. Obstet.*, 1999; **66**(1): 63–70.

82 Kleihauer, E., Braun, H. and Betke, K. [Demonstration of fetal hemoglobin in erythrocytes of a blood smear]. *Klin. Wochenschr.*, 1957; **35**(12): 637–8.

83 Bohra, U., Regan, C., O'Connell, M. P., *et al.* The role of investigations for term stillbirths. *J. Obstet. Gynaecol.*, 2004; **24**(2): 133–4.

84 Kennedy, G. A., Shaw, R., Just, S., *et al.* Quantification of feto-maternal haemorrhage (FMH) by flow cytometry: anti-fetal haemoglobin labelling potentially underestimates massive FMH in comparison to labelling with anti-D. *Transfus. Med.*, 2003; **13**(1): 25–33.

85 Ochsenbein-Imhof, N., Ochsenbein, A. F., Seifert, B., *et al.* Quantification of fetomaternal hemorrhage by fluorescence microscopy is equivalent to flow cytometry. *Transfusion*, 2002; **42**(7): 947–53.

86 Pelikan, D. M., Mesker, W. E., Scherjon, S. A., *et al.* Improvement of the Kleihauer-Betke test by automated detection of fetal erythrocytes in maternal blood. *Cytometry*, 2003; **54B**(1): 1–9.

87 Janssen, W. C. and Hoffmann, J. J. Evaluation of flow cytometric enumeration of foetal erythrocytes in maternal blood. *Clin. Lab. Haematol.*, 2002; **24**(2): 89–92.

88 Mundee, Y., Bigelow, N. C., Davis, B. H., *et al.* Flow cytometric method for simultaneous assay of foetal haemoglobin containing red cells, reticulocytes and foetal haemoglobin containing reticulocytes. *Clin. Lab. Haematol.*, 2001; **23**(3): 149–54.

89 Davis, B. H., Olsen, S., Bigelow, N. C., *et al.* Detection of fetal red cells in fetomaternal hemorrhage using a fetal hemoglobin monoclonal antibody by flow cytometry. *Transfusion*, 1998; **38**(8): 749–56.

90 Detti, L., Akiyama, M. and Mari, G. Doppler blood flow in obstetrics. *Curr. Opin. Obstet. Gynecol.*, 2002; **14**(6): 587–93.

91 Segata, M. and Mari, G. Fetal anemia: new technologies. *Curr. Opin. Obstet. Gynecol.*, 2004; **16**(2): 153–8.

92 Mari, G., Deter, R. L., Carpenter, R. L., *et al.* Noninvasive diagnosis by Doppler ultrasonography of fetal anemia due to maternal red-cell alloimmunization. Collaborative Group for Doppler Assessment of the Blood Velocity in Anemic Fetuses. *N. Engl. J. Med.*, 2000; **342**(1): 9–14.

93 Bahado-Singh, R., Oz, U., Deren, O., *et al.* Splenic artery Doppler peak systolic velocity predicts severe fetal anemia in rhesus disease. *Am. J. Obstet. Gynecol.*, 2000; **182**(5): 1222–6.

94 Detti, L. and Mari, G. Noninvasive diagnosis of fetal anemia. *Clin. Obstet. Gynecol.*, 2003; **46**(4): 923–30.

95 Moise, K. J., Jr. Management of rhesus alloimmunization in pregnancy. *Obstet. Gynecol.*, 2002; **100**(3): 600–11.

96 Urbaniak, S. J. and Greiss, M. A. RhD haemolytic disease of the fetus and the newborn. *Blood Rev.*, 2000; **14**(1): 44–61.

97 Bowman, J. The management of hemolytic disease in the fetus and newborn. *Semin. Perinatol.*, 1997; **21**(1): 39–44.

98 Liley, A. W. Liquor amnil analysis in the management of the pregnancy complicated by rhesus sensitization. *Am. J. Obstet. Gynecol.*, 1961; **82**: 1359–70.

99 Queenan, J. T., Tomai, T. P., Ural, S. H., *et al.* Deviation in amniotic fluid optical density at a wavelength of 450 nm in Rh-immunized pregnancies from 14 to 40 weeks' gestation: a proposal for clinical management. *Am. J. Obstet. Gynecol.*, 1993; **168**(5): 1370–6.

100 Liley, A. W. Intrauterine Transfusion of Foetus in Haemolytic Disease. *Br. Med. J.*, 1963; **5365**: 1107–9.

101 Schumacher, B. and Moise, K. J., Jr. Fetal transfusion for red blood cell alloimmunization in pregnancy. *Obstet. Gynecol.*, 1996; **88**(1): 137–50.

102 Ghi, T., Brondelli, L., Simonazzi, G., *et al.* Sonographic demonstration of brain injury in fetuses with severe red blood cell alloimmunization undergoing intrauterine transfusions. *Ultrasound Obstet. Gynecol.*, 2004; **23**(5): 428–31.

103 Cheong, Y. C., Goodrick, J., Kyle, P. M., *et al.* Management of anti-Rhesus-D antibodies in pregnancy: a review from 1994 to 1998. *Fetal Diagn. Ther.*, 2001; **16**(5): 294–8.

104 Mari, G., Detti, L., Oz, U., *et al.* Accurate prediction of fetal hemoglobin by Doppler ultrasonography. *Obstet. Gynecol.*, 2002; **99**(4): 589–93.

105 Whitecar, P. W. and Moise, K. J., Jr. Sonographic methods to detect fetal anemia in red blood cell alloimmunization. *Obstet. Gynecol. Surv.*, 2000; **55**(4): 240–50.

106 Hillyer, C. D., Emmens, R. K., Zago-Novaretti, M., *et al.* Methods for the reduction of transfusion-transmitted cytomegalovirus infection: filtration versus the use of seronegative donor units. *Transfusion*, 1994; **34**(10): 929–34.

107 Eisenfeld, L., Silver, H., McLaughlin, J., *et al.* Prevention of transfusion-associated cytomegalovirus infection in neonatal patients by the removal of white cells from blood. *Transfusion*, 1992; **32**(3): 205–9.

108 Adler, S. P. Transfusion-associated cytomegalovirus infections. *Rev. Infect. Dis.*, 1983; **5**(6): 977–93.

109 Nichols, W. G., Price, T. H., Gooley, T., *et al.* Transfusion-transmitted cytomegalovirus infection after receipt of leukoreduced blood products. *Blood*, 2003; **101**(10): 4195–200.

110 Triulzi, D. *Blood Transfusion Therapy*, 7th edn. Bethesda, MD: American Association of Blood Banks; 2002.

111 Schwoebel, A. and Sakraida, S. Hyperbilirubinemia: new approaches to an old problem. *J. Perinat. Neonatal Nurs.*, 1997; **11**(3): 78–97.

112 Dennery, P. A., Rhine, W. D. and Stevenson, D. K. Neonatal jaundice – what now? *Clin. Pediatr. (Phila)*, 1995; **34**(2): 103–7.

113 Toy, P. T., Reid, M. E., Papenfus, L., *et al.* Prevalence of ABO maternal–infant incompatibility in Asians, Blacks, Hispanics and Caucasians. *Vox Sang*, 1988; **54**(3): 181–3.

114 Panagopoulos, G., Valaes, T. and Doxiadis, S. A. Morbidity and mortality related to exchange transfusions. *J. Pediatr.*, 1969; **74**(2): 247–54.

115 Dikshit, S. K. and Gupta, P. K. Exchange transfusion in neonatal hyperbilirubinemia. *Indian Pediatr.*, 1989; **26**(11): 1139–45.

116 Visconti, M. R., Pennington, J., Garner, S. F., *et al.* Assessment of removal of human cytomegalovirus from blood components by leukocyte depletion filters using real-time quantitative PCR. *Blood*, 2004; **103**(3): 1137–9.

117 Strauss, R. G. Leukocyte-reduction to prevent transfusion-transmitted cytomegalovirus infections. *Pediatr. Transplant.*, 1999; **3** (Suppl 1): 19–22.

118 Yeager, A. S., Grumet, F. C., Hafleigh, E. B., *et al.* Prevention of transfusion-acquired cytomegalovirus infections in newborn infants. *J. Pediatr.*, 1981; **98**(2): 281–7.

119 Pamphilon, D. H., Rider, J. R., Barbara, J. A., *et al.* Prevention of transfusion-transmitted cytomegalovirus infection. *Transfus. Med.*, 1999; **9**(2): 115–23.

120 Hume, H. A. and Preiksaitis, J. B. Transfusion associated graft-versus-host disease, cytomegalovirus infection and HLA alloimmunization in neonatal and pediatric patients. *Transfus. Sci.*, 1999; **21**(1): 73–95.

121 Guidelines on gamma irradiation of blood components for the prevention of transfusion-associated graft-versus-host disease. BCSH Blood Transfusion Task Force. *Transfus. Med.*, 1996; **6**(3): 261–71.

122 Hansen, T. W. Therapeutic approaches to neonatal jaundice: an international survey. *Clin. Pediatr. (Phila)*, 1996; **35**(6): 309–16.

123 Patra, K., Storfer-Isser, A., Siner, B., *et al.* Adverse events associated with neonatal exchange transfusion in the 1990s. *J. Pediatr.*, 2004; **144**(5): 626–31.

124 Jackson, J. C. Adverse events associated with exchange transfusion in healthy and ill newborns. *Pediatrics*, 1997; **99**(5): E7.

125 Tan, K. L., Phua, K. B. and Ang, P. L. The mortality of exchange transfusions. *Med. J. Aust.*, 1976; **1**(14): 473–6.

5

Hereditary and acquired thrombophilia in pregnancy

Rodger L. Bick, M.D., Ph.D., F.A.C.P.[1] and
William F. Baker, Jr., M.D., F.A.C.P.[2]

[1]Professor of Medicine and Pathology, University of Texas Southwestern Medical Center; Director: Dallas Thrombosis Clinical Center, Dallas, Texas; Director: Pacific Thrombosis Clinical Center, Southern California, USA, email: rbick@thrombosis.com

[2]Associate Clinical Professor of Medicine, Center for Health Sciences, David Geffen School of Medicine at University of California-Los Angeles, Los Angeles, CA, USA Thrombosis, Hemostasis, and Special Hematology Clinic, Kern Medical Center, Bakersfield; California Clinical Thrombosis Center, Bakersfield, California, USA

Introduction

Thrombophilia in pregnancy represents a challenging problem for obstetricians, reproductive medicine specialists and hematologists. Normal pregnancy is known to be associated with an enhanced risk of deep vein thrombosis (DVT) and pulmonary embolus (PE). When combined with a thrombophilic disorder, this risk is significantly enhanced, usually considered to about 5–8-fold elevated in normal pregnant women, and addition of a thrombophilia, or other clinically significant risk factor, requires particular attention to avoid unnecessary fetal loss and maternal morbidity and mortality. Thrombophilia in obstetrics and pregnancy is known to be associated with not only enhanced risks of DVT and PE, but also recurrent miscarriage syndrome, infertility, stillborn births, eclampsia intrauterine growth retardation, pre-eclampsia, frank eclampsia, HELLP syndrome[1] and abruption, with the additional usual thrombohemorrhagic complications, such as disseminated intravascular coagulation.[2,3,4,5] Indeed many women with undiagnosed thrombophilia will experience their first clinical manifestation when pregnant – usually miscarriage or DVT with or without PE. In addition, many pregnancy patients who have had a prior DVT/PE harbor an undiagnosed thrombophilic disorder, thus emphasizing the importance of adequate investigation when a suggestive personal or family history warrants. This chapter summarizes (1) antithrombotic approaches to pregnant women with thrombophilia and other risk factors, and (2) the particular thrombophilias of concern to the obstetrician, reproductive medicine specialist and hematologist. In addition,

Hematological Complications in Obstetrics, Pregnancy, and Gynecology, ed. R. L. Bick *et al.* Published by Cambridge University Press.

treatment discussions and recommendations will be discussed in general and then, when necessary, for any particular disorder. It must be appreciated the clinical course of thrombophilic patients, particularly during pregnancy, is highly dynamic. When the response to therapy is not as expected, it must be remembered that more than one cause or type of thrombophilia or additional risk factor(s) may be present in any individual patient. Treatment must address the primary coagulopathy as well as any precipitating clinical risk factors, such as obesity, prior thrombosis or thromboembolic disease, prolonged immobility, pelvic or leg trauma, stasis or varicosities.[3,6] Furthermore, over the course of pregnancy, the clinical course may change. In general, the primary antithrombotics used in thrombophilic pregnancies are low-dose ASA and heparin/low molecular weight (LMW) heparin. Now that significant experience has been accumulated with use of LMW heparin, these are generally felt to be preferable over unfractionated heparin because of convenience of once a day dosing and a lower incidence of hemorrhage, heparin induced thrombocytopenia (HIT/T), and osteoporosis. Clearly, thromboprophylactic doses of heparin/LMW heparin should be used in those with a prior history of DVT or PE with or without pregnancy; what is less clear is the asymptomatic patient who is known to harbor a thrombophilia. We prefer to treat this later population with thromboprophylactic doses of LMW heparin (dalteparin) +/− low-dose ASA, however guidelines remain undefined. Also clear is the recommendation that those with an active thrombotic event during pregnancy need thrombotherapeutic doses of heparin/LMW heparin. It is also known that even with as yet limited data, some of the thrombophilias, such as Factor V Leiden, Prothrombin G20210A mutation, Protein C, S and antithrombin deficiency, hyperhomocysteinemia, and antiphospholipid syndrome render pregnant women particularly susceptible to recurrent miscarriage syndrome (RMS), thromboembolic events and other pregnancy-related complications, compared to some of the other thrombophilic disorders.[7,8]

The decision to treat, in patients with both inherited and acquired thrombophilia, will depend upon several factors. The critical information for each disorder should include: (1) the incidence of thrombosis for the disorder, (2) past medical and family history (3) additional clinical risk factors in an individual patient (4) the proportion of idiopathic versus secondary thrombotic events, (5) risks and benefits to the fetus and (6) the probability of a fatal outcome or significant morbidity to mother or neonate.[6,9] For pregnancy and thrombophilia randomized, blinded, controlled studies are rarely available. Thus many recommendations come from experience and available published information. As blinded, controlled trials become available, the indications for therapy and the therapeutic agent(s) of choice will more clearly evolve. The hereditary and acquired

Table 5.1 Thrombophilias: hereditary and acquired.

Approximate descending order of prevalence
Antiphospholipid syndrome
Sticky platelet syndrome
APC resistance
Factor V Leiden
MTHFR mutations
PAI-1 defects / mutations
Prothrombin G20210A
Protein S defects
Protein C defects
Antithrombin defects
Heparin cofactor II defects
Plasminogen defects
TPA defects
Factor XII defects
Dysfibrinogenemia
Homocysteinemia
Factor V Cambridge
Factor V Hong Kong
Factor V HR2 mutation

MTHFR: Methylenetetrahydrofolate Reductase
APC: Activated Protein C
PAI-1: Plasminogen Activator Inhibitor Type 1
TPA: Tissue Plasminogen Activator

thrombophilias are depicted in Table 5.1 in approximate descending order of prevalence.

Antithrombotic intervention in pregnancy

The choice(s) and dose(s) of therapeutic agent(s) will be guided by the clinical setting. Warfarins are not used during pregnancy as they cross the placenta and are associated with teratogenicity and excessive hemorrhage in mother and fetus. Thus, the choices are unfractionated (UF) heparin or low-molecular-weight (LMW) heparin either one often used in association with low-dose ASA, depending upon the clinical situation. Doses of UF heparin or LMW heparin depend upon the need for thromboprophylaxis or thrombotherapeutic effect. If using UF heparin, the thromboprophylactic dose used in pregnancy is generally 5,000 Units q 12 hours, subcutaneously; if treating an active event then either subcutaneous or intravenous heparin is used, using usual calibrated[10] activated partial thromboplastin time (aPTT) dose-adjusted regimens. When using LMW heparin, the dose is dependent upon the product used. In this regard, in January 2002 the FDA MedWatch Drug-Alert Adverse Reaction website issued a warning about the use of enoxaparin in pregnancy or women of childbearing age, so we do not recommend it be used in pregnancy, and all clinicians caring for pregnant women or women of child-bearing age should become thoroughly familiar with these warnings. The aforementioned FDA warning, issued in January 2002 (http://www.fda.gov/medwatch/SAFETY/2002/jan02.htm#lovenox), has alerted physicians to potential teratogenicity, and potential excessive fetal and maternal hemorrhage. Also, very little data yet exists regarding use of tinzaparin in pregnancy; therefore we use dalteparin (Fragmin) in pregnancy. The dose, when requiring thromboprophylaxis is 5000 U q 24 hours subcutaneously or dose-adjusted subcutaneous injections to keep the anti-Xa level, ideally drawn 4 hours after a subcutaneous dose, at 0.2–0.45 Units/ml. Some individuals advocate increasing the dose of thromboprophylactic UF heparin or LMW heparin during the third trimester, to "adjust for maternal weight gain", an average of 12.5 kg. However, this is usually an unnecessary effort as when analyzing distribution of maternal weight gain (27% = fetus, 5.2% = placenta, 6.4% = amniotic fluid, 7.5% = uterus, 3.2% = breasts, and 12% = extravascular fluid [= total of 61% of weight gain]); all of these parameters are fundamentally unaffected by thromboprophylactic therapy. Thus, we rarely find it necessary to increase doses later in pregnancy. Although we routinely monitor anti-Xa levels throughout pregnancy, it is extremely rare that a thromboprophylactic dose ever needs to be adjusted upward, as the desired thromboprophylactic anti-Xa level almost always remains in the desired range (0.2–0.45 units/ml) during the third trimester. The rare reasons are excessive obesity in conjunction with a low anti-Xa level and suggestion of a placental thrombus or early infarct, clearly seen in less than 20% of our patient population. Thus >80% of thrombophilic patients are not adjusted upward during later stages (third trimester) of pregnancy.

Women who have or develop an active thrombotic event during pregnancy are in need of thrombotherapeutic doses of heparin or LMW heparin during pregnancy. This is accomplished in one of several ways. The use of intravenous UF heparin for 5–7 days, then a change to thromboprophylactic doses may be considered. In this instance a therapeutic dose using a calibrated[10] aPTT dose-adjusted regimen to keep the aPTT at 1.5–2.5 times normal (or correlated to an anti-Xa level of 0.45–1.1 Units/ml). is used and then at 5–7 days a thromboprophylactic dose using UF heparin at 5,000 units every 12 hours or dalteparin (Fragmin) at 5,000 units per 24 hours is initiated and continued to term if clinically warranted. Alternatively, the thrombotherapeutic approach may be UF heparin used subcutaneously by every 12-hour injection using a calibrated[10] aPTT adjusted dose to keep the aPTT therapeutic (defined as an aPTT 1.5–2.5 times normal or correlating to an anti-Xa level of 0.45–1.1 U/ml for 5–7 days, then the patient changed to thromboprophylactic doses of UF heparin or dalteparin (Fragmin) for the duration of pregnancy is clinically warranted. A third, and in our opinion best and easiest approach to thrombotherapeutic treatment of an active thrombotic event during pregnancy is to use therapeutic doses of dalteparin (Fragmin) at 200 units/kg/24 hours for 5–7 days (usually may be done as an outpatient) then to change the patient to thromboprophylactic doses of 5,000 units/24 hours for the duration of pregnancy if clinically warranted.

Bridging therapy

Pregnant women with atrial fibrillation (AF) or prosthetic heart valves, or women with these conditions considering conception, if on full dose warfarin therapy, will require "bridging therapy" in the form of heparin or LMW heparin. One must recall that "full dose" warfarin anticoagulant therapy for prosthetic cardiac valves or AF is, in fact, thromboprophylactic therapy – not "therapeutic" (for an existing fresh thrombus). The goals of bridging therapy are prevention of arterial or venous thrombosis or extension/embolization of arterial or venous thrombosis. There are several approaches to bridging therapy in pregnancy. One such approach, usually unnecessary and usually inappropriate for nine months of pregnancy is to use intravenous thrombotherapeutic doses of porcine mucosal heparin in the usual doses of a bolus of 5,000 units followed by a dose adjusted calibrated aPTT to render an aPTT of 1.5–2.5 times normal. We generally disagree with and do not use this approach. Another is to use thrombotherapeutic doses of subcutaneous porcine mucosal heparin, again using twice a day or once a day subcutaneous heparin to render a calibrated aPTT which is 1.5–2.5 times normal. This approach is likewise unnecessary and not used by us. Another approach is to use thrombotherapeutic levels of dalteparin (Fragmin) at 200 Units/24 hours, subcutaneously. This approach is popular among some and has been shown to be generally safe and effective. A new approach has recently been published[11] using dalteparin at 100 units/kg twice daily, with excellent success in 650 patients. The most reasonable approach, and the one recommended by us, is to use dalteparin (Fragmin) at a fixed subcutaneous dose of 5,000 units every 24 hours by subcutaneous injection throughout pregnancy. One of the authors (RLB) has used this approach in over 300 thrombophilic pregnancies and in over 30 patients with prosthetic heart valves. No patient, as yet, has had a thrombotic or embolic event or a significant hemorrhage. For those clinicians considering use of LMW heparin as bridging therapy in pregnancy, it is mandatory to be familiar with the FDA MedWatch warnings regarding the use of the particular LMW heparin enoxaparin

(Lovenox) in pregnancy or in patients with prosthetic valves. The issues of potential problems with enoxaparin have been covered above. However, in January of 2002 the FDA, through its MedWatch adverse reaction reporting system posted the following warning regarding the use of enoxaparin in patients with prosthetic heart valves:

Warnings

Prosthetic Heart Valves

The use of Lovenox Injection is not recommended for thromboprophylaxis in patients with prosthetic heart valves. Cases of prosthetic heart valve thrombosis have been reported in patients with prosthetic valves who have received enoxaparin for thromboprophylaxis. Some of these cases were pregnant women in whom thrombosis led to maternal deaths and fetal deaths. Pregnant women with prosthetic heart valves may be at higher risk for thromboembolism.

To read this FDA MedWatch alert, the reader should go to: http://www.fda.gov/medwatch/SAFETY/2002/jan02.htm#lovenox.[12]

Bridging therapy for patients with AF or prosthetic heart valves should ideally be started as conception is being planned. However, more often pregnancy is “unplanned” and bridging therapy should be started as soon after conception as possible.

Monitoring of heparin/LMW heparin therapy during pregnancy

All patients should be counseled on the potential side effects of heparin/LMW heparin therapy. These will be discussed subsequently. All patients being placed in heparin/LMW heparin should have a pre-heparin/LMW heparin CBC and platelet count.[13] After initiating heparin/LMW heparin therapy a CBC/Platelet count should be done every other day for 14 days. Following this, assuming no significant decreases in the platelet count, pregnant women should have a CBC/platelet count done weekly for the first trimester, then monthly for the second and third trimester.[14] Obviously, if there is a significant decrease (discussed below), the heparin should be stopped or monitored more frequently. We, and others, advocate performing anti-Xa levels throughout pregnancy as well. These are drawn at the same frequency as the CBC/Platelet count. Anti-Xa levels should ideally be drawn approximately 4 hours after a subcutaneous injection. thromboprophylactic anti-Xa levels are 0.2–0.45 Units/ml and thrombotherapeutic anti-Xa levels are 0.45–1.1 Units/ml.

Table 5.2 Adverse effects of heparin/LMW heparin therapy.

Heparin-induced thrombocytopenia Type II (Immunologic)
Hemorrhage and bruising (usually mild)
Osteoporosis
Abnormal liver function tests (Benign)
Eosinophilia (Benign)
Hyperkalemia
Hypoaldosteronism
Priapism
Alopecia (usually mild)
Skin reactions:
Urticaria
Erythematous papules
Skin necrosis (may be severe)
Pruritus
Acute anaphylaxis

Side effects of heparin/LMW heparin therapy which should be discussed with the pregnant woman

Heparin has been the most important anticoagulant in clinical use over the past half century. It is effective, relatively inexpensive, and readily available. Even today it represents the most common agent for the treatment of acute thrombosis. Its extensive clinical use has commonly led to complacency and even disregard of the potential complications that relate to its use in the therapeutic or prophylactic setting. Although bleeding is the most obvious potential complication of heparin therapy, a very common sequalae is heparin-induced thrombocytopenia, which further can be complicated by the advent of thrombosis. Less common complications include osteoporosis, skin reactions, eosinophilia, alopecia, liver dysfunction and hyperkalemia. This review characterizes these potential, sometimes quite serious, sequelae (Table 5.2). Heparin Induced Thrombocytopenia (HIT/T) is discussed in a separate chapter.

Bleeding

The most common and more regularly anticipated complication of heparin/LMW heparin therapy is bleeding.[15–21] The true incidence of major bleeding has been sought, but is only an estimate commonly ranging between 6–14%, and is significantly less with LMW heparin.[18,19] Hirsch and colleagues have emphasized important variables relative to heparin related bleeding.[19,20,22] These are (1) the dose of heparin administered, (2) the method of administration (i.e. continuous vs. intermittent, etc.) and (3) the comorbid and concomitant therapy administered. Thus, heparin therapy is more commonly associated with bleeding when given to chronic alcoholics.[16] More complex and not completely resolved is the consideration that bleeding is more commonly seen in patients on aspirin.[16,19–21] Since this is a not uncommon treatment combination in patients with high risk pregnancy/thrombophilia in pregnancy, clinical vigilance for bleeding is the only intelligent approach.[23]

Acute heparin reaction (?anaphylaxis)

A rare, but potentially lethal acute reaction to heparin can occur. The event is abrupt and clinically dramatic.[24] It has been seen only in patients previously treated with heparin. It again merits emphasis that the heparin exposure need not be a quantitative one, since it has occurred with heparin exposure as minimal as heparin flush or use of a heparin coated catheter. Symptoms occur dramatically within 5 to 10 minutes of institution of the heparin bolus and include abrupt onset of chills and fever, tachycardia, diaphoreses and nausea. Hypotension may be noted, although most patients have become abruptly and transiently hypertensive. Retrosterned chest pain with the pattern of an acute myocardial infarction is common. Finally, a global amnesia syndrome has been linked to the crisis event. This anaphylaxis-like reaction has all of the features of an immunoglobulin E stimulated response. Immediate cessation of the heparin is critical. Other non-heparin antithrombotic agents should be used to treat the patient. We have seen four cases of anaphylaxis associated with enoxaparin.[25]

Heparin associated osteoporosis

Prolonged heparin exposure has been correlated with the development of osteoporosis.[26,27] The clinical findings that led to the evaluation of this finding were the unexpected development of bone pain or the identification of vertebral body or rib or fractures. The clinical correlate was that the patient had been on long-term heparin (in excess of 6 months) and usually at daily doses in excess of 15,000 anti-Xa units.[28] Limited epidemiologic and controlled studies are available to define the incidence of heparin associated osteoporosis. In addition, many of the studies have focused on pregnant patients, since such patients represent a group likely to have a long duration of therapy. However, since pregnancy itself is commonly associated with osteoporosis, such data must be cautiously interpreted. Howell *et al.* in randomized trials, identified a 5% incidence of vertebral fractures in women treated during their pregnancy with unfractionated heparin.[29] Monreal, *et al.* in a randomized study of 40 men and 40 women (mean age of 68) on long-term heparin therapy identified a 10% incidence of vertebral fractures.[30] Six of the seven occurred with unfractionated heparin the seventh with low molecular weight heparin (Fragmin). A very interesting finding in this study was that there was no difference in bone density between the group developing fractures compared to those without fractures. This study did not show a correlation between the lumbar bone density and the dose or duration of therapy.[30] Barbour and associates evaluated the subclinical occurrence of heparin associated osteoporosis in pregnancy by means of bone densitometry in a prospective, consecutive cohort of 14 pregnant women requiring heparin therapy and 14 pregnant controls matched for age, race and smoking status.[31] Proximal femur bone density measurements were taken at baseline, immediately post-partum, and 6 months post-partum in the cases and controls. Vertebral measurements were also obtained on both groups immediately post-partum and 6 months post-partum. Bone density relative to heparin dose and duration was examined. Five of 14 cases (36%) had a 10% decrease from their baseline proximal femur measurements to their immediate post-partum values, whereas none occurred in the 14 matched controls ($p = 0.04$). Mean proximal femur bone density measurements also decreased and this difference was still statistically significant 6 months post-partum ($p = 0.03$). This study concluded that no clear dose-response relationship could be demonstrated, and that unfractionated heparin adversely affected bone density in about 33% of exposed patients.[31] Dahlman studied the effect of long-term heparin treatment during pregnancy and the incidence of osteoporotic fractures and thromboembolic recurrence.[32] Long-term subcutaneous prophylaxis with heparin twice daily in pregnancy was used in 184 individuals. The dose of heparin was adjusted to anti-factor Xa activity or the activated partial thromboplastin time; and, different regimens were given depending upon risk stratification. Symptomatic osteoporotic fractures of the spine occurred post-partum in four women (2.2%). Their mean dosage of heparin ranged from 15,000 to 30,000 IU per 24 hours (mean 24,500 IU per 24 hours), and their duration of treatment was from 7 to 27 weeks (mean 17 weeks). It is of interest that in spite of prophylaxis with heparin, thromboembolic complications occurred in five women. Thus, osteoporotic vertebral fractures were found in 2.2% and these did correlate with the amount of heparin administered. There were no thrombocytopenias or excessive hemorrhage. Hunt *et al.*, during a study of low molecular weight heparin (Fragmin) for thromboprophylaxis in 34 high risk pregnancies identified one woman who developed an osteoporotic vertebral collapse post-partum.[33] This woman had no other risk factors for osteoporosis. Parenthetically, this study did support the efficacy of low molecular weight heparin in preventing recurrent thromboembolic disease in pregnant women at high risk. In this study, the incidence of osteoporotic fracture was 3%; however, bone density studies, to assess asymptomatic osteoporosis were not reported.

Doukets *et al.* in a prospective matched cohort studied the effects of long-term (>1 month) unfractionated heparin therapy on lumbar spine bone density.[34] Twenty-five women who received heparin during pregnancy, and 25 matched controls underwent dual photon absorptiometry of the lumbar spine in the post-partum period. None of 25 heparin-treated patients developed fractures. Heparin-treated patients had a 0.082 g/cm^2 lower bone density compared to untreated controls, which was statistically significant ($p = 0.0077$). There were six matched pairs in which only the heparin-treated patient had a bone density below 1.0 g/cm^2, compared to only one pair in which only the control patient had a bone density below this level ($p = 0.089$). The duration of heparin therapy, the mean daily dose, and the total dose of heparin were not at levels of independent significance. They concluded that long-term heparin therapy was associated with a significant reduction in bone density, although fractures are uncommon. They could not show a correlation between the lumber bone density and the dose or duration of heparin therapy. This is in contradistinction to the generally held views that heparin-induced osteoporosis is related to the dose and duration of therapy.[35,36]

A variety of studies have focused on the mechanism whereby heparin affects bone metabolism and structure. Muir *et al.* treated rats with once daily subcutaneous injections of unfractionated heparin or saline for 8 to 32 days and monitored the effects on bone histomorphometrically and measured urinary type 1 collagen cross-linked-pyridinoline (PYD) and serum alkaline phosphatase as surrogate markers of bone resorption and formation.[37] Biochemical markers of bone turnover showed that heparin produced a dose-dependent decrease in serum alkaline phosphatase and a transient increase in urinary PYD, thus confirming the histomorphometric data. They concluded that heparin decreases trabecular bone volume both by decreasing the rate of bone formation and increasing the rate of bone resorption.[37] In a subsequent study, this group evaluated the effect of low molecular weight heparin in a similar model system.[38] It was found both unfractionated and low molecular weight heparin decreased cancellous bone volume in a dose-dependent fashion, but unfractionated heparin caused significantly more bone loss than did the low molecular weight heparin. The biochemical markers of bone turnover demonstrated that both forms of heparins produced a dose-dependent decrease in serum alkaline phosphatase, consistent with reduced bone formation; whereas, only the unfractionated heparin caused an increase in urinary PYD, consistent with increased bone resorption. They concluded that unfractionated heparin decreases cancellous bone volume both by decreasing the rate of bone formation and increasing the rate of bone resorption; in contrast low molecular weight heparin causes less osteopenia because it only decreases the rate of bone formation.[38] Panagakos *et al.* have demonstrated that heparin induces osteoporosis by enhancing the effects of other bone resorbing factors particularly parathyroid hormone.[39] Shaughnessy *et al.* further examined the issue of calcium loss by an in vitro calcium release assay and demonstrated that size and sulfation of the heparins were the major determinants of the promotion of bone resorption.[40] Their extrapolation was that low molecular weight heparini preparations would, therefore, reduce the risk of the expected heparin associated osteoporosis. Murray and associates examined bone density in a rabbit model.[41] A reduction in cortical and trabecular bone density was seen with unfractionated heparin ($p < 0.05$) and high molecular weight heparin ($p < 0.01$), but not with low molecular weight heparin.

Thus, heparin associated osteoporosis is a clinically uncommon event occurring in less than 5% of long-term heparin treated patients. The evidence supports a lesser risk with low molecular weight heparin than with unfractionated heparin. The mechanisms appear related to impaired bone deposition and formation plus enhanced bone resorption with unfractionated heparin. A change in new bone deposition appears to be the major mechanism with low molecular weight heparin. Most clinical evidence supports the view that a long duration of therapy (i.e. greater than 6 months) and a higher dose of heparin increases the risk of bone changes.

From these observations, we currently recommend that bone density studies be done in patients whose duration of therapy will be greater than 6 months at an equivalent of 20,000 anti-Xa units per day, or at 3 months if the dose will exceed 20,000 anti-X U per day.[42] In addition, we encourage calcium supplements. If the patient is going to be on low-dose subcutaneous unfractionated or low-molecular-weight heparin for one year or more, baseline bone density studies are recommended and repeat comparative studies should be done yearly; if a significant change occurs and continued heparin is required, alendronate, or a similar medication should be started.[42]

Heparin-related skin reactions

Three general types of skin reactions can occur with heparin therapy.[35,42,43] The most common are those seen in patients being treated with subcutaneous heparin. These are small ecchymotic or erythematous papular or nodular lesions which are slightly tender and generally less than 1 cm in size. These occur at the sites of injection. Although at times these are the result of violated sterile technique and therefore, represent infections, most are sterile and require no change in therapy except the selection of an alternate site. The exact mechanism is not certain, but local cytokine release is the current working concept.

A second skin reaction is that of urticarial, often pruritic, lesions; again largely at the sites of subcutaneous injection. These allergic reactions have commonly been associated with the vehicle for the heparin and can often be avoided by either a change in the brand of heparin or the use of an anti-histamine at the time of the injections.

Heparin-induced skin necrosis is the most serious form of dermal reaction and fortunately the least common.[43,44,45,46,47] These lesions have many features similar to coumadin necrosis, but the pathophysiology is distinctly different. The route and form of heparin is unrelated to this occurrence. Commonly these begin 5 to 10 days into the heparin therapy and are manifest on the extremities, abdominal wall or nose; and, several of the case reports highlight their occurrence on the dorsum of the hand.[44,46] The onset is abrupt with a dusky or erythematous plaque-like lesion that can rapidly evolve into a hemorrhagic bullae with necrosis. The exact pathophysiologic basis for these necrotic lesions is not clear. The antibodies found in heparin induced thrombocytopenia have been seen in many of the patients in whom it has been sought, yet only about 25% of them will actually develop HIT II. These lesions signal an acute need to discontinue the heparin/LMW heparin therapy and select an appropriate alternative agent.

Altered liver function tests

Abnormal liver function studies, primarily a transaminasemia of minimal degree, have been correlated with long-term heparin administration. The finding is uncommon and the pathophysiologic mechanisms have never been defined. These changes revert to normal when the heparin is discontinued.[35,42]

Heparin and eosinophilia

Eosinophilia occurs in 5 to 10% of patients receiving either unfractionated or low molecular weight heparin therapy.[35,42,48] The eosinophilia is asymptomatic. In almost all of the patients it is unrelated to systemic allergic reactions, dermal allergic reactions, skin necrosis or any other evident symptom complex. It is not associated with any physiologic changes or sequelae. The eosinophilia abates 4 to 8 weeks after cessation of the heparin therapy. The current hypothesis relative to this occurrence is the activation of CD4 cells with the subsequent release of GM-CSF, IL-3 and IL-5, which can induce eosinophilia.[42]

Hyperkalemia, hypoaldosteronism, and related metabolic abnormalities

Prolonged heparin therapy has been recognized to be associated with functional hypoaldosteronism, hyperkalemia and allied metabolic abnormalities.[28,42,49] Although rare, the evidence supports heparin suppression of synthesis of aldosterone.[67] Cessation of the heparin results in resolution of the metabolic abnormalities and return to normal.

Alopecia

Alopecia, almost always mild, has been related to long-term heparin therapy.[28,35,42] Neither its occurrence nor potential pathophysiologic mechanisms have been well defined. However, pregnancy alone may be associated with mild alopecia, in the absence of heparin/LMW heparin therapy.

Thrombophilias in pregnancy

It must be remembered and emphasized that a diagnosis of thrombosis is similar to and as generic as a diagnosis of "anemia"; one must, in all instances, as in anemia, ask next: WHAT IS THE ETIOLOGY OF THE THROMBOSIS? Like anemia, the specific and appropriate therapy is highly dependent upon defining the etiology. Thrombosis, be it arterial or venous, can no longer be viewed as a generic diagnosis; approaching thrombosis in this manner probably accounts for not only many treatment failures, but also for often confusing and conflicting results of clinical trials. Most Clinicians and most trialists approaching thrombosis as a generic diagnosis fail to note that a very heterogeneous population is likely to be present and outcomes will depend upon designing therapy specific for a given etiology. As a simple example, it would not make sense to treat a patient with thrombosis and harboring sticky platelet syndrome with heparin or coumadin when they actually need aspirin; nor would it make sense to treat a patient with antiphospholipid syndrome and thrombosis with aspirin (no response) or warfarin (65% failure rate) when they respond most ideally to heparin. Some 65% of patients with recurrent miscarriage harbor a hereditary or acquired thrombophilia.[50,51]

In the rapidly changing field of thrombosis and hemostasis, diagnosis has become increasingly challenging, as new disorders are discovered and an array of new laboratory studies are developed. Thus, if a pregnant patient develops thrombosis, it cannot be assumed the thrombosis is simply secondary to pregnancy and a thrombophilic disorder must be strongly considered. Therapy is no less complex, as clinical studies continue to identify more effective treatment regimens.

Inherited disorders

Factor V Leiden As many as 5%–17% of Caucasians[52] and 20%–50% of unselected patients with deep vein thrombosis[53,54] are demonstrated to have a single point mutation (at point 1691) in the gene responsible for the production of factor V. As a result, the factor V produced is abnormal, with a glutamine (Q) for arginine (R) substitution at position 506 (FV:R506Q, factor V Leiden). Inactivation of factor Va by activated protein C is impaired, resulting in a lifelong hypercoagulable state.[53,54,55,56,57,58,59,60] APC resistance may also be acquired, as occurs with the use of oral contraceptives or in the presence of elevated factor VIII: C.[61] Regardless of the source of the APC abnormality, the clinical manifestations are similar. Since a hypercoagulable state is present, patients present either with venous or arterial thrombosis[83,84] or recurrent miscarriage syndrome (RMS).[14,62,63] In addition, FV Leiden is also associated with pregnancy associated DVT and PE, pre-eclampsia, and fetal growth retardation syndrome.[64] An important issue is the question of primary and secondary prophylaxis outside the clinical setting of pregnancy. Although there is a 5 to 10 times increased risk of thrombosis in heterozygous carriers of FV:R506Q, there is not yet a demonstrable major effect on life expectancy. Additionally, since there may be long intervals between episodes of thrombosis, it is unclear if lifelong primary prophylactic anticoagulation is indicated.[65,66] For the same reasons, screening of family members of patients with the mutation is also not recommended, until they are of an age where other risks, such as contact sports, surgery, trauma, oral contraceptives or hormone replacement therapy is contemplated.[67] Proper management becomes more critical in homozygous individuals, who may be at 50 to 100 times greater risk of thrombosis than the general population.[68] One recent study of 355 FV:R506Q patients with an initial episode of symptomatic DVT detected a recurrence rate of 30.3% after 8 years.[69] Factor V Leiden mutation patients, in another study, have been demonstrated to be four times more likely to have a recurrent event than first DVT patients without the mutation. Recurrences often follow discontinuation of anticoagulation.[70] A prospective trial of 251 patients following first DVT detected a FV:R506Q rate of 16.3%. Over an 8 year follow-up period, factor V Leiden mutation patients had a recurrence rate of 39.7%, compared to 18.3% for those without the mutation.[71] An additional study comparing homozygous and heterozygous individuals determined that the rate of recurrence was 9.5% per patient per year for homozygotes and 4.8% for heterozygotes.[72]

Lifelong anticoagulation with warfarin or heparin may be considered in selected heterozygous individuals with recurrent thrombotic events. Homozygotes suffering an initial episode of DVT may be considered for long-term anticoagulation on a case by case basis. Treatment of acute episodes of thrombosis should follow accepted recommendations, which include six weeks of anticoagulation following DVT associated with a reversible risk factor and 3 to 6 months of anticoagulation in idiopathic disease.[73] Patients with inherited or acquired thrombophilia who have recurrent, unprovoked venous thromboembolism should be considered for long-term anticoagulation.[74] Those with pregnancy, obviously, need therapeutic heparin or LMW heparin for 5–7 days, followed by thromboprophylactic doses of heparin or LMW heparin for the remainder of pregnancy and for at least two weeks following delivery, as previously outlined. The risk of thrombosis in individuals with FV:R506Q is compounded by the presence of other thrombophilic conditions. The risk associated with the use of oral contraceptives is increased from fourfold in genetically unaffected persons to 30-fold in FV:R506Q patients.[75,76,77] In symptomatic patients with protein C deficiency the prevalence of factor V Leiden was 14%.[78] Analysis of families with the concomitant presence of factor V Leiden mutation and protein S deficiency, detected a history of thrombosis in 72% of individuals with both abnormalities and 19% with either defect alone.[79] Patients with both hyperhomocyst(e)inemia and FV:R506Q are at 20 times increased risk of idiopathic venous thrombosis compared to those with neither defect. The likelihood of thrombosis was significantly greater in the presence of both abnormalities than with either in isolation.[80] Management of patients with more than one thrombophilic disorder must consider the enhanced risk and be adapted accordingly. Furthermore, therapy should target both disorders.

Patients with FV:R506Q who also experience a high risk of recurrent miscarriage syndrome (RMS) and have been effectively treated with UFH or LMWH + low-dose ASA, when therapy begins from first diagnosis and is continued to delivery or beyond.[81,82,83,84] Homozygous patients in high risk settings, particularly in the presence of additional risk factors such as oral contraceptive use, hormone replacement therapy or pregnancy should be treated with a prophylactic dose of LMWH during pregnancy and the puerperium (at least 14 days) wherein the risk of venous thromboembolism is also substantially increased.[67,85,86,87,88] One small study of pregnant women with acute thromboembolism detected a 40% to 59% incidence of APC resistance or FV:R506Q, thus heparin or LMW heparin prophylaxis is strongly recommended.[89] Controlled follow-up studies are, however, lacking.

Monitoring of patients with factor V Leiden mutation or with other forms of APC resistance who are not pregnant focuses primarily on the form of therapy utilized. Anti-platelet therapy with aspirin or clopidogrel requires no monitoring. Anticoagulation with warfarin should achieve a target international normalized ratio (INR) of 2.0 to 3.0.[73] Anti-thrombotic therapy with LMWH requires no monitoring except for a platelet count at least every two days during the first two weeks of treatment to assist in the early detection of heparin-induced thrombocytopenia (HIT/HITT).[90,91] The primary objective and clinical goals of treatment are avoidance of additional thrombotic events and, in the case of pregnancy, delivery of a healthy newborn to a healthy mother. Our approach to these patients is to use preconception low-dose ASA (81 mg/day) and immediately add post-conception dalteparin at 5,000 units, subcutaneously, every 24 hours. We also strongly encourage these patients to refrain from using oral contraceptives or hormone replacement therapy.

Factor V Cambridge The recent characterization of another genetic mutation in factor V as a cause of activated protein C resistance emphasizes the notion that a variety of genetic mutations are responsible for a propensity to both venous and arterial thrombosis. In this mutation the arginine (AGG) at position 306 was changed to threonine (ACG). This was found to result in removal of the recognition site for the restriction enzyme BstNI. Factor V Cambridge raises the risk for thrombosis and RMS in a similar manner as factor V Leiden. Both mutations exhibit the same clinical manifestations and the same degree of APC resistance in the laboratory.[92,93]

Treatment of patients with the factor V Cambridge mutation is the same as with FV:R506Q. Intervention in acute thrombosis with antithrombotic therapy followed by anticoagulation with warfarin is indicated. Long-term secondary prophylaxis with warfarin or heparin may be appropriate in selected patients. The pharmacological agent chosen guides monitoring.

Factor V HR2 haplotype The HR2 haplotype represents a defect of 6 base substitutions in exons 13 and 16, with two amino acid changes. This mutation is associated with activated Protein C resistance in both carriers and non-carriers of Factor V Leiden. The mutation, when found in association with Factor V Leiden imparts an additional 3X–4X-fold increase of venous thrombosis over carriers of Factor V Leiden alone.[106] Patients with the Factor V haplotype are also prone to thrombosis in individuals without Factor V Leiden. Unlike Factor V Leiden, which is predominately found in Caucasian populations, the Factor V HR2 haplotype has been found with about equal frequency in individuals of Caucasian, Italian, Indian and Somalian individuals.[107]

Factor V Hong Kong This phenotype, thus far only found in Hong Kong Chinese, actually represents two different genotypes, referred to as Factor V Hong Kong 1 and 2. The first mutation is an Arg 485 to Lys mutation at exon 10; this is the result of a G1691 A mutation. The second genotype (Factor V Hong Kong 2) is an Arg 306 to Gly substitution, resulting from an A1090G mutation. Both appear to lead to thrombosis. The first mutation is associated with a high tendency for thrombosis, but the second has not been assessed long enough to know the prevalence of thrombosis.

In patients with pregnancy and any type of APC resistance, based upon a mutation (Leiden, Cambridge, Hong Kong or HR2 haplotype), our approach to these patients is to use preconception low-dose ASA (81 mg/day) and immediately add post-conception dalteparin at 5,000 units, subcutaneously, every 24 hours. We also strongly encourage these patients to refrain from using oral contraceptives or hormone replacement therapy.

Prothrombin G20210A mutation Presence of a replacement of guanidine with adenine at position 20210 in the sequence of the 3′-untranslated region of the prothrombin gene (20210 G/A or 20210A) has been identified as a common genetic defect predisposing to thrombosis. The risk of venous thrombosis is nearly three times that of a control population.[94] Clinical manifestations include both venous thromboembolism, arterial thrombosis, recurrent miscarriage, and other complications of pregnancy. The risk of arterial disease in patients with the prothrombin G20210A mutation is debated. A Brazilian study of 116 patients with venous disease and 71 with arterial disease (compared to 295 controls) demonstrated an allele frequency of 4.3% in DVT patients, 5.7% in arterial disease patients and 0.33% among controls. Arterial disease patients were those with a history of myocardial infarction, cerebral arterial occlusive disease or occlusive peripheral arterial disease, in the absence of the accepted risk factors of hyper-lipoproteinemia, hypertension and diabetes mellitus.[95] An Italian study of 132 patients with venous thrombosis and 195 patients with cerebrovascular or coronary artery disease was compared to 161 controls. Whereas 16% of patients with venous thrombosis were found to have the GA genotype (4% of controls), the GA allele frequency was not increased in arterial disease patients.[96] It is clear from several studies that the risk of venous thrombosis rises significantly in patients with other concomitant thrombophilic defects. Makris *et al.* have demonstrated that in the presence of protein C or S deficiency, antithrombin deficiency or factor V Leiden the likelihood of thrombosis greatly increases.[97] Double heterozygotes have a much greater frequency of events and younger age at onset. Oral contraceptive use in patients with prothrombin G20210A greatly increases the risk of thrombosis, including of the cerebral venous system[98,99] and the celiac artery.[100]

Management includes the discontinuation of oral contraceptives and appropriate intervention for acute thrombosis. Since, in as many as 40% of patients, factor V Leiden is also present,[94] therapy must consider the enhanced thrombophilia associated with the concomitant presence of both disorders. Treatment with antithrombotic agents for acute venous thrombosis, as well as for acute cerebrovascular or coronary arterial thrombosis should follow accepted protocol.[73,101] Since the risk for recurrent thrombosis is high, patients heterozygous for factor V Leiden or other mutations and G20210A must be considered for long-term therapy with warfarin or heparin. No long-term, controlled trials are available to confirm this approach, however, Ferraresi *et al.*, note that 70% of their study population with more than one genetic defect experienced recurrent thrombosis.[96]

Although the prothrombin level is significantly increased in some, but not all, patients with the prothrombin mutation, measurement of the PT and other global clotting tests are not useful for diagnosis or surveillance of the disorder.[96,97,100,101] Prothrombin G20210 A is associated with complications of pregnancy, including not only DVT, PE, arterial thrombosis, but also eclampsia and fetal growth retardation syndrome.[5,14,87,88,102,103,104] Our approach to these patients is to use preconception low-dose ASA (81 mg/day) and immediately add post-conception dalteparin at 5,000 units, subcutaneously, every 24 hours.[102] We also strongly encourage these patients to refrain from using oral contraceptives or hormone replacement therapy following pregnancy.[102]

Factor XII (Hageman trait) Deficiency of factor XII (Hageman trait)[106] may result from either autosomal recessive or dominant inheritance.[107] While heterozygous individuals possess approximately 50% of normal factor XII levels, homozygous patients have very low levels.[108] Clinical manifestations vary from mild hemorrhage (rarely serious or fatal) to fatal venous thromboembolism or myocardial infarction.[109–112] Factor XII deficiency is also associated with RMS and DVT. Since patients rarely bleed, factor replacement is not generally required. If major hemorrhage does occur, hemostasis can be readily achieved with the infusion of fresh frozen plasma. In view of the defect in surface-mediated activation of fibrinolysis which is associated with the Hageman trait, there is some question as to whether treatment with a medication such as stanozolol to enhance fibrinolysis is indicated prophylactically.[108] Clearly, in the setting of increased thrombotic risk associated with a variety of medical and surgical disorders, LMWH or other prophylaxis is indicated. When thrombosis occurs, treatment should proceed according to accepted guidelines.[73,113] Our approach to these patients is to use preconception low-dose ASA (81 mg/day) and immediately add post-conception dalteparin at 5,000 units, subcutaneously, every 24 hours to or beyond delivery. We also strongly encourage these patients to refrain from using oral contraceptives or hormone replacement therapy following pregnancy.

Fibrinogen Congenital dysfibrinogenemia[114] is identified in over 100 specific molecular variants.[115,116] The usual consequence of dysfibrinogenemia is mild to moderate hemorrhage. Only about 10% of patients develop thrombosis,[114] mostly venous, but also arterial.[117] Although most of the dysfibrinogenemias associated with thrombosis have not been fully characterized, some defects appear to involve abnormal fibrin monomer polymerization, impaired activation of fibrinolysis or resistance to fibrinolysis.[118,119] We have not yet seen RMS or DVT in pregnancy in these patients, however, complications of pregnancy have been reported by others.[120,121,122]

Homocyst(e)inemia Homocyst(e)inemia refers to the combined pool of homocysteine, homocystine, mixed disulfides involving homocysteine and homocysteine thiolactone.[123] Homocysteinuria is a rare, autosomal recessive disorder in which the activity of cystathione beta-synthetase is decreased, resulting in disordered methionine metabolism. The result is homocysteinemia, methioninemia and homocystinuria. Patients with congenital deficiency exhibit typical features of ectopia lentis, mental retardation, and skeletal deformities.[124,125,126] As described by McCully in 1969, severe atherosclerosis develops at a young age.[119] Venous and arterial thrombosis are also common.[128] High total levels of homocyst(e)ine have recently been identified as the result of a mutation in the methylenetetrahydrofolate reductase (MTHFR) gene(C-to-T mutation at nucleotide 677),[129,130] rendering the enzyme thermolabile.[130,131,132,133]

While severe hyperhomocyst(e)inemia is rare, mild elevations of homocyst(e)ine are present in 5% to 7% of adults.[134,135] A study of 212 North American coronary disease patients, detected 17% with decreased activity of MTHFR, compared to 5% of 202 controls.[136] Estimates of incidence in arterial vascular disease have varied from 13% to 47% of patients.[134,137,138,139,140] The manifestations of recurrent venous and arterial thrombosis and precocious coronary and peripheral vascular disease develop in the third and fourth decade of life. While the pathophysiologic influence of homocyst(e)ine on hemostasis is poorly characterized, it is clear that hyperhomocyst(e)inemia is associated with both arterial[120,141] and venous[142,143,144,145] thrombosis.[145] Accelerated and severe atherosclerosis involves coronary,[133,146,147,148,149,150] cerebral[151,152,153] and peripheral arteries.[154,155] Marchant and colleagues have performed coagulation profiles as well as homocyst(e)ine levels in patients with a history of thrombosis. An elevated homocyst(e)ine level was confirmed as an independent risk factor for thrombosis.[156] Presentation is with deep vein thrombosis, angina or an acute coronary syndrome, stroke or claudication.

Hyperhomocyst(e)inemia and MTHFR mutations are managed primarily by the administration of high-dose folic acid with or without pyridoxine (B-6).[137,138,150,157,158,159,160,161,162,163,164,165] Our approach to these patients is to use preconception low-dose ASA (81 mg/day) and immediately add post-conception dalteparin at 5,000 units, subcutaneously, every 24 hours. We also use 5 mg/day folate and 50 mg/day of Pyridoxine (B6) during pregnancy due to the risks of miscarriage, thrombotic or thromboembolic problems and the increased incidence of birth defects. We also strongly encourage these patients to refrain from using oral contraceptives or hormone replacement therapy following pregnancy.[14,102]

Antithrombin Antithrombin (AT) deficiency may be both inherited and acquired. Antithrombin is an essential inhibitor of thrombin,[166] factors Xa, IXa, XIa and XIIa, plasmin, kallikrein and has activity against protein C and protein S.[167,168,169,170,171,172,173,174] While the etiologies of AT deficiency may differ, the clinical and laboratory consequences are similar. Likewise, therapy is the same for both inherited and acquired forms.

Hereditary deficiency of antithrombin is an autosomal dominant disorder characterized by either absence of antithrombin or the presence of a dysfunctional form. The majority of affected individuals are heterozygotes.[175] While a functional antithrombin level of above 50% to 70% of normal human plasma appears to be required to avoid thrombosis, some patients with lower levels may be unaffected.[176,177,178,179,180] Venous thrombosis is the primary presentation, usually begins in adolescence and is frequently accompanied by pulmonary emboli.[181] High risk events such as surgery, trauma, pregnancy and oral contraceptive use may initiate the first thrombotic event.[182] Patients with acquired deficiency who develop recurrent thrombotic events require lifelong anticoagulation.

Our approach to these patients is to use preconception low dose ASA (81 mg/day) and immediately add post-conception dalteparin at 5,000 units, subcutaneously, every 24 hours.[14,102] We also strongly encourage these patients to refrain from using oral contraceptives or hormone replacement therapy following pregnancy.

In an acute thrombotic episode, the management of patients with both inherited and acquired antithrombin deficiency may require antithrombin concentrates.[183] Since patients with AT deficiency lack the available site of action for heparin, anticoagulation of patients with congenital deficiency who present with acute venous thrombosis or pulmonary embolism, with heparin alone, is often ineffective. Administration of antithrombin concentrates must accompany anticoagulation with heparin/LMW heparin. Antithrombin concentrates may also be efficacious in patients with inherited deficiency, even without heparin.[184] Prophylaxis with AT for congenitally deficient patients in high risk settings may be indicated, however, controlled studies are not available to confirm this. Pregnancy represents a special risk for deficient patients. Subcutaneous heparin or LMWH is recommended throughout pregnancy. Warfarin is contraindicated due to teratogenicity. Antithrombin concentrates may be indicated at the time of greatest risk, during the puerperium and for obstetrical emergencies.[185]

Vinazzer and others have demonstrated the efficacy of antithrombin concentrates.[186] The formula for administration of therapeutic antithrombin concentrates is as follows:

$$\textit{Units required} = \frac{(\textit{desired-baseline AT level*}) \times \textit{weight (kg)}}{1.4}$$

*expressed as % normal level based on functional AT assay

Dosing frequency is generally every 6–12 hours, guided by repeat AT assays.[181,187]

Generally, a dose of 50 U/kg is recommended for a patient with a baseline functional level of 50%. Repeat administration of 60% of the loading dose every 24 hours will usually maintain adequate levels in patients with congenital deficiency.[187] The dose requirement may be much higher in patients with DIC and similar conditions which actively deplete AT.

Monitoring of patients with AT deficiency varies considerably between inherited and acquired states. Patients with the inherited disorder who experience recurrent thrombosis require lifelong anticoagulation, usually with warfarin and the determination of the PT at regular intervals (goal to maintain INR 2.0 to 3.0). As the clinical circumstance changes, the intervals of follow-up and monitoring may change. For clinical purposes, the assay of choice is the functional antithrombin assay, reported as % normal human plasma. Immunologic assays of AT are of no clinical value. In the acutely ill patient receiving antithrombin concentrates, repeat AT levels may be required at intervals of 6 to 12 hours.

Heparin cofactor II Heparin cofactor II (HC-II) directly inactivates the activity of thrombin on fibrinogen[188] and inhibits thrombin-induced platelet activation.[189] Congenital deficiency of HC-II appears to be very rare and is associated with an increased risk of both arterial and venous thrombosis.[190,191,192,193,194,195,196,197,198] Heterozygous individuals have 50% of normal levels and thrombotic risk appears to increase when levels decrease below 60%.[192] Treatment is based upon the clinical circumstances. We have seen only three pregnancy patients with HC-II deficiency; our approach to these patients is to use preconception low-dose ASA (81 mg/day) and immediately add post-conception dalteparin at 5,000 units, subcutaneously, every 24 hours. We also strongly encourage these patients to refrain from using oral contraceptives or hormone replacement therapy following pregnancy.[14,102]

Protein C Protein C is a vitamin K-dependent protein which inhibits the coagulation system primarily through inactivation of factors V and VIII: C, the cofactors required for activation of thrombin and factor Xa.[199] This serine protease is inhibited by AT[200] and enhanced by protein S.[201] The presence of protein C is essential to maintain hemostatic balance. Deficiencies of protein C may be either congenital or acquired.[202]

Congenital deficiency is autosomal dominant and characterized by recurrent venous thrombosis and thromboembolism beginning in adolescence.[203,204,205] Most homozygous patients die of thromboembolic disease in infancy.[206,207] Both absence and dysfunctional forms of the disorder are observed. Type I disease is characterized by reduction in both antigenic and functional levels and type II, in which functional levels are decreased much more than antigenic levels.[208,209,210,211,212,213]

Homozygous patients have been successfully managed with infusions of fresh frozen plasma or certain factor IX concentrates (those containing large amounts of protein C and S), together with heparin.[203,206,214] Maintenance of an INR of 3.5 or higher may be necessary to prevent recurrence of severe skin necrosis.[215] Considering the need for lifelong anticoagulation, the need for high-dose warfarin, the difficulties attendant to maintenance of a consistent level of anticoagulation and the risks of major hemorrhage, LMWH appears to be preferred for long-term management.[216]

Anticoagulation is the treatment of choice in patients with heterozygous protein C deficiency. Heparin or LMWH are used according to accepted guidelines for acute thrombotic events.[17,109] Long-term anticoagulation with warfarin is indicated following an acute event and as prophylaxis. Warfarin-induced skin necrosis is a major therapeutic problem.[217,218,219] With the institution of warfarin, the reduction of protein C (half-life 6 hours) occurs at a faster rate than the reduction in the other vitamin K-dependent factors II (half-life 72 hours), VII and X. This results in a transient hypercoagulable state, predisposing to thrombosis, including skin necrosis.[17] Recent studies have demonstrated that this problem can be controlled by maintaining full anticoagulation with heparin until the PT is well into the therapeutic range (target INR 3.0 to 3.5). Maintaining a therapeutic PT is, subsequently, essential to avoiding recurrent thrombosis. Despite therapeutic anticoagulation with warfarin, there are treatment failures. Long term therapy with heparin/LMWH may be required. Protein C concentrates are now available for treatment failures.[220]

Therapy is monitored with the appropriate laboratory test depending upon the pharmacological agent selected. The target INR for warfarin therapy is 3.0 to 3.5. Therapy with LMWH is weight adjusted and does not require monitoring, except for a platelet count every two to three days for the first two weeks of treatment. While the measurement of the biologic and immunologic activity of protein C is required for diagnosis,[221] follow-up analysis is not required. When evaluating a patient with unexplained thrombosis, however, it is essential to obtain the laboratory tests for protein C deficiency before therapy is initiated, since warfarin immediately reduces the vitamin K-dependent hepatic production of protein C. The levels of both protein C and S decrease to 40% to 60% of normal immediately and return to about 70% of normal after several weeks of therapy. Measurement of the protein C and S levels should wait for several weeks after initiation of warfarin therapy. On repeat evaluation of protein C and S, if levels above 60% are not detected, congenital deficiency should be considered.[220] Like other thrombophilias, Protein C deficiency is strongly associated with RMS, pre-eclampsia, eclampsia, fetal growth retardation syndrome, arterial and venous thrombosis and PE. In Protein C deficient pregnancy patients, our approach to these patients is to use preconception low-dose ASA (81 mg/day) and immediately add post-conception dalteparin at 5,000 units, subcutaneously, every 24 hours. We also strongly encourage these patients to refrain from using oral contraceptives or hormone replacement therapy following pregnancy.

Protein S Protein S is a cofactor for the protein C-induced inactivation of factor V[222] and the protein C-induced inactivation of factor VIII:C.[222] Protein S is also a cofactor in the protein C acceleration of fibrinolysis.[223] and appears to have anticoagulant functions independent of protein C by direct inhibition of procoagulant enzyme complexes.[224,225] Congenital protein S deficiency is autosomal dominant and is fairly common, identified in as many as 10% of patients under 45 presenting with deep vein thrombosis.[226] Incidence in other selected groups has varied from to 1.5% to 7%.[227,228] Simmonds *et al.* have recently reported analysis of a 122 member family in which 44 members were identified with the protein S gene mutation substitution, Gly-295 to Val. The probability of remaining thrombosis free was 0.97 for unaffected family members and 0.5 for those with the mutation.[218] Homozygotes have a severe propensity to thrombosis and may present with purpura fulminans soon after birth.[230] Heterozygous patients are at high risk for thrombosis throughout life. An asymptomatic variant may also exist.[231,232] Management of patients with protein S deficiency is similar to those with protein C deficiency. Acute thrombosis is managed with heparin anticoagulation according to accepted guidelines dependent upon the site and severity of disease. Long-term anticoagulation with warfarin is indicated post heparin therapy for an acute event and for prophylaxis. Follow-up of patients involves repeated clinical evaluation in the acute setting and monitoring is dependent upon the form of anticoagulation selected. LMWH requires only periodic evaluation of the platelet count. Warfarin is monitored with the PT to maintain a target INR of 2.0 to 3.0. Repeat analysis of the protein S level is usually not required if evaluation is performed before initiation of warfarin therapy. Subsequent measurement should wait for several weeks, as discussed with protein C. In warfarin failures, long-term therapy with UFH or LMWH may be required. As with other thrombophilic disorders, the patient and family members should be counseled regarding the need for diagnostic screening and the need to intervene in high risk circumstances. These include but are not limited to the avoidance of oral contraceptives, control of obesity and prophylactic anticoagulation at the time of surgery, prolonged immobility, pregnancy and the puerperium. As in other thrombophilias, Protein S deficiency is strongly associated with RMS, pre-eclampsia, eclampsia, fetal growth retardation syndrome, arterial and venous thrombosis and PE. In Protein S deficient pregnancy patients, our approach to these patients is to use preconception low-dose ASA (81 mg/day) and immediately add post-conception dalteparin at 5,000 units, subcutaneously, every 24 hours. We also strongly encourage these patients to refrain from using oral contraceptives or hormone replacement therapy following pregnancy.[14,102]

Fibrinolytic defects and thrombosis A variety of abnormalities of the fibrinolytic system predispose to thrombosis, RMS and DVT/PE. Plasminogen may be decreased due to impaired synthesis. Tissue plasminogen activator (tPA) may be decreased or there be abnormal factor XII activation. Tissue plasminogen activator inhibitor type I (PAI-1) may be present in increased amounts, with or without PAI-1 polymorphisms, or there may be an increase in fibrinolytic inhibitors, alpha-2-antiplasmin, alpha-2-macroglobulin and alpha-1-antitrypsin. A variety of clinical conditions are associated with elevated levels of fibrinolytic inhibitors, including diabetes mellitus,[233] thrombotic thrombocytopenic purpura,[234] myocardial infarction,[235,236] malignancy, deep vein thrombosis and pulmonary embolism,[237] scleroderma, pulmonary fibrosis, pregnancy, oral contraceptive use,[238] serious infections and surgery.[239,240] Patients with generalized atherosclerosis may exhibit decreased plasminogen activity due to damage to the vascular intima.[241,242] Treatment of impaired fibrinolysis must include treatment of the underlying disease with the appropriate modalities, as well as anticoagulation. Caution must be exercised in the application of thrombolytic agents since, in the absence of adequate levels of plasminogen, tissue plasminogen activator, streptokinase and urokinase may be less effective than expected.

Patients with congenital plasminogen deficiency have clinical features similar to patients with congenital protein C, protein S and antithrombin deficiency. Symptomatic patients generally present with DVT or PE.[243] We have not yet seen a pregnancy patient with plasminogen deficiency. The disorder is of autosomal recessive inheritance and is characterized by the onset of deep vein thrombosis and pulmonary embolism in adolescence.[244] As many as 2%–3% of young patients with idiopathic DVT may be so affected.[245] Both the absence form and dysfunctional form exist, with the dysfunctional form most common.[243,244,246] While the significance of congenital plasminogen deficiency has been disputed as a risk factor for thrombosis[1] both forms have been correlated with some increased risk, particularly when associated with other thrombophilic abnormalities or circumstantial risk factors.[247,248] Thrombosis is primarily venous and usually is correlated with a plasminogen level below 40% of normal.[246]

Treatment in patients with acute thrombosis should follow accepted guidelines for DVT and PE. Warfarin therapy should target an INR of 2.0 to 3.0. Acute intervention may include urokinase, when clinically indicated in the setting of massive pulmonary embolization and severe or recurrent iliofemoral thrombosis.[246,249] Antiplatelet therapy may also play a role in management.[246,249]

Monitoring must rely on clinical parameters and evaluation of the plasminogen level. In patients with the dysfunctional form rather than the absence form of the disorder, the biologic functional assay will be abnormal, while the immunologic quantitative assay will be normal.[250]

Patients with congenital tPA deficiency and with congenitally elevated levels of PAI are rare, and are characterized by the same increased risk of thrombosis as seen with congenital deficiency of plasminogen.[251,252,253] Three polymorphic alterations in the human PAI-1 gene have been associated with elevated plasma PAI-1 levels; these are (1) a Hind III restriction fragment length polymorphism (2) a (C-A)n dinucleotide repeat polymorphism; and (3) a single nucleotide insertion/deletion polymorphism (4G/5G). The Hind III polymorphism develops due to a base change in the 3′-untranslated region; the 1/1 genotype exhibits higher PAI-1 levels than 1/2 or 2/2 genotypes. The smaller alleles of an eight-allele dinucleotide repeat polymorphism are also noted to be associated with increased PAI-1 activity.[254,255] Regarding the sequence length polymorphism, which occurs in the promoter region of the PAI-1 gene, the 4G/4G genotype correlates with higher PAI-1 activity compared to genotypes possessing a 5G allele. Both the 4G and 5G alleles bind a transcriptional activator, but only the 5G allele binds a repressor protein; as a result, the 4G/4G genotype has a higher basal PAI-1 transcription rate and higher plasma PAI-1 levels. The association of the 4G/4G PAI-1 polymorphism with arterial thrombosis has rendered conflicting results. In an evaluation of 94 men with acute myocardial infarction before the age of 45 an increased prevalence of the 4G allele compared to a healthy control population was noted.[256] However, although another study confirmed an association between PAI-1 elevation and 4G/4G genotype, there were no differences in 4G allele prevalence between patients with myocardial infarction and controls.[257] The Physicians Health Study did not find an increased prevalence of the 4G allele in those with myocardial infarction or venous thrombosis.[258] Thus, although suggestive, more studies are needed to clearly define the association between these polymorphisms and thrombosis. However, the homozygous state (4G/4G) and heterozygous state (4G/5G) are clearly associated with venous thrombosis. This topic is extensively reviewed by Kwaan.[259]

Like other thrombophilias, fibrinolytic system defects are strongly associated with RMS, pre-eclampsia, eclampsia, fetal growth retardation syndrome, arterial and venous thrombosis and PE. The most commonly seen of these defects is clearly PAI-1 polymorphisms and this defect is clearly associated with all of the previously mentioned complications of pregnancy, including thrombosis, RMS, infertility, fetal growth retardation syndrome, and eclampsia. In pregnancy patients with any of the thrombophilic fibrinolytic system defects, our approach is to use preconception low dose ASA (81 mg/day) and immediately add post-conception dalteparin at 5,000 units, subcutaneously, every 24 hours. We also strongly encourage these patients to refrain from using oral contraceptives or hormone replacement therapy following pregnancy.[14,102]

Sticky platelet syndrome (SPS) A platelet defect which (1) appears quite common, (2) accounts for many episodes of arterial and venous thrombosis and significant morbidity and mortality (3) is easy to diagnose and (4) is easy to treat is Sticky Platelet Syndrome (SPS). Sticky platelet syndrome was first described by Mammen and associates in 1983 at the Ninth International Joint Conference on Stroke and Cerebral Circulation.[260] Subsequently Mammen and associates described 41 patients with coronary artery disease and SPS; this was followed by a report in 1986 delineating this syndrome in a number of individuals with cerebrovascular disease; the inheritance was noted to be autosomal dominant.[261,262] Finally in 1995 over 200 families, with a wide variety of arterial and venous thrombotic events due to SPS were described.[263] Although these publications have clearly delineated SPS as a common inherited and easily diagnosed and treated syndrome leading to significant, and often preventable, arterial and venous thrombosis, most clinicians and laboratory scientists are still unfamiliar with the prevalence of SPS and fail to consider this diagnosis in appropriate patient populations.[264] In addition, the actual prevalence remains unclear, especially as relates to venous versus arterial events. A more recent study[265] assessed the prevalence of SPS in a wide variety of patients with various types of arterial and venous events. One-hundred and fifty patients were referred for evaluation to determine the etiology, if possible, for unexplained arterial or venous events; 78 had suffered venous events consisting of deep vein thrombosis (DVT) with or without pulmonary embolus (PE). Seventy-five patients were referred for evaluation of arterial events; these patients suffered coronary artery thrombosis (21%), cerebrovascular thrombosis (50.6%), transient cerebral ischemic attacks (TIAS) (13.3%), retinal vascular thrombosis (6.6%) or peripheral arterial thrombosis (8%). Peripheral arterial thrombotic events consisted of unexplained thrombosis of renal (2), radial (1), popliteal (1) and mesenteric arteries (1). All patients referred for determining the etiology of an unexplained thrombotic event were subjected to a complete history and physical examination and then were studied for hypercoagulability syndromes, including SPS. Sticky platelet syndrome is the second most common thrombophilia, the most common being antiphospholipid syndrome, accounting for recurrent miscarriage syndrome and infertility.[14,102,265]

Based upon these studies, it appears Sticky Platelet Syndrome is a common cause of both arterial and venous events. A similar study was performed by Anderson and associates; this was also a prospective study wherein 195 patients with arterial, venous or arterial plus venous thrombosis were assessed for hypercoagulability; SPS was the singular most common defect found, being detected in 28% of the entire population. The authors also concluded, as in the previous study that SPS is a common inherited prothrombotic disorder leading to arterial and venous thrombosis.[266] The association of Sticky Platelet Syndrome as a cause of young age cerebrovascular thrombosis has also recently been noted by German investigators.[267] Given that it appears SPS accounts for about 14% of unexplained venous thrombotic events and between 12% (peripheral arterial thrombosis) and 33% (TIAS) of arterial events, this hereditary platelet function defect should be strongly suspected, and searched for, in any individual with an otherwise unexplained arterial or venous event. If one assumes, based upon prevalence studies, that the congenital blood coagulation protein defects, including antithrombin defects, Protein S, Protein C and other rare defects account for about 20% of all venous events, and APC resistance (Factor V Leiden) accounts for another 20% of unexplained venous events, then, when adding Sticky Platelet Syndrome (at 14%) it may be concluded that congenital defects account for about 50%–60% of unexplained venous events. If it is then considered that antiphospholipid syndrome, based upon prevalence studies, accounts for another 25% of venous events, then it may be reasonably concluded that about 80% to 90% of venous events, and a somewhat lesser number of arterial events can be defined as to cause. Since the treatment(s) for these disorders may differ and since about half are hereditary, it is important to define the presence of hereditary and acquired coagulation protein or platelet defects whenever possible. This leads to the inescapable conclusion that a diagnosis of thrombosis, like a diagnosis of anemia, is only a partial diagnosis and the precise nature and cause must next be defined. In the case of SPS, warfarin or heparin therapy would not generally be indicated, and ASA appears to be the treatment of choice.

In pregnancy patients with SPS, the defect is strongly associated with RMS, infertility, pre-eclampsia, arterial and venous thrombosis and PE. In SPS pregnancy patients, our approach to these patients is to use preconception low dose ASA (81 mg/day) and immediately add post-conception dalteparin at 5,000 units, subcutaneously, every 24 hours. We also strongly encourage these patients to refrain from using oral contraceptives or hormone replacement therapy following pregnancy.[14,102]

Antiphospholipid syndrome

Antiphospholipid Thrombosis Syndromes (APL-TS), which include not only the lupus anticoagulant (LA) and anticardiolipin antibodies (ACLA), but also more recently recognized "subgroups" of antiphospholipid antibodies (antibodies against Beta-2-Glycoprotein-1 (B-2-GP-1), and antibodies to phosphatidylserine. phosphatidylethanolamine, phosphatidylglycerol, phosphatidylinositol, phosphatidylcholine and anti-annexin-V, all comprise the "Antiphospholipid Thrombosis (APL-TS) Syndromes". Antiphospholipid syndrome is the most common acquired blood protein defect(s) associated with either venous or arterial thrombosis or both.[268] It is also the most common cause of RMS, infertility or thrombosis during pregnancy.[14,102] The thrombotic and thrombo-occlusive events associated with these antiphospholipid antibodies include thrombosis of the venous system, the arterial system, coronary artery thrombosis, cerebrovascular thrombosis, transient cerebral ischemic attacks (TIAs), retinal vascular thrombosis and placental vascular thrombosis (leading to recurrent miscarriage syndrome); these antibodies may also be associated with related clinical syndromes, as discussed.[269]

The antiphospholipid thrombosis syndrome consists of closely related but clearly distinct clinical syndromes that often are discordant with respect to types of antiphospholipid antibodies found: these are (1) the lupus anticoagulant thrombosis syndrome (2) the anticardiolipin antibody thrombosis syndrome and (3) thrombosis associated with subgroups of antiphospholipid antibodies. There is poor correlation between thrombosis patients harboring anticardiolipin antibodies and those harboring lupus anticoagulants, and stronger, but still not concordant, correlation between thrombosis patients with anticardiolipin antibodies and those with antibodies to B-2-GP-1, or antibodies to phosphatidylserine. phosphatidylethanolamine, phosphatidylglycerol, phosphatidylinositol, annexin-V and phosphatidylcholine. Although there are similarities, there are, at times, clinical, laboratory and biochemical differences, particularly regarding prevalence, etiology, possible mechanisms of thrombosis, clinical presentations, diagnosis and, at times, management.[270,271] The anticardiolipin antibody-thrombosis antiphospholipid syndrome is much more common than is the lupus anticoagulant-thrombosis antiphospholipid syndrome, the ratio being about 5 to 1.[269,272,273,274] All of these syndromes may be associated with (1) arterial and venous thrombosis (2) recurrent miscarriage and (3) thrombocytopenia in descending order of prevalence, however, the anticardiolipin syndrome is more commonly associated with both arterial and venous thrombosis, including typical deep vein thrombosis and pulmonary embolus, premature coronary artery disease, premature cerebrovascular disease (including TIAs, small stoke syndrome and cerebrovascular thrombotic stroke) and retinal arterial and venous occlusive disease. The lupus anticoagulant, although sometimes associated with arterial disease is more commonly associated with venous thrombosis with or without pulmonary embolus. Also, patients with anticardiolipin thrombosis syndrome develop more predictable types of thrombosis than do those with the lupus anticoagulant thrombosis syndrome and management of thrombotic problems can be quite different between the two syndromes. Thrombosis patients harboring antibodies to B-2-GP-1, or antibodies to phosphatidylserine. phosphatidylethanolamine, phosphatidylglycerol, phosphatidylinositol, annexin-V or phosphatidylcholine tend to more closely resemble patients with anticardiolipin antibodies than patients with isolated lupus anticoagulant. Although all of these antiphospholipid antibody thrombosis syndromes may be seen in association with systemic lupus erythematosus, other connective tissue and autoimmune disorders and other selected medical conditions such as lymphomas, the majority of individuals, about 90%, developing any of the antiphospholipid thrombosis syndromes, are otherwise healthy individuals and harbor no other underlying medical condition and are classified as having *Primary*, rather than *Secondary* antiphospholipid thrombosis syndrome.[274,275] This distinction is of significance, as those with secondary antiphospholipid syndromes generally have heterogeneous antibodies which react with a variety of phospholipid moieties, including anticardiolipin, lupus anticoagulant tests or antibodies to B-2-GP-1, phosphatidylserine, phosphatidylethanolamine, phosphatidylglycerol, phosphatidylinositol, annexin-V or phosphatidylcholine and render biological false positive tests for syphilis, whereas those with primary antiphospholipid thrombosis syndrome more commonly have homogeneous antibodies reacting with only one particular phospholipid moiety.[274,275] Thus, when evaluating published studies, one must carefully assess the population being studied for antiphospholipid antibodies. The findings and results of studies in patients with autoimmune disorders may not necessarily be extrapolated to studies or clinical and laboratory findings in patients with primary antiphospholipid thrombosis syndromes. These antiphospholipid thrombosis syndromes, including etiology, pathophysiology, clinical and laboratory diagnosis and management principles are herein discussed.

Lupus anticoagulants and thrombosis

In 1952 Conley and Hartmann described a coagulation disorder in two patients with systemic lupus erythematosus; the patients exhibited anticoagulant activity by in-vitro testing, which was manifested by a prolonged whole blood clotting time and prothrombin time.[265,276] It is now known that patients with systemic lupus or other autoimmune diseases may develop an immunoglobulin that has the ability to prolong phospholipid-dependent coagulation tests.[274,277,278] About 10% of patients with systemic lupus harbor a lupus anticoagulant (LA); however, the LA is commonly seen in other conditions as well, including malignancy, lymphoproliferative disorders, and viral infections, especially human immunodeficiency (HIV) virus infection.[279,280,281] Most commonly the lupus anticoagulant develops in otherwise healthy individuals (Primary Lupus Anticoagulant Thrombosis Syndrome). There is also an association with drug ingestion; commonly associated drugs include chlorpromazine, procainamide, quinidine, hydralazine, Dilantin, interferon, Fansidar and cocaine.[272,273,274,282,283,284] A common misconception is that patients with drug-induced lupus anticoagulant, usually IgM idiotype, do not suffer thrombosis, but in fact these patients also have an increased risk of thrombotic disease. The frequency of hemorrhage resulting from the lupus anticoagulant is clearly less than 1%; however, it is important to recognize conditions that may predispose lupus patients harboring a lupus anticoagulant to hemorrhage.[285,286] Twenty-five percent of patients with systemic lupus have concomitant prothrombin deficiency, and more than 40% may have thrombocytopenia; these accompanying defects are particularly noted in those with secondary LA-thrombosis syndromes.[274,285,286,287]

Of greater clinical significance, patients with the lupus anticoagulant are at increased risk for thromboembolic disease, most commonly deep vein thrombosis, pulmonary emboli, and thrombosis of other large vessels.[288,289] Thromboembolism occurs in about 10% of patients with systemic lupus; however, in patients with systemic lupus and the lupus anticoagulant, thromboembolism occurs in up to 50% of patients. In patients harboring a primary LA, the lupus anticoagulant is estimated to account for about 6% to 8% of thrombosis in otherwise healthy individuals. There have also been associations with primary lupus anticoagulant syndrome and recurrent miscarriage, neuropsychiatric disorders, renal vascular thrombosis, thrombosis of dermal vessels, and thrombocytopenia.[274,284,287,290,291]

Primary lupus anticoagulant thrombosis syndrome is much more common than the secondary type and consists of patients with lupus anticoagulant and thrombosis who harbor no other underlying disease; secondary lupus anticoagulant thrombosis syndrome consists of those patients with lupus anticoagulant and thrombosis with an underlying disease, such as lupus or other autoimmune disorders, malignancy, infection, inflammation or ingestion of drugs inducing the lupus anticoagulant.[274]

Patients with primary lupus anticoagulant phospholipid syndrome primarily suffer venous thrombosis and pulmonary emboli. A wide variety of venous systems may become involved, including not only the extremities (most common presentation) but also mesenteric, renal, hepatic, portal and superior and inferior vena cava.[274,275,279] Although patients may also suffer arterial events, this is uncommon in primary lupus anticoagulant thrombosis syndrome, as opposed to primary anticardiolipin antibody thrombosis syndrome where arterial events are almost as common as venous events. This is in distinction to patients with secondary lupus anticoagulant thrombosis syndrome wherein patients, especially those with systemic lupus and the lupus anticoagulant more commonly suffer arterial events than do those with primary lupus anticoagulant thrombosis syndrome. However, even in secondary lupus anticoagulant thrombosis syndrome, venous events are more common than arterial events. Arteries commonly involved include coronary, cerebral, carotid, aorta, mesenteric, renal and extremities.[274,275,292,293,294,298]

Purified lupus anticoagulant inhibits the Ca^{++}-dependent binding of prothrombin and Factor Xa to phospholipids, therefore inhibiting the activity of the phospholipid complex required for conversion of prothrombin to thrombin.[278,285] Of interest, biologic false-positive tests for syphilis are seen in up to 40% of patients with systemic lupus; the number increases to 90% in patients with systemic lupus plus the LA.[286,290,295] An abnormality often (theoretically) exists in the phospholipid-dependent coagulation reactions, including the prothrombin time, the activated partial thromboplastin time (aPTT), and the Russell's viper venom time, as the lupus anticoagulant is not directed against a specific factor, but to phospholipids. The inhibitor usually does not exert an increasing effect with prolonged incubation with normal plasma, and thus this simple screen can often be used to distinguish the lupus inhibitor from inhibitors that neutralize specific clotting factors. About 15% to 25% of lupus anticoagulants can, however, be time dependent, so this is not an absolute or definitive test. Incubation of the patients' plasma with normal plasma does not generally cause a sensitivity of the partial thromboplastin time to the inhibitor's effect and one-stage assays for factors XII, XI, IX, and VII may yield low values when the standard dilutions of test plasma are used. Usually further dilution of the test plasma causes the measured level of these factors to approach the normal range; an exception occurs in rare patients with decreased concentration of prothrombin resulting from accelerated removal of prothrombin antigen-antibody complexes.[296,297]

Multiple lupus anticoagulant assays are currently in use.[296] Sensitivity of the aPTT to the presence or absence of the lupus anticoagulant is highly dependent upon the reagents used. Many patients with thrombosis and the lupus anticoagulant have normal aPTTs, even with the newer allegedly more "sensitive" reagents, thus, the aPTT is *not* an appropriate screening test for lupus anticoagulants and when suspecting the presence of a lupus anticoagulant, a more definitive test, preferably the dRVVT, should immediately be performed regardless of the PTT.[272,273,274,298,299] The lupus inhibitor is identified by an ability to bind phospholipid and inhibit phospholipid-dependent coagulant reactions. The assays are based upon the use of limiting amounts of phospholipid, and therefore sensitized, in platelet-poor plasma. Initially, a prothrombin time was performed with dilute tissue thromboplastin and a reduced number of platelets in the mixture; however, IgM inhibitors were missed.[19] A "modified" Russell's viper venom time was developed in which the venom is diluted to give a "normal" time of 23 to 27 seconds, and the phospholipid is then diluted down to a minimal level that continues to support this range. A prolongation of this system will not correct with a mixture of patient and normal plasma and this system detects both IgG and IgM anticoagulants.[300] This assay is known as the dilute Russell's viper venom time (dRVVT) and is the most sensitive of all assays purported to be useful in the screening or diagnosis of lupus anticoagulants.[299] The kaolin clotting time test (KCT) has been modified to detect lupus anticoagulants. In this assay, platelet-poor plasma is mixed with varying proportions of test plasma and normal plasma. Kaolin is added and the time required for clotting is determined.[301] The KCT is then plotted against proportions of patients' plasma with normal plasma; an inhibitor is assumed to be present when a small portion of test plasma in comparison with normal plasma prolongs the assay system. A kaolin activated partial thromboplastin time, with rabbit brain phospholipid in a standard and four-fold increased "high" lipid concentration to normalize or "out-inhibit" the abnormal "standard" aPTT, has also been utilized in diagnosis of the lupus inhibitor.[302] The best test at present is the dRVVT; if this test is prolonged, the confirmation of a lupus inhibitor, by noting correction of the prolonged dRVV time by adding phospholipid in some form (preferably void of platelet membrane material) is recommended, especially if the patient is on warfarin or heparin therapy. Both heparin and warfarin are also capable of prolonging the dRVVT. In our experience, the most sensitive and specific is the dRVVT available from American Diagnostics.

There is a correlation between elevated anticardiolipin antibodies and the lupus anticoagulant in secondary antiphospholipid syndromes (those associated with other autoimmune diseases); however, the lupus anticoagulant, anticardiolipin antibodies and subgroups are separate entities, and most of the time anticardiolipin antibodies are found in the absence of the lupus anticoagulant in the *primary* antiphospholipid thrombosis syndromes.[285,303] The lupus anticoagulant has a stronger association with binding phospholipids of a hexagonal composition such as phosphocholine, or after membrane damage by infection, Interleukin-1 (IL-1), or other mechanisms leading to change from the lamellar to hexagonal form, whereas anticardiolipin antibodies usually have an affinity to lamellar phospholipids in a bilayer (lamellar) composition.[274,278,304,305] IgG and IgM anticardiolipin antibodies are the most frequent idiotypes and can be detected by ELISA; IgA anticardiolipin antibodies occur slightly less frequently and are also detected by ELISA. Although the lupus anticoagulant is associated with thrombosis, the mechanism(s) whereby thrombosis occurs remains unclear. It has been proposed that there might be an interaction with the vasculature, thereby altering prostaglandin release. There may be activation of platelets and changes in prostaglandin metabolism, or the antibodies block protein C, or the activated protein C pathway, or alter phospholipid interactions with activated factor V.[306] It has also been proposed that there may be hyperactivity of the fibrinolytic system and increased levels of plasminogen activation inhibitor.[307] Despite many proposed mechanisms, to date there remains no consensus on the precise mechanism(s) of action of lupus anticoagulants.[308,309]

The clinical sub-classification of types of thrombosis and lupus anticoagulant and anticardiolipin antibody patients into groups may be important for choosing therapy.[272,273,274,303] Patients can generally be divided into one of six clinical subgroups. Type I syndrome includes deep venous thrombosis of the upper and lower extremities, inferior vena cava, hepatic, portal, and renal veins, and pulmonary embolus. Type II syndrome includes patients with arterial thrombosis including the coronary arteries, peripheral (extremity) arteries, extracranial carotid arteries and aorta. Type III syndrome includes patients with retinal or cerebral vascular thrombosis/ischemia, including those with transient cerebral ischemia (TIAs). Several neurologic syndromes may be manifested including transient cerebral ischemic attacks, migraine headaches, and optic neuritis.[291] Type IV syndrome includes patients with combinations of the aforementioned types of thrombosis. Like anticardiolipin antibodies and other antiphospholipid subgroups, the lupus anticoagulant has been associated with a recurrent miscarriage syndrome; this is Type V. Abortion occurs frequently in the first, and less frequently in the second or third trimester. Placental vasculitis and vascular thrombosis may be apparent, and there may occasionally be an associated maternal thrombocytopenia.[14,102,268,286,310] Type VI patients are those harboring LA with no apparent disease, including thrombosis.

Although patients with lupus anticoagulant thrombosis syndrome can be classified similar to those with anticardiolipin thrombosis syndrome, most patients with *primary* lupus anticoagulant thrombosis syndrome will fit into Type I. In secondary lupus anticoagulant thrombosis syndrome, however, there will be more patients falling into Types II, III and V than is seen in the primary syndrome.[274,308]

The lupus inhibitor usually persists in patients with primary antiphospholipid thrombosis syndrome, although it may sometimes disappear spontaneously. In the secondary lupus anticoagulant thrombosis antiphospholipid syndrome treatment of the underlying autoimmune disorder frequently results in reduction or disappearance of inhibitor activity. Corticosteroids may have a suppressive effect on the titer of the lupus anticoagulant, and to a lesser degree on anticardiolipin antibodies, but they do not appear to decrease thrombotic risk. Thus, there is no role for immunosuppressive therapy, including steroids, cyclophosphamide or azathioprine, in patients with the primary lupus anticoagulant thrombosis syndrome. When steroids or other immunosuppressive therapy is warranted in the patient with an autoimmune disease and lupus anticoagulant thrombosis syndrome, the immunosuppression, while perhaps benefiting the underlying autoimmune disorder, will generally not alleviate propensity to thrombosis. Discovery of a lupus anticoagulant, in the absence of underlying disease, and without evidence of thrombosis (Type VI) does not necessarily require treatment, but current evidence suggests these individuals to have about a 40% chance of eventually suffering a thrombotic event over a three year follow-up period. Thus, the decision to anticoagulate an asymptomatic patient with the lupus anticoagulant requires individualization and judgment, as no clear guidelines yet exist. However, patients with the lupus anticoagulant or anticardiolipin antibodies and a history of thrombosis need to be on long-term anticoagulant therapy. If untreated, there is a high incidence of thromboembolic recurrence.[272,273,274,311,312] Patients with deep venous thrombosis or arterial thrombosis are generally best managed with long-term low-molecular weight heparin (LMWH) therapy, as they are notoriously resistant to warfarin therapy (≈50%–65% of patients with antiphospholipid thrombosis syndrome eventually fail warfarin therapy).[274,313,314] Over the past twenty-four months, we have assessed 111 patients with thrombosis and antiphospholipid syndrome (exclusive of recurrent miscarriage patients); of these, 59 patients were referred because of recurrent thrombosis on adequate doses of warfarin and on evaluation were found to harbor antiphospholipid antibodies or were known antiphospholipid thrombosis syndrome patients and gave a history of recurrence on adequate doses of warfarin. The failure rate to warfarin in this group was 59/111 patients or 53%. In contrast, less than 2% of patients will fail fixed low-dose unfractionated porcine mucosal heparin and we have not yet seen a DVT failure to LMWH therapy (dalteparin) in patients with antiphospholipid syndrome. After patients with DVT/PE are stable for a period of time on LMW heparin, consideration of changing to long-term clopidogrel may be entertained, as this agent has been effective in stable patients not failing LMW heparin. Patients with Type II thrombosis (coronary artery, large peripheral arteries) are successfully treated with LMWH. Like those with Type I, if the patient remains free of thrombotic events for a long period, clopidogrel may be successfully substituted, particularly if osteoporosis becomes a consideration. In patients with retinal or cerebral vascular thrombosis (Type III) fixed dose long-term low-molecular weight heparin plus clopidogrel for intracranial/cerebral vascular thrombosis is usually effective. If the patient remains symptom free for 6–12 months, consideration of stopping the LMW heparin and continuing with clopidogrel may be reasonable. Clopidogrel at 75 mg/day is usually effective for retinal vascular thrombosis and if failure occurs, LMWH is added to the clopidogrel therapy. In those with mixtures of thrombotic sites (Type IV) therapy is individualized based on predominant sites and severity of thrombosis.[272,273,274,310] The recurrent miscarriage syndrome (RMS) (Type V) is successfully treated, allowing full-term delivery, with initiation of low-dose ASA at 81 mg/day) preconception and the addition of fixed low-dose UFH at 5,000 units every 12 hours, both used to term. Using this regimen, our population of recurrent miscarriage syndrome patients with antiphospholipid syndrome have experienced a 97% pregnancy success outcome.[14,102,310] There is little or no role for prednisone in recurrent miscarriage syndrome due to the lupus anticoagulant if there is no underlying autoimmune disease.

Anticardiolipin antibodies, "subgroup" antibodies and thrombosis

Interest in antiphospholipids began with discovery of the Lupus Anticoagulant in about 10% of patients with systemic lupus in 1952[276] and shortly thereafter, it was recognized that presence of the lupus anticoagulant was associated with thrombosis, instead of bleeding.[315] It was also soon recognized that many patients without autoimmune disorders harbored lupus anticoagulants and these antiphospholipid antibodies have now been reported in many conditions including malignancy, immune thrombocytopenia purpura, leukemias, infections, in individuals ingesting chlorpromazine, dilantin, Fansidar, hydralazine, quinidine, cocaine, interferon or procainamide (Secondary Syndrome), and in many otherwise normal individuals (Primary Syndrome).[274,297,316,317,318,319,320] Because of a noted association between lupus, a biological false positive test for syphilis, and the presence of the lupus anticoagulant, Harris and coworkers in 1983 devised a new test for antiphospholipids using cardiolipin.[321] This, and subsequent modifications have now become known as the anticardiolipin antibody test; generally, IgG, IgA and IgM anticardiolipin idiotypes are currently assessed.[322] Shortly after development of the anticardiolipin antibody assay, it became apparent that these antibodies were not limited to the lupus patient population, but were found in non-lupus patients as well. Of particular importance, these anticardiolipin antibodies are associated with (1) thrombosis and thromboembolus of both arterial and venous systems[274,275,308,323,324,325] (2) recurrent miscarriage syndrome,[14,102,274,310,326,327] and (3) thrombocytopenia in descending order of prevalence.[328,329] More recently, it has become apparent that antibodies (all three idiotypes: IgG, IgA, and IgM) to B-2-GP-I, phosphatidylserine, phosphatidylethanolamine, phosphatidylglycerol, phosphatidylinositol, annexin-V or phosphatidylcholine are independent risk factors for thrombosis of all types (Types I–V).[274,330] Although there is an association between the lupus anticoagulant and anticardiolipin antibodies and an association between lupus anticoagulants and the aforementioned syndromes, it has become clear that lupus anticoagulants, anticardiolipin antibodies and antibodies to B-2-GP-I, phosphatidylserine, phosphatidylethanolamine, phosphatidylglycerol, phosphatidylinositol, phosphatidylcholine or annexin-V are separate entities; most individuals with anticardiolipin antibodies do not have a lupus anticoagulant and most with the lupus anticoagulant do not have anticardiolipin antibodies.[331] However, many with subgroups harbor anticardiolipin antibodies, but 10% to 20% of patients demonstrate discordance[332] and subgroups are present in the absence of positive ELISA assays for anticardiolipin antibodies or Lupus anticoagulant. In our experience, discordance is noted in about the same percentages. In particular, in patients with Type I about 7% are discordant, in Type II 14% are discordant, in Type III 15% are discordant and in Type V, 22% are discordant.[274,333] Thus, when suspecting antiphospholipid syndrome in a patient with thrombosis of any type and negative lupus anticoagulant assays and negative anticardiolipin assays, the presence of isolated antibodies to B-2-GP-I, phosphatidylserine, phosphatidylethanolamine, phosphatidylglycerol, phosphatidylinositol, annexin-V or phosphatidylcholine should be suspected and tested for.[274,330]

Regarding the primary antiphospholipid thrombosis syndrome, the anticardiolipin thrombosis syndrome is at least five-fold more common than is the lupus anticoagulant thrombosis syndrome.[272,274,275] Other differences between lupus anticoagulants and anticardiolipin antibodies include not only (1) differing clinical presentations, but also (2) the noting that anticardiolipins are usually, but not always, dependent upon a cofactor, Beta-2-Glycoprotein I (apolipoprotein H) in-vitro, whereas in-vitro lupus anticoagulant activity appears independent of Beta-2-glycoprotein I, (3) anticardiolipin antibodies and lupus anticoagulants have different isoelectric points on chromatofocusing separation, (4) both appear to be directed against different combinations of phospholipid moieties and complexes and (5) purified anticardiolipin antibodies do not generally prolong any of the phospholipid-dependent coagulation test, such as the aPTT, dRVVT, PNP, or KCT unless there is concomitant presence of a lupus anticoagulant.[334,335]

Initially, it was assumed that only IgG anticardiolipin antibody was associated with thrombosis however, it is now clear that IgA and IgM anticardiolipin antibodies are also associated with thrombosis.[274] The presence of any one anticardiolipin antibody, a combination of two or indeed, all three together may be associated with thrombosis and thromboembolus.[274,336] Also, although different types of thrombosis occur, there is no apparent association between the type of thrombotic event and the type or titer of anticardiolipin antibody present.[272,273,274] The mechanism of action of anticardiolipin antibodies, or subgroups, in causing thrombosis is unknown, but several plausible theories have been proposed. Anticardiolipin antibodies have affinity for important phospholipids involved at many points in the hemostasis system; they are directed primarily against phosphatidylserine and phosphatidylinositol, but not phosphatidylcholine, another important phospholipid in hemostasis.[274,337] The proposed mechanisms of action of anticardiolipin antibodies in interfering with hemostasis to induce thrombosis include (1) interference with endothelial release of prostacyclin[338] (2) interference with activation, via thrombomodulin, of Protein C activation or interference with Protein S activity as a cofactor for Protein C[339] (3) interference with antithrombin activity[340] (4) by interaction with platelet membrane phospholipids, leading to platelet activation[341] (5) by interference of prekallikrein activation to kallikrein,[342] (6) by interference with endothelial plasminogen activator release.[343] or (7) by interference with the APC system.[344] All these components of normal hemostasis are dependent upon phospholipid, except possibly antithrombin activity.

Anticardiolipins and venous/arterial thrombosis

Anticardiolipin antibodies are associated with many types of venous thrombotic problems including deep venous thrombosis of the upper and lower extremities, pulmonary embolus, intracranial veins, inferior and superior vena cava, hepatic vein (Budd-Chiari syndrome),[273,274,275,345] portal vein, renal vein and retinal veins.[346,347,348] Arterial thrombotic sites associated with anticardiolipin antibodies have included the coronary arteries, carotid arteries, cerebral arteries, retinal arteries, subclavian and/or axillary artery (aortic arch syndrome)[349] brachial arteries, mesenteric arteries,[350] peripheral (extremity) arteries, and both proximal and distal aorta.[351,352,353]

Anticardiolipins and cardiac disease

In an early study, it was found that 33% of coronary artery bypass (CABG) patients suffering late graft occlusion (as determined by coronary angiography 12 months post coronary artery bypass graft surgery) had preoperative anticardiolipin antibody levels over 2 standard deviations above control values, strongly suggesting an association between graft occlusion and antiphospholipid antibodies. In 80% of patients the anticardiolipin antibody levels rose to levels greater than the preoperative levels at some point in time. The observed increase in anticardiolipin antibody levels was greater in patients having suffered an acute myocardial infarction than those who had not.[274,354,355] Another study has revealed over 20% of young (less than 45 years of age) survivors of acute myocardial infarction to harbor anticardiolipin antibodies; in those surviving, 61% having these antibodies experienced a later thromboembolic event.[356] No association was found between the presence of anticardiolipin antibodies and antinuclear antibody or other clinical features which would have suggested the presence of systemic lupus erythematosus. Anticardiolipin antibodies are suggested as an indicator of increased risk for post-myocardial infarction thrombotic events and an indication for prophylactic anticoagulation or antiplatelet therapy.[356] Despite continuous prophylactic treatment with aspirin and warfarin, acute myocardial infarction has been documented in a patient with previously documented normal coronary arteries, treated successfully with tissue plasminogen activator.[357] In analyzing the relative frequency of acute myocardial infarction in patients with anticardiolipin antibodies, a study published in 1989 noted myocardial infarction in only 5 of 70 patients (significantly fewer than those experiencing cerebral arterial thromboses).[358] Another study has revealed a very high percentage of young individuals (those under 50 years of age) who suffer acute myocardial infarction, or who experience re-stenosis after coronary angioplasty (PTCA) or coronary artery bypass (CABG) harbor anticardiolipin antibodies.[359] Thus, anticardiolipin antibodies appear to play a significant and probable major role in premature/precocious coronary artery disease; this may approach almost 70% of young age patients with coronary artery disease.[294,359]

Anticardiolipin antibodies are also associated with cardiac valvular abnormalities. Cardiac disease in patients with systemic lupus erythematosus has been associated with valvular vegetations, regurgitation and stenosis. Almost 89 percent of patients with systemic lupus erythematosus and valvular disease have been found to have antiphospholipid antibodies, compared to only 44% of patients without valvular involvement. Although only 18% of all patients with lupus have valvular disease, cardiac valvular abnormalities are found in 36% of patients with the primary antiphospholipid syndrome. The valvular abnormalities of the primary antiphospholipid syndrome are characterized by significant, irregular thickening of the mitral and aortic valves, valvular regurgitation (but not stenosis), the potential for severe hemodynamic compromise and, surprisingly, an absence of valvular thrombi.[360] Patients with concomitant systemic lupus erythematosus and antiphospholipid antibodies have been found to have aortic and mitral valvulitis, including typical Libman-Sacks verrucous endocarditis.[361,362] Additionally, in patients with systemic lupus erythematosus, the presence of antiphospholipid antibodies is associated with isolated left ventricular dysfunction.[363] An isolated instance has been reported of an intracardiac mass in the right ventricle, presumably resulting from the combined effects of abnormal intracardiac flow resulting from anomalous muscle bundles combined with enhanced thrombogenesis associated with antiphospholipid antibodies.[364] In view of the high incidence of valvular abnormalities in patients with antiphospholipid antibodies and arterial thromboembolism, Doppler-echocardiography should routinely be considered.[365]

Anticardiolipins and cutaneous manifestations

Anticardiolipin antibodies are associated with livido reticularis, an unusual manifestation of cutaneous vascular stasis characterized by a distinctive pattern of cyanosis.[274,323,366,367] This cutaneous finding has been associated with recurrent arterial and venous thromboses, valvular abnormalities and cerebrovascular thromboses with concomitant essential hypertension ("Sneddon's syndrome").[274,323] Other cutaneous manifestations include a syndrome of recurrent deep venous thrombosis, necrotizing purpura, and stasis ulcers of the ankles.[274,323,366,367] Skin lesions of Dego's disease (a rare multisystem vasculopathy), characterized pathologically by cutaneous collagen necrosis, atrophy of the epidermis with an absence of inflammatory cells have been linked to the other consequences of the disease such as cerebral and bowel infarction and anticardiolipin antibodies or a lupus anticoagulant.[368] Vascular thromboses may be manifest as ischemia or necrosis of entire extremities as demonstrated in association with disseminated intravascular coagulation[369] with resultant cutaneous necrosis or more patchy, widespread, demarcated areas of cutaneous necrosis, manifest by areas of painful purpura and necrosis with underlying dermal necrosis.[370] Other common cutaneous manifestations include livido vasculitis/reticularis, unfading acral microlivido, peripheral gangrene, necrotizing purpura, hemorrhage (ecchymosis and hematoma formation),[370] and crusted ulcers about the nail beds.[371]

Anticardiolipins and neurologic syndromes

The neurological syndromes associated with anticardiolipin antibodies include transient cerebral ischemic attacks (TIAs), small stroke syndrome, arterial and venous retinal occlusive disease, cerebral arterial and venous thrombosis, migraine headaches, Dego's disease, Sneddon's syndrome,[274,362] Guillain-Barré syndrome,[363] chorea, seizures and optic neuritis.[368,374,375] The central nervous system manifestations of systemic lupus erythematosus are commonly, but not always, associated with positive antiphospholipid antibodies.[376,377] While it is clear that lupus patients with antiphospholipid antibodies may experience cerebrovascular thromboses, cerebral ischemia and infarction, these events occur more commonly in patients with the primary anticardiolipin thrombosis syndrome and absence of an underlying autoimmune disease. Multiple cerebral infarctions in patients with antiphospholipid antibodies may result in dementia.[378]

The primary phospholipid syndrome is often present in patients with a constellation of concomitant arterial occlusions, strokes, transient ischemic attacks leading to multiple infarct dementia, deep venous thrombosis associated with pulmonary embolization and resultant pulmonary hypertension, recurrent miscarriage, thrombocytopenia, positive Coomb's test and chorea.[291,379] The primary distinction between patients with primary phospholipid syndrome and Sneddon's syndrome is the involvement of large vessels in the former and exclusively medium sized arteries in the latter.[372,380,381] Patients with antiphospholipid antibodies are more likely to experience cerebral ischemic or thrombotic events when also harboring primary hypertension or coronary disease respectively.[382] Anticardiolipin antibodies and recurrent stroke have also been associated with thymoma.[383] Recent studies have found that antiphospholipid antibodies, including subgroups, particularly antiphosphatidyl serine, are important etiological factors. This is of major importance with respect to appropriate antithrombotic therapy and these patients cannot be treated with simple antiplatelet therapy or warfarin therapy with success, as they require LMWH or UFH with or without an antiplatelet agent for adequate protection against recurrence. One recent study found that 46% of young age individuals (age ≤50) with cerebral ischemic events harbored antiphospholipid antibodies;[384] another found 44% of young age individuals (age ≤51) to have antiphospholipid antibodies,[385] but another study found only 18% of patients under age 44 to harbor antiphospholipid antibodies.[386] Subgroups only of antiphospholipid antibodies have been noted in up to 23% of young age patients with cerebral thrombotic events; thus it is of extreme importance to consider these.[385] Antiphospholipid antibodies are also associated with cerebral venous events.[387] Another recent study noted 65% of patients with cerebrovascular thrombosis under the age of 60 to harbor antiphospholipid antibodies and in the same study, 28% of patients with only TIAs harbored antiphospholipid antibodies.[388] Studies have also noted that those with antiphospholipid antibodies tend to have the cerebrovascular occlusive/ischemic event about a decade earlier than those having cerebrovascular thrombotic or ischemic events in the absence of antiphospholipid antibodies.[389] Thus, it is clear that antiphospholipid antibodies are important in the etiology of cerebrovascular ischemic events.[274,291,390] The primary importance of these findings is in making an appropriate diagnosis so that effective therapy may be instituted (LMWH or UFH) to afford effectual secondary prevention. The complicated topic of neurological manifestations in APL-T syndromes has recently been reviewed.[291,390]

Anticardiolipins and autoimmune collagen disease

While much of the initial research and many of the first descriptions of antiphospholipid antibodies resulted from investigation of the lupus anticoagulant in populations with systemic lupus, it is now well established that antiphospholipid antibodies occur in patients without systemic lupus erythematosus much more frequently than in those with lupus or other autoimmune disorders. In patients with lupus, the presence of livido reticularis may represent an important cutaneous marker for the presence, or the later development of antiphospholipid antibodies.[366]Antiphospholipid antibodies may occur with increased frequency in individuals with other autoimmune disorders and have been reported in patients with mixed connective tissue disease, rheumatoid arthritis,[370] Sjogren's syndrome,[362] Behcet's syndrome (possible role in the pathogenesis of the multisystem manifestations of the syndrome)[391] and autoimmune thrombocytopenic purpura.[328] Most patients with anticardiolipin antibody thrombosis syndrome, however, have a *primary* syndrome with no underlying autoimmune disorder. Less than 10% of patients with thrombosis and antiphospholipid antibodies have, or will ever develop, an autoimmune disease such as systemic lupus, rheumatoid arthritis, mixed connective disease or related syndrome. The clinical manifestations can be varied and substantial.[290,381]

Anticardiolipins and obstetric syndromes

Anticardiolipin antibodies are associated with a high incidence of recurrent miscarriage; the characteristics of this syndrome are (1) frequent abortion in the first trimester due to placental thrombosis/vasculitis (2) recurrent fetal loss in the second and third trimesters, also due to placental thrombosis/vasculitis, and (3) maternal thrombocytopenia in descending order of prevalence.[274] This is especially likely in the presence of moderate or high IgG anticardiolipin levels.[392] This syndrome has been successfully treated to normal term by institution of aspirin, low-dose heparin, or plasma exchange.[14,102,274,327,392,393,394,395] Women harboring anticardiolipin antibodies have about a 50%–75% chance of fetal loss and successful anticoagulant therapy can increase the chances of normal term delivery to about 97%.[14,102,274,310]

Optimal therapy for the recurrent miscarriage syndrome (RMS) has not yet been defined but we have noted a 97% normal delivery outcome in 123 patients with recurrent miscarriage syndrome treated with preconception ASA at 81 mg/day with the immediate post-conception addition of UFH at 5,000 units q 12 hours and both agents used to term.[14,102,274] A variety of heparin doses have been used with significant success in carrying patients to term and most of these have been in combination with aspirin therapy. It is clear that in the primary antiphospholipid syndrome (absence of an underlying autoimmune disorder such as SLE), the use of corticosteroids or other immunosuppressive therapy is not warranted and only enhances side effects. However, immunosuppressive therapy may be useful in those with anticardiolipin syndrome and lupus. Also, a variety of vigorous antibody removing/eradicating modes of therapy have been attempted with varying degrees of success including plasmapheresis, plasma exchange, immunoadsorption column treatment, and intravenous immunoglobulin (IVIG). Based upon available reports and our own experience, the use of low-dose aspirin (about 81 mg per day) in combination with low-dose porcine mucosal heparin (5,000 units subcutaneously q 12 or Dalteparin at 5,000 units/24 hours) appears to consistently be the most effective therapy for term delivery at the present time. Our approach in treating the RMS is to start a patient on low-dose aspirin (81 mg/day) at the time a diagnosis of RMS is made: the demonstration of anticardiolipin antibody, lupus anticoagulant or antiphospholipid subgroups (seen in 22% of our patients with recurrent miscarriage syndrome and antiphospholipid antibodies) and a history of recurrent abortion.[14,100,102,274] Subgroup analysis, including anti-annexin-V antibodies, is particularly important in recurrent miscarriage syndrome.[14,102,274] As soon as pregnancy is achieved, fixed low-dose porcine mucosal heparin

(5,000 units every 12 hours) or Dalteparin (5,000 units/24 hours, subcutaneously) is added to the aspirin and used to term.[14,102] The low-dose heparin/LMW heparin need not be stopped during delivery as it is extremely unlikely to be associated with significant hemorrhage and affords peripartum and postpartum protection against thrombosis and thromboembolic disease. Thus far our success rate using this regimen has been 97%.[14,102] LMWH may also be used, but in view of reported cases of perispinal/epidural bleeding with epidural anesthetics reported with enoxaparin, antiphospholipid antibody patients on the LMWH, enoxaparin, during pregnancy should be changed to UFH during the last trimester.

The incidence of antiphospholipid antibodies in recurrent miscarriage syndrome has been studied by a number of groups. Most studies, however, have not utilized control pregnant populations. Lin studied a population of 245 women with RMS and found 13.5% to have anticardiolipin antibodies.[396] Parazzini studied 220 patients with $\geq$2 spontaneous abortions and found 19% to harbor anticardiolipin antibodies.[387] Grandone[388] assessed 32 patients with RMS and found 28% to have ACLAs and Birdsall[389] studied 81 patients with RMS, finding 41% to harbor ACLAs. Maclean assessed 243 patients with RMS ($\geq$2 spontaneous ABs) and found 17% to have ACLAs, 7% to have LAs, and 2% to harbor both.[400] Howard assessed 29 non-lupus patients with RMS and found 48% to have LAs.[401] Taylor,[402] in a study of 189 women with unexplained miscarriage found lupus anticoagulants in 7% and anticardiolipin antibodies in 15%. The only two studies assessing matched controls were those of Parke,[393] who found 7% of pregnant women without RMS and 16% of those with RMS to have antiphospholipid antibodies and Parazzini,[387] who found an incidence of 3% ACLAs in control women. Thus, it appears a small population of normal pregnant females without symptoms of RMS will also harbor antiphospholipid antibodies. This, of course raises the question of treatment in the pregnant female harboring antiphospholipid antibodies but no prior history of spontaneous miscarriage; at present no data provide adequate direction for this dilemma.

Anticardiolipin antibodies are also associated with a peculiar postpartum syndrome of spiking fevers, pleuritic chest pain, dyspnea and pleural effusion, patchy pulmonary infiltrates, cardiomyopathy, and ventricular arrhythmias. This syndrome characteristically occurs two to ten days postpartum.[404] Since the majority of patients with postpartum syndrome recover spontaneously, most require no therapy other than symptomatic treatment. It is unclear if any type of antithrombotic therapy is warranted in this population since recovery almost always occurs spontaneously.

Miscellaneous disorders and anticardiolipin thrombosis syndrome

Anticardiolipin antibodies have recently been reported in patients with human immunodeficiency virus infection, with or without immune thrombocytopenic purpura.[405] Particularly elevated are IgG isotypes, however, there is no correlation between antiphospholipid antibody level and disease progression or the incidence of thrombosis, despite a correlation with the titer and presence of thrombocytopenia.[405,406,407,408] Elevations of one or more of the anticardiolipin isotypes has been observed following a number of acute infections, including ornithosis, Mycoplasma infection, adenovirus infection, rubella, varicella, mumps, malaria, and Lyme disease.[409] Abnormalities of the activated partial thromboplastin time in patients with hepatic cirrhosis have recently been attributed to the presence of antiphospholipid antibodies.[410] Drugs associated with the development of anticardiolipin antibodies include phenytoin,[411] quinidine, Fansidar, hydralazine, procainamide, cocaine, interferon and phenothiazines (with a predisposition to thrombosis- which does occur in drug-associated antiphospholipid syndrome).[272,273,274,412] The anticardiolipin thrombosis syndrome can be divided into those which are primary and those which are secondary. Primary anticardiolipin thrombosis syndrome is much more common and consists of patients with anticardiolipin antibody and thrombosis who harbor no other underlying disease; secondary anticardiolipin thrombosis syndrome consists of those patients with anticardiolipin antibody and thrombosis with an underlying disease, such as lupus or other autoimmune disorder, malignancy, infection, inflammation or ingestion of drugs inducing an anticardiolipin antibody.

Classification of antiphospholipid thrombosis syndromes

The finding of anticardiolipin antibodies, subgroups of antiphospholipid antibodies or lupus anticoagulants in association with thrombosis is referred to as the Antiphospholipid Thrombosis Syndrome. Patients with LA don't tend to have thromboses that are as predictable as those with ACLA or the subgroups of antibodies to B-2-GP-1, phosphatidylserine, phosphatidylethanolamine, phosphatidylglycerol, phosphatidylinositol, phosphatidylcholine or annexin-V; however, management principles, as far as is currently known, apply equally to all.[274,330]

The antiphospholipid thrombosis syndrome, associated with anticardiolipin or subgroup antibodies, can be divided into one of *six* subgroups; *Type I* syndrome comprises patients with deep venous thrombosis and pulmonary embolus, *Type II* syndrome comprises patients with coronary artery or peripheral arterial (including aorta and carotid artery) thrombosis, *Type III* syndrome comprises patients with retinal or cerebrovascular (intracranial) thrombosis and *Type IV* patients are those with admixtures of the first three types. Type IV patients are uncommon, with most patients fitting into one of the first three types. *Type V* patients are those with RMS and *Type VI* patients are those harboring antiphospholipid syndromes without any (as yet) clinical expression, including thrombosis. There is little overlap (about 10% or less) between these sub-types and

Table 5.3 Antiphospholipid antibodies: Syndromes of thrombosis.

Type I Syndrome
Deep vein thrombosis/Pulmonary embolus
Other large vein thrombosis
Type II Syndrome
Coronary artery thrombosis
Peripheral artery thrombosis
Aortic thrombosis
Carotid artery thrombosis (Extracranial)
Type III Syndrome
Retinal vascular thrombosis
Cerebrovascular thrombosis
Transient cerebral ischemic attack (TIA)
Type IV Syndrome
Mixtures of all syndrome types
(these are rare)
Type V Syndrome
Recurrent miscarriage syndrome
Placental vascular thrombosis
Maternal thrombocytopenia (rare)
Type VI Syndrome
APLS with no apparent clinical disorders

patients usually conveniently fit into only one of these clinical types. The types of antiphospholipid and thrombosis syndromes associated with anticardiolipin antibodies are summarized in Table 5.3.[269,271,272,333] Although there appears to be no correlation with the type, or titer, of anticardiolipin antibody and type of syndrome (I through VI), the sub-classification of thrombosis and anticardiolipin antibody patients into these groups is important from the therapy standpoint.[269,271,274,333] Type I patients are best managed by use of long-term fixed-dose LMWH or fixed-dose subcutaneous UFH therapy. If the patient remains thrombus free for 6–12 months or if osteoporosis becomes a consideration, long-term clopidogrel may eventually be substituted for the heparin. Type II patients are also best managed by long-term fixed-dose LMWH (about 5,000 units/24 hours) or fixed-dose subcutaneous UFH therapy (usually 5,000 units every 12 hours) and after long-term stability clopidogrel may be an alternative, and Type III patients, those with cerebrovascular disease or retinal vascular disease should be treated with fixed dose long-term low-molecular weight heparin plus clopidogrel for intracranial/cerebral vessel thrombosis/TIA; long-term stability can usually be achieved by stopping the heparin/LMW heparin and continuing clopidogrel. Clopidogrel (at 75 mg/day) is usually effective for retinal vascular thrombosis and if failure occurs, LMWH is added to the clopidogrel therapy. Therapy of Type IV depends upon types and sites of thrombosis present.[269,271,274,333] Patients with Type V, Recurrent miscarriage syndrome, are best treated with pre-conception initiation of low-dose ASA (81 mg/day) as soon as the diagnosis is made and then started on fixed low-dose porcine mucosal heparin (5,000 units, subcutaneously every 12 hours) or Dalteparin (at 5,000 units subcutaneously every 24 hours) immediately post-conception, with both drugs being used to term delivery.[14,102] Patients with Type V syndrome are usually encouraged to stop the heparin following delivery (depending upon the individual clinical situation), but to continue on long-term low-dose ASA indefinitely. The decision to continue ASA after delivery in these patients is empirical, but might ward off other minor thrombotic manifestations of antiphospholipid syndrome. There are no guidelines available to know how to best treat these patients following delivery, as most (<10%) will not develop a non-placental thrombosis.

Obviously, patients with thrombosis and anticardiolipin antibodies require long-term antithrombotic therapy and treatment should only be stopped if the anticardiolipin antibody is persistently absent for at least six months before considering cessation of antithrombotic therapy.[269,271,274,333] After persistent absence of their antiphospholipid antibody for at least six months, we usually discuss the risks and benefits of continuing antithrombotic therapy and encourage patients to take one low-dose ASA (81 mg/day) or long-term clopidogrel (depending upon the seriousness of the initial thrombotic event(s)), in hopes the antibody and thrombosis will not return. Obviously, patients with antiphospholipid syndrome who are going to be on long-term fixed low-dose UFH or LMWH therapy should have initial bone density studies and should be cautioned about heparin-induced thrombocytopenia, mild alopecia, mild allergic reactions, osteoporosis, benign transaminasemia (seen in about 5% treated with UFH and in about 10% treated with LMWH) and the development of benign eosinophilia.[413,414] Patients should be monitored with weekly heparin levels (anti-Xa method) and CBC/platelet counts for the first month of therapy and monthly thereafter; this also applies to patients with Type V syndrome. Since most patients with thrombosis and antiphospholipid antibodies fail warfarin therapy, the clinician should always suspect and search for antiphospholipid antibodies when evaluating a patient for warfarin failure.[274]

Clinical presentations

It is becoming increasingly clear with increased experience in utilizing the anticardiolipin assay in clinical practice, primary antiphospholipid syndromes are much more common than suspected. Diagnostic evaluation of the patient to determine the etiology of a wide variety of thrombotic problems must now include assays for anticardiolipin antibodies, lupus anticoagulants and, when indicated, subgroups. Although it is appropriate to suspect antiphospholipid antibodies in virtually any clinical problem complicated by thrombosis, certain presentations are stronger indicators than others.

In patients with Type I disease, a strong index of suspicion is appropriate, particularly in individuals with deep venous thrombosis unaccompanied by another potential risk factor, such as exogenous estrogen administration, surgery, prolonged immobility, malignancy or another hypercoagulable state. Likewise, patients may present with recurrent deep venous thrombosis with or without a significant clinical risk factor. As is frequently observed in clinical practice, patients may only be referred for evaluation after a second episode of thrombosis. The initial thrombotic event may have appeared to result from a recognizable predisposing problem, only later proven to be present concomitantly with anticardiolipin antibodies. Although the severity or location (iliofemoral, popliteal calf vein or other sites) of thrombosis or the presence of pulmonary embolization does not correlate with the presence of anticardiolipin antibodies, recurrent thromboembolic events or multiple sites of thrombosis should strongly suggest an anticardiolipin antibody. Another very common presentation is a patient referred because of failure (re-thrombosis) while on warfarin therapy. Failure to apparently adequate doses of warfarin should immediately alert the physician to strongly consider APL-T syndrome.

Patients with Type II disease frequently present with catastrophic illness. A history of myocardial infarction at a young age, recurrent myocardial infarction, early graft occlusion following coronary artery bypass graft surgery and early re-occlusion post transluminal angioplasty is typical. Aorta, subclavian, mesenteric, femoral or other large vessel thrombosis may present with complete occlusion and acute symptoms of ischemia and threatened limb loss. Emergent diagnosis and appropriate therapy may decrease unnecessary morbidity and be life-saving.

Type III patients may be referred for a variety of problems. Acute loss or distortion of vision may lead to ophthalmologic confirmation of retinal arterial or venous thrombosis. Focal neurologic symptoms may suggest the presence of cerebrovascular thrombosis resulting in symptoms of stroke or transient ischemic attack. Alternatively, multiple infarct dementia may present more gradually, without clearly defined acute ischemic events. Early diagnosis is critical in Type III patients, since failure to treat may result in irreversible cerebral or retinal injury.

Type IV patients, having a mixture of the aforementioned types are extremely rare and comprise only about ten percent of patients with anticardiolipin thrombosis syndrome. A strong index of suspicion is required for the diagnosis, and therapy must be individualized depending upon the particular combination of thromboses.

Table 5.4 Drugs associated with APLS.

Phenytoin
Fansidar
Quinidine
Quinine
Hydralazine
Procainamide
Phenothiazines
Alpha-interferon
Cocaine

Type V patients are usually those with one or more spontaneous miscarriages and are most often referred by the obstetrician or high-risk reproductive experts. Most women relate a history of spontaneous miscarriage in the first trimester (most commonly the 6th to 12th week), but some also spontaneously miscarry in the second and third trimester.

Drugs associated with antiphospholipid thrombosis syndrome are listed in Table 5.4.

Prevalence of the antiphospholipid thrombosis syndrome

Unfortunately, very little information is available on prevalence of antiphospholipid antibodies, especially in asymptomatic individuals. Additionally, nothing is known about the potential propensity to develop thrombosis or other clinical manifestations when seemingly health individuals are found to harbor these antibodies. Two recent studies have addressed this issue. The first such study was the Montpellier Antiphospholipid (MAP) study[415] wherein 1014 patients (488 males and 526 females) admitted to a general internal medicine department for a variety of reasons were assessed for IgG, IgA, and IgM ACLAs. Lupus anticoagulant assays were not performed. Of the patients tested, 72 (7.1%) were positive for at least one idiotype. When assessing these 72 patients, 20 (28%) were determined to have clinical manifestations of the APL-T syndrome. Fifty-two patients, when questioned, had not yet demonstrated any manifestations of APL-T syndrome, suggesting a false positive incidence of 5.1%. However, long-term follow-up of the thus far asymptomatic patients has not occurred and a follow-up report of the MAP study will be awaited with interest. In another recent study[416] 552 healthy blood donors were screened for study; IgG and IgM idiotypes and lupus anticoagulant were assessed. It was found 6.5% (28 donors) of the population harbored IgG and 9.4% (38 donors) of the population harbored IgM ACLAs and 5 donors had both idiotypes. No donor was positive for Lupus anticoagulant. The donors were followed for twelve months; during the follow-up time, no ACLA positive patient developed a thrombotic event. However, nine ACLA positive donors had a positive family history for thrombosis and three of the ACLA positive donors had a history of unexplained miscarriage.[416] In a recent survey of 100 consecutive patients presenting with deep vein thrombosis or pulmonary embolus, 24% of patients were found to have ACLAs.[313] It is suggested that ACLAs are common in patients presenting with unexplained DVT or PE and certainly any patient presenting with unexplained DVT or PE should be evaluated for presence of antiphospholipid antibodies.

Laboratory diagnosis of antiphospholipid syndromes

Detection of anticardiolipin antibodies

The detection of anticardiolipin antibodies is straightforward and there is general agreement that solid-phase ELISA is the method of choice.[274,417,418,419] In the past, only IgG and IgA idiotypes have been assayed; however, with current recognition that IgM idiotypes, whether primary or secondary (especially drug-induced) are also associated with thrombosis, most laboratories are, or should be, assaying all three idiotypes. Thus, the appropriate assay for detecting anticardiolipins is solid-phase ELISA, measuring all three (IgG, IgA and IgM) idiotypes.[274,295,298,420]

Detection of lupus anticoagulants

In the presence of the lupus anticoagulant an abnormality exists in the phospholipid-dependent coagulation reactions including the prothrombin time, the activated partial thromboplastin time (aPTT), and the Russell's viper venom time.[273,274,278] The lupus anticoagulant is not directed against a specific factor, but to phospholipids. The inhibitor does not exert an increasing effect with prolonged incubation with normal plasma, and thus this simple screen can be used to distinguish the lupus inhibitor from inhibitors that neutralize specific clotting factors. Incubation of the patients' plasma with normal plasma does not cause a sensitivity of the partial thromboplastin time to the inhibitor's effect, and one-stage assays for factors XII, XI, IX, and VII may yield low values when the standard dilutions of test plasma are used.[278] Usually further dilution of the test plasma causes the measured level of these factors to approach the normal range; the exception occurs in rare patients with a decreased concentration of prothrombin, resulting from accelerated removal of prothrombin antigen-antibody complexes, sometimes seen in patients with systemic lupus.

Multiple lupus anticoagulant assays are currently in use. Sensitivity of the aPTT to the presence or absence of the lupus anticoagulant is highly dependent upon the reagents used. Many patients with thrombosis and the lupus anticoagulant have normal aPTT's, even with the newer allegedly more "sensitive" reagents, thus, the aPTT is *not* a reliable screening test for lupus anticoagulants and should not be used for this purpose.[273,274,278,298,299,421,422,423] When suspecting the presence of a lupus anticoagulant, a more definitive test, preferably the dRVVT, should immediately be performed regardless of the aPTT. The lupus inhibitor is identified by the ability to bind phospholipid and inhibit phospholipid-dependent coagulant reactions. The assays available are based upon the use of limiting amounts of phospholipid and therefore sensitized in platelet-poor plasma. Initially, a prothrombin time was performed with dilute tissue thromboplastin and a reduced number of platelets in the mixture; however, IgM inhibitors were missed. Subsequently, a "modified" Russell's viper venom time was developed in which the venom is diluted to give a "normal" time of 23 to 27 seconds, and the phospholipid is then diluted down to a minimal level that continues to support this range. A prolongation of this system will not correct with a mixture of patient and normal plasma; this system detects both IgG and IgM lupus anticoagulants.[300] This assay is generally known as the dilute Russell's Viper Venom Time (dRVVT) and appears the most sensitive of all assays for the lupus anticoagulant.[307] The kaolin clotting time test (KCT) has also been modified to assay for the lupus anticoagulant inhibitor. In the KCT, platelet-poor plasma is mixed with varying proportions of test plasma and normal plasma. Kaolin is added and time required for clotting is determined.[278] The KCT is then plotted against proportions of patients' plasma with normal plasma; an inhibitor is assumed to be present when a small portion of test serum, in comparison with normal serum, prolongs the assay. A kaolin activated partial thromboplastin time, with rabbit brain phospholipid in a standard and fourfold increased "high" lipid concentration to normalize or "out-inhibit" the abnormal "standard" aPTT, has also been utilized in diagnosis of the lupus inhibitor.[278] This is known as the rabbit brain neutralization procedure, and although specific (due to rabbit brain neutralization), lacks sensitivity comparable to the dRVVT. The best test to detect the lupus anticoagulant at present is the dRVVT; if this test is prolonged, the confirmation of a lupus inhibitor, by noting correction of the prolonged dRVV time by adding phospholipid in some form (unfortunately often platelet membrane-derived) is required, especially if the patient is on warfarin or heparin therapy.[274] Both heparin and warfarin are capable of also prolonging the dRVVT. Confirmation of a lupus anticoagulant in the above assays is by phospholipid neutralization (shortening) of the prolonged test.[273,274,278] As a practical matter, most clinicians and laboratories are asked to evaluate patients for the lupus anticoagulant after they have been placed on anticoagulant therapy. Both heparin and warfarin prolong most of the above tests, including the most sensitive test, the dRVVT. If the patient is on warfarin and the dRVVT is prolonged and then neutralized by appropriate phospholipid, a lupus anticoagulant is confirmed.[273,274,278] However, if the patient is on heparin and the dRVVT is prolonged, the neutralization by platelet-derived phospholipid is not confirmatory, as large amounts of platelet-derived platelet factor 4 may inhibit the heparin effect to correct the test. For example, a commercially available platelet extract for the platelet neutralization procedure was found to contain about 100 International Units per ml of platelet factor 4 and normal male freeze-thaw platelet extract, commonly prepared for "platelet or phospholipid neutralization procedures" in the clinical laboratory, contains about 95 International Units per ml of platelet factor 4, enough to neutralize heparin and shorten a prolonged clotting test and render a false positive result in the dRVVT or platelet neutralization procedure for a lupus anticoagulant.[273,274,278,413] As a practical matter, therefore, use of the dRVVT offers the most sensitive assay for detection of a lupus anticoagulant and neutralization of this test by a non-platelet-derived phospholipid, in particular cephalin (Bell-Alton extract),[263] which contains no platelet factor 4, makes this test the most specific as well.

Due to marked heterogeneity of antiphospholipid antibodies especially in the secondary antiphospholipid syndromes, there is a correlation between elevated anticardiolipin antibodies and the lupus anticoagulant in secondary APL-T syndromes. However, the lupus anticoagulant and anticardiolipin antibodies are two separate entities, and most of the time one occurs without the other being present, especially in the primary antiphospholipid thrombosis syndromes.[272,274] The lupus anticoagulant has a stronger association with binding phospholipids of a hexagonal composition such as phosphatidylcholine, or after membrane damage by infection, IL-1, or other mechanisms leading to change from the lamellar to hexagonal form, whereas anticardiolipin antibodies have an affinity to lamellar phospholipids in a bilayer (lamellar) composition.[263]

Detection of "subtypes" of antiphospholipid antibodies

When suspecting thrombosis or recurrent miscarriage patients of harboring antiphospholipid antibodies and noting negative assays for anticardiolipin antibodies or lupus anticoagulants, the clinician should suspect discordant subgroups and order assays for anti-B-2-GP-I, and antibodies to phosphatidylserine, phosphatidylethanolamine, phosphatidylglycerol, phosphatidylinositol, annexin-V, and phosphatidylcholine. These are all available by EIA assay. It must be remembered that there is significant discordance between these subgroups and lupus anticoagulants or the three idiotypes of anticardiolipin antibodies, thus they must be recalled and tested for in the appropriate clinical situations discussed previously.[263,274,320,378]

As mentioned above, discordance will be seen in a significant number of patients. In particular, many patients will have subgroups of antiphospholipid

Table 5.5 Types of antiphospholipid antibodies.

Most common
Anticardiolipin antibodies (IgG, IgA, IgM)
Lupus anticoagulants
Hexagonal phospholipid
Subgroups
Antiphosphatidylserine (IgG, IgA, IgM)
Antiphosphatidylinositol (IgG, IgA, IgM)
Antiphosphatidylcholine (IgG, IgA, IgM)
Antiphosphatidylethanolamine (IgG, IgA, IgM)
Antiphosphatidic acid (IgG, IgA, IgM)
Antiphosphatidylglycerol (IgG, IgA, IgM)
Anti-annexin V antibody (IgG, IgA, IgM)

antibody (Beta-2-Glycoprotein-1, antiphosphatidylserine, antiphosphatidylcholine, antiphosphatidylglycerol, antiphosphatidylinositol, and antiphosphatidylethanolamine) in the absence of anticardiolipin antibodies (IgG, IgA or IgM) or Lupus Anticoagulant. Specifically, this will be seen in 7% of patients with antiphospholipid thrombosis syndrome and DVT/PE (Type I), 15% of those with coronary artery or peripheral arterial thrombosis (Type II), 15%–24% of those with cerebrovascular or retinal vascular thrombosis (Type III), and in 22% of those with recurrent miscarriage syndrome (Type V). All antiphospholipid antibodies of importance, to date, are depicted in Table 5.5. The tests at the top are ordered first and those at the bottom ordered if clinical suspicion of a subgroup is present. Figure 5.1 depicts an approach to the laboratory diagnosis of antiphospholipid thrombosis syndrome.

In summary, antiphospholipid antibodies are strongly associated with thrombosis and are the most common of the acquired blood protein defects causing thrombosis. Antiphospholipid antibodies are clearly the most common thrombophilia associated with complications of pregnancy: RMS, infertility, fetal growth retardation syndrome, and thrombosis. Although the precise mechanism(s) whereby antiphospholipid antibodies alter hemostasis to induce a hypercoagulable state remain unclear, numerous theories, as previously discussed, have been advanced. The most common thrombotic events associated with ACLAs are deep vein thrombosis and pulmonary embolus (Type I Syndrome), coronary or peripheral artery thrombosis (Type II Syndrome) or cerebrovascular/retinal vessel thrombosis (Type III Syndrome), and occasionally patients present with mixtures (Type IV Syndrome). Type V patients are those with antiphospholipid antibodies and recurrent miscarriage syndrome (RMS). It is as yet unclear how many seemingly normal individuals who may never develop manifestations of antiphospholipid

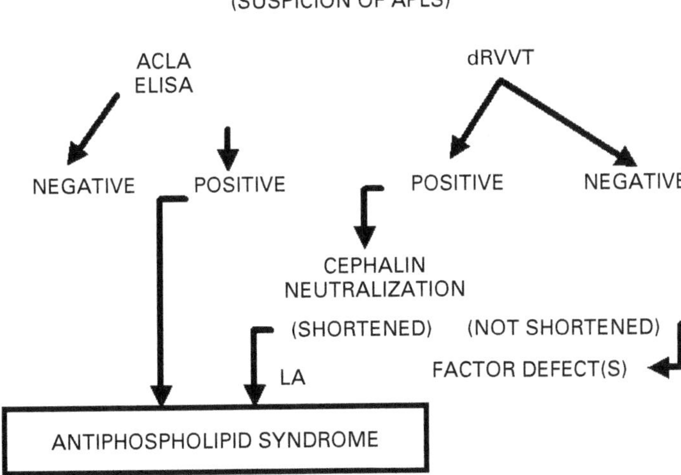

Figure 5.1 Laboratory diagnosis of APLS.

syndrome (Type VI) harbor asymptomatic antiphospholipid antibodies. The relative frequency of ACLA's in association with arterial and venous thrombosis strongly suggests that these should be looked for in any individual with unexplained thrombosis; all three idiotypes (IgG, IgA, and IgM) should be assessed. Also, the Type of syndrome (I through VI) should be defined if possible, as this may dictate both type and duration of both immediate and long-term anticoagulant therapy. Unlike those with ACLA's, patients with primary lupus anticoagulant thrombosis syndrome usually suffer venous thrombosis. Since the aPTT is unreliable in patients with lupus anticoagulant (prolonged in only about 40% to 50% of patients) and is not usually prolonged in patients with anticardiolipin antibodies, definitive tests including ELISA for ACLA, the dRVVT for lupus anticoagulant, hexagonal phospholipid neutralization procedure and B-2-GP-I (IgG, IgA and IgM) should be immediately ordered when suspecting antiphospholipid syndrome or in individuals with otherwise unexplained thrombotic or thromboembolic events. If these are negative, in the appropriate clinical setting, subgroups should also be assessed. Finally, most patients with antiphospholipid thrombosis syndrome will fail warfarin therapy and, except for retinal vascular thrombosis, may fail some types of antiplatelet therapy, thus it is of major importance to make this diagnosis in order that patients can be treated with the most effective therapy for secondary prevention – LMWH or UFH in most instances and clopidogrel in some instances.

Like other thrombophilias, antiphospholipid syndrome is strongly associated with RMS, pre-eclampsia, eclampsia, fetal growth retardation syndrome, arterial and venous thrombosis and PE. Thus, a detailed work-up and prophylactic therapy are strongly warranted. In antiphospholipid syndrome pregnancy patients, our approach is to use preconception low-dose ASA (81 mg/day) and immediately add post-conception dalteparin at 5,000 units, subcutaneously, every 24 hours. We also strongly encourage these patients to refrain from using oral contraceptives or hormone replacement therapy following pregnancy.

Summary

In this chapter we have covered hereditary and acquired thrombophilia disorders which may be encountered in obstetrics and gynecology. The hematologist, obstetrician, gynecologist, reproductive endocrinologist and reproductive specialists must be aware of these, including their clinical manifestations, mode of inheritance, and potential complications, including complications in neonates. Tables 5.6, 5.7,

Table 5.6 Unexplained DVT /PE or venous thromboembolic disease: Causative/Contributory defects in descending order of probability of abnormalities.

More Common	Less Common
Antiphospholipid syndrome	5,10 MTHFR mutations
Anticardiolipin antibodies (IgG, IgA, IgM)	Hyperhomocysteinemia
Beta-2-glycoprotein-1 (IgG, IgA, IgM)	Lipoprotein (a)
Antiphosphatidylserine (IgG, IgA, IgM)	TPA deficiency
Antiphosphatidylinositol (IgG, IgA, IgM)	Heparin cofactor II deficiency
Antiphosphatidylcholine (IgG, IgA, IgM)	Dysfibrinogenemia
Antiphosphatidic acid (IgG, IgA, IgM)	Hypoplasminogenemia
Antiphosphatidylethanolamine (IgG, IgA, IgM)	
Antiphosphatidylglycerol (IgG, IgA, IgM)	
Anti-annexin-V-antibody (IgG, IgA, IgM)	
Lupus anticoagulant	
Hexagonal phospholipid	
Sticky platelet syndrome	
APC resistance (many types)	
Factor V Leiden	
Prothrombin G20210A mutation	
PAI-1 Polymorphisms/Elevation	
Antithrombin deficiency	
Protein S deficiency	

DVT = Deep Vein Thrombosis
PE = Pulmonary Embolus

Table 5.7 Premature coronary artery thrombosis: Causative/Contributory defects.

Common	Less Common
Antiphospholipid syndrome	TPA deficiency
Anticardiolipin antibodies (IgG, IgA, IgM)	Immune vasculitis
Beta-2-glycoprotein-1 (IgG, IgA, IgM)	Prothrombin G20210A mutation
Antiphosphatidylserine (IgG, IgA, IgM)	Antithrombin deficiency
Antiphosphatidylinositol (IgG, IgA, IgM)	Protein S deficiency
Antiphosphatidylcholine (IgG, IgA, IgM)	Protein C deficiency
Antiphosphatidic acid (IgG, IgA, IgM)	Heparin cofactor II deficiency
Antiphosphatidylethanolamine (IgG, IgA, IgM)	Dysfibrinogenemia
Antiphosphatidylglycerol (IgG, IgA, IgM)	Hypoplasminogenemia
Anti-annexin-V-antibody (IgG, IgA, IgM)	Elevated VIII??
Lupus Anticoagulant	Elevated fibrinogen??
Hexagonal phospholipid	Elevated VII??
Sticky Platelet Syndrome	
5,10 MTHFR Mutations	
Hyperhomocysteinemia	
PAI-1 Polymorphisms/Elevation	
Hyperlipoprotein (a)	

Table 5.8 Premature cerebrovascular thrombosis/TIAs: Causative/Contributory defects.

Descending Probability of Defects	
More Common	Less Common
Antiphospholipid syndrome	TPA deficiency
Anticardiolipin antibodies (IgG, IgA, IgM)	Immune vasculitis
Beta-2-Glycoprotein-1 (IgG, IgA, IgM)	Chlamydia Pneumoniae titers
Antiphosphatidylserine (IgG, IgA, IgM)	Antithrombin deficiency
Antiphosphatidylinositol (IgG, IgA, IgM)	Protein S deficiency
Antiphosphatidylcholine (IgG, IgA, IgM)	Protein C deficiency
Antiphosphatidic acid (IgG, IgA, IgM)	Heparin cofactor II deficiency
Antiphosphatidylethanolamine (IgG, IgA, IgM)	Dysfibrinogenemia
Antiphosphatidylglycerol (IgG, IgA, IgM)	Hypoplasminogenemia
Anti-Annexin-V-antibody (IgG, IgA, IgM)	
Lupus Anticoagulant	
Hexagonal phospholipid	
Sticky platelet syndrome	
PAI-1 Elevation	
5,10 MTHFR mutations	
Prothrombin G20210A mutation	

Table 5.8 (*cont.*)

Descending Probability of Defects	
More Common	Less Common
Hyperhomocysteinemia	
Hyperlipoprotein (a)	
Factor V Leiden/APC resistance	

Table 5.9 Thrombotic disorders associated with recurrent miscarriage syndrome (common).

Antiphospholipid syndrome
Sticky platelet syndrome
MTHFR mutations
Hyperhomocysteinemia
PAI-1 Elevation/Polymorphisms
Protein S deficiency
Factor V Leiden
Prothrombin G20210A
Protein C deficiency
Antithrombin deficiency
Heparin-cofactor II deficiency
TPA deficiency
Elevated lipoprotein (a)
Immune vasculitis

5.8 and 5.9 depict the prevalence of thrombophilic disorder associated with DVT/PE (Table 5.6), coronary artery thrombosis (Table 5.7), cerebrovascular disease (Table 5.8) and recurrent miscarriage/infertility (Table 5.9).

REFERENCES

1 Brandenburg, V. M., Frank, R. D., Heintz, B., *et al.* HELLP syndrome, multifactorial thrombophilia and postpartum myocardial infarction. *J. Perinat. Med.*, **32**: 181, 2004.

2 Bick, R. L. Disseminated intravascular coagulation: current concepts of etiology, pathophysiology, diagnosis and management. (Chapter 8) In *Hematology Oncology Clinics North America*, **17**: 149, 2003.

3 Colman-Brochu, S. Deep vein thrombosis in pregnancy. *Am. J. Maternal Child. Nursing*, **29**: 186, 2004.

4 Anteby, E. Y., Musalam, B., Milwidsky, A. Fetal inherited thrombophilias influence the severity of preeclampsia, IUGR and placental abruption. *Eur. J. Obstet Gynecol. Reprod. Biol.*, **113**: 31, 2004.
5 Bick, R. L. Disseminated intravascular coagulation: objective criteria for clinical and laboratory diagnosis and assessment of therapeutic response. *Clinical & Applied Thrombosis Hemostasis*, **1**: 3, 1995.
6 Bick, R. L. and Haas, S. Thromboprophylaxis and thrombosis in medical, surgical, trauma and obstetric/gynecologic patients. (Chapter 11) In *Hematology Oncology Clinics North America*, **17**: 217, 2003.
7 De Stefano, V., Rossi, E. and Leone, G. Inherited thrombophilia, pregnancy, and oral contraceptive use: clinical implications. *Semin. Vasc. Med.*, **3**: 47, 2003.
8 Ducloy-Bouthors, A. S. and Trillot, N. Risk factors of thromboembolism associated with pregnancy and the puerperium. Role of inherited and acquired thrombophilia. *Ann. Med. Interne*, (Paris) **154**: 295, 2003.
9 Van den Belt, A. G. M., Prins, M., Huisman, M. H., *et al.* Familial thrombophilia: a review analysis. *Clin. Appl. Thromb. Hemostas.*, **2**: 227, 1996.
10 Laposata, M., Green, D., Van Cott, E. M., *et al.* The clinical use and laboratory monitoring of low-molecular-weight heparin, danaparoid, hirudin and related compounds, and argatroban. College of American Pathologists Conference XXXI on laboratory monitoring of anticoagulant therapy. *Arch. Path. Lab. Med.*, **122**: 799, 1998.
11 Douiketis, I. J. D., Johnson, J. A. and Turpie, A. G. Low molecular weight heparin as bridging anticoagulation during interruption of warfarin. *Archives Internal Medicine*, **164**: 1319, 2004.
12 FDA MEDWATCH ADVERSE REACTION ALERT, JANUARY, 2002: LOVENOX (enoxaparin sodium) injection: Pregnancy and heart valves. http://www.fda.gov/medwatch/SAFETY/2002/jan02.htm#lovenox.
13 Bick, R. L. Heparin therapy and monitoring: Guidelines and practice parameters for clinical and laboratory approaches. *Clin. Appl. Thrombosis Hemostas.*, **2**: 12, 1996.
14 Bick, R. L. Recurrent miscarriage syndrome and infertility caused by blood coagulation protein or platelet defects. *Hematology Oncology Clinics North America*, **14**: 1131, 2000.
15 Thomas, D. P. Heparin prophylaxis and treatment of venous thromboembolism. *Semin. Hematol.*, **15**: 1, 1978.
16 Yett, H. S., Skillman, J. J. and Salzman, E. W. The hazards of aspirin plus heparin. *N. Engl. J. Med.*, **298**: 1092, 1978.
17 Warkentin, T. E., Soutar, R. L. and Panju, A. Acute systemic reactions to intravenous bolus heparin therapy: characterization and relationship to heparin induced thrombocytopenia. *Blood*, **80**: 160 (Abst). 1992.
18 Jaffe, M. D. and Willis, P. W. Multiple fractures associated with long-term sodium heparin therapy. *JAMA*, **193**: 152, 1965.
19 Levine, M. Non-hemorrhagic complications of anticoagulant therapy. *Semin. Thromb. Hemost.*, **12**: 63, 1986.
20 Howell, R., Fidler, J., Letsky, E., *et al.* The risks of antenatal subcutaneous heparin prophylaxis: a controlled trial. *Br. J. Obstet. Gynaecol.*, **90**: 1124, 1983.

21 Monreal, M., Lafoz, E., Olive, A., *et al.* Comparison of subcutaneous unfractionated heparin with low molecular weight heparin (fragmin) in patients with venous thromboembolism and contraindications. *Thrombosis Haemostasis*, **71**: 7, 1994.
22 Morabia, A. Heparin doses and major bleedings. *Lancet*, **1**: 1278, 1986.
23 Bick, R. L. and Frenkel, E. P. Clinical aspects of heparin-induced thrombocytopenia and thrombosis and other side effects of heparin therapy. *J. Clin. Appl. Thrombosis Hemostasis*, **5** (Suppl 1): 7, 1999.
24 Warkentin, T. E., Soutar, R. L. and Panju, A. Acute systemic reactions to intravenous bolus heparin therapy: characterization and relationship to heparin induced thrombocytopenia. *Blood*, **80**: 160 (Abst). 1992.
25 Bick, R. L. Four cases of anaphylaxis with first or second dose of low-molecular-weight heparin therapy. FDA: Adverse Reaction Report – on file.
26 Jaffe, M. D. and Willis, P. W. Multiple fractures associated with long-term sodium heparin therapy. *JAMA*, **193**: 152, 1965.
27 Levine, M. Non-hemorrhagic complications of anticoagulant therapy. *Semin. Thromb. Hemost.*, **12**: 63, 1986.
28 Hirsh, J., Raschke, R., Warkentin, T. E., *et al.* Heparin: mechanism of action, pharmacokinetics, dosing considerations, monitoring, efficacy, and safety. *Chest*, **108**: 259S, 1995.
29 Howell, R., Fidler, J., Letsky, E., *et al.* The risks of antenatal subcutaneous heparin prophylaxis: a controlled trial. *Br. J. Obstet. Gynaecol.*, **90**: 1124, 1983.
30 Monreal, M., Lafoz, E., Olive, A., *et al.* Comparison of subcutaneous unfractionated heparin with a low molecular weight heparin (fragmin) in patients with venous thromboembolism and contraindications to coumarin. *Thromb. Haemost.*, **71**: 7, 1994.
31 Barbour, L. A., Kick, S. D., Steiner, J. F., *et al.* A prospective study of heparin-induced osteoporosis in pregnancy using bone densitometry. *Am. J. Obst. Gyn.*, **170**: 862, 1994.
32 Dahlman, T. C. Osteoporotic fractures and the recurrence of thromboembolism during pregnancy and the puerperium in 184 women undergoing thromboprophylaxis with heparin *Am. J. Obst. Gyn.*, **168**: 1265, 1993.
33 Hunt, B. J., Doughty, H., Majumdar, G., *et al.* Thromboprophylaxis with low molecular weight heparin (Fragmin) in high risk pregnancies. *Thromb. Haemost.*, **77**: 39, 1997.
34 Douketis, J., Ginsberg, J. S., Burrows, R. F., *et al.* The effects of long-term heparin therapy during pregnancy on bone density. A prospective matched cohort study. *Thromb. Haemost.*, **75**: 254, 1996.
35 Walenga, J. M. and Bick, R. L. Heparin-induced thrombocytopenia, paradoxical thromboembolism, and other side effects of heparin therapy. *Med. Clin. North. Am.*, **82**: 635, 1998.
36 Walenga, J. M. and Bick, R. L. Heparin-induced thrombocytopenia, paradoxical thromboembolism, and other side effects of heparin therapy. *Card Clinics: Annual Drug Therapy*, **2**: 123, 1998.
37 Muir, J. M., Andrew, M., Hirsh, J., *et al.* Histomorphometric analysis of the effects of standard heparin on trabecular bone in vivo. *Blood*, **88**: 1314, 1996.
38 Muir, J. M., Hirsh, J., Weitz, J. I., *et al.* A histomorphometric comparison of the effects of heparin and low-molecular-weight heparin on cancellous bone in rats. *Blood*, **89**: 3236, 1997.
39 Panagakos, F. S., Jandinski, J. J., Feder, L., *et al.* Heparin fails to potentiate the effects of IL-1 beta-mediated bone resorption of fetal rat long bones in vitro. *Biochimie*, **77**: 915, 1995.

40 Shaughnesy, S. G., Young, E., Deschamps, *et al.* The effects of low molecular weight and standard heparin on calcium loss from fetal rat calvoria. *Blood*, **86**: 1368, 1995.

41 Murray, W. J., Clinical pesentations of heparin induced thrombocytopenia. *Seminars Hematology*, **35** (Suppl) 9, 1998.

42 Bick, R. L. Heparin and low molecular weight heparins. (Chapter 17) In *Disorders of Thrombosis and Hemostasis*, Bick, R. L., ed. Philadelphia, PA; Lippincott, Williams and Wilkins, 2002, p. 359.

43 Warkentin, T. E. Heparin-induced skin lesions. *Br. J. Haematol.*, **92**: 494, 1996.

44 Hall, J. C., McConahay, D., Gibson, D., *et al.* Heparin necrosis and anticoagulation syndrome. *JAMA*, **244**: 1831, 1980.

45 Hill, J., Caprini, J. A. and Robbins, J. L. An unusual complication of minidose heparin therapy. *Clin. Orthop.*, **118**: 130, 1976.

46 White, P. W., Sadd, J. R. and Wensel, R. E. Thrombotic complications of heparin therapy. *Ann. Surg.*, **190**: 595, 1979.

47 Levine, L. E., Bernstein, J. E. and Soltani, K. Heparin-induced cutaneous necrosis unrelated to injection sites. *Arch. Derm.*, **119**: 400, 1983.

48 Bircher, A. J., Itin, P. H. and Buchner, S. A. Skin lesions, hypereosinophilia and subcutaneous heparin. *N. Engl. J. Med.*, **343**: 861 (letter), 1994.

49 Aull, L., Chao, H. and Coy, K. Heparin-induced hyperkalemia. *Ann. Pharmacotherapy*, **24**: 244, 1990.

50 Bick, R. L. Introduction to thrombosis: proficient and cost-effective approaches to thrombosis. *Hematology Oncology Clinics North America*, **17**: 1, 2003.

51 Krabbendam, I. and Dekker, G. Pregnancy outcome in patients with a history of recurrent spontaneous miscarriages and documented thrombophilias. *Obstet. Gynecol. Surv.*, **59**: 651, 2004.

52 Rees, D. S., Cox, M. and Clegg, J. B. World distribution of factor V Leiden. *Lancet*, **346**: 1133, 1995.

53 Svensson, P. and Dahlback, B. Resistance to activated protein C as a basis for venous thrombosis. *N. Engl. J. Med.*, **330**: 517, 1994.

54 Koster, T., Rosendaal, F. R., de Ronde, H., *et al.* Venous thrombosis due to poor anticoagulant response to activated protein C: Leiden Thrombophilia Study. *Lancet*, **342**: 1503, 1993.

55 Dahlback, B., Carlsson, M. and Svensson, P. J. Familial thrombophilia due to a previously unrecognized mechanism characterized by poor anticoagulant response to activated protein C: prediction of a cofactor to activated protein C. *Proc. Natl. Acad. Sci. USA*, **90**: 1004, 1993.

56 Bertina, R. M. Factor V Leiden and other coagulation factor mutations affecting thrombotic risk. *Clin. Chem.*, **43**: 1678, 1997.

57 Bertina, R. M., Reitsma, P. H., Rosendaal, F. R., *et al.* Resistance to activated protein C and factor V Leiden as risk factors for venous thrombosis. *Thromb. Haemostas.*, **74**: 449, 1995.

58 Greengard, J. S., Fisher, C. L., Villoutreix, B., *et al.* Structural basis for type I and type II deficiencies of antithrombotic plasma protein C: patterns revealed by three-dimensional molecular modeling of mutations of the protease domain. *Proteins*, **18**: 367, 1994.

59 Voorberg, J., Roelse, J., Koopman, R., *et al.* Association of idiopathic venous thromboembolism with single-point mutation at Arg506 of factor V. *Lancet*, **343**: 1535, 1994.

60 Zoller, B., Hillarp, A., Berntorp, E. Activated protein C resistance due to a common factor V gene mutation is a major risk factor for venous thrombosis. *Annu. Rev. Med.*, **48**: 45, 1997.
61 Laffan, M. A. and Manning, T. The influence of factor VIII on measurement of activated protein C resistance. *Blood Coag. Fibrinol.*, **7**: 761, 1996.
62 Bontempo, F. A. The factor V Leiden mutation: spectrum of thrombotic events and laboratory evaluation. *J. Vasc. Surg.*, **2**: 271, 1997.
63 Simioni, P., Scalia, D., Tormene, D., *et al.* Intra-arterial thrombosis and homozygous factor V Leiden mutation. *Clin. Appl. Thromb. Hemostas.*, **3**: 215, 1997.
64 Vefring, H., Lie, R., Odegard, R., *et al.* Maternal and fetal variants of genetic thrombophilias and the risk of preeclampsia. *Epidemiology,* **15**: 317, 2004.
65 Samama, M. M., Simon, D., Horellou, M. H., *et al.* Diagnosis and clinical characteristics of inherited activated protein C resistance. *Haemostasis,* **26**, Suppl 4: 315, 1996.
66 Hile, E. T., Westendorp, R. G., Vandenbroucke, J. P., *et al.* Mortality and causes of death in families with the factor V Leiden mutation (resistance to activated protein C). *Blood,* **89**: 1963, 1997.
67 Middeldorp, S., Henkens, C. M., Koopman, M. M., *et al.* The incidence of venous thromboembolism in family members of patients with factor V Leiden mutation and venous thrombosis. *Ann. Int. Med.*, **128**: 15, 1998.
68 Bick, R. L. Syndromes of thrombosis and hypercoagulability. In Cullen, J. H., (ed.): *Current Concepts of Thrombosis*, vol. 82. Philadelphia, PA; W. B. Saunders Co., 1998, p. 409.
69 Prandoni, P., Lensing, A. W., Cogo, A., *et al.* The long-term clinical course of acute deep venous thrombosis. *Ann. Int. Med.*, **125**: 1, 1996.
70 Miletich, J. P., Stampfer, M. J., Goldhaber, S. Z., *et al.* Factor V Leiden and recurrent idiopathic venous thromboembolism. *Circulation,* **92**: 2800, 1995.
71 Simioni, P., Prandoni, P., Lensing, A. W., *et al.* The risk of recurrent venous thromboembolism in patients with an Arg506 → Gln mutation in the gene for factor V (factor V Leiden). *N. Engl. J. Med.*, **336**: 399, 1997.
72 Rintelen, C., Pabinger, I., Knobl, P., *et al.* Probability of recurrence of thrombosis in patients with and without factor V Leiden. *Thromb. Haemostas.*, **75**: 229, 1996.
73 Levine, M. N., Hirsh, J., Gent, M., *et al.* Optimal duration of oral anticoagulant therapy: a randomized trial comparing four weeks with three months of warfarin in patients with proximal deep vein thrombosis. *Thromb. Haemostas.*, **74**: 606, 1995.
74 Vandenbroucke, J. P., Koster, T., Briet, E., *et al.* Increased risk of venous thrombosis in oral-contraceprive users who are carriers of factor V Leiden mutation. *Lancet,* **344**: 1453, 1994.
75 Bloemenkamp, K. W., Rosendaal, F. R., Helmerhorst, F. M., *et al.* Enhancement by factor V Leiden mutation of risk of deep-vein thrombosis associated with oral contraceptives containing a third-generation progestagen. *Lancet,* **346**: 1593, 1995.
76 Rintelen, C., Mannhalter, C., Ireland, H., *et al.* Oral contraceptives enhance the risk of clinical manifestation of venous thrombosis at a young age in females homozygous for factor V Leiden. *Br. J. Haematol.*, **93**: 487, 1996.
77 Gandrille, S., Greengard, J. S., Alhenc-Gelac, M., *et al.* Incidence of activated protein C resistance caused by the ARG 506 GLN mutation in factor V in 113 unrelated symptomatic protein C-deficient patients. The French Network on the behalf of INSERM. *Blood,* **86**: 219, 1995.

78 Zoller, B., Berntsdotter, A., Garcia de Frutos, P., *et al.* Resistance to activated protein C as an additional genetic risk factor in hereditary deficiency of protein S. *Blood,* **85**: 3518, 1955.
79 Ridker, P. M., Hennekens, C. H., Selhub, J., *et al.* Interrelation of hyperhomocyst(e)inemia, factor V Leiden, and risks of future venous thromboembolism. *Circulation,* **95**, 1777, 1997.
80 Bick, R. L., Laughlin, H. R., Cohen, B., *et al.* Fetal wastage syndrome due to blood protein/platelet defects: results of prevalence studies and treatment outcome with low-dose heparin and low-dose aspirin. *Clin. Appl. Thromb. Hemostas.*, **1**: 286, 1995.
81 Bick, R. L. and Hoppensteadt, D. Thrombohemorrhagic defects and recurrent miscarriage syndrome. *Blood,* **104**: 712A, 2004.
82 Dudding, T. and Attia, J. The asociation between adverse pregnancy outcomes and maternal factor V Leiden genotype: a meta-analysis. *Thromb. Haemostasis.*, **91**: 700, 2004.
83 Gebhardt, G. and Hall, D. Inherited and acquired thrombophilias and poor pregnancy outcome: should we be treating with heparin? *Curr. Opinion Obstet. Gynecol.*, **15**: 501, 2003.
84 Sonmezer, M., Aytac, R., Demirel, L., *et al.* Mesenteric vein thrombosis in a pregnant patient heterozygous for the factor VG (1691 G to A) Leiden mutation. *European J. Obstet. Gynaecol. Reproductive Bio.*, **114**: 234, 2004.
85 Camilleri, R., Peebles, D., Portmann, C., *et al.* 455G/A beta fibrinogen gene polymorphism factor V Leiden, prothrombin G 20210 A mutation and MTHFR C677T, and placental vascular complications. *Blood Coagulation Fibrinolysis,* **15**: 139, 2004.
86 Kovalevsky, G., Gracia, C., Berlin, J., *et al.* Evaluation of the asociation between hereditary thrombophilias and recurrent miscarriage loss: a meta-analysis. *Arch. Int. Med.*, **164**: 558, 2004.
87 Yilmazer, M., Kurtay, G., Sonmezer, M., *et al.* Factor V Leiden and prothrombin G20210A G-A mutations in controls and in patients with thromboembolic events during pregnancy or the puerperium. *Arch. Gynecol. Obstet.*, **268**: 304, 2003.
88 Bokarewa, M. I., Bremme, K. and Blomback, M. Arg506-Gln mutation in factor V and risk of thrombosis during pregnancy. *Br. J. Haematol.*, **92**: 473, 1996.
89 Kibbe, M. R. and Rhee, R. Y. Heparin-induced thrombocytopenia: pathophysiology. *Semin. Vasc. Surg.*, **9**: 284, 1996.
90 Wallis, D. E., Lewis, B. E., Messmore, H., *et al.* Heparin-induced thrombocytopenia and thrombosis syndrome. *Clin. Appl. Thromb. Hemostas.*, **4**: 160, 1998.
91 Williamson, D., Brown, K., Luddingtonm, R., *et al.* Factor V Cambridge: a new mutation (Arg306→Thr) associated with resistance to activated protein C. *Blood,* **91**: 1140, 1998.
92 Chan, W. P., Lee, C. K., Kwong, Y. L., *et al.* A novel mutation of Arg306 of factor V gene in Hong Kong Chinese. *Blood,* **91**: 1135, 1998.
93 Poort, S. R., Rosendaal, F. R., Reitsma, P. H., *et al.* A common genetic variation in the 3′-untranslated region of the prothrombin gene is associated with elevated plasma prothrombin levels and an increase in venous thrombosis. *Blood,* **88**: 3698, 1996.
94 Arruda, V. R., Annichino-Bizacchi, J. M., Goncalves, M. S., *et al.* Prevalence of the prothrombin gene variant (nt20201A) in venous thrombosis and arterial disease. *Thromb. Haemostas.*, **78**: 1430, 1997.
95 Ferraresi, P., Marchetti, G., Legnani, C., *et al.* The heterozygous 20210 G/A prothrombin genotype is associated with early venous thrombosis in inherited thrombophilias and is not increased in frequency in artery disease. *Arterioscler. Thromb. Vasc. Biol.*, **17**: 2418, 1997.

96 Makris, M., Preston, F. E., Beauchamp, N. J., *et al.* Co-inheritance of the 20210 A allele of the prothrombin gene increases the risk of thrombosis in subjects with familial thrombophilia. *Thromb. Haemost.*, **78**: 1426, 1997.

97 Bloem, B. R., van Putten, M. J., van der Meer, J. M., *et al.* Superior saggital sinus thrombosis in a patient heterozygous for the novel 20210 A allele of the prothrombin gene. *Thromb. Haemostas.*, **79**: 235, 1997.

98 Martinelli, I., Sacchi, E., Landi, G., *et al.* High risk of cerebral-vein thrombosis in carriers of a prothrombin-gene mutation and in users of oral contraceptives. *NEJM*, **338**: 1793, 1998.

99 Gould, J., Deam, S. and Dolan, G. Prothrombin 20210: A polymorphism and third generation oral conraceptives – a case report of coeliac axis thrombosis and splenic infarction. *Thromb. Haemostas.*, **79**: 1214, 1998.

100 Poort, S. R., Rosendaal, F. R., Reitsma, P. H., *et al.* A common genetic variation in the 3′-untranslated region of the prothrombin gene is associated with elevated plasma prothrombin levels and an increase in venous thrombosis. *Blood*, **88**: 3698, 1996.

101 Ratnoff, O. D. and Colopy, J. E. A familial hemorrhagic trait associated with a deficiency of clot-promoting fraction of plasma. *J. Clin. Invest.*, **34**: 602, 1955.

102 Seegers, W. H. Factor X (autoprothrombin III). *Semin. Thromb. Hemostas.*, **7**: 233, 1981.

103 Bick, R. *Disorders of Thrombosis and Hemostasis: Clinical and Laboratory Practice.* Chicago, IL, ASCP Press, 1992, p. 109.

104 Mcpherson, R. A. Thromboembolism in Hageman trait. *Am. J. Clin. Pathol.*, **68**: 240, 1977.

105 Baker, W. F., Jr. and Bick, R. L. Deep vein thrombosis: diagnosis and management. *Med. Clin. N. Am.*, **78**: 685, 1994.

106 Hoak, J. C., Swanson, L. W., Warner, E. D., *et al.* Myocardial infarction associated with severe factor XI deficiency. *Lancet*, **2**: 884, 1966.

107 Ratnoff, O. D., Busse, R. J. and Sheon, R. P. The demise of John Hageman. *N. Engl. J. Med.*, **279**: 760, 1968.

108 Goodnough, L. T., Saito, H. and Ratnoff, O. Thrombosis or myocardial infarction in congenital clotting factor abnormalities and chronic thrombocytopenias: a report of 21 patients and a review of 50 previously reported cases. *Medicine*, **62**: 248, 1983.

109 Di Imperato, D. and Dettori, A. G. Ipofibrinogenemia congenita con fibrinoastenia. *Helvitica Pediatrica Acta*, **13**: 380, 1958.

110 Bithell, T. C. Hereditary dysfibrinogenemia. *Clin. Chem.*, **31**: 509, 1985.

111 Mammen, E. F. Fibrinogen abnormalities. *Semin. Hemostas. Thromb.*, **9**: 1, 1983.

112 Al Mondhiry, H. and Galanakis, D. Dysfibrinogenemia and lupus anticoagulant in a patient with recurrent thrombosis. *J. Lab. Clin. Med.*, **110**: 726, 1987.

113 Lijnen, H. R., Soria, J. and Soria, C. Dysfibrinogenemia (Fibrinogen Dusard) associated with impaired fibrin-enhanced plasminogen activation. *Thromb. Haemostas.*, **51**: 108, 1984.

114 Reber, P., Furlan, M. and Henschen, A. Three abnormal fibrinogen variants with the same amino acid substitution (gamma-275 Arg-His): Fibrinogens Bergamo II, Essen and Perugia. *Thromb. Haemostas.*, **56**: 401, 1986.

115 Welch, G. N. and Loscalzo, J. Homocysteine and atherothrombosis. *N. Engl. J. Med.*, **338**: 1042, 1998.

116 Carson, N. A. J. and Neill, D. W. Metabolic abnormalities detected in a survey of mentally backward individuals in Northern Ireland. *Arch. Dis. Child*, **37**: 505, 1962.

117 Mudd, S. H., Finkelstein, J. D., Irreverre, F., *et al.* Homocystinuria: an enzymatic defect. *Science*, **143**: 1443, 1964.

118 Valle, D., Pai, G. S., Thomas, G. H., *et al.* Homocystinuria due to cystathione beta-synthetase deficiency: clinical manifestations and therapy. *Johns Hopkins Med. J.*, **146**: 110, 1980.

119 McCully, K. S. Vascular pathology of homocysteinemia: implications for the pathogenesis of arteriosclerosis. *Am. J. Pathol.*, **56**: 111, 1969.

120 Carey, M. C., Donovan, D. E., Fitzgerald, O., *et al.* Homocystinuria, I: a clinical and pathologic study of nine subjects in six families. *Am. J. Med.*, **45**: 17, 1968.

121 Goyette, P., Sumner, J. S., Milos, R., *et al.* Human methylenetetrahydrofolate reductase: isolation of cDNA, mapping and mutation identification. *Natural Genetics*, **7**: 195, 1994.

122 Frosst, P., Blom, H. J., Milos, R., *et al.* A candidate genetic risk factor for vascular disease: a common mutation in methylenetetrahydrofolate reductase. *Natural Genetics*, **10**: 111, 1995.

123 Van der Put, N. M. J., Steegers-Theunissen, R. P. M., Frosst, P., *et al.* Mutated methylene-tetrahydrofolate reductase as a risk factor for spina bifida. *Lancet*, **346**: 1070, 1995.

124 Jacques, P. F., Bostom, A. G., Williams, R. R., *et al.* Relation between folate status, a common mutation in methylenetetrahydrofolate reductase, and plasma homocysteine concentrations. *Circulation*, **93**: 7, 1996.

125 Rozen, R. Molecular genetic aspects of hyperhomocysteinemia and its relation to folic acid. *Clin. Investig. Med.*, **19**: 171, 1996.

126 Kang, S. S., Wong, P. W. and Malinow, M. R. Hyperhomocyst(e)inemia as a risk factor for occlusive vascular disease. *Ann. Rev. Nutr.*, **12**: 279, 1992.

127 Stampfer, M. J., Malinow, M. R., Wilett, W. C., *et al.* A prospective study of plasma homocyst(e)ine and risk of myocardial infarction in US physicians. *JAMA*, **268**: 877, 1992.

128 Kang, S. S., Wong, P. W. K., Susmano, A., *et al.* Thermolabile methylenetetrahydrofolate reductase: an inherited risk factor for coronary artery disease. *Am. J. Hum. Genetics*, **48**: 536, 1991.

129 Malinow, M. R. Hyperhomocyst(e)inemia: a common and easily reversible risk factor for occlusive atherosclerosis. *Circulation*, **81**: 2004, 1990.

130 Boushey, C. J., Beresford, A. A., Omenn, G. S., *et al.* A quantitative assessment of plasma homocysteine as a risk factor for vascular disease: probable benefits of increasing folic acid intake. *JAMA*, **274**: 1049, 1995.

131 Duell, P. B. and Malinow, M. R. Plasma homocyst(e)ine: an important risk factor for atherosclerotic vascular disease. *Curr. Opin. Lipidol.*, **8**: 28, 1997.

132 Mayer, E. L., Jacobsen, D. W. and Robinson, K. Homocysteine and coronary athero-sclerosis. *J. Am. Coll. Cardiol.*, **27**: 517, 1996.

133 Nygard, O., Nordrehaug, J. E., Refsum, H., *et al.* Plasma homocysteine levels and mortality in patients with coronary artery disease. *N. Engl. J. Med.*, **337**: 230, 1997.

134 Cattaneo, M., Martinelli, I. and Manucci, P. M. Hyperhomocysteinemia as a risk factor for deep-vein thrombosis. *N. Engl. J. Med.*, **336**: 1399, 1997.

135 Falcon, C. R., Cattaneo, M., Panzeri, D., *et al.* High prevalence of hyperhomocyst(e)inemia in patients with juvenile venous thrombosis. *Arterioscl. Thromb.*, **14**: 1080, 1994.

136 Den Heijer, M., Koster, T., Blom, H. U., *et al.* Hyperhomocysteinemia as a risk factor for deep-vein thrombosis. *N. Engl. J. Med.*, **334**: 759, 1996.

137 Fermo, I., Vigano, D., Angelo, S., Paroni, R., *et al.* Prevalence of moderate hyperhomocysteinemia in patients with early-onset venous and arterial occlusive disease. *Ann. Intern. Med.*, **123**: 747, 1995.

138 Moghadasian, M. H., McManus, B. M. and Frohlich, J. J. Homocyst(e)ine and coronary artery disease: clinical evidence and genetic and metabolic background. *Arch. Int. Med.*, **157**: 2299, 1997.

139 Robinson, K., Mayer, E. L., Miller, D. P., *et al.* Hyperhomocysteinemia and low pyridoxal phosphate: common and independent reversible risk factors for coronary artery disease. *Circulation,* **92:** 2825, 1995.

140 Israelsson, B., Brattstorm, L. E. and Hultberg, B. L. Homocysteine and myocardial infarction. *Atherosclerosis,* **71**: 227, 1988.

141 Wu, L. L., Wu, J., Hunt, S. C., *et al.* Plasma homocyst(e)ine as a risk factor for early familial coronary artery disease. *Clin. Chem.*, **40**: 1361, 1994.

142 Wald, N. J., Watt, H. C., Law, M. R., *et al.* Homocysteine and ischemic heart disease: results of a prospective study with implications regarding prevention. *Arch. Int. Med.*, **158**: 862, 1998.

143 Araki, A., Sako, Y., Fukushima, Y., *et al.* Plasma sulfhydryl-containing amino acids in patients with cerebral infarction and in hypertensive subjects. *Atherosclerosis,* **79**: 139, 1989.

144 Brattstrom, L., Lindgren, A., Israelsson, B., *et al.* Hyperhomocysteinemia in stroke: prevalence, cause and relationship to type of stroke and stroke risk factors. *Eur. J. Clin. Invest.*, **22**: 214, 1992.

145 Coull, B. M., Malinow, M. R., Beamer, N., *et al.* Elevated plasma homocyst(e)ine concentration as a possible independent risk factor for stroke. *Stroke,* **21**: 572, 1990.

146 Molgaard, J., Malinow, M. R., Lassvik, C., *et al.* Hyperhomocyst(e)inaemia: an independent risk factor for intermittent claudication. *J. Int. Med.*, **231**: 273, 1992.

147 Van den Berg, M., Stehouwer, D. A., Biedrager, E., *et al.* Plasma homocysteine and severity of atherosclerosis in young patients with lower-limb atherosclerotic disease. *Arterioscl. Thromb. Vasc. Biol.*, **16**: 165, 1996.

148 Kottke-Marchant, K., Green, R., Jacobsen, D. W., *et al.* High plasma homocysteine: a risk factor for arterial and venous thrombosis in patients with normal coagulation profiles. *Clin. Appl. Thromb. Hemostas.*, **3**: 239, 1997.

149 Franken, D. G., Boers, G. H., Blom, H. J., *et al.* Treatment of mild hyperhomocysteinemia in vascular disease patients. *Arterioscl. Thromb.*, **14**: 465, 1994.

150 Brattstrom, L., Israelsson, B., Norving, B., *et al.* Impaired homocysteine metabolism in early onset cerebral and peripheral occlusive arterial disease: effect of pyridoxine and folic acid treatment. *Atherosclerosis,* **81**: 51, 1990.

151 Brattsrom, L. E., Israelsson, B., Jeppsson, J. O., *et al.* Folic acid: an innocuous means to reduce plasma homocysteine. *Scandin. J. Clin. Lab. Invest.*, **48**: 215, 1988.

152 Ubbink, J. B., Hayward Vermaak, W. J., van der Merwe, A., *et al.* Vitamin requirements for the treatment of hypercysteinemia in humans. *J. Nutr.*, **124**: 1927, 1994.
153 Naurath, H. J., Joosten, E., Riezler, R., *et al.* Effects of vitamin B12, folate, and vitamin B6 supplements in elderly people with normal serum vitamin concentrations. *Lancet*, **346**: 85, 1995.
154 Landgren, P., Israelsson, B., Lindgren, A., *et al.* Plasma homocysteine in acute myocardial infarction: homocysteine lowering effect of folic acid. *J. Int. Med.*, **237**: 381, 1995.
155 Ward, M., McNulty, H., McPartlin, J., *et al.* Plasma homocysteine, a risk factor for cardiovascular disease, is lowered by physiological doses of folic acid. *Quart. J. Med.*, **909**: 519, 1997.
156 Cuskelly, G. J., McNulty, H., McPartlin, J. M., *et al.* Plasma homocysteine response to folate intervention in young women. *Irish J. Med. Science*, **164**: 3, 1995.
157 Malinow, M. R., Duell, P. B., Hess, D. L., *et al.* Reduction of plasma homocyst(e)ine levels by breakfast cereal fortified with folic acid in patients with coronary heart disease. *N. Engl. J. Med.*, **338**: 1009, 1998.
158 Abidgaard, U. Purification of two progressive antithrombins of human plasma. *Scan. J. Clin. Lab. Invest.*, **19**: 190, 1967.
159 Kurachi, K., Schmer, G. and Hermodson, M. Inhibition of bovine factor IXa and factor Xa by anti-thrombin-III. *Biochemistry*, **15**: 368, 1976.
160 Lahiri, K., Rosenberg, R. D. and Talamo, R. C. Antithrombin-III: an inhibitor of human plasma kallikrein. *Fed. Proc.*, **33**: 642, 1974.
161 Seegers, W. H., Cole, E. R. and, Harmison, C. R. Neutralization of autoprothrombin-C activity with antithrombin. *Can. J. Biochem.*, **42**: 359, 1964.
162 Walker, F. and Esmon, C. The molecular mechanism of heparin action: II. Separation of functionally different heparins by affinity chromatography. *Thromb. Res.*, **14**: 219, 1979.
163 Abildgaard, U. Binding of thrombin to antithrombin III. *Scan. J. Clin. Lab. Invest.*, **24**: 23, 1969.
164 Seegers, W. H., Schroer, H. and, Kagami, M. Interactivation of purified autoprothrombin I with antithrombin. *Can. J. Biochem.*, **42**: 1425, 1964.
165 Stead, N., Kaplan, A. P. and, Rosenberg, R. D. Inhibition of activated factor XII by antithrombin-heparin cofactor. *J. Biol. Chem.*, **251**: 6481, 1976.
166 Vennerod, A. M., Laake, K. and Soleberg, A. K. Inactivation and binding of human plasma kallikrein by antithrombin III and heparin. *Thromb. Res.*, **9**: 457, 1976.
167 Fischer, A. M., Cornu, P., Sternberg, C., *et al.* Antithrombin III Alger: a new homozygous ATIII variant. *Thromb. Haemostas.*, **55**: 218, 1986.
168 Fagerhol, M. and Abildgaard, U. Immunologic studies in human antithrombin III. Influence of age, sex, and use of oral contraceptives on serum concentration. *Scan. J. Haematol.*, **7**: 10, 1970.
169 Howie, P., Mallinson, A. and Prentice, C. Effect of combined oestrogen–progesterone contraceptives, oestrogen, and progesterone on antiplasmin and antithrombin activity. *Lancet*, **2**: 1329, 1990.
170 McKay, E. Immunochemical analysis of active and inactive antithrombin III. *Br. J. Haematol.*, **46**: 277, 1980.

171 Peterson, C., Kelley, R. and Minard, B. Antithrombin III. Comparison of functional and immunologic assays. *Am. J. Clin. Pathol.*, **69**: 500, 1978.
172 Sveger, T. Antithrombin III in adolescents. *Thromb. Res.*, **15**: 885, 1979.
173 Bick, R. L. Clinical relevance of antithrombin III. *Semin. Hemostas. Thromb.*, **8**: 276, 1982.
174 Candrina, R. and Goppini, A. Antithrombin III deficiency. *Blood Rev.*, **2**: 239, 1988.
175 Menache, D., O'Malley, J. P., Schorr, J. B., *et al.* Evaluation of the safety, recovery, half-life, and clinical efficacy of Antithrombin III (Human) in patients with hereditary antithrombin III deficiency. *Blood*, **75**: 33, 1990.
176 Menache, D. Replacement therapy in patients with hereditary antithrombin III deficiency. *Semin. Hematol.*, **28**: 31, 1991.
177 Owen, J. Antithrombin III replacement therapy in pregnancy. *Semin. Hematol.*, **28**: 46, 1991.
178 Vinnazer, H. Antithrombin III in shock and disseminated intravascular coagulation. *Clin. Appl. Thromb. Hemostas.*, **1**: 62, 1995.
179 Schwartz, R. S., Bauer, K. A., Rosenberg, R. D., *et al.* Clinical experience with Antithrombin III concentrate in treatment of congenital and acquired deficiency of antithrombin. *Am. J. Med.*, **87**: 53S, 1989.
180 Tollefson, D. M., Majerus, D. W. and Blank, M. K. Heparin cofactor II: purification and properties of a heparin-dependent inhibitor of thrombin in human plasma. *J. Biol. Chem.*, **257**: 2162, 1982.
181 Sie, P., Fernandez, F. and Caranobe, C. Inhibition of thrombin-induced platelet aggregation and serotonin release by antithrombin III and heparin cofactor II in the presence of standard heparin, dermatan sulfate and pentosan polysulfate. *Thromb. Res.*, **35**: 231, 1984.
182 Sie, P., Dupouy, D. and Pichon, J. Constitutional heparin cofactor II deficiency associated with recurrent thrombosis. *Lancet*, **2**: 414, 1985.
183 Anderson, T., Larsen, M. and Abildgaard, U. Low heparin cofactor II associated with abnormal crossed immunoelectrophoresis pattern in two Norwegian families. *Thromb. Res.*, **47**: 243, 1987.
184 Bertina, R. M., Van der, L., I. K., Engesser, L., *et al.* Hereditary cofactor-II deficiency and the risk of development of thrombosis. *Thromb. Haemostas.*, **57**: 196, 1987.
185 Chaunsumrit, A., Manco-Johnson, M. J. and Hathaway, W. E. Heparin cofactor II in adults and infants with thrombosis and DIC. *Am. J. Hematol.*, **31**: 109, 1989.
186 Toulin, P., Vitoux, J. F. and Capron, L. Heparin cofactor II in patients with deep venous thrombosis under heparin and oral anticoagulant therapy. *Thromb. Res.*, **49**: 479, 1988.
187 Grau, E., Oliver, A. and Felez, J. Plasma and urinary heparin cofactor II levels in patients with nephrotic syndrome. *Thromb. Haemostas.*, **60**: 137, 1988.
188 Stenflo, J. Structure and function of protein C. *Semin. Thromb. Hemostas.*, **10**: 109, 1984.
189 Esmon, C. T. and Esmon, N. L. Protein C activation. *Semin. Thromb. Hemostas.*, **10**: 122, 1984.
190 Walker, F. J. Protein S and the regulation of activated protein C: *Semin. Thromb. Hemostas.*, **10**: 131, 1984.
191 Dahlback, B. The protein C anticoagulant system: inherited defects as a basis for venous thrombosis. *Thromb. Res.*, **77**: 1, 1995.
192 Griffin, J. H. Clinical studies on protein C. *Semin. Thromb. Hemostas.*, **10**: 162, 1984.

193 Marlar, R. A. and Endres-Brooks, J. Recurrent thromboembolic disease due to heterozygous protein C deficiency. *Thromb. Haemostas.*, **50**: 351, 1983.
194 Broekmans, A. W. Hereditary protein C deficiency. *Haemostasis*, **15**: 233, 1985.
195 Seligsohn, U., Berger, A. and Abend, M. Homozygous protein C deficiency manifested by massive venous thrombosis in the newborn. *N. Engl. J. Med.*, **310**: 559, 1984.
196 Marciniak, E., Wilson, H. O. and Marlar, R. A. Neonatal purpura fulminans: a genetic disorder related to the absence of protein C in blood. *Blood*, **65**: 15, 198.
197 Mammen, E. F. Inhibitor abnormalities. *Semin. Thromb. Hemostas.*, **9**: 42, 198.
198 Reitsma, P. H., Poort, S. R., Allaart, C. F., *et al.* The spectrum of genetic defects in a panel of 40 Dutch families with symptomatic protein C deficiency type I: heterogeneity and founder effects. *Blood*, **78**: 890, 199.
199 Comp, P. C., Nixon, R. and Esmon, C. T. Determination of functional levels of protein C, an antithrombotic protein, using thrombin/thrombomodulin complex. *Blood*, **63**: 15, 198.
200 Griffin, J. H., Bezeaud, A. and Evatt, B. Functional and immunologic studies of protein C in thromboembolic disease. *Blood*, **62**: 301a, 1987.
201 Miletich, J. P. Laboratory diagnosis of protein C. *Semin. Thromb. Hemostas.*, **16**: 169, 1998.
202 Bick, R. L. Hypercoagulability and thrombosis. In Bick, R. L., Bennett, J. M., Byrnes, R. K. (eds.): *Hematology: Clinical and Laboratory Practice*, St. Louis, MO; CV Mosby Publishers, 1993, p. 155.
203 Marlar, R. A., Sills, R. H. and Montgomery, R. R. Protein C in commercial factor IX (F IX) concentrations (CONC) and its use in the treatment of "homozygous" protein C deficiency. *Blood*, **62**: 303, 1998.
204 Pescatore, P., Horellou, H., Conard, J., *et al.* Problems of oral anticoagulation in an adult with homozygous protein C deficiency and late onset of thrombosis. *Thromb. Haemostas.*, **69**: 311, 1993.
205 Monagle, P., Andrew, M., Halton, J., *et al.* Homozygous protein C deficiency: description of a new mutation and successful treatment with low molecular weight heparin. *Thromb. Haemostas.*, **79**: 756, 1998.
206 Broekmans, A. W., Bertina, R. M., Loeliger, E. A., *et al.* Protein C and the development of skin necrosis during anticoagulant therapy. *Thromb. Haemostas.*, **49**: 251, 1983.
207 Zauber, N. P. and Stark, M. W. Successful warfarin anticoagulation despite protein C deficiency and a history of warfarin necrosis. *Ann. Int. Med.*, **104**: 659, 1986.
208 Samama, M., Horellou, M. H., Soria, J., *et al.* Successful progressive anticoagulation in a severe protein C deficiency and previous skin necrosis at the initiation of oral anticoagulation treatment. *Thromb. Haemostas.*, **51**: 132 (letter), 1984.
209 Bick, R. L. and Kaplan, H. Syndromes of thrombosis and hypercoagulability: congenital and acquired thrombophilias. *Clin. Appl. Thromb. Hemostas.*, **4**: 25, 1998.
210 Nilsson, I. M. and Pandofi, M. Fibrinolytic response of the vascular wall. *Thrombosis Diathesis Hemorrhagica*, **40**: 231, 1970.
211 Gardiner, J. E., McGann, M. A. and Berridge, C. W. Protein S as a cofactor for activated protein C in plasma and the inactivation of purified factor VIII: C. *Circulation*, **70**: 205, 1984.

212 De Fouw, N. J., Haverkate, F. and Bertina, R. M. The cofactor role of protein S in the acceleration of whole blood clot lysis by activated protein C in vitro. *Blood,* **67**: 1189, 1986.

213 Hackeng, T. M., van't Veer, C., Meijers, J. C., *et al.* Human protein S inhibits prothrombinase complex activity on endothelial cells and platelets via direct interactions with factors Va and Xa. *J. Biol. Chem.*, **269**: 21051, 1994.

214 Koppelman, S. J., Hackeng, T. M., Sixma, J. J., *et al.* Inhibition of the intrinsic factor X activating complex by protein S: evidence for specific binding of protein S to factor VIII. *Blood,* **86**: 1062, 1995.

215 Gladson, K. H., Griffin, J. H. and Hach, V. The incidence of protein C and protein S deficiency in 139 young thrombotic patients. *Thromb. Hemostas.*, **59**: 18, 1988.

216 Heijboer, H., Brandjes, D. P., Buller, H. R., *et al.* Deficiencies of coagulation-inhibiting and fibrinolytic proteins in outpatients with deep-vein thrombosis. *N. Engl. J. Med.*, **323**: 1512, 1990.

217 Tabernero, M. D., Tomas, J. F., Alberca, I., *et al.* Incidence and clinical characteristics of hereditary disorders associated with venous thrombosis. *Am. J. Hematol.*, **36**: 249, 1991.

218 Simmonds, R. E., Ireland, H., Lane, D., *et al.* Clarification of the risk for venous thrombosis associated with hereditary protein S deficiency by investigation of a large kindred with a characterized gene defect. *Ann. Int. Med.*, **128**: 8, 1998.

219 Mahasandana, C., Suvatte, V., Marlar, R. A., *et al.* Neonatal purpura fulminans associated with homozygous protein S deficiency. *Lancet,* **335**: 61, 1990.

220 Broekmans, M. A., Engesser, L. and Briet, E. Clinical manifestations of hereditary protein S deficiency. *Thromb. Haemostas.*, **54**: 57, 1985.

221 Engesser, L., Broekmans, A. W., Briet, E., *et al.* Hereditary protein S deficiency: clinical manifestations. *Ann. Int. Med.*, **106**: 677, 1987.

222 Juhan-Vague, I., Roul, C., Alessi, M. C., *et al.* Increased plasminogen activator inhibitor activity in non-insulin dependent diabetic patients – relationship with plasma insulin. *Thromb. Haemostas.*, **61**: 370, 1989.

223 Nalbandian, R. M., Henry, R. L. and Bick, R. L. Thrombotic thrombocytopenic purpura: an extended editorial. *Semin. Thromb. Hemostas.*, **5**: 216, 1979.

224 Bick, R. L., Bishop, R. C. and Shanbrom, E. Fibrinolytic activity in acute myocardial infarction. *Am. J. Clin. Pathol.*, **57**: 359, 1972.

225 Collen, D. and Juhan-Vague, I. Fibrinolysis and atherosclerosis. *Semin. Thromb. Hemostas.*, **14**: 180, 1988.

226 Mansfield, M. O. Alterations in fibrinolysis associated with surgery and venous thrombosis. *Br. J. Surg.*, **59**: 754, 1972.

227 Bick, R. L. and Thompson, W. B. Fibrinolytic activity: changes induced with oral contraceptives. *Obstet. Gynecol.*, **39**: 213, 1972.

228 Marsh, N. Fibrinolysis in disease. In Bick, R. L. (ed.): *Fibrinolysis*. New York, NY: John Wiley and Sons, 1981, p. 125.

229 Hedner, U. and Nilsson, I. M. Urokinase in serum in a clinical series. *Acta Medica Scandin.*, **4**: 185, 1971.

230 Stemerman, M. B. Vascular intimal components: precursors of thrombosis. *Prog. Hemostas. Thromb.*, **2**: 1, 1974.

231 Wight, T. Vessel proteoglycans and thrombogenesis. *Prog. Hemostas. Thromb.*, **5**: 1, 1980.
232 Mammen, E. F. Plasminogen abnormalities. *Semin. Hemostas. Thromb.*, **9**: 50, 1983.
233 Aoki, N., Moroi, M. and Sakata, Y. Abnormal plasminogen. A hereditary molecular abnormality found in a patient with recurrent thrombosis. *J. Clin. Invest.*, **61**: 1186, 1978.
234 Blaisdell, W. Acquired and congenital clotting syndromes. *World J. Surg.*, **14**: 664, 1990.
235 Hasegawa, D. K., Tyler, B. J. and Edson, J. R. Thrombotic disease in three families with inherited plasminogen deficiency. *Blood,* **60**: 213, 1982.
236 Sartori, M. T., Patrassi, G. M., Girolami, B., *et al.* Type I plasminogen deficiency should be included among familial thrombophilias. Letter. *Clin. Appl. Thromb. Hemostas.*, **3**: 218, 1997.
237 Biasutti, F. D., Sulzer, I., Stucki, B., *et al.* Is plasminogen deficiency a thrombotic risk factor? A study on 23 thrombophilic patients and their family members. *Thromb. Haemostas.*, **80**: 167, 1998.
238 Kazama, M., Tahara, C. and Suzki, Z. Abnormal plasminogen: a case of recurrent thrombosis. *Thromb. Res.*, **21**: 517, 1981.
239 Bick, R. L. Clinical hemostasis practice: The major impact of laboratory automation. *Semin. Thromb. Hemostas.*, **9**: 139, 1983.
240 Nilsson, I. M. and Tehgborn, L. A. A family with thrombosis associated with high level of tissue plasminogen activator inhibitor. *Haemostasis,* **14**: 24, 1984.
241 Petaja, M., Rasi, V. and Myllyla, G. Familial hypofibrinolysis and venous thrombosis. *Br. J. Haematol.*, **71**: 393, 1989.
242 Tabernero, M. D., Estelles, A. and Vincente, V. Incidence of increased plasminogen activator inhibitor in patients with deep venous thrombosis and/or pulmonary embolism. *Thromb. Res.*, **56**: 565, 1989.
243 Dawson, S., Hamsten, A. and Wiman, B. Genetic variation at the plasminogen activator inhibitor-1 locus is associated with altered levels of plasma plasminogen activator inhibitor activity. *Athersclerosis Thrombosis,* **11**: 183, 1991.
244 Li, X. N., Grtenett, H. E. and Benza, R. L. Genotype-specific transcriptional regulation of PAI-1 expression by hypertriglyceridemic VLDL and LP(a) in cultured human endothelial cells. *Atherosclerosis Thrombosis Vascular Biol.*, **17**: 3215, 1997.
245 Eriksson, P., Kallin, B. and Van Hooft, F. M. Allele-specific increase in basal transcription of the plasminogen-activator inhibitor 1 gene is associated with myocardial infarction. *National Acad. Science, USA,* **92**: 1851, 1995.
246 Ye, S., Green, F. R. and Scarabin, P. Y. The 4G/5G genetic polymorphism in the promoter of the plasminogen activator inhibitor 1 (PAI-1) gene is associated with differences in plasma PAI-1 activity but not with the risk of myocardial infarction in the ECTIM study. *Thromb. Haemosta.*, **74**: 837, 1995.
247 Ridker, P. M., Hennekens, C. H. and Lindpaintner, K. Arterial and venous thrombosis is not associated with the 4G/5G polymorphism in the promoter of the plasminogen activator inhibitor gene in a large cohort of US men. *Circulation,* **95**: 59, 1997.
248 Hong, J. J. and Kwaan, H. C. Hereditary defects in fibrinolysis associated with thrombosis. *Seminars Thrombosis Hemostasis,* **25**: 321, 1999.
249 Mammen, E. F., Barnhart, M. I., Selik, N. R., *et al.*: "Sticky Platelet Syndrome": a congenital platelet abnormality predisposing to thrombosis. *Folia Haematologica,* **115**: 361, 1988.

250 Rubenfire, M., Blevens, R. D., Barnhart, M. I., *et al.* Platelet hyperaggregability in patients with chest pain and angiographically normal coronary arteries. *Am. J. Cardiol.*, **57**: 657, 1986.

251 Chittoor, S., Elsehety, A. E., Roberts, G. F., *et al.* Sticky platelet syndrome: a case report and review of the literature. *J. Clinical Applied Thrombosis Hemostasis*, **4**: 280, 1998.

252 Mammen, E. F. Ten year's experience with the "Sticky Platelet Syndrome". *J. Clin. Appl. Thromb. Hemostas.*, **1**: 66, 1995.

253 Mammen, E. F. Sticky platelet syndrome. *Seminars Thrombosis Hemostasis*, **25**: 361, 1999.

254 Bick, R. L. Sticky Platelet Syndrome: a common cause of unexplained venous and arterial thrombosis – results of prevalence and treatment outcome. *J. Clin. Appl. Thromb. Hemostas.*, **4**: 77, 1998.

255 Anderson, J. A., Bleeding and thrombosis in women. *Biomedical Prog.*, **12**: 40, 1999.

256 Berg-Damer, E., Henkes, E., Trobisch, H., *et al.* Sticky platelet syndrome: a cause of neurovascular thrombosis and thromboembolism. *Interventional Neuroradiology*, **3**: 145, 1997.

257 Bick, R. L. Hypercoagulability and thrombosis. *Medical Clinics North America*, **78**: 635, 1994.

258 Bick, R. L. Antiphospholipid thrombosis syndromes: etiology, pathophysiology, diagnosis and management. *International J. Hematology*, **65**: 193, 1997.

259 Oosting, J. D., Derksen, R. H. and Bobbink, I. W. G. Antiphospholipid antibodies directed against a combination of phospholipids with prothrombin, protein C or protein S: an explanation for their pathogenic mechanism? *Blood*, **81**: 2618, 1993.

260 Bick, R. L. The antiphospholipid thrombosis syndromes: a common multidisciplinary medical problem. *J. Clinical Applied Thrombosis Hemostasis*, **3**: 270, 1997.

261 Bick, R. L. and Baker, W. F. Anticardiolipin antibodies and thrombosis. *Hematology Oncology Clinics North America*, **6**: 1287, 1992.

262 Bick, R. L. and Baker, W. F. Antiphospholipid syndrome and thrombosis. *Seminars Thrombosis Hemostasis*, **25**: 333, 1999.

263 Bick, R. L. Antiphospholipid thrombosis syndromes. *Hematology Oncology Clinics North America*, **17**: 115, 2003.

264 Bick, R. L. and Baker, W. F. The antiphospholipid and thrombosis syndromes. *Medical Clinics North America*, **78**: 667, 1994.

265 Conley, C. L. and Hartmann, R. C. A hemorrhagic disorder caused by circulating anticoagulant in patients with disseminated lupus erythematosus. *J. Clin. Invest.*, **31**: 621, 1952.

266 Criel, A., Collen, D. and Masson, P. L. A case of IgM antibodies which inhibit the contact activation of blood coagulation. *Thromb. Research.*, **12**: 833, 1978.

267 Kunkel, L. Acquired circulating anticoagulants. *Hematology Oncology Clinics North America*, **6**: 1341, 1992.

268 Coller, B. S., Hultin, M. B. and Hoyer, L. W. Normal pregnancy in a patient with a prior postpartum factor VIII inhibitor: with observations on pathogenesis and prognosis. *Blood*, **58**: 619, 1981.

269 LeFrere, J. J., Gozin, D. and Lerable, J. Circulating anticoagulant in asymptomatic persons seropositive for human immunodeficiency virus. *Ann. Internal Med.*, **108**: 771 (letter), 1988.

270 Taillan, B., Roul, C. and Fuzibet, J. G. Circulating anticoagulant in patients seropositive for human immunodeficiency virus. *Ann. Internal Med. (France)*, **87**: 405, 1989.

271 Davis, S., Furie, B. and Griffin, J. H. Circulating inhibitors of blood coagulation associated with procainamide-induced lupus anticoagulants. *Am. J. Hematology*, **4**: 401, 1978.

272 Jeffrey, R. F. Transient lupus anticoagulant with fansidar therapy. *Postgrad. Med. J.*, **62**: 893, 1986.

273 Morgan, M., Downs, K., Chesterman, C. N., *et al.* Clinical analysis of 125 patients with the lupus anticoagulant. *Aust. N. Z. J. Med.*, **23**: 151, 1993.

274 Bick, R. L. and Ucar, K. Hypercoagulability and thrombosis. *Hematology Oncology Clinics North America*, **6**: 1421, 1992.

275 Schleider, M. A., Nachman, R. L. and Jaffe, E. A. A clinical study of the lupus anticoagulant. *Blood*, **48**: 499, 1976.

276 Regan, M. G., Lackner, H. and Karpatkin, S. Platelet function and coagulation profile in lupus erythematosus. *Ann. Internal Med.*, **81**: 462, 1974.

277 Mueh, J. R., Herbst, K. D. and Rapaport, S. I. Thrombosis in patients with the "lupus"-type circulating anticoagulant. *Ann. Internal Med.*, **92**: 156, 1980.

278 Shapiro, S. S. and Rajagopalon, V. Hemorrhagic disorders associated with circulating inhibitors. (chapter 7) In Ratnoff, O. D. and Forbes, C. D. (eds.), *Disorders of Hemostasis*. Philadelphia, PA; W. B. Saunders, 1996, p. 208.

279 Kampe, C. E. Clinical syndromes associated with lupus anticoagulants. *Seminars Thrombosis Hemostasis*, **20**: 16, 1994.

280 Hinton, R. C. Neurological syndromes associated with antiphospholipid antibodies. *Seminars Thrombosis Hemostasis*, **20**: 46, 1994.

281 Kleinknecht, D., Bobrie, G., Meyer, O., *et al.* Recurrent thrombosis and renal vascular disease in a patient with lupus anticoagulant. *Nephrology, Dialysis, Transplantation*, **4**: 854, 1989.

282 Pope, J. M., Canny, C. L. and Bell, D. A. Cerebral ischemic events associated with endocarditis, retinal vascular disease and lupus anticoagulant. *Am. J. Medicine*, **90**: 299–309, 1991.

283 Baker, W. F. and Bick, R. L. Antiphospholipid antibodies in coronary artery disease. *Seminars Thrombosis Hemostasis*, **20**: 27, 1994.

284 Reyes, H., Dearing, L. and Shoenfeld, Y. Antiphospholipid antibodies: a critique of their heterogeneity and hegemony. *Seminars Thrombosis Hemostasis*, **20**: 89, 1994.

285 Kaczor, N. A., Bickford, N. N. and Triplett, D. A. Evaluation of different mixing study reagents and dilution effect in lupus anticoagulant testing. *J. Clin. Pathol.*, **95**: 408, 1991.

286 Shapiro, S. S. and Thiagarajan, P. Lupus anticoagulants. *Prog. Hemostas. Thrombosis*, **6**: 263, 1982.

287 Ko, J., Guaglianone, P., Wolin, M., *et al.* Variation in the sensitivity of an activated thromboplasin time reagent to the lupus anticoagulant. *Am. J. Clin. Pathology*, **99**: 333 (abstract), 1993.

288 Bick, R. L. The antiphospholipid thrombosis syndromes: fact, fiction, confusion & controversy. *Am. J. Clin. Path.*, **100**: 477, 1993.

289 Thiagarajan, P., Pengo, V. and Shapiro, S. S. The use of the dilute Russel viper venom time for the diagnosis of lupus anticoagulants. *Blood*, **68**: 869, 1986.

290 McGehee, W. G., Patch, M. J. and Lingao, J. U. Detection of the lupus anticoagulant: a comparison of the kaolin clotting time with the tissue thromboplastin inhibition test. *Blood*, (Suppl) **62**: 276a (abstract), 1983.

291 Rosove, M. H., Ismail, M. and Koziol, B. J. Lupus anticoagulants: improved diagnosis with a kaolin clotting time using rabbit brain phospholipid in standard and high concentrations. *Blood*, **68**: 472, 1986.

292 Bick, R. L. Hypercoagulability and thrombosis (Chapter 13). In *Disorders of Thrombosis and Hemostasis: Clinical and Laboratory Practice*, Chicago, IL; ASCP Press, 1992, p. 261.

293 Harris, E. N. Immunology of antiphospholipid antibodies. In Lahita, R. (ed.), *Systemic Lupus Erythematosus, 2nd edn.*, London, Churchill Livingstone, 1992, p. 305.

294 Rauch, J. and Janoff, A. S. The nature of antiphospholipid antibodies. *J. Rheumatology*, **19**: 1782, 1992.

295 De Castellarnau, C., Vila, C. L. and Sancho, M. J. Lupus anticoagulant, recurrent abortion, and prostacyclin production by cultured smooth muscle cells. *Lancet*, **2**: 1137, 1983.

296 Sanfelippo, M. J. and Drayna, C. J. Prekallikrein inhibition associated with the lupus anticoagulant: a mechanism for thrombosis. *Am. J. Clin. Pathol.*, **77**: 275, 1982.

297 Bick, R. L. and Baker, W. F. Antiphospholipid and thrombosis syndromes. *Seminars Thrombosis Hemostasis*, **20**: 3, 1994.

298 Roubey, R. A. S. Autoantibodies to phospholipid-bonding plasma proteins: a new view of lupus anticoagulants and other "antiphospholipid" antibodies. *Blood*, **84**: 2854, 1994.

299 Bick, R. L., Laughlin, H. R., Cohen, B., *et al.* Fetal wastage syndrome due to blood protein/platelet defects: results of prevalence studies and treatment outcome with low-dose heparin and low-dose aspirin. *Clin. Applied Thrombosis Hemostasis*, **1**: 286, 1995.

300 Bick, R. L. The antiphospholipid thrombosis (APL-T) syndromes: Characteristics and recommendations for classification and treatment. *Am. J. Clin. Pathol.*, **96**: 424, 1991.

301 Rosove, M. H. and Brewer, P. M. C. Antiphospholipid thrombosis: clinical course after the first thrombotic event in 70 patients. *Ann. Internal Med.*, **117**: 303, 1992.

302 Bick, R. L. and Baker, W. F. Deep vein thrombosis: Prevalence of etiologic factors and results of management in 100 consecutive patients. *Seminars Thrombosis Hemostasis*, **18**: 267, 1992.

303 Bick, R. L., Madden, J., Heller, K. B., *et al.* Recurrent miscarriage: causes, evaluation, and treatment. *Medscape Women's Health*, **3**: 1, 1998.

304 Bick, R. L. and Toofanian, A. Recurrent miscarriage syndrome: outcome in 133 patients with thrombotic disorders treatd with heparin and aspirin. *J. Clinical Applied Thrombosis Hemostasis*, 5 (2005), in press.

305 Bowie, E. J. W., Thompson, J. H., Pascuzzi, C. A. Thrombosis in systemic lupus erythematosus despite circulating anticoagulant. *J. Lab. Clin. Med.*, **162**: 417, 1963.

306 Bell, W. R., Boss, G. R. and J. S. Wolfson. Circulating anticoagulant in the procainamide-induced lupus syndrome. *Arch. Int. Med.*, **137**: 1471, 1977.

307 Bick, R. L. The antiphospholipid thrombosis syndromes: Lupus anticoagulants & anticardiolipin antibodies (Chapter 14). In *Advances in Pathology and Laboratory Medicine*, Vol. 8, Mosby, Saint Louis, MO; **8**: 391,1995.

308 Espinoza, L. R., Hartmann, R. C. Significance of the lupus anticoagulant. *Am. J. Hematology*, **22**: 331, 1986.

309 Manoussakis, M. N., Tzioufas, A. G., Silis, M. P. High prevalence of anticardiolipin and other autoantibodies in a healthy elderly population. *Clin. Exp. Immunology*, **69**: 557, 1987.

310 Zarrabi, M. H., Zucker, S., Miller, F. Immunologic and coagulation disorders in chlorpromazine-treated patients. *Ann. Internal Med.*, **91**: 914, 1979.

311 Harris, E. N., Gharavi, A. E., Boey, M. L. Anticardiolipin antibodies: detection by radioimmunoassay and association with thrombosis in systemic lupus erythematosus. *Lancet*, **II**: 1211, 1983.

312 Weidmann, C. E., Wallace, D., Peter, J. Studies of IgG, IgM and IgA antiphospholipid antibody isotypes in systemic lupus erythematosus. *J. Rheumatol.*, **15**: 74, 1988.

313 Asherson, R. A., Harris, E. N. Anticardiolipin antibodies: clinical associations. *Postgrad. Med. J.*, **62**: 1081, 1986.

314 Hughes, G. V. R., Harris, E. N. and Gharavi, A. E. The anticardiolipin syndrome. *J. Rheumatol.*, **13**: 486, 1986.

315 Triplett, D. A. Clinical Significance of Antiphospholipid Antibodies. *Am. Soc. Clin. Pathol. Press: Hemostasis Thrombosis Check Sample*, **10**: 1, 1988.

316 Derue, G., Englert, H., Harris, E. Fetal loss in systemic lupus: association with anticardiolipin antibodies. *Brit. J. Obstet. Gynecol.*, **5**: 207, 1985.

317 Lubbe, W. F., Palmer, S. J., Butler, W. S. Fetal survival after prednisolone suppression of maternal lupus anticoagulant. *Lancet*, **I**: 1361, 1983.

318 Harris, E. N., Gharavi, A. E., Hedge, U. Anticardiolipin antibodies in autoimmune thrombocytopenia purpura. *Brit. J. Haematol.*, **59**: 231, 1985.

319 Harris, E. N., Asherson, R. A., Gharavi, A. E. Thrombocytopenia in SLE and related autoimmune disorders: association with anticardiolipin antibodies. *Brit. J. Haematol.*, **59**: 227, 1985.

320 Bick, R. L. and Kaplan, H. Syndromes of thrombosis and hypercoagulability: congenital and acquired thrombophilias. *Medical Clinics North America*, **82**: 409, 1998.

321 Rosove, M. H., Brewer, P. and Runge, A. Simultaneous lupus anticoagulant and anticardiolipin assays and clinical detection of antiphospholipids. *Am. J. Hematol.*, **32**: 148, 1989.

322 Tanne, D. T., Triplett, D. A. and Levine, S. R. Antiphospholipid-protein antibodies and ischemic stroke: not just cardiolipin any more. *Stroke*, **29**: 1755, 1998.

323 Bick, R. L. Discordance in antiphospholipid types in patients with arterial and venous thrombosis. *J. Clinical Applied Thrombosis Hemostasis*, 2005, in press.

324 McNeil, H. P., Chesterman, C. N., and Krilis, S. A. Anticardiolipin antibodies and lupus anticoagulants comprise separate antibody subgroups with different phospholipid binding characteriastics. *Brit. J. Haematol.*, **73**: 506, 1989.

325 Shi, B. S., Chong, B. H. and Chesterman, C. N. Beta-2-Glycoprotein I is a requirement for anticardiolipin antibodies binding to activated platelets: differences with lupus anticoagulants. *Blood*, **81**: 1255, 1993.

326 Harris, E. N., Hughes, G. R. V., Gharavi, A. E. Antiphospholipid antibodies: an elderly statesman dons new garments. *J. Rheumatol.*, **14**: 208, 1987.

327 Gharavi, A. E., Harris, E. N., Asherson, R. A. Anticardiolipin antibodies: isotype distribution and phospholipid specificity. *Ann. Rheumatic Dis.*, **46**: 1, 1987.

328 Carreras, L., Defreyn, G. and Manchin, S. Arterial thrombosis, intrauterine death and lupus anticoagulant: detection of immunoglobulin interfering with prostacyclin formation. *Lancet*, **1**: 244, 1981.

329 Cariou, R., Tobelem, G. and Bellucci, S. Effect of lupus anticoagulant on antithrombogenic properties of endothelial cells: inhibition of thrombomodulin-dependent protein C activation. *Thromb. Haemostas.*, **60**: 54, 1988.

330 Cosgriff, T. M., Martin, B. A. Low functional and high antigenic antithrombin III level in a patient with the lupus anticoagulant. *Arthritis Rheum.*, **24**: 94, 1981.

331 Khamashta, M. A., Harris, E. N. and Gharavi, A. E. Immune mediated mechanism for thrombosis: antiphospholipid antibody binding to platelet membranes. *Ann. Rheum. Dis.*, **47**: 849, 1988.

332 Sanfellipo, M. J., Drayna, C. J. Prekallikrein inhibition associated with the lupus anticoagulant. *Am. J. Clin. Pathol.*, **77**: 275, 1982.

333 Angeles-Cano, E., Sultan, Y. and Clauvel, J. P. Predisposing factors to thrombosis in systemic lupus erythematosus. Possible relationship to endothelial cell damage. *J. Lab. Clin. Med.*, **94**: 312, 1979.

334 Ruiz-Arguelles, G. The activated protein C resistance phenotype of the antiphospholipid syndrome may follow a relapsing course. *Clinical Applied Thrombosis Hemostasis*, **4**: 277, 1998.

335 Ginsburg, K. S., Liang, M. H., Newcomer, L. *et al.* Anticardiolipin antibodies and the risk for ischemic stroke and venous thrombosis. *Ann. Int. Med.*, **117**: 997, 1992.

336 Boey, M. L., Colaco, C. B. and Gharavi, A. E. Thrombosis in SLE: striking association with the presence of circulating "lupus anticoagulant". *Br. Med. J.*, **287**: 1021, 1983.

337 Elias, M. and Eldor, A. Thromboembolism in patients with the "lupus-like" circulating anticoagulant. *Arch. Int. Med.*, **144**: 510, 1984.

338 Hall, S., Buettner, H. and Luthra, H. S. Occlusive retinal vascular disease in systemic lupus erythematosus. *J. Rheumatol.*, **11**: 96, 1984.

339 Asherson, R. A., Harris, E. N. and Gharavi, A. E. Arterial occlusions associated with antibodies to anticardiolipin. *Arthritis Rheumatism*, **28**: s89 (abstr.), 1985.

340 Hamilton, M. E. Superior mesenteric artery thrombosis associated with antiphospholipid syndrome. *Western J. Medicine*, **155**: 174, 1991.

341 Asherson, R. A., Harris, E. N. and Gharavi, A. E. Aortic arch syndrome associated with anticardiolipin antibodies and the lupus anticoagulant. *Arthritis Rheumatism*, **28**: 594, 1985.

342 Asherson, R. A., Morgan, S. H. and Harris, E. N. Arterial occlusion causing large bowel infarction: a reflection of clotting diathesis in SLE. *Clin. Rheumatol.*, **5**: 102, 1986.

343 Asherson, R. A., MacKay, I. R. and Harris, E. N. Myocardial infarction in a young male with systemic lupus erythematosus, deep vein thrombosis and antiphospholipid antibodies. *Br. Heart J.*, **56**: 190, 1986.

344 Gavaghan, T. P., Krilis, S. A. and Daggard, G. E. Anticardiolipin antibodies and occlusion of coronary artery bypass grafts. *Lancet*, **II**: 977, 1987.

345 Morton, K. T., Gavaghan, S., Krilis, G. Coronary artery bypass graft failure: an autoimmune phenomenon? *Lancet*, **I**: 1353, 1986.

346 Hamsten, A., Norberg, R. and Bjorkholm, M. Antibodies to cardiolipin in young survivors of myocardial infarction: an association with recurrent cardiovascular events. *Lancet*, **I**: 113, 1986.

347 Harpaz, D. and Sidi, Y. Successful thrombolytic therapy for acute myocardial infarction in a patient with the antiphospholipid antibody syndrome. *American Heart J.*, **122**: 1492, 1991.

348 Asherson, R. A., Khamashta, M. A. and Ordi-Ros, J. The "primary" antiphospholipid syndrome: major clinical and serological features. *Medicine*, **68**: 366, 1989.

349 Bick, R. L., Ismail, Y. and Baker, W. F. Coagulation abnormalities in patients with precocious coronary artery thrombosis and patients failing coronary artery bypass grafting and percutaneous transcoronary angioplasty. *Seminars Thrombosis Hemostasis*, **19**: 411, 1993.

350 Galve, E., Ordi, J. and Barquinero, J. Valvular heart disease in the primary antiphospholipid syndrome. *Ann. Internal Medicine*, **116**: 293, 1992.

351 Chartash, E. K., Lans, D. M. and Paget, S. A. Aortic insufficiency and mitral regurgitation in patients wirh systemic lupus erythematosus and the antiphospholipid syndrome. *American J. Medicine*, **86**: 406, 1989.

352 Chartash, E. K., Paget, S. A. and Lockshin, M. D. Lupus anticoagulant associated with aortic and mitral valve insufficiency. *Arthritis Rheumatism*, **29**: 95, 1986.

353 Leung, W. H., Wong, K. L. and Wong, C. K. Association between antiphospholipid antibodies and cardiac abnormalities in patients with systemic lupus erythematosus. *American J. Medicine*, **89**: 411, 1990.

354 Coppock, M. A., Safford, R. E. and Danielson, G. K. Intracardiac thrombosis, phospholipid antibodies, and two-chambered right ventricle. *British Heart J.*, **60**: 455, 1988.

355 Reisner, S. A., Blumenfeld, Z. and Brenner, B. Cardiac involvement in patients with primary antiphospholipid syndrome. *Circulation (Suppl III)*, **82**: 398, 1990.

356 Weinstein, C., Miller, M. and Axtens, R. Livido reticularis associated with increased titers of anticardiolipin antibodies in systemic lupus erythematosus. *Arch. Dermatol.*, **123**: 596, 1987.

357 Eng, A. M. Cutaneous expressions of antiphospholipid syndromes. *Seminars Thrombosis Hemostasis*, **20**: 71, 1994.

358 Englert, H., Hawkes, C. and Boey, M. Dagos' Disease: association with anticardiolipin antibodies and the lupus anticoagulant. *Brit. Med. J.*, **289**, 576, 1984.

359 Bird, A. G., Lendrum, R. and Asherson, R. A. Disseminated intravascular coagulation, antiphospholipid antibodies, and ischemic necrosis of extremities. *Ann. Rheumatic Diseases*, **46**: 251, 1987.

360 Wolf, P., Peter-Soyer, H. and Auer-Grumbach, P. Widespread cutaneous necrosis in a patient with rheumatoid arthritis associated with anticardiolipin antibodies. *Arch. Dermatology*, **127**: 1739, 1991.

361 Ingram, S. B., Goodnight, S. H. and Bennett, R. M. An unusual syndrome of a devastating non-inflammatory vasculopathy associated with anticardiolipin antibodies: report of two cases. *Arthritis and Rheumatism*, **30**: 1167, 1987.

362 Levine, S. R., Langer, S. L. and Albers, J. W. Sneddon's syndrome: an antiphospholipid antibody syndrome? *Neurology*, **38**: 798, 1988.

363 Frampton, G., Winer, J. B. and Cameron, J. S. Severe Guillain-Barré syndrome: an association with IgA anti-cardiolipin antibody in a series of 92 patients. *J. Neuroimmunology*, **19**: 133, 1988.

364 Levine, S. and Welch, K. The spectrum of neurologic disease associated with anticardiolipin antibodies. *Arch. Neurol.*, **44**: 876, 1987.

365 Oppenheimer, S. and Hoffbrand, B. Optic neuritis and myelopathy in systemic lupus erythematosus. *Can. J. Neurol. Sci.*, **13**: 129, 1986.

366 Harris, E. N., Gharavi, A. E. and Asherson, R. A. Cerebral infarction in systemic lupus: association with anticardiolipin antibodies. *Clin. Exp. Rheumatology*, **2**: 471, 1984.

367 Williams, R. C. Cerebral infarction in systemic lupus: association with anticardiolipin antibodies. *Clin. Exp. Rheumatology*, **2**: 3, 1984.

368 Coull, B. M., Bourdette, D. N. and Goodnight, S. H. Multiple cerebral infarctions and dementia associated with anticardiolipin antibodies. *Stroke*, **18**: 1107, 1987.

369 Asherson, R. A., Khamashta, M. A. and Hughes, G. R. V. Sneddon's syndrome. *Neurology* **39**: 1138 (letter), 1989.

370 Moral, A. Sneddon's syndrome with antiphospholipid antibodies and arteriopathy. *Stroke*, **22**: 1327, 1991.

371 Sohngen, D., Wehmeier, A. and Specker, C. Antiphospholipid antibodies in systemic lupus erythematosus and Sneddon's syndrome. *Seminars Thrombosis Hemostasis*, **20**: 55, 1994.

372 Levine, S. R., Brey, R. L. and Joseph, C. L. M. Risk of recurrent thromboembolic events in patients with focal cerebral ischemia and antiphospholipid antibodies. *Stroke*, **23** (Suppl. I), 29, 1992.

373 Levine, S. R., Diaczok, I. M. and Deegan, M. J. Recurrent stroke associated with thymoma and anticardiolipin antibodies. *Arch. Neurology*, **44**: 678, 1987.

374 Brey, R. L., Hart, R. G., Sherman, D. G., *et al.* Antiphospholipid antibodies and cerebral ischemia in young people. *Neurology*, **40**: 1190, 1990.

375 Toschi, V., Motta, A., Castelli, C., *et al.* High prevalence of antiphosphatidylinositol antibodies in young patients with cerebral ischemia of undetermined cause. *Stroke*, **29**: 1759, 1998.

376 Nencini, P., Baruffi, M. C., Abbate, R., *et al.* Lupus anticoagulant and anticardiolipin antibodies in young adults with cerebral ischemia. *Stroke*, **23**: 189, 1992.

377 Carhaupoma, J. R., Mitsias, P. and Levine, S. R. Cerebral venous thrombosis and anticardiolipin antibodies. *Stroke*, **28**: 2363, 1997.

378 Bick, R. L. and Hinton, R. C. Prevalence of hereditary and acquired coagulation protein/platelet defects in patients with cerebral ischemia. *Blood*, **92**: (Suppl 1, part 2) 114b (abstr. 3466), 1998.

379 Levine, S. R., Brey, R. L., Sawaya, K. L., *et al.* Recurrent stroke and thrombo-occlusive events in the antiphospholipid syndrome. *Ann. Neurology*, **38**: 119, 1995.

380 Brey, R. for the APASS Group. Anticardiolipin antibodies are an independent risk factor for first ischemic stroke. *Neurology*, **43**: 2069, 1993.

381 Hull, R. G., Harris, N. and Gharavi, A. E. Anticardiolipin antibodies: occurrence in Behcet's syndrome. *Ann. Rheumatic Diseases*, **43**: 746, 1984.

382 Harris, N. E. and Spinnato, J. A. Should anticardiolipin tests be performed in otherwise healthy pregnant women? *Am. J. Obstetrics Gynecology*, **165**: 1272, 1991.

383 Buchanan, N. M., Khamashta, M. A., Morton, K. E., *et al.* A study of 100 high-risk lupus pregnancies. *American J. Reproductive Immunology*, **28**: 192, 1992.

384 Editorial: Anticardiolipin antibodies – a risk factor for venous and arterial thrombosis. *Lancet*, **I**: 912, 1985.
385 Kwak, J. Y., Gilman-Sachs, A., Beaman, K. D., *et al.* Reproductive outcome in women with recurrent spontaneous abortions of alloimmune and autoimmune causes: preconception versus postconception treatment. *American J. Obstetrics Gynecology*, **166**: 1787, 1992.
386 Bick, R. L. Recurrent miscarriage syndrome and infertility caused by blood coagulation protein or platelet defects. *Hematology Oncology Clinics North America*, **14**: 1117, 2000; *Chin. J. Obstet. Gynecol.*, **28**: 674, 1993.
387 Parazzini, F., Acaia, B. and Faden, D. Antiphospholipid antibodies and recurrent abortion. *Obstet. Gynecol.*, **77**: 854, 1991.
388 Grandone, E., Margaglione, M. and Vecchione, G. Antiphospholipid antibodies and risk of fetal loss: a pilot report of a cross-sectional study. *Thrombosis Haemostasis*, **69**: 597 (abstract), 1993.
389 Birdsall, M., Pattison, N. and Chamley, L. Antiphospholipid antibodies in pregnancy. *Aust. N. Z. J. Obstet. Gynaecol.*, **32**: 328, 1992.
390 Maclean, M. A., Cumming, G. P. and McCall, F. The prevalence of lupus anticoagulant and anticardiolipin antibodies in women with a history of first trimester miscarriages. *Brit. J. Obstet. Gynaecol.*, **101**: 103, 1994.
391 Howard, M. A., Firkin, B. G. and Healy, D. L. Lupus anticoagulant in a woman with multiple spontaneous miscarriage. *Am. J. Hematology*, **26**: 175, 1987.
392 Taylor, M., Cauchi, M. N. and Buchanan, R. R. C. The lupus anticoagulant, anticardiolipin antibodies, and recurrent miscarriage. *Am. J. Reproductive Immunol.*, **23**: 33, 1990.
393 Parke, A. L., Wilson, D. and Maier, D. The prevalence of antiphospholipid antibodies in women with recurrent spontaneous abortion, women with successful pregnancies, and women who have never been pregnant. *Arthritis Rheumatism*, **34**: 1231, 1991.
394 Kochenour, N. K., Branch, D. W. and Rote, N. S. A new postpartum syndrome associated with antiphospholipid antibodies. *Obstet. Gynecol.*, **69**: 460, 1987.
395 Intrator, L., Oksenhendler, E. and Desforges, L. Anticardiolipin antibodies in HIV infected patients with or without immune thrombocytopenic purpura. *Brit. J. Haematol.*, **67**: 269, 1988.
396 Canoso, R. T., Zon, L. I. and Groopman, J. E. Anticardiolipin antibodies associated with HTLV-III infection. *Brit. J. Haematology*, **65**: 495, 1987.
397 Panzer, S., Stain, C. and Hartl, H. Anticardiolipin antibodies are elevated in HIV-1 infected haemophiliacs but do not predict for disease progression. *Thrombosis Haemostasis*, **61**: 81, 1989.
398 Stimmler, M. M., Quismorio, F. P. and McGehee, W. G. Anticardiolipin antibodies in acquired immunodeficiency syndrome. *Arch. Int. Medicine*, **149**: 1833, 1989.
399 Vaarala, O., Palosuo, T. and Kleemola, M. Anticardiolipin response in acute infections. *Clin. Immunology and Immunopathology*, **41**: 8, 1986.
400 Violi, F., Ferro, D. and Quintarelli, C. Dilute aPTT prolongation by antiphospholipid antibodies in patients with liver cirrhosis. *Thrombosis Haemostasis*, **63**: 183, 1990.
401 Harrison, R. L., Alperin, J. B. and Kumar, D. Concurrent lupus anticoagulants and prothrombin deficiency due to phenytoin use. *Arch. Pathology Laboratory Medicine*, **111**: 719, 1987.

402 Lillicrap, D. P., Pinto, M. and Benford, K. Heterogeneity of laboratory test results for antiphospholipid antibodies in patients treated with chlorpromazine and other phenothiazines. *Am. J. Clin. Pathology*, **93**: 771, 1990.

403 Walenga, J. M. and Bick, R. L. Heparin-induced thrombocytopenia, paradoxical thromboembolism and other side effects of heparin therapy. *Cardiology Clinics: Annual of Drug Therapy*, **2**: 123, 1998.

404 Girolami, B., Prandoni, P., Rossi, L., *et al.* Transaminase elevation in patients treated with unfractionated heparin or low molecular weight heparin for venous thromboembolism. *Clinical Applied Thrombosis Hemostasis*, **4**: 126, 1998.

405 Schved, J. F., Dupuy-Fons, C. and Biron, C. A prospective epidemiological study on the occurrence of antiphospholipid antibody: the Montpellier Antiphospholipid (MAP) Study. *Haemostasis*, **24**: 175, 1994.

406 Vila, P., Hernandez, M. C. and Lopez-Fernandez, M. F. Prevalence, follow-up and clinical significance of the anticardiolipin antibodies in normal subjects. *Thrombosis Haemostasis*, **72**: 209, 1994.

407 Bick, R. L. and Ancypa, D. The antiphospholipid and thrombosis syndromes: clinical and laboratory correlates. *Clinics Laboratory Medicine*, **15**: 63, 1995.

408 Falcon, C. R., Hoffer, A. M., Forastiero, R. R., *et al.* Clinical significance of various ELISA assays for detecting antiphospholipid antibodies. *Thrombosis Haemostasis*, **64**: 21, 1990.

409 Loizou, S., McCrea, J. D., Rudge, A. C., *et al.* Measurement of anti-cardiolipin antibodies by an enzyme-linked immunosorbent assay (ELISA): standardization and quantitation of results. *Clin. Exp. Immunology*, **62**: 738, 1985.

410 Reyes, H., Dearing, L., Bick, R. L., *et al.* Laboratory diagnosis of antiphospholipid syndromes. *Clinics Laboratory Medicine*, **15**: 85, 1995.

411 Triplett, D. A. Laboratory evaluation of circulating anticoagulants. (Chapter 98) In *Hematology: Clinical and Laboratory Practice*, ed. Bick, R. L., Bennett, R. M., Brynes, R. K., *et al.* St. Louis, MO, C. V. Mosby Publisher, 1993, pp. 1539–48.

412 Mannucci, P. M., Canciani, M. T., Mari, D., *et al.* The varied sensitivity of partial thromboplastin and prothrombin time reagents in the demonstration of the lupus-like inhibitor. *Scand. J. Haematology*, **22**: 423, 1979.

413 Bick, R. L., Pascoe, H. R. and Laughlin, W. R. Efficacy of four common activated partial thromboplastin times in screening for the lupus anticoagulant. *Blood*, **84**: 82 (abstract), 1994.

414 Saxena, R., Saraya, A. K., Kotte, V. K., *et al.* Evaluation of four coagulation tests to detect plasma lupus anticoagulants. *Am. J. Clinical Pathology*, **96**: 755, 1991.

415 Exner, T., Triplett, D. A., Taberner, D., *et al.* Guidelines for testing and revised criteria for lupus anticoagulants. *Thrombosis Haemostasis*, **65**: 320, 1991.

416 Bell, H. G. and Alton, H. G. A brain extract as a substitute for platelet suspensions in the thromboplastin generation test. *Nature*, **174**: 880, 1954.

417 Rauch, J., Tannenbaum, M. and Janoff, A. S. Distinguishing plasma lupus anticoagulants from anti-factor antibodies using hexagonal (II) phase phospholipids. *Thrombosis Haemostasis*, **62**: 892, 1989.

418 Cabral, A. R., Amigo, M. C., Cabiedes, J., *et al.* The antiphospholipid/cofactor syndromes: a primary variant with antibodies to beta-2-glycoprotein-1 but no antibodies detectable in standard antiphospholipid assays. *American J. Medicine*, **101**: 472, 1996.

419 Falcon, C. R., Hoffer, A. M. and Carreras, L. O. Antiphosphatidylinositol antibodies as markers of the antiphospholipid syndrome. *Thrombosis Haemostasis,* **63**: 321, 1990.

420 Falcon, C. R., Hoffer, A. M. and Carreras, L. O. Evaluation of the clinical and laboratory associations of antiphosphatidylethanolamine antibodies. *Thrombosis Research,* **59**: 383, 1990.

421 Sorice, M., Circella, A., Garofalo, G. T., *et al.* Anticardiolipin and anti-beta-2-GPI are two distinct populations of antibodies. *Thrombosis Haemostasis,* **75**: 303, 1996.

422 Martinuzzo, M. E., Forastiero, R. R. and Carreras, L. O. Anti-beta-2-glycoprotein I antibodies: detection and association with thrombosis. *Br. J. Haematology,* **89**: 397, 1995.

423 Staub, H. L., Harris, E. N., Khamashta, M. A., *et al.* Antibody to phosphatidylethanolamine in a patient with lupus anticoagulant and thrombosis. *Ann. Rheumatic Diseases,* **48**: 166, 1989.

6

Thromboprophylaxis and treatment of thrombosis in pregnancy

L. Heilmann,[1] W. Rath[2] and R. L. Bick[3]

[1]Professor of Obstetrics and Gynaecology, City Hospital, Rüsselsheim
[2]Professor of Obstetrics and Gynaecology, University of Aachen, Aachen, Germany
[3]Clinical Professor of Medicine and Pathology, University of Texas Southwestern Medical Center; Director: Dallas Thrombosis Hemostasis and Vascular Medicine Clinical Center, Dallas, Texas, USA

Introduction

The true incidence of thromboembolic complications in pregnancy and the distribution of these events between the antenatal and postnatal periods are unknown.[3,27] Early studies have estimated an incidence of symptomatic venous thrombosis during pregnancy using radiographic investigations between 0.5 and 3.0 per 1,000 deliveries.[8,75] Lindqvist *et al.*[57] used the Swedish national registries of births to investigate the number of objectively confirmed DVT between 1990 and 1993. The overall incidence of venous thromboembolic events was 1.3 per 1,000 deliveries in contrast to McColl *et al.*[61,62] with 0.8 per 1,000 deliveries, Gherman *et al.*[34] with 0.6 per 1,000 deliveries and Simpson *et al.*[78] with 0.85 per 1,000 deliveries. More recent studies have demonstrated that antepartum deep vein thrombosis (DVT) is at least as common as postpartum DVT (Fig. 6.1) and can occur at any time during gestation, although pulmonary emboli (PE) remains more common postpartum.[31,74] Earlier postpartum ambulation and discharge of patients from the hospital may have resulted in a relative decrease in postpartum events as compared to antepartum period, but the daily risk of thromboembolic complication was therefore highest in the postpartum period.

In a retrospective study McColl *et al.*[61] described an incidence of DVT at 0.5 per 1,000 deliveries in the antenatal period and 0.21 in the puerperium. The incidence of pulmonary embolism was 0.07 per 1,000 deliveries and 0.08 in the puerperium respectively.

Ray and Chan[73] summarized the available data of DVT during pregnancy and puerperium and found no evidence for significant difference between the trimester events. This study also found that 82.2% of pregnancy-related events affected the left leg.

Hematological Complications in Obstetrics, Pregnancy, and Gynecology, ed. R. L. Bick *et al.* Published by Cambridge University Press.

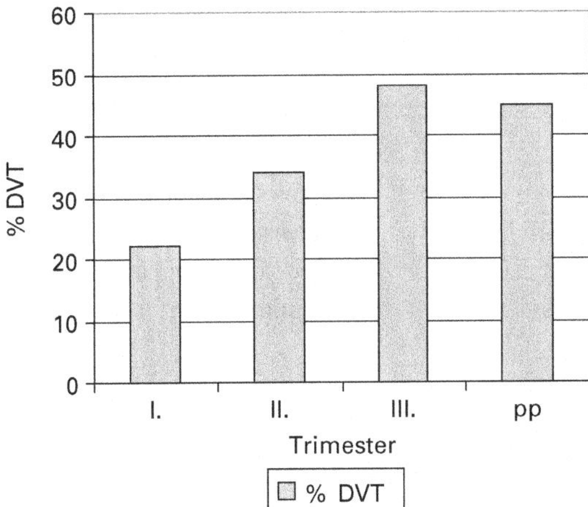

Figure 6.1 Distribution of DVT in pregnancy and postpartum. Data from Ray and Chan.[73]

Although the estimated rates are low, DVT and its associated complications remain a leading cause of maternal mortality and morbidity. Pulmonary emboli will occur in 16% of patients with untreated DVT, with 13% mortality.[79] An important cause of maternal death in UK between 1994 and 1996 were thrombosis and hypertension.[24] The confidential enquiries into maternal deaths in the UK described 46 deaths caused by pulmonary embolism. Ten antenatal deaths occurred in the first trimester, three other deaths in the second trimester, and two deaths took place after 24 weeks of gestation. Additional risk factors were surgery, prolonged bed rest and previous thromboembolism. Fifteen deaths occurred after cesarean section and 10 deaths after vaginal delivery.

An important clinical problem is the indication for thrombosis prophylaxis and management in pregnancy and when venous thrombosis is suspected in pregnancy it is important to obtain an objective diagnosis. This review focuses on prophylaxis and treatment of DVT in pregnancy and includes studies on thrombophilia and pregnancy complications.

Pathogenesis of deep venous thrombosis in pregnancy

An increasing trend towards hypercoagulability is physiologically present during pregnancy. Important factors for the regulation of the coagulation system consist of inhibitors that inactivate coagulation factors and the fibrinolytic system. These factors are displayed in Table 6.1.

Control of the coagulation cascade depends on maintaining a balance between prothrombotic factors and the natural anticoagulants, antithrombin and activated

Table 6.1 Hemostatic changes in pregnancy: Comparison conditions pro and against thrombosis.

Conditions pro thrombosis	Conditions against thrombosis
Decreases in fibrinolytic activity	Decreased factors XI and XIII
Activation of factors V, VII, VIII, IX, X, XII and fibrinogen	Expansion of plasma volume
Increased activation of platelets	Thrombin neutralization by antithrombin
Hereditary thrombophilia	
Decreases in protein S	
Antiphospholipid antibodies	
Endothelial damage associated with labor	
Venous stasis of the lower extremities	

protein C (APC). Activated protein C and its cofactor protein S catalyze the inactivation of factors Va and VIIIa, decreasing coagulation and reducing thrombin and fibrin generation.[72] Protein S decreases of more than 50% are regarded as normal and the resistance to activated protein C increases probably as a function of increases in factors V and VIII. Activated protein C may also stimulate fibrinolysis (increased PAI-1 and PAI-2, the latter being produced by the placenta). Additional factors that are involved in other anticoagulant mechanisms and may be involved in this process are tissue-factor pathway inhibitor (TFPI), thrombomodulin, and annexin V. The glycoprotein thrombomodulin is located on the surface of the endothelium as a part of the affinity to anionic membrane phospholipids and thus prevents the coagulation on the phospholipids' surface. The lack or destruction of this shield is probably involved in the development of the antiphospholipid syndrome.[46,70]

The individual risk of DVT or pulmonary embolism (PE) varies depending on the presence of additional clinical risk factors such as a history of DVT, operative delivery, bed rest, obesity, age, and inherited or acquired coagulation defects.

Clinical risk factors

Cesarean section

The incidence of postpartum DVT is affected by the mode of delivery. According to Macklon and Greer,[59] cesarean section was complicated by DVT with a rate of 0.4 per 1,000, compared with a rate of 0.173 per 1,000 following vaginal delivery

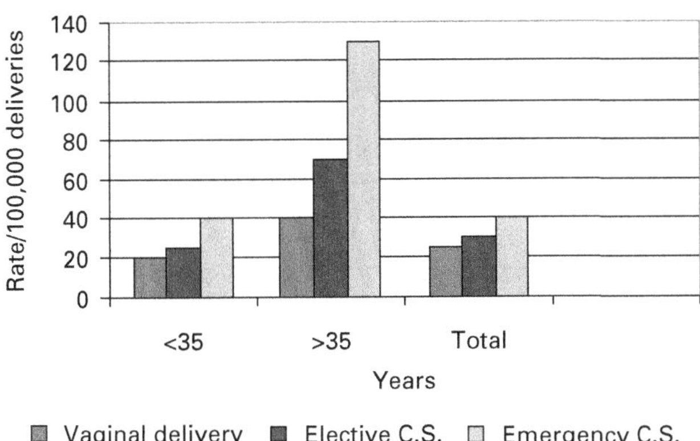

Figure 6.2 Incidence of postpartum DVT (C.S.: Cesarean Section).

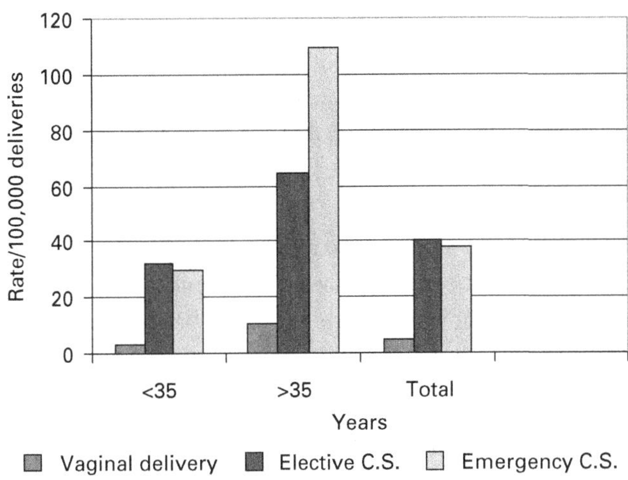

Figure 6.3 Incidence of postpartum PE (C.S.: Cesarean Section).

(Fig. 6.2). Women older than 35 years having an emergency cesarean section had a higher rate of postpartum DVT but not a higher rate of PE than women undergoing elective cesarean section (Fig. 6.3). It is clinically important that most instances of DVT and PE were diagnosed after discharge from hospital (38% and 22% respectively). In a cohort study of about 395.335 women with live births between 1988 and 1997 the annual incidence rate ranked from 60 per 100,000 maternities in 1995 to 117 per 100,000 maternities in 1997.[78] Incidence rate increased with increased age and following cesarean section (178 per 100,000 c.s.), approximately four times that following vaginal deliveries.

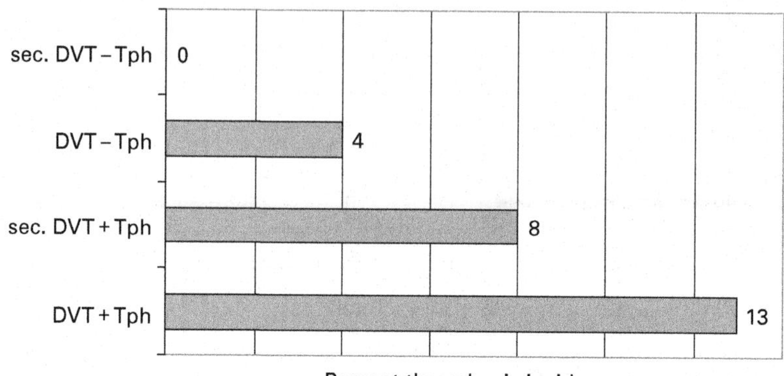

Figure 6.4 Distribution of recurrent DVT (%) according to causes (Tph: thrombophilia, +: thrombophilia present, –: without thrombophilia, sec. DVT: secondary DVT). Data from ref. 14.

Previous history of deep vein thrombosis and pulmonary embolism

Patients with a history of DVT have an increased risk of DVT. In retrospective studies the recurrence rate was as high as 15%.[23] In contrast, in 59 women with single previous episodes of DVT during pregnancy, none experienced thrombosis in the next pregnancy despite the lack of antenatal prophylaxis.[43] The same authors calculated that the risk of recurrent thrombosis for women after single episode of DVT is lower than 5%. However, these studies have some limitation; objective testing was not used in all cases, some of the studies were retrospective and the prospective studies had a relatively small number of cases. Brill-Edwards *et al.*[14] performed a prospective study of 125 pregnant women with a single previous DVT episode. The antepartum recurrence rate was 2.4%. In a subgroup analysis of 81 pregnant women with thrombophilia the recurrence rate was 5.9% (95% CI 1.2–16%). Based on these results, the absolute risk of antepartum recurrent thrombosis in women without thrombophilia but idiopathic thrombosis is 7.7% (95% CI 0.01–25.1) or very low in patients with prior DVT associated with a transient risk factor (0% (95% CI 0.0–8.0)). In patients with idiopathic or DVT with temporary risk the recurrence rate were 20% (95% CI 2.5–55.6) and 13.9% (95% CI 1.7–40.5) respectively (Fig. 6.4).

The authors recommend the antepartum prophylaxis for pregnant women with idiopathic DVT and thrombophilia and women with idiopathic DVT without thrombophilia. The data of a subgroup of pregnant women with prior DVT associated with a transient risk factor (oral contraceptive use, DVT prior pregnancy or post surgery) are insufficient for a clear recommendation. Pabinger *et al.*[67] described a relative risk of recurrent DVT of 3.5 (95% CI 1.6–7.8, $p = 0.002$) and believe (Fig. 6.5) – in agreement with other experts[1,35,36,37,45,84] – that a significant high risk exists for recurrent DVT and favor prophylactic anticoagulation during pregnancy and postpartum.

Table 6.2 Incidence of DVT according to age (data from ref. 78).

Age	Incidence/ 100,000 deliveries
>25	76
25–34	83
>34	115

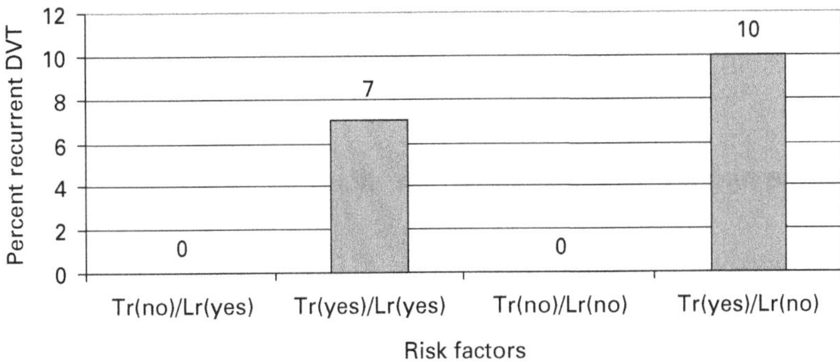

Figure 6.5 Recurrent DVT during pregnancy and variable risk factors (N = 109 women with a history of DVT). Tr: Temporary risk factor yes (Oral contraceptive use, pregnancy, surgery, trauma, immobilization) or no. Lr: Laboratory risk factor yes (thrombophilia) or no. Data from ref. 67.

Age at delivery

The incidence of antenatal and postnatal DVT in women older than 35 years is significantly higher ($p = 0.005$) than in those younger than 35 years. An age over 35 years is also associated with a significantly greater risk of PE (Fig. 6.3), with an incidence of 0.4 per 1,000 maternities as opposed to 0.11 per 1,000 in women younger than 35 years. In summary, an age over 35 years doubles the risk for thrombosis and PE.[41,42]

In a great cohort study the DVT and PE events increased with increased age (Table 6.2).

Bed rest and obesity

The Royal College of Obstetricians and Gynaecologists has recently published standards for thromboprophylaxis in obstetrics.[43,81] These standards also include additional risk factors for DVT, such as age greater than 35 years, weight above 80 kg at booking or >90 kg at delivery, more than 4 pregnancies, varicose veins, preeclampsia (OR: 2.2, 95% CI 1.3–3.7), immobilization for longer than 4 days before delivery and surgery. According to Nelson-Piercy,[65] obese women over the age of 37 years should use thromboprophylaxis not only for cesarean section but also for a normal delivery and for the following 3 to 4 days postpartum.

The influence of prolonged bed rest (>3 days) on thrombotic events was investigated in a retrospective study from Kovacevich *et al.*[50] A cohort group of 192 patients with preterm labour or preterm rupture of membranes were compared with 6,164, which were not treated with extended bed rest. The incidence of thromboembolic events were 15.6 per 1,000 deliveries in the group with extended bed rest and 0.8 per 1,000 deliveries in the control group. In contrast Carr *et al.*[15] investigate 48,525 deliveries over 5.5 years and 266 (0.5%) women received prolonged antepartum bed rest. The authors observed no cases of DVT and recommended no anticoagulation during prolonged bed rest unless other risk factors for DVT are present.

Thrombophilia and thromboemboembolic disease

Inherited thrombophilia

In the recent years, evidence supporting a genetic predisposition to thromboembolic disease has increased. In summary two groups of thrombophilic states are associated with thromboembolic events:[19] Group I disorders are the inhibitors of the coagulation cascade and the group II disorders are associated with increased levels or function of coagulation factors (Table 6.3).

Antithrombin and protein C and protein S deficiency

Early studies[17,18,21,68] suggested a high rate of DVT during pregnancy and postpartum in women with inherited inhibitor deficiencies. In contrast Vincente *et al.*[82] found an antenatal thrombosis in 1.8% of the protein-S-deficient

Table 6.3 The major hereditary prothrombotic conditions in pregnancy.

Groups	Thrombophilia
Group I	Antithrombin deficiencies
	Protein C deficiencies
	Protein S deficiencies
Group II	Activated protein C resistance without Factor V Leiden mutation
	Factor V Leiden mutation
	Prothrombin mutation
	Elevated levels of factors VIII, IX, and XI
	Elevated levels of lipoprotein (a)

Table 6.4 Relative risk of deep vein thrombosis associated with deficiencies of antithrombin, protein C, and protein S.

Study	Study-design	Deficiency	RR (95% CI)
Friedrich *et al.* (1996)	Family study	Antithrombin, protein C and S	8.0 (1.2–184)
McColl *et al.* (2000)	Case control study	Antithrombin Type I	282 (31–2,532)
		Antithrombin Type II	28 (5.5–142)
Gerhardt *et al.* (2000)	Case control study	Antithrombin	10.4 (12.2–62.5)
		Protein C	2.2 (0.8–6.1)

women. In a recent study by McColl *et al.*[60] Antithrombin or protein C deficiency was associated with an incidence of DVT in 12% and 2% of women respectively (Table 6.4). The authors calculated the relative risk of thrombosis for pregnant women with Antithrombin deficiency type I to be 1 in 2.8 and for type II to be 1 in 42 and for protein C deficiency to be 1 in 113. Friedrich *et al.*[30] estimated the relative risk for asymptomatic pregnant women with Thrombophilia (Antithrombin, protein C and S-deficiency) to 8.0 (95% CI: 1.2–184).

Data from Gerhardt *et al.*[32] shows a prevalence of inherited thrombophilic risk factors of 24.8% compared with 11.4% in the control group, but only the Antithrombin deficiency could be identified as an independent risk factor for DVT. The same authors[33] published a new study with more consecutive enrolled cases and found a prevalence of antithrombin, protein C and S deficiency of 5.6%, 7.0%, and 6.7% vs. 0.6%, 1.4%, and 3.3% in a control population. Only the severe cases of Antithrombin and protein C deficiencies were statistically associated with increased risk for DVT with an Odds Ratio of 64 and 7.2, respectively.

Activated protein C resistance, Factor V Leiden (FVL) and prothrombin-mutation

Activated protein C resistance was first described by Dahlback *et al.*[20] in 1993. Factor V Leiden mutation is very common and is present in about 3–7% of healthy Caucasians in contrast to the Prothrombin mutation with an incidence in 2–3% of healthy individuals.[38]

In two studies of pregnant women with FVL mutation, 15% and 28% respectively, were complicated by thrombosis.[25,26] Almost 30% of the thrombosis episodes occurred in the puerperium. In a study by Gerhardt *et al.*[32] in women with DVT, the prevalence of the FVL mutation was 43.7% compared with 7.7% in no pregnant controls (Table 6.5). The association of DVT and FVL in the early state of pregnancy was investigated by Hirsch *et al.*[47] First trimester thromboembolic complications was observed in 6 of 10 women with the mutation and 3 of 40 without mutations. In two prospective studies by Lindqvist *et al.*[58] and Tormene *et al.*[80]

Table 6.5 Factor V Leiden mutation in association with DVT.

Authors	DVT (N)	Controls (N)	FVL-mutation (%)	Controls (%)	OR (95% CI)
Bokarewa *et al.* (1996)[5]	70	n.d.	46	n.d.	n.d.
Dilley *et al.* (2000)	41	76	29.6	2.4	18.3 (2.7–432)
Gerhardt *et al.* (2000)	119	233	43.7	7.7	6.9 (3.3–15.2)
Grandone *et al.* (1998)	42	213	23.8	1.9	16.3 (4.8–54.9)
Hallak *et al.* (1997)	15	n.d.	46.6	n.d.	n.d.
McColl *et al.* (2000)	75	224	9.3	2.2	4.5 (2.1–14.5)
Murphy *et al.* (2000)	33	527	12.1	2.4	n.d.

n.d.: not determined, OR: odds ratio, 95% CI: 95% confidence intervals.

Table 6.6 Prevalence of prothrombin-mutation in women with DVT compared with non-DVT-patients.

Authors	OR	95% CI
Grandone *et al.* (1998)	10.2	4.0–25.9
Gerhard *et al.* (2000)	9.5	2.1–66.7
Gerhard *et al.* (2003)	6.1	1.7–22
McColl *et al.* (2000)	4.4	1.2–16

the authors observed an increased risk of DVT in FVL-Mutations (OR: 8.3, 95% CI: 1.7–41.2, and OR: 5.3, 95% CI: 0.6–43.9); homozygous carriers had a relative risk of RR 15.4 (95% CI: 1.4–164) respectively.

Prothrombin-Mutation is associated with an increased Prothrombin-level and is more common in southern Europe.[66] Recent studies in no-pregnant cases failed to demonstrate that the Prothrombin-Mutation is a risk factor for patients with one thrombotic event. Four studies relating to pregnancy (Table 6.6) show a statistical association between Prothrombin-Mutation and DVT. In the recent study of Gerhard *et al.*[32] the combination of FVL and Prothrombin-Mutation leads to a further significant increase of thrombotic risk (OR: 88, 95% CI 40.7–166).

Other defects

The antiphospholipid syndrome (APLS)

APLS is defined by the association of vascular thrombosis and/or pregnancy complications with the laboratory evidence of anticardiolipin antibodies (ACA) and/or lupus anticoagulant (LA). According to international consensus, APLS has a clear definition with one clinical criterion and at least one of two laboratory

Table 6.7 International consensus statement on criteria for the classification of the APLS.[83]

Clinical criteria	Clinical and laboratory events
Thrombosis	Venous, arterial or small vessel
Pregnancy morbidity	2 and more unexplained fetal loss (<10 weeks of gestation)
	1 and more unexplained fetal loss (<10 weeks of gestation)
	1 and more premature births of morphologically normal neonates at/before 34th week of gestation
Laboratory criteria	Anticardiolipin antibodies IgG or IgM present in moderate or high titres on two occasions at least 6 weeks apart
	Lupus anticoagulant on two occasions at least 6 weeks apart

Table 6.8 Late pregnancy complications in women with APLS.

Authors	N	Preeclampsia (%)	IUGR (%)	Prematurity (%)
Branch *et al.* (1992)	82	51	31	37
Lima *et al.* (1996)	60	18	31	43
Granger and Farquharson (1997)	53	3	11	8
Backos *et al.* (1999)	150	11	15	24

criteria (Table 6.7). The incidence of ACA and LA in the normal obstetric population is about 2 %, compared with 11–61% in women with complicated pregnancy outcome.[11,12,52,48]

Women with APA have an unusually high proportion of pregnancy loss in the pre-embryonic and embryonic period and severe complications in late pregnancies such as preeclampsia, intrauterine growth retardation, and prematurity (Table 6.8). The association between elevated titres of APA and recurrent miscarriage is well known. Nearly 10% of patients with early recurrent fetal loss have LA and nearly the same percentage have ACA.[49] The rate of fetal loss in untreated women with positive APA and previous pregnancy failure may be higher than 80%.[69]

Venous thrombosis occurred during pregnancy in 30.2% of women with APLS.[51,78] Arterial thrombosis is less common than venous thrombosis but in both cases thrombosis tends to be recurrent.[63,77] The general opinion of the experts was to treat with low molecular weight heparin (LMWH), leaving unfractionated heparin (UFH) for emergency situations such as the delivery day. The dosage should be adjusted according to the body weight in cases with recurrent thrombosis and for severe arterial thrombosis. In patients with recurrent abortion or late pregnancy complications the additional use of 100 mg Aspirin daily is recommended.[13]

Elevated factors VIII, IX, and XI, lipoprotein (a) and acquired APC-resistance

Factor VIII is an important cofactor in the activation of factor X by the tenase complex. Elevated factor VIII could be potentially prothrombotic by increasing stability of the tenase complex or by conferring a relative resistance to APC degradation. Moderately high plasma levels of coagulation factors FVIII, FIX or FXI have been associated with marked risk of first and recurrent venous thrombosis by 2- to 4-fold.[53] Factor VIII levels are known to vary depending on blood group type and a genetic association is likely.

Lipoprotein (a) is essentially an LDL-cholesterol particle with an additional protein covalently attached, called apolipoprotein (a) and an independent risk factor for DVD. APC resistance without factor V Leiden mutation was found to be related to the increased risk of DVD.[23]

Prophylactic treatment of pregnant women with risk of DVT

A number of publications have suggested guidelines for the management of asymptomatic women with prior DVT or laboratory abnormalities (thrombophilia factors) with increased risk of pregnancy related thrombosis.[1] A study of British obstetricians found that 90% would employ antenatal prophylaxis for patients with recurrent thrombosis, 81% for patients with a previous single episode of DVT, 54% for patients with previous DVT and family history, 52% for patients with previous DVT without risk, and 37% for thrombophilia.[41] In cases with prior DVT, the grade of risk and prophylactic regimes can be calculated according to the observed clinical risk factors (Table 6.9). Clinical risks associated

Table 6.9 Recommendations about prophylaxis in women with prior DVT.

Risk	USA[2,35]	Australasia[1]	Germany[45]	UK[62]
Idiopathic DVT with clinical risk	LMWH	LMWH	LMWH	LMWH
Idiopathic DVT without clinical risk	Clinical observation	Need for prophylaxis negotiable	LMWH	LMWH
Secondary DVT with clinical risk	LMWH	Need for prophylaxis negotiable	LMWH	LMWH
Secondary DVT without clinical risk	Clinical observation (LMWH, if DVT is related to a highly thrombogenic event (*ACOG Pract. Bull.*, 2000)	Clinical observation	LMWH	LMWH

Table 6.10 Risk groups for pregnancy-related DVT and prophylactic regimes (according to the working group on behalf of the Obstetric medicine group of the German Society for Thrombosis and Haemostasis Research).

Risk	Patients	Management
Low	Family history, heterozygous FVL, PII Protein C or S	Clinical observation, LMWH postpartum over 6 weeks
Moderate	Homozygous FVL, prior idiopathic DVT, antiphospholipid syndrome, family history and thrombophilia	LMWH during pregnancy and 6 weeks postpartum
High	Antithrombin deficiency, prosthetic heart valves (Enoxaparin contraindicated), current DVT, combined thrombophilic defects	Therapeutic doses of LMWH (initial doses: 2 × 40 mg Enoxaparin to achieve a peak anti-Xa activity of 0.35–0.7 mlh 3 h after injection and later 1 mg/kg twice daily

with thrombotic risk are conditions after surgery, pregnancy, oral contraceptive use, immobilization, and trauma included also women with family risk. Family risk is defined by thrombotic findings in the same family or in one or more first-degree relatives. Laboratory risks include deficiencies of protein C, protein S or Antithrombin and the presence of APLA, FVL, and Prothrombin mutation.

Patients with DVT in a current pregnancy or those with Antithrombin deficiency, or women with prosthetic heart valves, women with recurrent DVT (2 and more DVT in history) and patients on long-term anticoagulant therapy should be considered as high risk patients. Patients with a history of previous DVT (see Table 6.9) or family history in combination with Thrombophilia; homozygous FVL and Prothrombin mutation are considered to be at moderate risk for DVT (Table 6.10). Women with a protein C or S deficiency or heterozygous FVL/Pro-thrombin mutation are considered to be at low risk for DVT. These patients are treated with LMWH or oral anticoagulation in the postpartum period (six weeks after delivery).

Heparin dosage in prophylactic regimes

Low molecular weight heparin is an attractive alternative to UFH because of ease of administration, less frequent need for laboratory monitoring, and ability to continue anticoagulation during delivery. Although the optimal dosage is not known, most clinicians use an unchanged dose during pregnancy.[22] Another possibility is the weight-adjusted dosage increasing to the end of pregnancy with monitoring by anti-Xa-level monthly to achieve a concentration of 0.5–1.2 U/ml. In Germany and/or the USA the following preparations are available (Table 6.11).

Table 6.11 Application and dosages of LMWH available in Germany and the United States.

Agent	Moderate Risk	High risk	Treatment of DVT	Available in
Enoxaparin	40 mg/die	2 × 40 mg	2 × 1 mg/kg	USA, Germany
Dalteparin	5000 U/die	2 × 5000 U/die	200 U/(kg daily)	USA, Germany
Nadroparin	0.3 ml/daily	40–60 U/(kg daily)	200 U/(kg daily)	Germany
Tinzaparin	3500 U/daily 4500 U/daily (USA)	50–75 U/(kg daily)	175 U/(kg daily)	USA, Germany
Certoparin	3000 U/daily	3000 U/daily	2 × 8000 U/daily	Germany
Reviparin	1750 U/daily	4200 U/2 × daily	35–40 kg:3500 U 45–60 kg:4200 U >60 kg:6300 U	Germany

Prevention of thrombosis in women with prosthetic heart valves

Patients with bio prosthetic valves have a high risk of thromboembolism and should receive anticoagulation in therapeutic doses. At present there are insufficient data to make definitive recommendations about the optimal prevention. The American College of Chest Physicians[36] recommends any options for the use of UFH, LMWH, and oral anticoagulation during pregnancy. Therapeutic UFH can be given throughout pregnancy or in the first trimester and in the last trimester in combination with warfarin given during weeks 14 to 34. Unfractionated heparin (adjusted to prolong a 6-hour postinjection-aPTT into therapeutic range) is being replaced by LMWH. Recently, Aventis Pharmaceutical warned that Enoxaparin should not be used in patients with prosthetic heart valves.

Long-term outcome of DVT

Venous thromboembolism during pregnancy carries not only an increased risk of recurrence but also often of post-thrombotic syndrome. According to Bergqvist *et al.*,[7,8] 75% of patients with DVT during pregnancy developed at least one symptom related to post-thrombotic syndrome, and 4% develop leg ulcerations. Lindhagen *et al.*[56] studied 23 women after DVT in pregnancy and found signs of chronic venous insufficiency (CVI) in 65%. The incidence of CVI in pregnancy is higher than in non-pregnant patients after postoperative DVT. In these cases compression stockings may be useful.

Safety of LMWH in pregnancy

Several studies[46,54,76] have demonstrated that LMWH is effective and safe for the prevention and treatment of venous thromboembolism in pregnancy (Table 6.12).

Table 6.12 Safety of LMWH in pregnancy (clinically important side effects).

Complication	Sanson *et al.*[76]	Heilmann *et al.*[46]	Lepercq *et al.*[54]
DVT	0.6%	1.7%	1.3%
HIT	none	0.05%	1.6%
Major bleeding	none	none	1.8%
Minor bleeding	2.7%	3.2%	1.3%
Allergic reaction	0.6%	0.5%	none
Osteopenia	0.6%	no data	no data
Fractures	none	0.1%	none
Total of adverse effects	8.3%	12.6%	38.1%

The most common complications are thrombocytopenia (HIT II), osteopenia, and hemorrhage. In practice the risk of bleeding does seem to be reduced because LMWH has very little anticoagulant activity (anti IIa) and a higher antithrombotic activity (anti Xa) compared to UFH. HIT II may occur mostly in the first three weeks of treatment, but is rare[29] and can be prevented by measurement of platelets one to two times weekly. The risk of osteopenia and osteoporosis is less in pregnant women treated with LMWH and osteoporotic fractures are observed in two women with a higher than usual dosage of LMWH.[28]

Diagnosis of DVT and pulmonary embolism (PE) in pregnancy

Diagnosis of DVT or PE in pregnant women has major implications for their care, and the problems with current diagnostic tests are potential risks to the fetus. The first diagnostic step in patients with a high probability for DVT is the use of Compression Ultrasound (CUS). Impedance plethysmography (IPG) is insensitive to calf vein DVT and some non-occlusive proximal DVT and is less sensitive compared with CUS in non-pregnant patients with a suspected first DVT. A normal CUS does not exclude calf DVT. If the test remains negative, a serial non-invasive testing or venography with abdominal shielding can be used. If pelvic vein thrombosis is suspected MRI can be used (Fig. 6.6).

For the diagnosis of PE, a ventilation-perfusion scan should be performed first. A recent study of Chan *et al.*[16] concerning pregnant women with suspected PE who underwent lung scanning showed a low prevalence of positive lung scans. If necessary, spiral CT or pulmonary arteriography should be performed. Spiral CT is sensitive for large central emboli but less sensitive for smaller peripheral PE. The use of D-Dimer testing to exclude DVT in pregnancy has not been evaluated. D-Dimer levels are increased with the progression of normal pregnancy

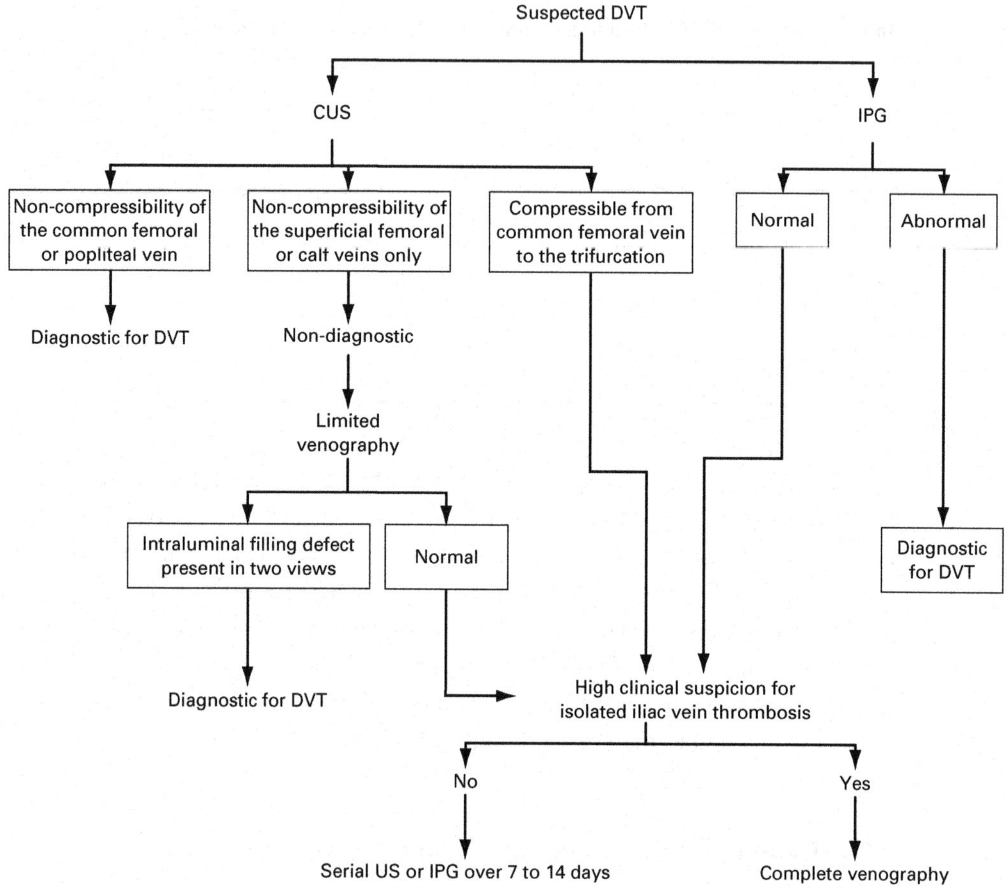

Figure 6.6 Recommendations for diagnosing DVT during pregnancy.

and in cases with preeclampsia, and the estimation of a specific cut-off level must be required in further studies.[5,6]

Management of DVT in pregnancy

Although unfractionated heparin (UFH) has been used during pregnancy for many years there are many examples of LMWH replacing UFH. Most experts believe that pregnant women with DVT can be treated with either unfractionated heparin or low molecular weight heparin. When an intravenous route of UFH is used for acute treatment (Table 6.13) the initial dose of UFH is about 40,000 IU/24 hours given by continuous intravenous infusion. After about 1 week the risk of recurrence is low and the IV route will be replaced by low-dose heparin 10,000 IU given subcutaneously, twice daily or LMWH. Postpartum the use of oral anticoagulants or low molecular weight heparin is recommended. Oral

Table 6.13 Protocol for adjustment of the dose of intravenous heparin.

aPTT (s)	Repeat bolus	Stop infusion	New rate of infusion	Repeat aPTT
<50	Yes (5000 U)	No	+3 ml/h (+2,880 U/24h)	6 h
50–59	No	No	+3 ml/h (+2,880/24 h)	6 h
60–85	No	No	Unchanged	Next morning
86–95	No	No	−2 ml/h (−1,920 U/24 h)	Next morning
96–120	No	Yes (for 30 min)	−2 ml/h (−1,920/24 h)	6 h
>120	No	Yes (for 60 min)	−4 ml/h (−3,840 U/24 h)	6 h

Adapted from Toglia, M. R., Weg, J. G. *NEJM* (1996) **335**, 108–14.

anticoagulants such as Coumarin derivatives cross the placenta with the risk of bleeding in any trimester and Embryopathie in the first trimester. The use of oral anticoagulants is contraindicated in the pregnancy and only recommended in rare cases in patients who are allergic to heparin or have mechanical heart valves.

After a period of continuous infusion, a subcutaneous heparin therapy is initiated. The treatment is controlled by aPTT measurement until it reaches a range of 1.5–2.5 of normal value. Changes in metabolism and clearance of UFH during pregnancy complicate adequate dosing and equivalent doses of subcutaneous heparin produce lower plasma concentration (measure with anti-Xa-activity) than in non-pregnant women and it is unclear if increased level of anti-Xa-activities (ranges of 0.5–1.2 U/ml) are associated with more bleeding and subnormal levels are associated with rethrombosis.[71] Suboptimal dosage of UFH and the difficulties in the monitoring leads to limited use of UFH in pregnancy. Based upon safety and effectiveness, LMWH is the preferred drug for the treatment of DVT during pregnancy. After therapeutic administration for 10–14 days (see Table 6.11) a prophylactic dose of LMWH should be continued through the pregnancy and for 6 weeks postpartum. Prophylactic regimes after acute treatment are to compare with a dosage in moderate risk (40–80 mg Enoxaparin/daily or 5,000–10,000 U Dalteparin/daily). Monitoring of LMWH is not usually required, but the measurement of anti-Xa-level (0.4–0.6 U/ml) is useful in cases with obesity and with high risk for bleeding. Epidural anesthesia should be avoided after 4 hours with UFH and 10–12 hours[24] with LMWH. Unfractionated heparin can be restarted 2 hours and LMWH 4–6 hours after catheter removal.

Management of anticoagulant therapy at the time of delivery

In normal cases with moderate risk most centers stop the LMWH therapy 24 hours before delivery and continue the treatment 12 hours postpartum.

In cases with high thrombotic risk (e.g. proximal DVT or PE within 4 weeks) therapeutic doses of intravenously UFH replace LMWH and can be discontinued 4 to 6 hours prior to the expected delivery time. Anticoagulants should be given for at least 6 weeks following delivery and longer if DVT or PE was diagnosed shortly before delivery.

Summary

Thromboembolic complications in pregnancy are six times greater than in non-pregnant women. Maternal age, prior DVT (idiopathic or secondary), the mode of delivery, bed rest and obesity or both, and the diagnosis of thrombophilic defects significantly increase the risk of DVT and PE. Low molecular weight heparin is the drug of choice for treatment and prevention of thromboembolic complications in pregnancy. The diagnosis of DVT or PE presents special problems because of the multiple hemodynamic interactions with the usual tests. The monitoring of LMWH in moderate and high risk patients by determination of the platelet count is generally recommended. Adverse effects such as osteoporosis, HIT II or bleeding complications are rare. Low molecular weight heparin has been shown also to have therapeutic effects in patients with high risk for preeclampsia, intra-uterine growth retardation, antiphospholipid syndrome, and abruption placenta.

REFERENCES

1 A Working Group on behalf of the Obstetric Medicine Group of Australasia: Anticoagulation in pregnancy and the puerperium. *MJA*, **175**: 258, 2001.

2 *ACOG Practice Bulletin*: Thromboembolism in pregnancy. No 19, 2000.

3 Armour, R., Schwedler, M., Kerstein, M. D. Current assessment of thromboembolic disease and pregnancy. *Am. Surgeon*, **67**: 641, 2001.

4 Backos, M., Chilcott, I., Rai, R. Pregnancy complications in women with recurrent miscarriage and antiphospholipid-antibodies treated with aspirin and heparin. *Hum. Reprod.*, **12**: 61, 1997.

5 Bates, S. M., Ginsberg, J. S. How we manage venous thromboembolism during pregnancy. *Blood*, **100**: 3470, 2002.

6 Bates, S. M., Ginsberg, J. S. Pregnancy and deep vein thrombosis. *Seminars Vasc. Med.*, **1**: 97, 2001.

7 Bergqvist D, Bergqvist A, Lindhagen A. Longterm outcome of patients with venous thromboembolism during pregnancy. In Greer, I. A., Turpie, A. G. C., Forbes, C. O., (eds.). *Haemostasis and Thrombosis in Obstetrics and Gynecology*. London; Chapman & Hall, 1992.

8 Bergqvist, D., Hedner, U. Pregnancy and venous thromboembolism. *Acta Obstet. Gynecol. Scand.*, **62**: 449, 1983.

9 Bockarewa, M. I., Bremme, K., Blombäck, M. Arg 506-Gln mutation in factor V and risk of thrombosis during pregnancy. *Br. J. Haematol.*, **92**: 473, 1996.

10 Branch, D. W., Silver, R. M., Blackwell, J. L. Outcome of treated pregnancies in women with antiphosopholipid syndrome. An update of the Utah experience. *Obstet. Gynecol.*, **4**: 614, 1992.

11 Brenner, B., Blumenfeld, Z. Thrombophilia and fetal loss. *Blood Rev.*, **11**: 72, 1997.

12 Brenner, B., Kupferminc, M. J. Inherited thrombophilia and poor pregnancy outcome. *Best Practice & Research Clinical Obstetrics & Gynaecology*, **17**: 427, 2003.

13 Brenner, B. Antithrombotic prophylaxis for women with thrombophilia and pregnancy complications – Yes. *J. Thromb. Haemost.*, **1**: 2070, 2003.

14 Brill-Edwards, P., Ginsberg, J. S., Gent, M., *et al.* Safety of withholding heparin in pregnant women with a history of venous thromboembolism. *NEJM*, **343**: 1439, 2000.

15 Carr, M. H., Towers, C. V., Eastenson, A. R., *et al.* Prolonged bedrest during pregnancy: Does the risk of deep vein thrombosis warrant the use of routine heparin prophylaxis? *J. Maternal Fetal Med.*, **6**: 264, 1997.

16 Chan, W. S., Ray, J. G., Murray, S., *et al.* Suspected pulmonary embolism in pregnancy. *Arch. Intern. Med.*, **162**: 1170, 2002.

17 Conard, J., Horellou, M. H., van Dreden, P. Pregnancy and congenital deficiency in antithrombin III or protein C. *Thromb. Haemost.*, **58**: 39, 1987.

18 Conard, J., Horellou, M. H., van Dreden, P. Thrombosis and pregnancy in congenital deficiencies in AT III, protein C or protein S. *Thromb. Haemost.*, **63**: 319, 1990.

19 Crowther, M. A., Kelton, J. G. Congenital thrombophilic states associated with venous thrombosis: A qualitative overview and proposed classification system. *Ann. Intern. Med.*, **138**: 128, 2003.

20 Dahlback, B., Carlsson, M., Svensson, P. J. Familial thrombophilia due to a previously unrecognized mechanism characterized by poor anticoagulant response to activated protein C: prediction of a cofactor to activated protein C. *PNAS*, **90**: 1004, 1993.

21 De Stefano, V., Leone, G., Mastrangelo, S., *et al.* Thrombosis during pregnancy and surgery in patients with congenital deficiency of antithrombin III, protein C, protein S. *Thromb. Haemost.*, **71**: 799, 1994.

22 De Stefano, V., Mastrangelo, S., Paciaroni, K. Thrombotic risk during pregnancy and puerperium in women with APC resistance-effective subcutaneous heparin prophylaxis in a pregnant patient. *Thromb. Haemost.*, **74**: 793, 1995.

23 De Stefano, V., Rossi, E., Paciaroni, K., *et al.* Screening for inherited thrombophilia: indications and therapeutic implications. *Haematologica*, **87**: 1095, 2002.

24 De Swiet, M. Maternal mortality: Confidential enquiries into maternal deaths in the United Kingdom. *Am. J. Obstet. Gynecol.*, **182**: 760, 2000.

25 Dilley, A., Austin, H., El-Jamil, M., *et al.* Genetic factors associated with thrombosis in pregnancy in a United States population. *Am. J. Obstet. Gynecol.*, **183**: 1271, 2000.

26 Dizon-Townson, D. S., Nelson, L. M., Jang, H., *et al.* The incidence of the factor V Leiden mutation in an obstetric population and its relationship to deep vein thrombosis. *Am. J. Obstet. Gynecol.*, **176**: 883, 1997.

27 Eldor, A. Thrombophilia, thrombosis and pregnancy. *Thromb. Haemost.*, **86**: 104, 2001.

28 Ensom, M. H. H., Stephenson, M. D. Low-molecular-weight heparins in pregnancy. *Pharmacotherapy*, **19**: 1013, 1999.

29 Fausett, M. B., Vogtlander, M., Lee, R. M., *et al.* Heparin-induced thrombocytopenia is rare in pregnancy. *Am. J. Obstet. Gynecol.*, **185**: 148, 2001.

30 Friederich, P. W., Samson, B. J., Simioni, P. Frequency of pregnancy related thromboembolism in anticoagulant factor deficient women: Implications for prophylaxis. *Ann. Intern. Med.*, **125**: 955, 1996.

31 Gates, S. Thromboembolic disease in pregnancy. *Curr. Opin. Obstet. Gynecol.*, **12**: 117, 2000.

32 Gerhardt, A., Scharf, R. E., Beckmann, M. W., *et al.* Prothrombin and factor V mutations in women with a history of thrombosis during pregnancy and the puerperium. *NEJM*, **342**: 374, 2000.

33 Gerhardt, A., Scharf, R. E., Zotz, R. B. Effect of hemostatic risk factors on the individual probability of thrombosis during pregnancy and the puerperium. *Thromb. Haemost.*, **90**: 77, 2003.

34 Gherman, R. B., Goodwin, T. M., Leung, B., *et al.* Incidence, clinical characteristics, and timing of objectively diagnosed venous thromboembolism during pregnancy. *Obstet. Gynecol.*, **94**: 730, 1999.

35 Ginsberg, J. S., Bates, S. M. Management of venous thromboembolism during pregnancy. *J. Thromb. Haemost.*, **1**: 1435, 2003.

36 Ginsberg, J. S., Greer, I. A., Hirsh, J. Use of antithrombotic agents during pregnancy. *Chest*, **119**: 122, 2001.

37 Ginsberg, J. S. Thromboembolism and pregnancy. *Thromb. Haemost.*, **82**: 620, 1999.

38 Girling, J., deSwiet, M. Inherited thrombophilia and pregnancy. *Curr. Opin. Obstet. Gynecol.*, **10**: 135, 1998.

39 Grandone, E., Margaglione, M., Colaizzo, D., *et al.* Genetic susceptibility to pregnancy-related venous thromboembolism: Roles of factor V Leiden, prothrombin G20210 A, and methylenetetrahydrofolate reductase C677 T mutations. *Am. J. Obstet. Gynecol.*, **179**: 1324, 1998.

40 Granger, K. A., Farquharson, R. G. Obstetric outcome in antiphospholipid syndrome. *Lupus*, **6**: 509, 1997.

41 Greer, I. A. Epidemiology, risk factors and prophylaxis of venous thromboembolism in obstetrics and gynecology. *Baillieres Clin. Obstet. Gynecol.*, **11**: 403, 1997.

42 Greer, I. A. The special case of venous thromboembolism in pregnancy. *Haemostasis*, **28** (Suppl. 3): 22, 1998.

43 Greer, I. A., de Swiet, M. Thrombosis prophylaxis in obstetrics and gynecology. *BJOG*, **100**: 37, 1993.

44 Hallak, M., Senderowicz, J., Cassel, A. Activated protein C resistance (factor V Leiden) associated with thrombosis in pregnancy. *Am. J. Obstet. Gynecol.*, **176**: 889, 1997.

45 Heilmann, L., Rath, W., v. Tempelhoff, G. F., *et al.* The use of low molecular weight heparin (LMWH) in pregnancy. *Geburtsh Frauenheilk*, **61**: 355, 2001.

46 Heilmann, L., Rath, W. *Thrombophilia in Pregnancy*. Bremen, London, New York; Unimed, 2002.

47 Hirsch, D. R., Mikkola, K. M., Marks, P. W. Pulmonary embolism and deep venous thrombosis during pregnancy or oral contraceptive use. Prevalence of factor V Leiden. *Am. Heart J.*, **131**: 1145, 1996.
48 Katano, K., Aoki, K., Sasa, H. Beta-2-glycoprotein-1-dependent anticardiolipin antibodies as a predictor of adverse pregnancy outcomes in healthy pregnant women. *Hum. Reprod.*, **11**: 509, 1996.
49 Khare, M., Nelson-Piercy, C. Acquired thrombophilias and pregnancy. *Best Practice & Research Clinical Obstetrics & Gynaecology*, **17**: 491, 2003.
50 Kovacevich, G. J., Gaich, S. A., Lavin, J. P., *et al.* The prevalence of thromboembolic events among women with extended bed rest prescribed as part of the treatment for premature labor or preterm premature rupture of membranes. *Am. J. Obstet. Gynecol.*, **182**: 1089, 2000.
51 Krnic-Barrie, S., O'Connor, C. R., Looney, S. W. A retrospective review of 61 patients with antiphospholipid syndrome. *Arch. Intern. Med.*, **157**: 2101, 1997.
52 Kupferminc, M. J., Eldor, A., Steinman, N. Increased frequency of genetic thrombophilia in women with complications of pregnancy. *NEJM*, **340**: 9, 1999.
53 Kyrle, P. A., Minar, E., Hirschl, M., *et al.* High plasma levels of factor VIII and the risk of recurrent venous thromboembolism. *NEJM*, **343**: 457, 2000.
54 Lepercq, J., Conard, J., Burel-Derlon, A., *et al.* Venous thromboembolism during pregnancy: a retrospective study of enoxaparin safety in 624 pregnancies. *BJOG*, **108**: 1134, 2001.
55 Lima, F., Khamashta, M. A., Buchanan, N. M. M. A study of sixty pregnancies in patients with the antiphospholipid syndrome. *Clin. Exp. Rheumatol.*, **14**: 131, 1996.
56 Lindhagen, A., Bergqvist, A., Bergqvist, D. Late venous function in the leg after deep venous thrombosis occurring in relation to pregnancy. *BJOG*, **93**: 348, 1986.
57 Lindqvist, P., Dahlback, B., Marsal, K. Thrombotic risk during pregnancy: A population study. *Obstet. Gynecol.*, **94**: 595, 1999.
58 Lindqvist, P. Risk estimation and prediction of preeclampsia, IUGR, and thrombosis in pregnancy (thesis). Malmö, Sweden, 1999.
59 Macklon, N. S., Greer, I. A. Venous thromboembolic disease in obstetrics and gynaecology. The Scottish experience. *Scott. Med. J.*, **41**: 83, 1996.
60 McColl, M. D., Ellison, J., Reid, F., *et al.* Prothrombin 202210 G–A, MTHFR C677 T mutations in women with venous thromboembolism associated with pregnancy. *BJOG*, **107**: 565, 2000.
61 McColl, M. D., Ramsay, J., Tait, R. Risk factors for pregnancy associated venous thromboembolism. *Thromb. Haemost.*, **78**: 1183, 1997.
62 McColl, M. D., Walker, I., Greer, I. A. The role of inherited thrombophilia in venous thromboembolism associated with pregnancy. *BJOG*, **106**: 756, 1999.
63 Meroni, P. L., Moia, M., Derksen, R. H. W. M., *et al.* Venous thromboembolism in the antiphospholipid syndrome: management guidelines for secondary prophylaxis. *Lupus*, **12**: 504, 2003.
64 Murphy, R. P., Donoghue, C., Nallen, R. J., *et al.* Prospective evaluation of the risk conferred by factor V Leiden and thermolabile methylene-tetrahydrofolate reductase polymorphisms in pregnancy. *Arterioscler. Thromb. Vasc. Biol.*, **20**: 266, 2000.

65 Nelson-Piercy, C. Prevention of thromboembolism in pregnancy. *Scand. J. Rheumatol.*, **27** (Suppl. 107): 92, 1998.

66 Nguyen, A. Prothrombin G20210 A polymorphism and thrombophilia. *Mayo Clin. Proc.*, **75**: 595, 2000.

67 Pabinger, I., Grafenhofer, A., Kyrle, P. A., *et al.* Temporary increase in the risk for recurrence during pregnancy in women with a history of venous thromboembolism. *Blood*, **100**: 1060, 2002.

68 Pabinger, I., Schneider, B., For the Gesellschaft für Thrombose- und Hämostaseforschung (GTH) Study Group on Natural Inhibitor: Thrombotic risk in hereditary antithrombin III, protein C, or protein S deficiency. *Arterioscler. Thromb. Vasc. Biol.*, **16**: 742, 1996.

69 Rai, R. S., Clifford, K., Cohen, H., *et al.* High prospective fetal loss rate in untreated pregnancies of women with recurrent miscarriage and antiphospholipid antibodies. *Hum. Reprod.*, **10**: 3301, 1995.

70 Rand, H. J., Wu, X. X., Guller, S. Reduction of annexin V (placental anti-coagulant protein I) on placental villi of women with antiphospholipid antibodies and recurrent spontaneous abortion. *Am. J. Obstet. Gynecol.*, **171**: 1566, 1994.

71 Raschke, R., Hirsh, J., Guidry, J. R. Suboptimal monitoring and dosing of unfractionated heparin in comparative studies with low molecular heparin. *Ann. Intern. Med.*, **138**: 720, 2003.

72 Rath, W., Heilmann, L. *Haemostatic Disorders in Obstetrics and Gynecology*. New York, NY; Thieme Stuttgart, 1999.

73 Ray, J. G., Chan, W. S. Deep vein thrombosis during pregnancy and the puerperium: A metaanalysis of the period of risk and the leg of presentation. *Obstet. Gynecol. Surv.*, **54**: 265, 1999.

74 Rosendaal, F. R. Risk factors for venous thrombotic disease. *Thromb. Haemost.*, **82**: 610, 1999.

75 Rutherford, S. W., Montero, M., McSchee, W. Thromboembolic disease associated with pregnancy: An 11 year review. *Am. J. Obstet. Gynecol.*, **164**: 286, 1991.

76 Sanson, B. J., Lensing, A. W. A., Prin, M. H. Safety of low molecular weight heparin in pregnancy: A systematic review. *Thromb. Haemost.*, **81**: 668, 1999.

77 Silver, R. M., Draper, M. J., Scott, J. R. Clinical consequences of antiphospholipid antibodies: An historic cohort study. *Obstet. Gynecol.*, **83**: 372, 1994.

78 Simpson, E. L., Lawrenson, R. A., Nightingale, A. L., *et al.* Venous thromboembolism in pregnancy and the puerperium: incidence and additional risk factors from a London perinatal database. *BJOG*, **108**: 56, 2001.

79 Toglia, M. R., Weg, J. D. Venous thromboembolism during pregnancy. *NEJM*, **335**: 108, 1996.

80 Tormene, D., Simioni, P., Prandoni, P., *et al.* Factor V Leiden mutation and the risk of venous thromboembolism in pregnant women. *Haematologica*, **86**: 1305, 2001.

81 Van Walraven, C., Mamdani, M., Cohn, A., *et al.* Risk of subsequent thomboembolism for patients with pre-eclampsia. *BMJ*, **326**: 791, 2003.

82 Vincente, V., Rodriguez, C., Soto, I. Risk of thrombosis during pregnancy and postpartum in hereditary thrombophilia. *Am. J. Haematol.*, **46**: 151, 1994.

83 Wilson, W. A., Gharavi, A. E., Koike, T., *et al.* International consensus statement on preliminary classification criteria for definite anti-phospholipid syndrome. *Arthritis & Rheumatism*, **42**: 1309, 1999.

84 Zotz, R. B., Gerhardt, A., Scharf, R. E. Prediction, prevention, and treatment of venous thromboembolic disease in pregnancy. *Seminars in Thromb. and Haemost.*, **29**: 143, 2003.

Address for correspondence:
Prof. Dr. Lothar Heilmann, Dept. Obstet. Gynec.
City Hospital, August-Bebel-Str. 59
D-65428 Rüsselsheim
Germany
Email: dr_lothar_heilmann@yahoo.de

Diagnosis of deep vein thrombosis and pulmonary embolism in pregnancy

William F. Baker, Jr., M.D., F.A.C.P.,[1] Eugene P. Frenkel, M.D., F.A.C.P.,[2] and Rodger L. Bick, M.D., Ph.D., F.A.C.P.[3]

[1]Associate Clinical Professor of Medicine, Center for Health Sciences, David Geffen School of Medicine at University of California-Los Angeles, Los Angeles, CA, USA Thrombosis, Hemostasis, and Special Hematology Clinic, Kern Medical Center, Bakersfield; California Clinical Thrombosis Center, Bakersfield, California, USA
[2]Professor of Medicine and Radiology Harold C. Simmons Comprehensive Cancer Center, University of Texas Southwestern Medical School, Dallas, Texas, USA
[3]Clinical Professor of Medicine and Pathology, University of Texas Southwestern Medical Center, Director: Dallas Thrombosis Hemostasis and Vascular Medicine Clinical Center, Dallas, Texas, USA

Venous thromboembolism (VTE) represents a major cause of morbidity and mortality during pregnancy, complicating from 0.5 to 3.0 of every 1000 pregnancies.[1] Pulmonary embolism (PE) has been the leading cause of maternal mortality in the United States and Great Britain for at least 20 years[1,2] and complicates approximately 1 in 1,000 pregnancies.[3,4] This represents a VTE risk of 3–4 times greater than age-matched non-pregnant controls.[5] Diagnosing venous thromboembolism is challenging because clinical findings are often misleading. When evaluated with objective testing, as many as 75% of patients suspected of having venous thromboembolism are found to have an alternative diagnosis.[2,6] This poses an even greater problem in the pregnant patient who experiences vasodilatation and intravascular volume expansion (20–25% increase)[7] with associated lower extremity edema.[3] The accuracy of many diagnostic tests used in the non-pregnant patient are either not useful at all or are potentially misleading. Diagnosis of VTE is critical since 24% of pregnant women with untreated deep vein thrombosis (DVT) develop PE, with a death rate of 15% to 30%.[1] Proper diagnosis and treatment reduces the mortality rate of PE to 1%[8]–3%.[9] In addition, postphlebitic syndrome in the affected leg occurs nearly 80% of the time following DVT in pregnancy,[10,11] compared to 30–40% in the non-pregnant patient. Although it is well recognized that the incidence of PE is greatly reduced with treatment for deep vein thrombosis (DVT), treatment is also problematic since anticoagulation regimens used in the non-pregnant patient may be highly teratogenic or in other ways hazardous to

Hematological Complications in Obstetrics, Pregnancy, and Gynecology, ed. R. L. Bick *et al.* Published by Cambridge University Press.

mother and/or fetus. This chapter will explore the features of history and physical examination, the laboratory studies and the various imaging modalities, which result in a precise diagnosis. Algorithms will be presented which reflect pretest clinical probability and the outcome of both laboratory and imaging studies.

Overview

The requirement for vigilance regarding VTE is never more evident than in the high-risk clinical condition of pregnancy. The risk of pregnancy-associated VTE also extends beyond delivery as 3–5 times more DVTs occur postpartum than antepartum and this risk is 3–16 times greater after delivery by cesarean section than with vaginal delivery.[2] Older studies indicate that the VTE risk is lowest during the first two trimesters and highest during the third trimester.[1] This incidence is disputed by a more recent report by Gherman and colleagues of 165 cases of VTE (127 with DVT and 38 with PE) among 286,000 pregnancies. Deep vein thrombosis was detected in 94 women antepartum and 33 postpartum. The diagnosis of DVT was made before 15 weeks gestation in over half (47) and after 20 weeks in 28. Of the 38 cases of PE, 23 occurred postpartum and 19 of these after cesarean section.[12] Gerhardt *et al.* reported on the characteristics of 119 women with pregnancy-associated VTE and found that 52% experienced DVT antepartum with 23% in the first trimester, 20% in the second trimester and 56% in the third trimester. Postpartum DVT occurred in 48%, with 68% of these occurring after vaginal delivery and 32% after cesarean section.[13]

Women who have previously experienced VTE during pregnancy or while on combination oral contraceptives are at a significantly increased risk of recurrence (7.5% to 12.5%).[14] Older women (over 40) are at ten times greater risk of VTE than women younger than 25, and the death rate is higher in black than white women.[15] Major VTE risk factors in pregnant women include: age greater than 35, higher parity, obesity, prolonged immobilization, pelvic trauma, surgery during pregnancy, cesarean section, multiple pregnancy, preeclampsia and hereditary thrombophilia (Table 7.1).[16] Farrell has proposed a three-tiered risk stratification for VTE in pregnancy (Table 7.2): (1) low risk: <35 years of age, uncomplicated pregnancy, and elective cesarean section, (2) moderate risk: >35 years of age, obesity, gross varicose veins, recurrent infections, immobility >4 days before delivery, preeclampsia, and emergency cesarean section, (3) high risk: three or more moderate risk factors, hereditary thrombophilic disease or antiphospholipid antibody syndrome, personal or family history of DVT, history of PE, and cesarean section hysterectomy.[17]

Just as in the non-pregnant patient, the pathophysiology of maternal VTE is well described with the application of Virchow's triad (hypercoagulability, venous

Table 7.1 Risk factors for venous thromboembolism (VTE) in pregnancy.

Clinical risk factors	
Age >35	
Multiparity	
Obesity	
Personal or family history of VTE	
Prolonged immobilization (bed rest, paralysis, travel including plane flight longer than 3 h 45 min.)	
Pelvic trauma	
Surgery during pregnancy	
Cesarean section	
Multiple pregnancy	
Preeclampsia	
Malignancy	
Thrombophilic disorders	
Inherited	Acquired
Factor V Leiden mutation	Antiphospholipid antibodies
Prothrombin G20210A mutation	Elevated factors
Antithrombin deficiency	Elevated PAI-1 and PAI-2
Protein C and S deficiencies	Others
Others	

stasis, and vascular injury). Measurable increases in fibrinogen, von Willebrand factor, clotting factors (I, II, V, VII, VIII, IX, X, XII),[2,3] increased inhibition of fibrinolysis (increased plasminogen activator inhibitor type I (PAI-1) and type II (PAI-2) (produced by the placenta)[18] and reduced levels of coagulation inhibitors (decreased protein S,[19] acquired resistance to activated protein C)[20] create a hypercoagulable state not typical of preconception. Maternal risk may also be elevated owing to underlying hereditary and acquired blood defects such as: protein C and S deficiency, antithrombin deficiency, hyperhomocysteinemia, Leiden and other factor V mutations,[21–24] prothrombin G20210A mutation,[25–27] antiphospholipid antibodies, lupus anticoagulant, heparin cofactor II deficiency, plasminogen deficiency, tissue plasminogen activator deficiency, sticky platelet syndrome, dysfibrinogenemia, and factor XII deficiency.[28,29] Increased VTE risk may also result from acquired resistance to protein C resulting from increased levels of factor V and factor VIII.[20] An eight-fold increased risk of VTE during pregnancy has been reported in pregnant women with an underlying inherited or acquired thrombophilic disorder.[30] The most common acquired thrombophilia is the antiphospholipid syndrome, for which the reported risk of VTE has varied

Table 7.2 Risk stratification for venous thromboembolism (VTE) in pregnancy.

Low risk
Age <35 years
Uncomplicated pregnancy
Elective cesarean section
Moderate risk
Age >35 years
Obesity
Gross varicose veins
Recurrent infections
Immobility >4 days before delivery
Preeclampsia
Emergency cesarean section
High risk
Three or more moderate risk factors
Hereditary thrombophilic disease
Antiphospholipid antibody syndrome
Personal or family history of DVT
History of PE
Cesarean section hysterectomy

Source: Farrell, S. E., *Emerg. Med. Clin. North Am.*, 2001. **19**: 1013–23.

from 5%[31] to 22%.[32] Recurrent thrombosis may occur in as many as 69% of antiphospholipid patients.[33]

Increased venous capacitance results in a measurable reduction of venous flow in the lower extremities beginning early in the first trimester.[34] Beginning with the second trimester, significant venous stasis is present owing to compression of the inferior vena cava, left iliac vein and pelvic veins by the gravid uterus.[35] Venous stasis may be accentuated by the presence of varicosities, immobility or surgery (especially cesarean section with or without hysterectomy). Vaginal and cesarean delivery both damage pelvic veins, adding vascular injury to the other components of Virchow's triad. Other clinical risk factors may also be present such as sepsis, or trauma. Disorders such as malignancy and severe cardiac disease, which also increase the risk of VTE, are however unusual in reproductive-age women. Successful diagnosis, treatment and secondary prevention requires definition and management of not only the thrombotic process but also the underlying risk factors. A summary of the pathophysiology of VTE during pregnancy is presented in Figure 7.1.

The location and presentation of maternal VTE is similar but not exactly the same as in the non-pregnant patient. Deep vein thrombosis and PE represent

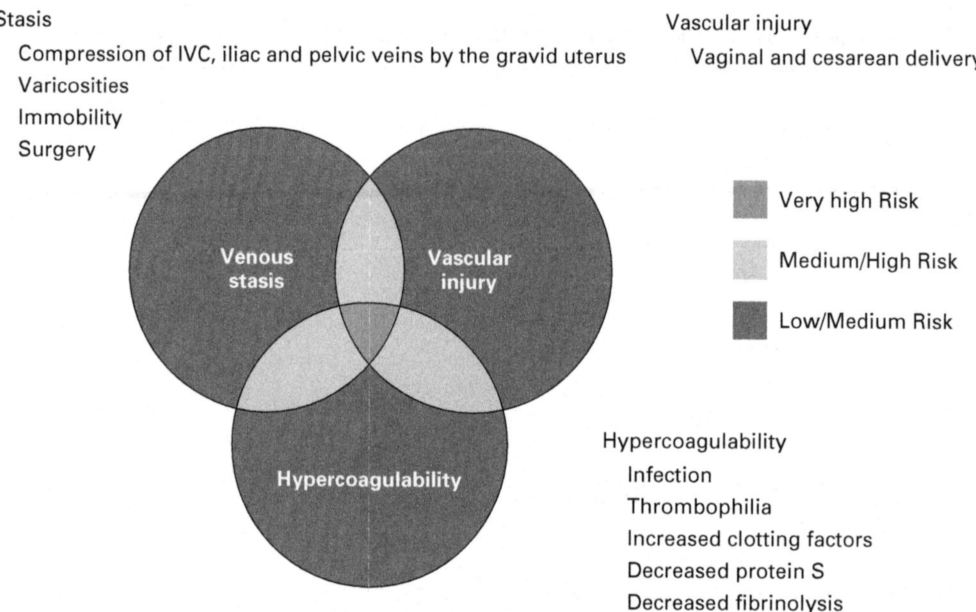

Figure 7.1 Pathophysiology of VTE in pregnancy.

manifestations of a continuum of disease. Over 50% of cases[36] of PE may not have recognized sources of DVT. Many patients with proximal DVT have clinically silent PE. Symptomatic thrombi are usually found in proximal veins[37,38] however; at least 50% of pulmonary emboli occur in asymptomatic patients.[39] In the non-pregnant patient the majority of all venous thrombi occur in infrapopliteal veins; however, the primary source of PE is proximal DVT.[40–42] Calf DVT propagates proximally in about 30% to 40% of cases. During pregnancy, DVT occurs more commonly in the iliofemoral veins (72%) than in the calf veins. Compression of the left iliac vein by the right iliac and the ovarian arteries (which only cross the iliac vein on the left side), may explain the 90% prevalence of left-sided DVT (compared to 55% in non-pregnant women). This anatomic asymmetry may also explain the predisposition for thrombosis to occur in the iliofemoral systems (72%) rather than the distal veins (9%).[43] Postpartum DVT, however, is more likely to occur in the popliteal veins (≥50%).

Clinical evaluation

The diagnosis of VTE is not possible on clinical grounds alone. Nonetheless, an understanding of the clinical features is essential to the selection of patients for objective diagnostic studies. The clinician must be ever mindful of the consequences of a missed diagnosis and maintain a high level of suspicion whenever the pregnant patient presents with symptoms or signs suggesting venous thrombosis. A variety of risk factors have been recognized and the clinician should have a heightened awareness of these in every pregnant patient. It is reported that 72% of pregnant women with VTE have some additional clinical risk factor.[44]

One particularly important risk factor is a previous history of venous thromboembolism. The previous episode must be evaluated to determine whether it was associated with a transient risk factor such as trauma, long-term immobility, or a previous pregnancy. For those patients who experienced VTE in the absence of a defined risk factor, a careful evaluation for inherited or acquired thrombophilia is required. This is particularly true for those patients who also have a family history of venous thromboembolism.

Other risk factors that should increase clinical vigilance include older maternal age, higher parity and obesity.[45] Since the risk of venous thromboembolism is greatest in the postpartum period (10 to 20 times greater than during pregnancy),[16,17] the clinician must be aware that the risk is many fold increased following cesarean section compared to vaginal delivery and there is a 10-fold higher risk of fatal pulmonary embolism during that period.[46] This risk is further increased in those patients in whom a hysterectomy is done during the procedure. In addition, women who have sustained VTE during a previous pregnancy or while taking combination oral contraception[14] are at significant risk of thrombosis during a subsequent pregnancy.[47]

The recent recognition that the ovarian hyperstimulation syndrome results in a very significant risk factor for venous thromboembolism has provided a new problem for the clinician. Several aspects of the clinical features that result from assisted reproductive treatment must be born in mind. It is now clear that thromboembolism is more common in those hyperstimulation cycles that result in pregnancy than those that do not.[48,49] It is of interest that an important systemic hypercoagulable state occurs with ovarian hyperstimulation. Thus, the site of thrombosis is as likely to be in the upper extremities or neck veins as in the lower extremities. As expected from an induced pathophysiologic event, the risk of venous thromboembolism in these patients is highest in the first trimester.

Clinical presentation of deep vein thrombosis

A classic clinical presenting triad has commonly been taught that includes calf pain, edema (particularly unilateral), and pain with dorsiflexion of the foot (Homan's sign). This description has long fallen by the wayside, since careful serial non-invasive studies have shown that only a small fraction (30%) of pregnant patients with deep vein thrombosis express this "triad",[50] and many consider the Homans' sign not only unreliable but potentially dangerous, since it

Table 7.3 Differential diagnosis of calf pain, redness or swelling.

DVT	Inguinal abcess
Superficial phlebitis	Erythema nodosum
Varicose veins	Gout
Congestive heart failure	Malignancy with venous or lymphatic obstruction
Trauma	Rheumatoid arthritis
Baker's cyst	Pregnancy
Cellulitis	Paralysis
Lymphangitis	

can occur with many clinical circumstances such as muscle strain, hematoma, or contusion. In addition, most now believe that some clinical risk exists for the brisk dorsiflexion examination, because a clot, if present, can become dislodged with resultant pulmonary embolization. A study by Gherman of 165 pregnant patients with VTE (127 DVT and 38 PE), revealed that while 85.7% of patients presented with pain, tenderness, and unilateral leg swelling, only 46.6% had a positive Homans' sign, 27.6% had erythema, 13.4% had increased warmth and 12.6% had a palpable cord.[12]

A common presentation in pregnancy is with the complaint of low back or flank pain, calf discomfort, or the clinical recognition of tenderness when the patient is examined. The presence of unilateral edema, especially with some associated calf tenderness, is particularly important, since the actual clinical presentation is often quite subtle. Since these findings may be very subtle the clinician must practice due diligence in the evaluation of the lower extremities during pregnancy. Table 7.3 illustrates the multiple diagnostic possibilities in evaluating the red, painful, swollen calf. In addition, since the first six to eight weeks postpartum are actually the time of greatest risk, the physician needs to be particularly vigilant after what may be even a simple, non-complicated delivery. The complexity and significance of the "high index of suspicion" in the pregnant patient who is found to have leg edema, dyspnea, back pain and/or chest pain has been carefully reviewed by Bates and Ginsberg,[51] who have shown that the actual prevalence of venous thromboembolism in pregnant women with these symptoms is less than in the general age-correlated population, because these findings are so very common during pregnancy.

Nevertheless, unilateral edema and/or pain in the lower extremity, especially in the iliofemoral region, continue to be the noteworthy presenting features of deep vein thrombosis. This is particularly true in the pregnant patient when the left leg is the edematous extremity. Certainly, clinical evidence of edema is most evident in the third trimester, although most studies demonstrate that the risk of venous thromboembolism is significant through all trimesters. The actual risk is significantly enhanced in the postpartum period, when the mechanisms for iliac vein compression no longer exist. Clinically, it is often easier to identify possible VTE patients with edema and/or pain during the earlier trimesters; whereas in the third trimester the large fetus-containing uterus is all too often regarded as the reasonable cause of compression of the iliac veins and thereby not regarded as a significant finding. The fact that significant proportions of pregnancy or postpartum patients who present with a pulmonary embolism have no physical findings and may not even recall symptoms, emphasizes the difficulty in the clinical diagnosis of venous thromboembolism. A study of patients with angiographically proven PE has demonstrated that over half had clinically asymptomatic DVT in the extremities.[52]

Clinical presentation of pulmonary embolism

Although the classical clinical features of pulmonary embolism have been extensively reviewed, all clinicians are aware that many episodes occur in the absence of the complete clinical picture. The usual presentation is unexpected dyspnea or chest pain, which may be pleuritic, or the presence of both symptoms simultaneously. The sudden onset of tachypnea and tachycardia provide a helpful diagnostic focus. A cough is common and, rarely, actual hemoptysis occurs; and its presence can serve as a very dramatic clinical focus. A feature commonly evident is anxiety, which needs to be acknowledged as an important symptom. All too often this symptom is ascribed to the mental status related to the pregnancy and its potential significance is overlooked. Unfortunately, some patients present with acute right-sided heart failure with the abrupt and progressive development of peripheral edema and even anasarca, prominent neck vein distension in the upright position, and extremity skin discoloration. Rarely, the presentation can be one of cardiovascular collapse and as many as 40% of patients with fatal PE present with syncope. The presenting symptoms and signs of PE are summarized in Tables 7.4 and 7.5.

Diagnostic modalities

Laboratory studies

The utility of the clinical laboratory in diagnosing VTE is greatly reduced owing to the intrinsic prothrombotic state inherent in pregnancy. The D-dimer assay elevates and becomes progressively more positive during the second and third trimester,[53] thrombin–antithrombin complexes become elevated, and protein S levels decrease. The high risk postpartum period is similarly a time of elevated

Table 7.4 Symptoms of pulmonary embolism (PE).

Cardiovascular collapse
Cardiopulmonary arrest, sudden death
Chest pain, sudden onset, typically pleuritic
Syncope
Hemoptysis
Diaphoresis
Anxiety
Unexplained shortness of breath
Stroke caused by paradoxical embolism
Fever of undetermined origin
(Clinical risk strongly influences interpretation of symptoms)

Table 7.5 Signs of pulmonary embolism (PE).

Apprehension
Diaphoresis
Tachycardia (rapid heart rate)
Tachypnea (rapid breathing rate)
Fever

D-dimers, regardless of the presence of thromboembolism. Since the primary usefulness of the D-dimer assay is for its negative predictive value, and since it is usually positive during uncomplicated pregnancy and postpartum, it is not a useful assay for this population. Even in the non-pregnant patient, few laboratory studies are particularly useful in confirming suspected DVT or PE. The complete blood count and chemistry analysis are of little value but may aid considerably in the identification of underlying illness predisposing to or initiating thrombosis.

The antithrombin level (AT) (normal 85% to 125% of normal human plasma (NHP)) is diminished to a degree corresponding to the severity of thrombosis, as AT binds to thrombin. The AT level should be obtained in patients suspected of having DVT as a diagnostic adjunct and to assess the suitability for heparin therapy.[54] The antithrombin level, however, cannot be relied upon as a useful diagnostic study for VTE in pregnancy.

An interesting laboratory finding has been the evidence that individuals with blood group O have a decreased risk of venous thromboembolic disease. The mean relative risk is one-half that of the population.[55] The biologic explanation for this is unclear.

Table 7.6 Diagnostic modalities for the diagnosis of DVT.

Non-invasive
Impedance plethysmography (IPG)
Compression ultrasound (CUS)
Compression ultrasound with color Doppler (Duplex)
Magnetic resonance imaging (MRI)
Invasive
Ascending contrast venography

Imaging studies

It is clear that in both pregnant and non-pregnant patients, clinical criteria alone are not adequate to establish the diagnosis of DVT or PE. Less than half of patients with suspicious clinical signs and symptoms are proven to have DVT by objective testing. The physiological changes of normal pregnancy render the diagnosis of lower extremity DVT especially difficult. Non-thrombotic etiologies of maternal leg pain and swelling are common. The enlarged uterus makes many of the newer diagnostic tests applicable in the non-pregnant patient difficult to use and interpret. The same criteria for diagnosis are applied; however, the preponderance of antepartum DVT in the pelvic and iliofemoral veins limits the utility of compression ultrasound (CUS), thus altering the approach to diagnosis. Diagnostic modalities useful in the diagnosis of DVT are summarized in Table 7.6.

The diagnostic evaluation of suspected PE is not changed by pregnancy. The Prospective Investigation of Pulmonary Embolism Diagnosis (PIOPED) study of patients with suspected PE determined that if the pretest clinical probability of PE was 80% to 100% (10% of patients), the diagnosis was correctly predicted in only 68%. When the clinical probability was 0% to 19% (26% of patients), PE was excluded in 91%. Unfortunately, in the majority of patients (64%) the clinical diagnosis was noncommittal (20% to 79% probability of PE). The PIOPED study clearly demonstrates that pretest probability correlates primarily with negative diagnostic studies.[56,57]

The imaging reference standards for diagnosis are ascending contrast venography for DVT and pulmonary angiography for PE. The primary modality for diagnosis of DVT is CUS with or without color flow Doppler. Owing to the limitations of CUS in pregnancy, magnetic resonance imaging (MRI) has emerged as a particularly useful technique for the diagnosis of pelvic and iliofemoral thrombosis.[58] Impedance plethysmography may be of value in diagnosis; however, is not widely available and has many limitations, particularly during pregnancy.[59] While ventilation/perfusion (V/Q) lung scans have been the primary modality for

Table 7.7 Diagnostic modalities for the diagnosis of PE.

Non-invasive
Ventilation/Perfusion lung scan (V/Q scan)
Spiral computerized tomography (spiral CT)
Echocardiography (2-D echo)
Invasive
Pulmonary angiography

diagnosis of PE, spiral computerized tomographic imaging has supplanted the V/Q scan in many institutions. Pregnancy results in a number of physiological changes, which alter the diagnostic utility of the imaging studies employed for diagnosis in the non-pregnant patient. Diagnostic modalities utilized for the diagnosis of PE are summarized in Table 7.7.

A great deal of study has been done to delineate the risks to the mother and fetus of the various imaging approaches. Ginsberg and colleagues[60] have defined the exposure risks to the fetus with the various imaging modalities. The ventilation lung scan with ^{99m}Tc results in an estimated fetal exposure of 20 to 30 m Rads. The addition of the perfusion lung scan with the ^{99m}Tc adds an estimated 10 to 18 m Rads. Thus, the full study provides an estimated fetal exposure of approximately 50 m Rads.[61] Since earlier estimates of the occurrence of adverse fetal affects have utilized the benchmark of 4,000 m Rads, this projected exposure appears reasonable and appropriate.

Diagnostic modalities for deep vein thrombosis

Impedance plethysmography

An older but diagnostically useful study is impedance plethysmography (IPG). It is non-invasive, sensitive and specific for proximal vein thrombosis, the anatomical site of greatest risk for pulmonary embolization and the site most difficult to evaluate in the pregnant patient.[59,62] However, IPG does not provide as good delineation of the status of the calf veins.[63] As a result, repeat testing has been proposed in equivocal cases or in circumstances where the clinical picture is highly suggestive but the IPG non-diagnostic. Hull and coworkers[59] have proposed repeating the IPG on days 2, 3, 5, 7, 10 and 14 in such circumstances to exclude the possibility of an inadequately recognized calf vein thrombosis that is extending. Importantly, they have shown such a sequential approach safe, so that in the absence of affirmative data, institution of anticoagulant therapy can be withheld.[55] Pseudothrombosis in pregnancy can produce a false positive test, particularly in the third trimester when compression of the iliac veins by a large uterus may occur. Repeating the study in the lateral decubitus position will often clarify this situation.[57] Unfortunately, impedance plethysmography is no longer widely available and has been replaced by ultrasound as the diagnostic study of choice for suspected DVT.[64]

Real-time B-mode compression ultrasound

In all patients, real-time B-mode compression ultrasound (CUS) is the imaging modality of choice for the diagnosis of proximal DVT. The primary diagnostic finding is the presence (normal) or absence (thrombosis) of compressibility of the vein. Useful findings also include the lack of movement of the venous valves and walls with direct pressure and maneuvers such as respiration and valsalva. The external iliac, common femoral, and popliteal veins are examined. Examination of the veins of the calf may be excluded from examination owing to the low sensitivity to calf thrombi.[38,65–68]

In the non-pregnant patient, CUS is nearly 100% sensitive and specific for the diagnosis of proximal DVT.[66,68–71] CUS fails to adequately identify calf thrombi (<50% sensitivity);[68,70,72] however, only 30% to 40% of calf thrombi extend proximally and these are rarely asymptomatic.[42] Follow-up studies performed seven days after an initially negative CUS have identified only 1% to 1.4%[71] of patients with the subsequent development of DVT. The incidence of PE in the patients who were treated without anticoagulation based upon the negative ultrasound was only 0.7% in the study by Cogo *et al.*[73] and 0.6% in the series of Birdwell *et al.*[71]

Compression ultrasonography is limited by the inaccuracy in detecting pelvic DVT and the relatively low sensitivity and specificity in asymptomatic patients. False negative CUS may occur as the result of: (a) thrombosis involving less than 3 cm of the distal popliteal vein; (b) a single lumen thrombosis of a duplicate popliteal vein; (c) edema; (d) distortion of the venous anatomy owing to malignancy or cellulitis; (e) common femoral vein involvement by a short tail of thrombus originating in the deep femoral vein and (f) unknown reasons.[69,74] Pregnant patients have physiologic changes resulting in dilatation of pelvic and lower extremity veins, varicose veins and overt venous insufficiency and edema of the lower extremities. This results in a significantly decreased specificity of CUS for the diagnosis of DVT. Furthermore, the significantly increased frequency of iliofemoral DVT (70%) versus popliteal and calf DVT (9%)[75] in pregnancy compared to the non-pregnant patient, presents a further limitation to reliance upon CUS.

Particularly in pregnancy, diagnosis may be challenging. Repeat CUS, after an initially negative study, may be indicated in symptomatic hospitalized patients[69,76] and in symptomatic outpatients,[74] particularly in the setting of high clinical probability (characteristic of pregnancy) and a positive D-dimer assay (as is usually the case during pregnancy). In clinical situations in which the diagnosis of pelvic or calf vein thrombosis is critical, or if there is particularly poor laboratory to clinical correlation, contrast venography or magnetic resonance imaging may be required. Magnetic resonance imaging or venography may be required for diagnosis in pregnancy. Compression ultrasound may also be included in the diagnostic evaluation of patients with intermediate probability ventilation perfusion lung scans (V/Q) or non-diagnostic spiral CT scans.

Real-time B-mode ultrasound with color Doppler (Duplex scanning)

Improvement in the diagnostic accuracy and specificity of standard CUS may result from enhancement of B-mode ultrasound with color Doppler (Duplex). Ultrasound analysis augmented by color Doppler analysis with a 3–5 megahertz Doppler transducer compares favorably with contrast venography.[69] The Doppler component allows the examiner to determine areas of abnormality and focus on changes in blood flow spontaneity, phasicity, and augmentation. Venous patency is confirmed by normal phasic flow signals and obliteration of the venous lumen by direct compression of the vein with the transducer. Thrombotic venous occlusion eliminates normal Doppler signals and the lumen is rendered non-compressible with direct pressure. Non-occlusive clots result in partial obliteration of the lumen with pressure and continuous (rather than phasic) venous signals. Evaluation of calf veins requires foot compression and monitoring of signals from the posterior tibial vein. Very recent thrombi resemble flowing blood with Doppler and are compressible with CUS. Older clots are incompressible and somewhat less echogenic. As with CUS, Duplex is 97% to 100% sensitive and specific in symptomatic non-pregnant patients with proximal DVT.[69] Numerous studies have also demonstrated that neither CUS nor Duplex scanning are cost effective for screening high-risk, asymptomatic patients and should primarily be applied for patients with symptoms.[77,78]

Ascending contrast venography

The radiocontrast venogram remains the reference standard for the diagnosis of DVT.[77,79] Venous thrombosis is diagnosed by an abrupt termination or redirection of blood flow, or an intravascular filling defect visible on more than one view. Although highly reliable, ascending contrast venography is an invasive procedure limited by the difficulty encountered in venous cannulation, a patient history of allergy to iodine or radiocontrast media, and relatively poor availability (compared to ultrasound). As many as 20% of hospitalized patients may not be suitable candidates for study.[80] In addition, thrombogenicity of iodinated radiocontrast results in a 2% to 4% risk of developing DVT from the procedure.[81] In the pregnant patient, radiation exposure is often raised as an objection to the use of venography. Fortunately, the radiation exposure to the fetus for unilateral imaging with spot films and without abdominal shielding is less than 1 Rad (0.0005Gy). This level of exposure is well below the minimum level regarded as teratogenic.[61]

Magnetic resonance imaging

Magnetic resonance imaging (MRI) is primarily utilized for the diagnosis of DVT in pregnant women. The diagnostic evaluation of lower extremity edema in this group is often difficult and the risk of DVT in pregnancy is high. Spitzer and associates have applied MRI and have determined sensitivity for detecting thrombi of 87% in the calf and 97% to 100% above the knee.[58] Magnetic resonance imaging may also be useful in the patient with suspected pelvic, iliac or calf thrombosis, in spite of a negative venous Duplex scan of the lower extremities.[82]

Diagnostic modalities for pulmonary embolism

Chest radiograph

Chest radiography is usually of little or no value in confirming the diagnosis of PE. Approximately 40% of patients with PE have a normal chest X-ray. Classical abnormalities include the "cut-off" sign of central pulmonary artery occlusion with increased lucency of the lung field, atelectasis, small pleural effusions and a pleural-based, wedge-shaped density of pulmonary infarction.[83] In the majority of patients, the chest X-ray is primarily of value in suggesting alternative diagnoses and in clarifying the etiology of matching defects on the V/Q scan.

Electrocardiogram

The electrocardiogram of a patient with PE is usually normal or reveals sinus tachycardia. The classic findings of "S_1-T_3", T inversion in the right precordial leads, right-axis deviation, and incomplete or complete bundle branch block owing to right ventricular enlargement and strain may be observed but are not diagnostic.[84] Most often, the electrocardiogram serves as an indicator of underlying illness and is infrequently of value in confirming the diagnosis of PE.

Arterial blood gas

Reliance upon the arterial blood gas for useful diagnostic information is perhaps the most common mistake in evaluating the patient with suspected PE. Patients with acute PE may have both matching and non-matching abnormalities of ventilation and perfusion, and many have underlying disease as a cause of an abnormal arterial blood gas. Characteristic findings include a decrease in the normal pO_2 and pCO_2, thus a widening of the arterial–alveolar oxygen gradient accompanied by an alkalotic pH. Among PE patients with no prior cardiopulmonary disease, 30% or more will have a $pO_2 > 80$ mmHg.[83] A normal blood gas does not exclude PE and an abnormal result does not confirm PE.

Ventilation/Perfusion lung scan

Ventilation/perfusion lung scanning (V/Q) is the diagnostic procedure of choice to confirm a suspected PE. Perfusion scanning is performed by venous administration of isotopically labeled macroaggregates of human albumin. Ventilation scanning involves the inhalation of aerosols of either ^{127}Xe or technetium. A normal scan exhibits homogenous and matching distribution of the aerosol and the macroaggregated albumin throughout both lungs.

The degree of ventilation–perfusion match guides interpretation. Scans consistent with PE exhibit areas of V/Q mismatch characterized by absence of perfusion in the presence of normal ventilation. Matching defects are typical of lung disease. Peripherally based, large perfusion defects in areas of normal ventilation are strongly suggestive of PE, while matching, small, central or ill-defined defects are less likely to represent PE. The scans are interpreted as: high probability, intermediate probability, low probability, very low probability or normal, as defined by PIOPED criteria.[56] Pretest clinical suspicion plays a major role in establishing the diagnosis. With a strong pretest suspicion for PE and a high probability scan, the V/Q is 96% accurate in identifying PE. A moderate clinical probability combined with a high probability scan confirms PE in only 80% to 88% of cases.[56,85,86] The primary challenge has been to develop management strategies for patients with intermediate probability scans, since patients with high to moderately high clinical suspicion and high-probability scans only represent 12% to 32% of patients with abnormal scans. Among patients with a low clinical suspicion and high-probability scan, only 56% are confirmed to have PE. Less than 6% of patients with low clinical suspicion of PE and a low-probability scan will be determined to have a PE.[56]

High pretest probability and a high-probability scan as well as low pretest probability and a low-probability scan reliably confirm the diagnosis and guide therapy. Remaining is the over 50% of patients for whom the diagnosis is not clear based upon the clinical findings and V/Q result.[87]

Pulmonary angiography

Pulmonary angiography (PA) is the primary reference standard for diagnosis of PE. Analysis of the PIOPED data has demonstrated that PA is about 98% accurate for the diagnosis of PE.[56] While the error rate is low, in the selected patient with ongoing clinical indications of thromboembolic disease further evaluation may be indicated.[82,83,88] As an invasive procedure, PA is not without risk of complications.[89] Accepted morbidity and mortality rates (caused by severe allergic reactions to radiocontrast, cardiac perforation and serious cardiac arrhythmias) are 0.2% and 1.9%, respectively.[90]

Clearly, the risk of failure to diagnose PE is great and the risk/benefit ratio of PA must be weighed in each patient. Numerous experts have concluded that the inclusion of pulmonary angiography in a diagnostic algorithm was important and cost-effective. Pulmonary angiography was most useful when performed in patients with non-high probability scans and normal leg CUS.[90] The consensus of most proposals has been that PA should be performed whenever the V/Q is interpreted as intermediate or low probability, the leg CUS is normal, the clinical probability is intermediate or high and the D-dimer assay is abnormal. Pulmonary angiography has also been recommended whenever there is a strong clinical indication of PE, even in the absence of a positive V/Q or CUS.[76,90,91]

Spiral computed tomographic angiography

Spiral computerized tomography with contrast (SCTA) is a non-invasive alternative to PA, which provides three-dimensional visualization of pulmonary thromboemboli. Sensitivity for diagnosis of PE with SCTA is 95.5% (range 64% to 100%), with a specificity of 97.6% (range 89% to 100%).[92,93] When PE are confined to subsegmental pulmonary arteries, sensitivity is lower (as low as 36%).[92,94] Subsegmental emboli have been demonstrated in as many as 30% of patients with intermediate probability V/Q scans.[92] Stein *et al.* resolved the concern regarding subsegmental emboli, noting that only 6% of PE detected among all PIOPED patients were subsegmental and that these corresponded to low-probability V/Q scans.[95]

Evaluation of a diagnostic algorithm for the diagnosis of PE, proposed by van Erkel and associates in 1996, confirmed that SCTA could be an important component of the best approach to diagnosis. D-dimer was used to exclude DVT and PE and SCTA was used to confirm PE in all patients with non-high probability V/Q scans. Both clinical outcome and cost effectiveness data were superior to other approaches.[92] Subsequent studies have confirmed the superiority of SCTA over V/Q scanning for the diagnosis of PE. Mayo and associates compared SCTA and V/Q scanning, determining sensitivity and specificity for SCTA of 95% and 94% versus 87% and 65% for V/Q scanning.[96] Garg *et al.* compared the two modalities and clearly demonstrated the superiority of SCTA over V/Q scanning. Spiral CT angiography exhibited greater accuracy and specificity and was recommended as the primary screening technique for PE. Notably, SCTA provided significant, clinically useful information not available from V/Q scanning as old clots were distinguishable from new and an alternative diagnosis was established in 31% of patients.[97] Cross and associates performed a similar analysis and recommended that SCTA replace V/Q scanning as the initial diagnostic study in patients with suspected PE.[98] The review by Perrier *et al.* has, however, demonstrated that SCTA should not be used alone to diagnose PE; rather it should be combined with other studies such as CUS/Doppler and D-dimer (non-pregnant patients) in diagnostic algorithms. It was advised that SCTA might replace pulmonary angiogrpahy in combined approaches which include CUS/Doppler and V/Q scanning.[99]

Echocardiography

Patients with PE who undergo echocardiography are found to have right ventricular enlargement or hypokinesis approximately 40% of the time.[100] These findings are non-specific but in the setting of acute submassive PE without shock or massive PE with shock may provide prognostic information which will guide the choice of therapy (anticoagulation alone or with thrombolytic therapy).[101] Evidence of pulmonary arterial hypertension or the finding of main pulmonary artery thrombus may also influence patient management. In addition, as a diagnostic tool in evaluating the patient who presents with unexplained chest pain and shortness of breath, other findings such as myocardial infarction, valvular heart disease, aortic dissection or cardiac tamponade may be identified.[102,103]

Diagnostic strategies

As has been emphasized, pregnancy provides a complex setting for diagnostic approaches.[51] The initial clinical features may be quite subtle. Critical issues of safety for the fetus and mother limit the diagnostic approaches available in the non-pregnant state. The currently recommended algorithms for evaluation of non-pregnant patients with suspected VTE emphasize: (a) clinical probability, (b) the D-dimer assay, (c) diagnostic imaging (compression ultrasound for DVT and V/Q lung scanning or spiral CT angiography for PE), (d) clinical reassessment and serial testing. In the pregnant patient the approach is much the same. The major differences are the inability to rely upon the D-dimer assay and difficulty in interpreting lower extremity compression ultrasound images owing to edema and obesity (the setting in which MRI is most useful). The evaluation of the patient with suspected DVT or PE begins with a thorough history and physical examination. A clinical probability (Tables 7.8 and 7.9)[104] is then developed to guide the selection of diagnostic studies. Test results are interpreted with knowledge of the clinical context and the outcome of other studies. Figures 7.2 through 7.4 illustrate various approaches to suspected DVT and PE.

Table 7.8 Pretest clinical probability of DVT.

Clinical features*	Score**
Cancer (treatment ongoing or within 6 months, or palliative)	1.0
Paralysis, paresis, plaster immobilization of the lower extremities	1.0
Bedridden for more than 3 days or major surgery within 4 weeks	1.0
Tenderness localized along the deep venous system	1.0
Entire leg swollen	1.0
Calf swelling >3 cm compared to asymptomatic leg (measure 10 cm below tibial tuberosity)	1.0
Pitting edema (greater in the symptomatic leg)	1.0
Collateral superficial veins (non-varicose)	1.0
Alternative diagnosis as likely or greater than DVT	−2.0
Low probability	≤0
Moderate probability	1.0–2.0
High probability	≥3.0

Sources: Wells, P. S. *et al.*, *Lancet*, 1997; **350**: 1795–8.

*In patients with symptoms in both legs, the more symptomatic leg is used.

**Analysis: Patients were categorized as being low, moderate or high pretest probability for deep vein thrombosis by the scoring model. A high score was one of three or more, a moderate score was one of two or more, and a low score was zero or less.

Table 7.9 Pretest clinical probability of PE.

Clinical features	Score**
Clinical signs and symptoms of DVT	3.0
Heart rate >100 beats/minute	1.5
Immobilization (for ≥3 consecutive days)	1.5
Surgery in the previous 4 weeks	1.5
Previous diagnosis of DVT or PE	1.5
Hemoptysis	1.0
Cancer (treatment ongoing or within 6 months, or palliative)	1.0
PE as likely or more likely than another diagnosis	3.0
Low probability	<2.0
Moderate probability	2.0–6.0
High probability	>6.0

Sources: Wells, P. S., Anderson, D. R., Rodger, M., *et al. Ann. Int. Med.*, 2001; **135**: 98–107.

**Analysis: The pretest probability of pulmonary embolism was considered low in patients whose score was less than 2.0, moderate in patients whose score was at least 2.0 but no higher than 6.0, and high in patients whose score was greater than 6.0.

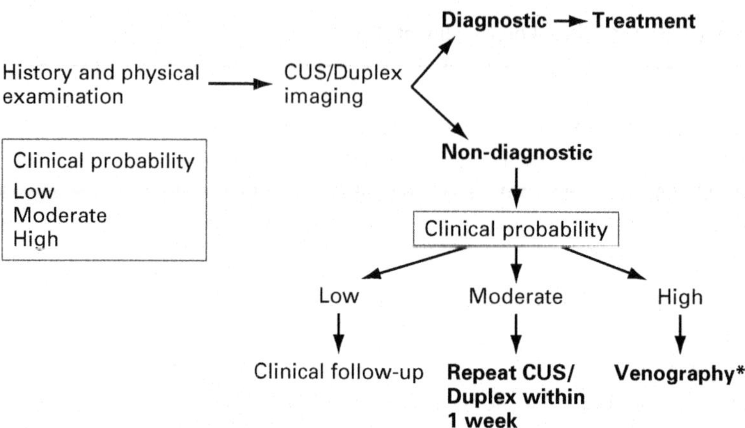

Figure 7.2 Evaluation for suspected DVT.
*An MRI may be considered; however, if it is non-diagnostic, contrast venography is required.

Diagnostic strategy for suspected deep vein thrombosis

Figure 7.2 is an algorithm which directs the approach to the pregnant patient presenting with signs and symptoms of DVT. Clinical probability is first calculated by considering details of the history and physical examination. Diagnostic imaging is then obtained in the hope of confirming or excluding the diagnosis. When the results of diagnostic imaging are not satisfactory or when there is poor clinical to radiographic correlation, additional studies may be indicated. Magnetic resonance imaging may be utilized, or in certain difficult circumstances in which the potential benefit is felt to outweigh the small risk, ascending contrast venography may be required. It must be emphasized that although Duplex scanning is the first-line diagnostic strategy,[10] it does not provide good visualization of the iliac vessels, which is a serious consideration during pregnancy. As the failure to diagnose DVT may have dire consequences, the diagnosis of DVT must be confidently excluded for treatment to be withheld. When the diagnosis remains truly uncertain, it is recommended that either anticoagulation be initiated pending the outcome of additional studies or the patient must be followed very closely with serial Duplex imaging or other studies.

In the algorithms, CUS may be used interchangeably with Duplex. The indication for repeat imaging with Duplex has been extensively reviewed.[71–73,76] Repeat imaging is primarily indicated in patients with high clinical probability, an initially negative Duplex and continuing symptoms. Venography or MRI is usually reserved for the 1% of cases for whom the clinical probability remains high and the diagnosis remains obscure.

Diagnostic strategy for suspected pulmonary embolism

The highest clinical probability of PE is present in patients with known risk factors who present with new onset pleuritic chest pain, shortness of breath or acute cardiovascular collapse. In the circumstances of a suspected pulmonary embolus it is clear that the potential risk of withholding treatment is significantly greater than the risk of an invasive diagnostic procedure. Although immediate anticoagulation in all suspected cases may be appropriate, it should be kept in mind that the risks of therapy are not trivial. As there are many potential etiologies for the "classic" symptom complex, "empiric therapy" is only indicated while awaiting the results of objective testing.

The diagnostic procedure of first choice when PE is suspected is the V/Q scan or SCTA (depending upon availability). The SCTA should now be preferred. Pulmonary radiocontrast angiography is only indicated when the basic studies are inadequate to establish a firm diagnosis and clinical probability is high. The algorithm presented in Figure 7.3 combines clinical probability, the V/Q scan and other studies. Patients with intermediate probability V/Q scans may require additional diagnostic studies, including CUS or Duplex and careful clinical follow-up. Figure 7.4 reflects the superiority of SCTA as the initial investigation for patients with suspected PE.

The major controversy focuses on the approach when non-diagnostic lung scans are found. Studies have shown that almost 12% of individuals with a "low probability" ventilation–perfusion scan have identifiable pulmonary emboli.[56] In those patients with documentation of an occlusive lesion in the leg or pelvis, an "indeterminate" ventilation–perfusion scan can be considered the basis to proceed with therapy. By contrast, such findings in patients who have no evidence of a lower extremity thrombosis and similarly non-diagnostic spiral CT angiography, may require radiocontrast pulmonary angiography, which continues to be the diagnostic gold standard for pulmonary embolism. When the pulmonary angiography is done via the brachial artery approach the estimated fetal radiation exposure is less than 50 m Rads, which sharply contrasts with the risks via the classical femoral route of well over 400 m Rads.[61]

Conclusion

Pregnancy represents a high-risk clinical condition for VTE. A precise diagnosis can be achieved in a timely manner if the clinician is aware of the presenting signs and symptoms and the available diagnostic studies. There are many potential pitfalls that may result in an incorrect or missed diagnosis. A few of these are outlined in Table 7.10. An algorithmic approach must guide evaluation.

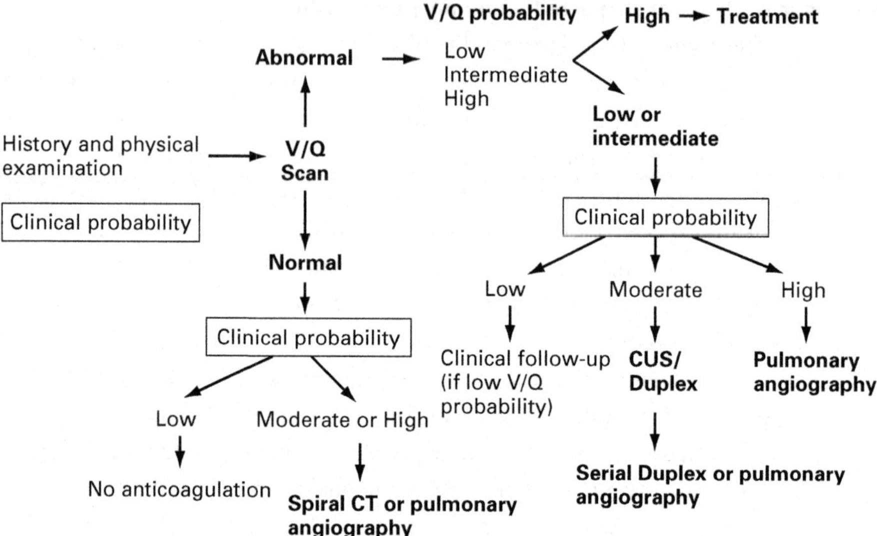

Figure 7.3 Evaluation for suspected PE with the V/Q scan.

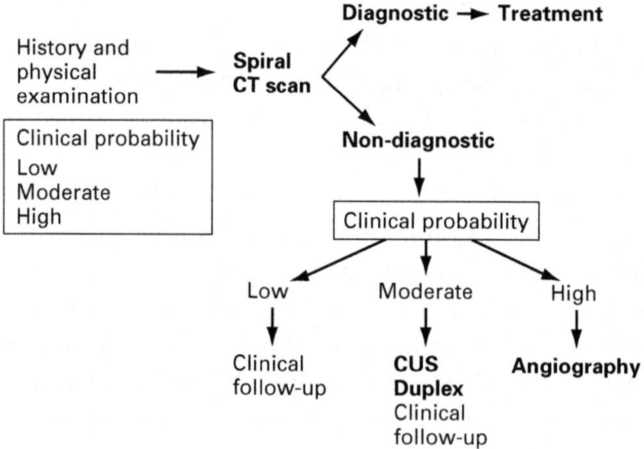

Figure 7.4 Evaluation for suspected PE with spiral CT scan.

Abstract

The diagnostic approach to suspected deep vein thrombosis (DVT) and pulmonary embolism (PE) is evolving. A greater understanding of the details of the history and physical examination now allows designation of clinical probability as a guide to the application of various diagnostic modalities. The traditional

Table 7.10 Pitfalls in the diagnosis of VTE in pregnancy.

Failure to consider pretest probability
Failure to risk stratify based on history and physical examination
Reliance on the physical examination alone
Failure to recognize subtle signs
Interpreting important findings as "normal in pregnancy"
Misinterpretation of elevated heart rate or respiratory rate
Reliance on a single test for diagnosis
ABG results misleading both in support of and exclusion of PE
CUS/Duplex may miss calf DVT
The CUS/Duplex in patients with prior DVT may lack sensitivity and specificity
V/Q scan may be normal in massive PE
Relying on the V/Q in patients with COPD
Failure to pursue a comprehensive approach to correct diagnosis
Failure to follow a structured algorithm

approaches to diagnosis are primarily based upon the results of compression ultrasonography (CUS) for DVT and the ventilation/perfusion lung scan (V/Q) for PE. Spiral computerized tomographic imaging (SCTA) may replace the V/Q scan and the need for pulmonary angiography is diminishing.

REFERENCES

1 Andres, R. L. and A. Miles, Venous thromboembolism and pregnancy. *Obstet. Gynecol. Clin. North. Am.*, 2001. **28**(3): 613–30.

2 Dizon-Townson, D., Pregnancy-related venous thromboembolism. *Clin. Obstet. Gynecol.*, 2002. **45**(2): 363–8.

3 Bates, S. M. and J. Ginsberg, Pregnancy and deep vein thrombosis. *Seminars in Vascular Medicine*, 2001(1): 97–104.

4 Anderson, B. S., *et al.*, The cumulative incidence of venous thromboembolism during pregnancy and the puerperium: an 11-year Danish population based study of 63,300 pregnancies. *Acta. Obstet. Gynecol. Scand.*, 1998. **77**: 110–13.

5 Nordstrom, M. and B. Lindblad, A prosective study of the incidence of deep-vein thrombosis within a defined urban population. *J. Intern. Med.*, 1992. **232**: 155–60.

6 Ginsberg, J., Management of venous thromboembolism. *N. Engl. J. Med.*, 1996. **334**: 1816.

7 Metcalfe, J. and K. Ueland, Maternal cardiovascular adjustments to pregnancy. *Prog. Cardiovasc. Dis.*, 1974. **16**: 363–74.

8 Rutherford, S., Monotoro, M., and W. McGhee, Thromboembolic disease associated with pregnancy: An 11 year review. *Am. J. Obstet. Gynecol.*, 1991. **164**(Suppl.): 286.

9 Toglia, M. R. and J. G. Weg, Venous thromboembolism during pregnancy. *N. Engl. J. Med.*, 1996. **335**: 109–14.

10 Greer, I. A., The acute management of venous thromboembolism in pregnancy. *Curr. Opin. Obstet. Gynecol.*, 2001. **13**(6): 569–75.

11 McColl, M. D., *et al.*, Prevalence of the post-thrombotic syndrome in young women wih previous venous thromboembolism. *Br. J. Haematol.*, 2000. **108**: 272–4.

12 Gherman, R. B., *et al.*, Incidence, clinical characteristics, and timing of objectively diagnosed venous thromboembolism during pregnancy. *Obstet. Gynecol.*, 1999. **94**: 730–4.

13 Gerhardt, A., *et al.*, Prothrombin and factor V mutations in women with a history of thrombosis during pregnancy and the puerperium. *N. Engl. J. Med.*, 2000. **342**: 374–80.

14 Bardaracco, M. A. and M. D. Vessey, Recurrence of venous thromboembolic disease and oral contraceptives. *Br. Med. J.*, 1974. **1**: 215–17.

15 Franks, A. L., *et al.*, Obstetrical pulmonary embolism mortality, United States, 1970–1985. *Am. J. Public Health*, 1990. **80**: 720–2.

16 Gei, A. F., Vadhera, R. B., and G. D. Hankins, Embolism during pregnancy: thrombus, air, and amniotic fluid. *Anesthesiol. Clin. North America*, 2003. **21**(1): 165–82.

17 Farrell, S. E., Special situations: pediatric, pregnant, and geriatric patients. *Emerg. Med. Clin. North. Am.*, 2001. **19**: 1013–23.

18 Bremme, K., *et al.*, Enhanced thrombin generation and fibrinolytic activity in normal pregnancy and the puerperium. *Obstet. Gynecol.*, 1992. **80**: 132–7.

19 Comp, P. C., Thurnau, G. R., and J. Welsh, Functional and immunological protein S levels are decreased during pregnancy. *Blood*, 1986. **68**: 881.

20 Clark, P., *et al.*, Activated protein C sensitivity, protein C, protein S, and coagulation in normal pregnancy. *Thromb. Haemost.*, 1998. **79**: 1166–70.

21 Manten, B., *et al.*, Risk factor profiles in patients with different clinical manifestations of venous thromboembolism: a focus on the factor V Leiden mutation. *Thromb. Haemost.*, 1996. **76**(4): 510–13.

22 Melichart, M., *et al.*, Thrombotic tendency in 75 symptomatic, unrelated patients with APC resistance. *Wien. Klin. Wochenschr.*, 1996. **108**(19): 607–10.

23 Simioni, P., *et al.*, The risk of recurrent venous thromboembolism in patients with an Arg506 -> Gln mutation in the gene for factor V (factor V Leiden). *N. Engl. J. Med.*, 1997. **336**: 399–403.

24 Williamson, D., *et al.*, Factor V Cambridge: a new mutation (Arg^{306}-> Thr) associated with resistance to activated protein C. *Blood*, 1998. **91**: 1140–4.

25 Arruda, V. R., *et al.*, Prevalence of the prothrombin gene variant (nt20201A) in venous thrombosis and arterial disease. *Thromb. Haemost.*, 1997. **78**: 1430–3.

26 Makris, M., *et al.*, Co-inheritance of the 20210A allele of the prothrombin gene increases the risk of thrombosis in subjects with familial thrombophilia. *Thromb. Haemost.*, 1997. **78**(6): 1426–9.

27 Martinelli, I., *et al.*, High risk of cerebral-vein thrombosis in carriers of a prothrombin-gene mutation and in users of oral contraceptives. *N. Engl. J. Med.*, 1998. **338**: 1793–7.

28 Bick, R. L. and H. Kaplan, Syndromes of thrombosis and hypercoagulability. Congenital and acquired causes of thrombosis. *Med. Clin. North. Am.*, 1998. **82**(3): 409–58.
29 Seligman, U. and A. Lubetsky, Genetic susceptibility to venous thrombosis. *N. Engl. J. Med.*, 2001. **344**: p. 12221231.
30 Girling, J. and M. de Swiet, Inherited thrombophilia and pregnancy. *Curr. Opin. Obstet. Gynecol.*, 1998. **10**: 135–55.
31 Branch, D. W., *et al.*, Outcome of treated pregnancies in women with antiphospholipid syndrome: An update of the Utah experience. *Obstet. Gynecol.*, 1992. **80**: 614–29.
32 Silver, R. M., *et al.*, Anticardiolipin antibodies: Clinical consequences of low titers. *Obstet. Gynecol.*, 1996. **87**: 494–500.
33 Khamashta, M. A., *et al.*, The management of thrombosis in the antiphospholipid-antibody syndrome. *N. Engl. J. Med.*, 1995. **332**: 993–7.
34 Ikard, R. W., Ueland, K., and R. Folse, Lower limb venous dynamics in pregnant women. *Surg. Gynecol. Obstet.*, 1971. **132**: 483.
35 Burns, M. M., Emerging concepts in the diagnosis and management of venous thromboembolism during pregnancy. *J. Thromb. Thrombolysis*, 2000. **10**(1): 59–68.
36 Eze, A. R., *et al.*, Is venous duplex imaging an appropriate initial screening test for patients with suspected pulmonary embolism? *Ann. Vasc. Surg.*, 1996. **10**(3): 220–3.
37 Heijboer, H., Brandjes, D., and A. W. Lensing, Efficacy of real-time B-mode ultrasonography in the diagnosis of deep vein thrombosis in symptomatic outpatients. 1991. **65**: 804.
38 Heijboer, H., *et al.*, Detection of deep vein thrombosis with impedance plethysmography and real-time compression ultrasonography in hospitalized patients. *Arch. Intern. Med.*, 1992. **152**(9): 1901–3.
39 Clagett, G. P. and E. W. Salzman, Prevention of venous thromboembolism in surgical patients. *N. Engl. J. Med.*, 1974. **290**(2): 93–6.
40 Kistner, R. L., *et al.*, Incidence of pulmonary embolism in the course of thrombophlebitis of the lower extremities. *Am. J. Surg.*, 1972. **124**(2): 169–76.
41 Moser, K. M., Brach, B. B., and G. F. Dolan, Clinically suspected deep venous thrombosis of the lower extremities. A comparison of venography, impedance plethysmography, and radiolabeled fibrinogen. *JAMA*, 1977. **237**(20): 2195–8.
42 Philbrick, J. T., *et al.*, Calf deep venous thrombosis. A wolf in sheep's clothing? *Arch. Intern. Med.*, 1988. **148**(10): 2131–8.
43 Greer, I. A., Thrombosis in pregnancy: maternal and fetal issues. *Lancet*, 1999. **353**: 1258–65.
44 McColl, M. D., *et al.*, Risk factors for pregnancy associated venous thromboembolism. *Thromb. Haemost.*, 1997. **78**: 1183–8.
45 Barbour, L. A., ACOG practice bulletin. Thrombembolism in pregnancy. *Int. J. Gynaecol. Obstet.*, 2001. **75**(2): 203–12.
46 Bonnar, J., Can more be done in obstetric and gynecologic practice to reduce morbidity and mortality associated with venous thromboembolism? *Am. J. Obstet. Gynecol.*, 1999. **180**(4): 784–91.
47 Tengborn, L., *et al.*, Recurrent thromboembolism in pregnancy and puerperium: Is there a need for thromboprophylaxis. *Am. J. Obstet. Gynecol.*, 1989. **160**: 90–4.

48 Stewart, J. A., *et al.*, Thromboembolic disease associated with ovarian stimulation and assisted conception techniques. *Hum. Reprod.*, 1997. **12**(10): 2167–73.

49 Baumann, P., *et al.*, Thromboembolic complications associated with reproductive endocrinologic procedures. *Hematol. Oncol. Clin. North Am.*, 2000. **14**(2): 431–43.

50 Grendys, E. C., Jr. and J. V. Fiorica, Advances in the prevention and treatment of deep vein thrombosis and pulmonary embolism. *Curr. Opin. Obstet. Gynecol.*, 1999. **11**(1): 71–9.

51 Bates, S. M. and J. S. Ginsberg, How we manage venous thromboembolism during pregnancy. *Blood*, 2002. **100**(10): 3470–8.

52 Hull, R., *et al.*, Pulmonary angiography, ventilation lung scanning and venography for clinically suspected pulmonary embolism with abnormal perfusion lung scan. *Ann. Intern. Med.*, 1983. **98**: 891–9.

53 Edelstam, G., *et al.*, New reference values on routine blood samples and human neutrophilic lipocalin during third trimester pregnancy. *Scand. J. Clin. Lab. Invest.*, 2001. **61**: 583–92.

54 Bick, R. L., Clinical relevance of antithrombin III. *Seminars in Hemostasis and Thrombosis*, 1982. **8**: 276.

55 Jick, H., *et al.*, Venous thromboembolic disease and ABO blood type. A cooperative study. *Lancet*, 1969. **1**(7594): 539–42.

56 Nicolaides, A. N., *et al.*, Value of the ventilation/perfusion scan in acute pulmonary embolism. *JAMA*, 1990. **263**(20): 2753–9.

57 Ginsberg, J., *et al.*, Pseudothrombosis in pregnancy. *CMAJ*, 1988. **139**(5): 409–10.

58 Spritzer, C. E., Evans, A. C., and H. H. Kay, Magnetic resonance imaging of deep venous thrombosis in pregnant women with lower extremity edema. *Obstet. Gynecol.*, 1995. **85**(4): 603–7.

59 Hull, R. D., Raskob, G. E., and C. J. Carter, Serial impedance plethysmography in pregnant patients with clinically suspected deep-vein thrombosis. Clinical validity of negative findings. *Ann. Intern. Med.*, 1990. **112**(9): 663–7.

60 Ginsberg, J. S., *et al.*, D-dimer in patients with clinically suspected pulmonary embolism. *Chest*, 1993. **104**(6): 1679–84.

61 Ginsberg, J. S., *et al.*, Risks to the fetus of radiologic procedures used in the diagnosis of maternal venous thromboembolic disease. *Thromb. Haemost.*, 1989. **61**(2): 189–96.

62 Cockett, F. B., Thomas, M. L., and D. Negus, Iliac vein compression. Its relation to iliofemoral thrombosis and the post-thrombotic syndrome. *BMJ*, 1967. **2**(543): 14–19.

63 Hull, R. D., *et al.*, Diagnostic efficacy of impedance plethysmography for clinically suspected deep-vein thrombosis. A randomized trial. *Ann. Intern. Med.*, 1985. **102**(1): 21–8.

64 Wheeler, H. B., *et al.*, Diagnostic tests for deep vein thrombosis: clinical usefulness depends on probability of disease. *Arch. Intern. Med.*, 1994. **154**: 1921–28.

65 Cronan, J. J., *et al.*, Deep venous thrombosis: US assessment using vein compression. *Radiology*, 1987. **162**(1.1): 191–4.

66 Appelman, P. T., *et al.*, Deep venous thrombosis of the leg: US findings. *Radiology*, 1987. **163**(3): 743–6.

67 Lensing, A. W., *et al.*, Detection of deep-vein thrombosis by real-time B-mode ultrasonography. *N. Engl. J. Med.*, 1989. **320**(6): 342–5.

68 Monreal, M., *et al.*, Real-time ultrasound for diagnosis of symptomatic venous thrombosis and for screening of patients at risk: correlation with ascending conventional venography. *Angiology*, 1989. **40**(6): 527–33.

69 Pedersen, O. M., *et al.*, Compression ultrasonography in hospitalized patients with suspected deep venous thrombosis. *Arch. Intern. Med.*, 1991. **151**(11): 2217–20.

70 Cogo, A., *et al.*, Distribution of thrombosis in patients with symptomatic deep vein thrombosis. Implications for simplifying the diagnostic process with compression ultrasound. *Arch. Intern. Med.*, 1993. **153**(24): 2777–80.

71 Birdwell, B. G., *et al.*, The clinical validity of normal compression ultrasonography in outpatients suspected of having deep venous thrombosis. *Ann. Intern. Med.*, 1998. **128**(1): 1–7.

72 Kearon, C., *et al.*, Noninvasive diagnosis of deep venous thrombosis. McMaster Diagnostic Imaging Practice Guidelines Initiative. *Ann. Intern. Med.*, 1998. **128**(8): 663–77.

73 Cogo, A., *et al.*, Compression ultrasonography for diagnostic management of patients with clinically suspected deep vein thrombosis: prospective cohort study. *BMJ*, 1998. **316**(7124): 17–20.

74 Raghavendra, B. N., *et al.*, Deep venous thrombosis: detection by high-resolution real-time ultrasonography. *Radiology*, 1984. **152**(3): 789–93.

75 Greer, I. A. and A. J. Thomson, Management of venous thromboembolism in pregnancy. *Best Pract. Res. Clin. Obstet. Gynaecol.*, 2001. **15**(4): 583–603.

76 Michiels, J. J., Rational diagnosis of pulmonary embolism (RADIA PE) in symptomatic outpatients with suspected PE: an improved strategy to exclude or diagnose venous thromboembolism by the sequential use of a clinical model, rapid ELISA D-dimer test, perfusion lung scan, ultrasonography, spiral CT, and pulmonary angiography. *Semin. Thromb. Hemost.*, 1998. **24**(4): 413–18.

77 Davidson, B. L., Elliott, C. G., and A. W. Lensing, Low accuracy of color Doppler ultrasound in the detection of proximal leg vein thrombosis in asymptomatic high-risk patients. The RD Heparin Arthroplasty Group. *Ann. Intern. Med.*, 1992. **117**(9): 735–8.

78 Barnes, R. W., *et al.*, Perioperative asymptomatic venous thrombosis: role of duplex scanning versus venography. *J. Vasc. Surg.*, 1989. **9**(2): 251–60.

79 Hull, R., *et al.*, Clinical validity of a negative venogram in patients with clinically suspected venous thrombosis. *Circulation*, 1981. **64**(3): 622–5.

80 Heijboer, H., *et al.*, A comparison of real-time compression ultrasonography with impedance plethysmography for the diagnosis of deep-vein thrombosis in symptomatic outpatients. *N. Engl. J. Med.*, 1993. **329**(19): 1365–9.

81 Albrechtsson, U. and C. G. Olsson, Thrombotic side-effects of lower-limb phlebography. *Lancet*, 1976. **1**(7962): 723–4.

82 Brown, H. L. and A. K. Hiett, Deep venous thrombosis and pulmonary embolism. *Clin. Obstet. Gynecol.*, 1996. **39**(1): 87–100.

83 Bergus, G. R., Barloon, T. S., and D. Kahn, An approach to diagnostic imaging of suspected pulmonary embolism. *Am. Fam. Physician*, 1996. **53**(4): 1259–66.

84 Georgopoulos, D. C., Diagnosis of pulmonary embolism. *Monaldi Arch. Chest Dis.*, 1996. **51**(4): 306–9.

85 Hirsh, J. and J. Hoak, Management of deep vein thrombosis and pulmonary embolism. A statement for healthcare professionals. Council on Thrombosis (in consultation with the Council on Cardiovascular Radiology), American Heart Association. *Circulation*, 1996. **93**(12): 2212–45.

86 Hull, R. D., *et al.*, Diagnostic value of ventilation–perfusion lung scanning in patients with suspected pulmonary embolism. *Chest*, 1985. **88**(6): 819–28.

87 Stein, P. D., Henry, J. W., and A. Gottschalk, The addition of clinical assessment to stratification according to prior cardiopulmonary disease further optimizes the interpretation of ventilation/perfusion lung scans in pulmonary embolism. *Chest*, 1993. **104**(5): 1472–6.

88 Janssen, M. C., *et al.*, Reliability of five rapid D-dimer assays compared to ELISA in the exclusion of deep venous thrombosis. *Thromb. Haemost.*, 1997. **77**(2): 262–6.

89 Brattstrom, L., *et al.*, Hyperhomocysteinemia in stroke: prevalence, cause and relationship to type of stroke and stroke risk factors. *European Journal of Clinical Investigation*, 1992. **22**: 214–21.

90 Oudkerk, M., *et al.*, Cost-effectiveness analysis of various strategies in the diagnostic management of pulmonary embolism. *Arch. Intern. Med.*, 1993. **153**(8): 947–54.

91 Hull, R. D., *et al.*, Cost-effectiveness of pulmonary embolism diagnosis. *Arch. Intern. Med.*, 1996. **156**(1): 68–72.

92 Van Erkel, A. R., *et al.*, Spiral CT angiography for suspected pulmonary embolism: a cost-effectiveness analysis. *Radiology*, 1996. **201**(1): 29–36.

93 Van Rossum, A. B., *et al.*, Role of spiral volumetric computed tomographic scanning in the assessment of patients with clinical suspicion of pulmonary embolism and an abnormal ventilation/perfusion lung scan. *Thorax*, 1996. **51**(1): 23–8.

94 Goodman, L. R., *et al.*, Detection of pulmonary embolism in patients with unresolved clinical and scintigraphic diagnosis: helical CT versus angiography. *AJR Am. J. Roentgenol.*, 1995. **164**(6): 1369–74.

95 Stein, P. D. and J. W. Henry, Prevalence of acute pulmonary embolism in central and subsegmental pulmonary arteries and relation to probability interpretation of ventilation/perfusion lung scans. *Chest*, 1997. **111**(5): 1246–8.

96 Mayo, J. R., *et al.*, Pulmonary embolism: prospective comparison of spiral CT with ventilation–perfusion scintigraphy. *Radiology*, 1997. **205**(2): 447–52.

97 Garg, K., *et al.*, Pulmonary embolism: diagnosis with spiral CT and ventilation–perfusion scanning: correlation with pulmonary angiographic results or clinical outcome. *Radiology*, 1998. **208**(1): 201–8.

98 Cross, J., Kemp, P. M., and Walsh, A randomized trial of spiral CT and ventilation–perfusion scintigraphy for the diagnosis of pulmonary embolism. 1998. **53**: 17.

99 Perrier, A., *et al.*, Performance of helical computed tomography in unselected outpatients with suspected pulmonary embolism. *Ann. Intern. Med.*, 2001. **135**: 88–97.

100 Goldhaber, S. Z., *et al.*, Alteplase versus heparin in acute pulmonary embolism: randomised trial assessing right-ventricular function and pulmonary perfusion. *Lancet*, 1993. **341**: 507–11.

101 Konstantinides, S., *et al.*, Heparin plus alteplase copared with heparin alone in submassive pulmonary embolism. *N. Engl. J. Med.*, 2002. **347**: 1143–50.

102 Tapson, V. F., *et al.*, The diagnostic approach to acute venous thromboembolism. Clinical practice guideline. *Am. J. Respir. Crit. Care Med.*, 1999. **160**: 1043–66.

103 Goldhaber, S. Z., Pulmonary embolism. *N. Engl. J. Med.*, 1998. **339**: 93–104.

104 Wells, P. S., *et al.*, Derivation of a simple clinical model to categorize patients probability of pulmonary embolism: Increasing the models utility with the SimpliRED d-dimer. *Thromb. Haemost.*, 2000. **83**: 416–20.

8

Hemorrhagic and thrombotic lesions of the placenta

Raymond W. Redline, M.D.

Professor of Pathology and Reproductive Biology, Case School of Medicine; Co-Director, Pediatric and Perinatal Pathology, University Hospitals of Cleveland, Cleveland, Ohio, USA

Introduction

The placenta has two important functions: absorption of substrates from the maternal circulation and protection of the fetus from harmful external forces. As an absorptive organ the placenta is essentially an interhemal membrane separating maternal blood in the intervillous space from fetal blood in the umbilical-villous circulation. Given the importance of both placental blood supplies it is not surprising that many external forces exert their harmful effects via hemorrhage and thrombosis. The pathologic sequelae of these processes in the placenta will be the primary focus of this chapter. Adaptations occur during placental development to maximize blood flow and minimize the diffusion distance that substrates must traverse. These developmental adjustments can predispose to later hemorrhage or thrombosis and this will be the second major emphasis of this chapter. A schematic diagram illustrating the spectrum and anatomical site of major thrombotic and hemorrhagic lesions in the placenta is provided in Figure 8.1.

Maternal perfusion of the interhemal membrane is augmented by several mechanisms. Cardiac output increases by approximately 40% over the course of pregnancy, largely due to a 50% increase in maternal plasma volume.[1] Large uterine arteries dilate two-fold under the influence of pregnancy hormones, many of which are secreted by the placenta.[2] Endometrial spiral arterioles are remodeled by invading trophoblast to form funnel shaped conduits that are incapable of restricting blood flow because of dissolution of their smooth muscle wall.[3] Blood enters the intervillous space of the placenta via 80–120 of these spiral arterioles. This blood flows upward in the area between the villous trees until it strikes the undersurface of the chorionic plate after which it percolates downward along the interstices of the villous tree where the bulk of substrate exchange occurs. Blood preferentially enters the placenta in the central 2/3 where spiral arteriolar

Hematological Complications in Obstetrics, Pregnancy, and Gynecology, ed. R. L. Bick *et al.* Published by Cambridge University Press.

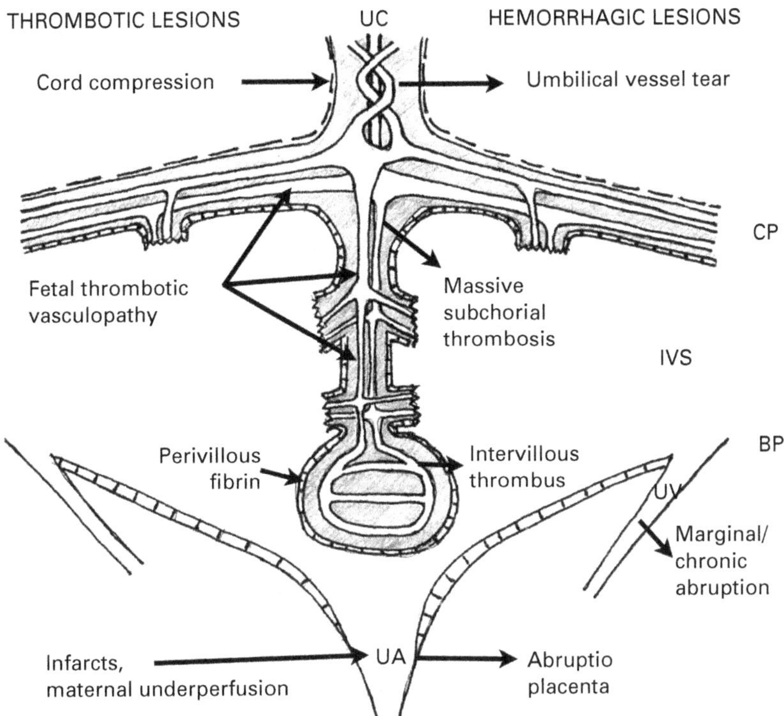

Figure 8.1 Schematic view of placental anatomic relationships with the types and anatomical site of major thrombotic and hemorrhagic lesions. Thrombotic lesions are listed on the left with arrows indicating their anatomic localization. Hemorrhagic lesions are listed on the right with arrows indicating the anatomic site of rupture. The fetus would be above the figure, the maternal uterus at the bottom. Shaded areas represent the chorionic plate and villous tree. Cross hatched areas are placental trophoblast. UC: umbilical cord; CP: chorionic plate; IVS: intervillous space; BP: basal plate; UV: uterine veins; UA: uterine artery.

remodeling is best developed.[4] Venous drainage preferentially occurs at the lateral margins. Lateral drainage is further accentuated by remodeling of marginal veins that occurs during lateral placental growth during the middle third of pregnancy.[5,6] These relationships are shown in schematic form in Figure 8.1. Failure of maternal volume expansion, deficiencies of placental hormones, obstructive lesions of any level of the uterine circulation, and obliteration of the intervillous space can all profoundly affect maternal perfusion of the interhemal membrane.

On the fetal side, the villous tree is lined by syncytiotrophoblast which expresses anticoagulant and pro-fibrinolytic proteins including thrombomodulin, annexin V, and PP5 TFPI-2 that prevent coagulation.[7,8] Growth and development of the villous tree is driven by elongation and branching of the fetal vasculature.[9] Only the distal tips of the villous tree, known as terminal villi have absorptive capacity which primarily occurs at specialized structures known as vasculosyncytial membranes where syncytiotrophoblast and fetal capillary endothelium are in unusually tight contact.[10] Terminal villi first develop in the third trimester and act to increase placental efficiency as growth relative to the fetus decreases. Structural support for the fetal circulation is provided by collagenization of larger villous trunks that arise from the chorionic plate and support the terminal villi. These larger villi and the chorionic plate contain muscularized veins and arteries that converge at the umbilical cord as two arteries and a single vein (see Figure 8.1). While not directly involved in gas exchange these larger vessels connecting the fetus to the interhemal membrane of the placenta are critically important for placental function and are susceptible to interruption by both intrinsic and extrinsic thromboocclusive lesions. The fetoplacental circulation is a low resistance circuit which normally receives about one third of the fetal cardiac output. Thrombosis, mechanical obstruction to venous return, primary myocardial dysfunction, fetal volume depletion, chronic hypoxia, and changes in both oxygen carrying capacity (anemia) and viscosity (polycythemia) can all cause profound circulatory changes affecting fetal perfusion of the interhemal membrane.

Maternal vasculature (Table 8.1)

Table 8.1 Outline of maternal vascular lesions of the placenta with clinical presentation and underlying associations with thrombophilia and other risk factors.*

Pathologic lesion	Clinical presentation	Association with thrombophilia?	Other associations
Developmental			
Decidual arteriopathy	Early onset preeclampsia	Yes	Chronic renal disease
			Connective tissue disease
Acute atherosis	Idiopathic IUGR		Type 1 diabetes mellitus
Hypertrophic	Abruptio placenta		Primigravida
,	Oligohydramnios		
Basal plate	(same)	Yes	(same)
Persistent arterial smooth muscle			
Excessive intermediate trophoblast			
Prematurely differentiated trophoblast			
Obstructive			
Uteroplacental underperfusion			
Distal villous hypoplasia			

Table 8.1 *(cont.)*

Pathologic lesion	Clinical presentation	Association with thrombophilia?	Other associations
Increased syncytial knots/intervillous fibrin			
Villous infarcts			
Intervillous space	Severe early onset IUGR	Yes	Connective tissue disease
Massive perivillous fibrinoid deposition ("Maternal floor infarction")			Fetal LCHAD deficiency
Loss of integrity			
Retroplacental hemorrhage		Yes	Hypertension, trauma, primigravida, smoking, cocaine
with placental indentation/rupture	Abruptio placenta		
with overlying villous infarction	Subacute or concealed abruption		
Marginal retroplacental and retromembranous hemorrhage		No	Oligohydramnios Multiparity
Acute peripheral separation	Marginal abruption		
Chronic peripheral separation	Chronic abruption		

*References in text.

Developmental lesions

Human pregnancy is characterized by deep interstitial implantation with arterial remodeling.[11] This implantation is mediated by placental trophoblast and involves both tissue invasion of the uterine wall and vascular invasion of the uterine arteries. The result of deep implantation is greater maternal blood flow allowing more fetal growth and a longer period of intrauterine development than in other species. A decrease in the depth of implantation occurs in *early onset preeclampsia* and some cases of *maternal thrombophilia, connective tissue disease, idiopathic intrauterine growth retardation, and abruptio placenta.*[12–17] The precise series of events leading to superficial implantation remains unclear. Early endometrial hypoxia, aberrations of the local renin-angiotensin system, abnormal maternal responses to paternal antigens, and deficiencies of trophoblast hormonal and adhesion molecule expression have all been implicated.[18–21]

Placental lesions indicative of superficial implantation include lack of normal arterial remodeling (**persistent smooth muscle in basal plate arteries**), accumulation of **excessive immature and prematurely differentiated trophoblast** near the base of the placenta, reduced placental weight for gestational age, and two forms of uterine arteriopathy.[22,23] Uterine arteries in the membranes and basal plate may undergo hypertrophy of the arterial vascular wall (**hypertrophic decidual vasculopathy**).[24] Mothers with the Thr235 allele of the angiotensinogen gene are at increased risk for hypertrophy.[25] This allele is also associated with essential hypertension in some populations. Late in pregnancy, usually in patients with clinical signs of *preeclampsia*, uterine arteries may also develop fibrinoid necrosis of the muscular wall (**acute atherosis**).[26] A similar lesion is also seen in some cases of hyperacute transplant rejection, Kawasaki's disease, hemolytic uremic syndrome, thrombotic thrombocytopenic purpura, and heparin-associated thrombocytopenia. All of these disorders are characterized by acute endothelial damage; in many cases associated with anti-endothelial antibodies. Patients with antiphospholipid antibodies commonly show acute atherosis and patients with preeclampsia have a high incidence of angiotensin II receptor antibodies.[27–29] Both antibodies bind endothelial cells. Arteries that lack normal remodelling and show the two forms of arteriopathy described above are associated with chronic underperfusion of the intervillous space and are at increased risk for thrombosis or rupture.

Obstructive lesions

Obstruction to uterine blood flow can be either chronic or acute. Severe and prolonged maternal underperfusion leads to truncated placental development. Histologically, these placentas are characterized by **distal villous hypoplasia** (numerically decreased and abnormally small nonbranching terminal villi with decreased capillaries).[30–34] Grossly, they are often extremely small for gestational age. The clinical syndrome that correlates with these placental findings is *severe IUGR with abnormal fetal pulsed flow doppler studies*. In this situation abnormal fetal blood flow, as reflected by doppler studies, indicates increased resistance due to decreased villous vascular development.

In less severe or longstanding cases of maternal underperfusion, the placenta is characterized by lesser decreases in weight for gestational age, **increased syncytial knots**, and **increased intervillous fibrin (fibrin-type fibrinoid)**. Syncytial knots are groups of degenerating trophoblastic nuclei on the surface of terminal villi.[35] Their presence is indicative of hypoxic damage and increased trophoblast turnover. Some evidence suggests that they may enhance villous absorption by narrowing the diffusion distance across nonaffected portions of the villous surface.[36,37] Increased intervillous and perivillous fibrin probably reflects both stasis of maternal blood flow due to underperfusion and abnormal coagulation due to trophoblast damage and the failure of normal anticoagulation mechanisms.[38,39]

A distinct variant of intervillous fibrin is **massive perivillous fibrin (matrix-type fibrinoid) deposition** (also known as **maternal floor infarction**). This idiopathic and rare placental lesion is associated with very high perinatal morbidity and mortality and tends to recur in subsequent pregnancies.[40–42] While superficially similar to increased intervillous fibrin, the fibrinoid material associated with this lesion contains matrix-type molecules (fibronectin, Type IV collagen, laminin), is infiltrated by trophoblast, and may cause severe secondary villous degenerative changes.[43] Matrix-type fibrinoid is produced by the trophoblast itself and may represent a phenotypic change secondary to decreased blood flow. A strong genetic component is suggested by a high recurrence rate and some investigators have described cases associated with maternal thrombophilic mutations.[44,45] One report has described an association with fetal LCHAD deficiency.[46]

Acute interruption of uterine blood flow, usually due to thrombosis, results in a **villous infarct.**[47] Since there is considerable overlap between the vascular distributions of individual spiral arterioles it is likely that villous infarcts result from occlusion of a larger uterine artery. Marginal villous infarcts with a diameter of less than 3 cm are common in term placentas.[48] All other infarcts are abnormal and often seen in the context of the developmental and chronic obstructive lesions described above. Extensively infarcted placentas may be seen with preeclampsia and maternal thrombophilia.[49,50] Their identification in multigravid women is one possible indication for considering genetic and immunologic studies of the coagulation system.

Sickle cell disease in pregnancy was historically associated with extremely high rates of fetal and maternal morbidity and mortality.[51] In more recent times aggressive antenatal management has dramatically improved the prognosis for both mother and infant.[52] While placentas from mothers with sickle cell disease are more likely to show changes attributable to mild chronic maternal underperfusion, no pathognomonic lesion of sickle cell disease has been identified. Sickling of maternal red blood cells in the intervillous space may be useful diagnostically, but is a formalin-induced artifact seen in both sickle cell trait and sickle cell disease.[53] It has no prognostic importance.

Disturbance of maternal vascular integrity

Hemorrhages arising from the maternal placental circulation can exit the gravid uterus as vaginal bleeding, accumulate between uterus and placenta, or can separate the placenta from the uterus leading to delivery. They may be subclassified into a number of pathophysiologically distinct categories. Acute rupture of a major artery is known as *acute abruption* or *abruptio placenta.*[54] The subset of these cases where only a portion of the placenta is affected and pregnancy persists is termed *partial, incomplete, or subacute abruption.* Acute rupture of a major marginal vein (acute peripheral separation) is known as *marginal abruption.*[55] Chronic or recurrent venous hemorrhage at the margin of the placenta (chronic peripheral separation) is referred to as *chronic abruption* or the *chronic abruption-oligohydramnio sequence.*[56,57]

Retroplacental hemorrhages are often linked to one of three factors: intrinsic abnormalities of the arterial wall, pathologic processes that secondarily involve blood vessels, or effects of direct mechanical shear force. The most common intrinsic abnormalities are the arteriopathies of preeclampsia and related conditions including the inherited and acquired thrombophilias, all of which are strong risk factors for *abruptio placenta.*[16,58,59] Hemorrhage in these situations may be either a direct result of vessel wall necrosis (acute atherosis) or an indirect result of thrombosis and downstream ischemic necrosis. Secondary damage to blood vessels leading to *abruptio placenta* may occur in patients who use vasoactive drugs such as cocaine or nicotine during pregnancy.[60–62] Acute inflammation at the periphery of the placenta can weaken vessels leading to *marginal abruption* in mothers with chorioamnionitis, particularly in the late second or early third trimester. Increased uterine venous pressure due to obstruction of the inferior vena cava may also lead to *marginal abruption.*[54] Distortion of the normal marginal venous anatomy due to excessively deep implantation or impaired lateral placental growth has been implicated in *chronic abruption.*[63] Direct mechanical shear forces resulting from motor vehicle accidents, physical abuse, or traumatic falls account for a minority of cases of *abruptio placenta.* Rupture of membranes can also introduce mechanical forces by altering the relationship of the placenta to the uterus resulting in rupture of marginal veins and the development of *marginal or chronic abruption.*[64] Much rarer causes of placental abruption include deficiencies of coagulation factors X, XIII, and fibrinogen.[65,66]

Classical studies comparing the clinical and pathologic diagnoses of placental abruption showed poor correlation with agreement in only one third of cases.[67] Increased awareness of the different subcategories of abruption and recognition of additional placental criteria have improved this agreement somewhat. Nevertheless, neither the clinical nor the pathologic criteria are foolproof and the only true gold standard for abruption is direct visualization of retroplacental blood clot at the time of C-section. Pathologic criteria strongly suggestive of acute abruption include central or paracentral **retroplacental hemorrhage with indentation or rupture of the overlying placenta**. Occult abruption is occasionally manifest as an irregularly shaped **basal intervillous thrombus. Interstitial hemorrhage of the decidua basalis** and **recent stromal hemorrhage** of overlying villi are supportive, but less specific findings.[68] Subacute abruption is diagnosed by **recent infarction** of the overlying villous parenchyma. Pathologic findings consistent with acute peripheral separation (marginal abruption) include adherent **recent marginal blood clot** with compression of the marginal anatomy and **retromembranous hemorrhage**. Chronic peripheral separation (chronic abruption) is characterized by **circumvallate membrane insertion, old marginal blood clot, chorioamnionic hemosiderosis**, and **green discoloration** of the chorionic plate due to biliverdin staining.[69] In all cases the greater the number of supporting pathologic features the greater the probability of the clinical diagnosis.

Fetal vasculature (Table 8.2)

Table 8.2 Outline of fetal vascular lesions of the placenta with clinical presentation and underlying associations with thrombophilia and other risk factors.*

Pathologic lesion	Clinical presentations	Associated with thrombophilia?	Other associations
Developmental			
Abnormal cord insertion	Fetal distress	No	Uterine anomalies
	Ruptured vasa previa		Multiple gestation
Marginal/membranous			
Anomalous membrane vessel			Prior instrumentation
Furcate			
Amniotic web			
Vascular tumors	Fetal hydrops	No	High altitudes
Chorangioma	Fetal DIC		Multiple gestation
Umbilical hemangioma/ angiomyxoma	Local hemorrhage		Beckwith–Weidmann syndrome
Obstructive			
Fetal thrombotic vasculopathy	Fetal thromboembolism	Yes	Chronic cord compression
Avascular villi	Cerebral palsy		Maternal diabetes
Villous stromal karyorrhexis and hemorrhage	IUFD, IUGR		Fetal cardiac dysfunction
Chorionic/umbilical vessel thrombi			
Fibromuscular sclerosis			
Intimal fibrin cushions			

Table 8.2 (*cont.*)

Pathologic lesion	Clinical presentations	Associated with thrombophilia?	Other associations
Disturbance of Integrity			
Distal villous circulation			
Acute villous stromal hemorrhage	Abruptio placenta	Yes	(see above)
Chronic villous stromal hemosiderosis	Congenital viral infection	No	
Intervillous thrombi	Fetomaternal hemorrhage	No	
Proximal villous circulation			
Massive subchorial thrombus	IUFD, abortion	Yes	
Umbilical/chorionic large vessels			
Traumatic hemorrhage	Ruptured vasa previa	No	(see above)
Iatrogenic hemorrhage	Traumatic amniocentesis/PUBS	No	

*References in text.

Developmental lesions

Thrombosis and hemorrhage involving the fetal vasculature may occur in the context of aberrant vascular development or within vascular tumors. Clinically significant developmental lesions usually involve the insertion site of the umbilical cord into the placenta. The umbilical cord initially forms at the center of the placental disc following implantation. Later reorientation of the disc to areas with a better maternal blood supply can lead to secondary atrophy at the initial implantation site. This placental migration, known as "trophotropism", can result in **marginal or membranous insertion of the umbilical cord** where the cord vessels are not well supported. In other cases the cord inserts in the placental disc, but one or more adjacent chorionic vessels traverse membranous areas of the placenta (**aberrant membranous vessel**). The umbilical cord can also terminate proximal to the insertion site leading to exposed umbilical vessels lacking a protective sheath of Wharton's jelly (**furcate cord**). Finally, folds of amnion can encircle the umbilical cord near its insertion site (**amnionic webs**) leading to acute angulation with changes in fetal position. All of these anatomic abnormalities can lead to obstruction or loss of integrity of cord vessels (*ruptured vasa previa*) as detailed below.

Vascular tumors of the villous circulation are known as **chorangiomas.**[70] Those of the umbilical or viteline circulation are known as **umbilical hemangiomas or**

angiomyxomas.[71] Chorangiomas contain a complex microcirculation that under some circumstances can be the nidus for a fetal microangiopathic hemolytic anemia or platelet sequestration leading to thrombocytopenia.[72,73] Cord hemangiomas are composed of large thin-walled vessels that can rupture leading to fetal blood loss into an **umbilical cord hematoma.**

Obstructive lesions

Fetal thromboocclusive processes in the placenta occur in two contexts. They can either be the local consequence of systemic fetal thrombophilia or isolated lesions resulting from local alterations in blood flow. Irrespective of etiology, they compromise placental function by decreasing the volume of the fetal vascular bed and by creating circulatory mismatch between the maternal and fetal circulations. In rare cases thromboemboli may travel from the placenta to systemic fetal circulation via the foramen ovale or ductus arteriosus to cause CNS or other organ damage. Inherited fetal thrombophilias have been postulated to be causes of fetal thromboocclusive disease of the placenta, but the degree of risk is controversial.[74–76] We found no increase in fetal thromboocclusive lesions in patients with documented fetal thrombophilia compared to those without,[94] but did find a 2–3 fold increase in the prevalence of Factor V Leiden, PT2015, and MTHFR mutations in patients with severe fetal thromboocclusive disease (Table 8.3, unpublished data). One interpretation is that such mutations decrease the threshold for thrombosis, but require additional stimuli. Other potential stimuli include maternal antiphospholipid and antiplatelet antibodies, maternal diabetes, vascular wall damage from prolonged meconium exposure or severe fetal chorioamnionitis, and obstruction to placental venous return blood flow due to compression of chorionic or umbilical vessels, increased fetal central venous pressure, or hyperviscosity secondary to polycythemia.[77–80]

Table 8.3 Fetal thrombophilia in Caucasian patients with extensive avascular villi in placenta.

		Thrombophilic Mutations* N (% positive)					
Avascular villi/Slide	Cases tested	Factor V Leiden	Prothrombin 20210A	MTHFR (homozygous)	MTHFR (heterozygous)	Any	More than one
>15	9	2 (22)	2 (22)	2 (22)	1 (11)	4 (44)	2 (11)
<15	6	0	0	0	2 (33)	2 (33)	0

*Evaluated by polymerase chain reaction using DNA extracted from deparaffinized umbilical cord sections. Unpublished data, E. Brandewie and R. Redline, University Hospitals of Cleveland, Ohio, USA.

The most sensitive indicator of fetal thromboocclusive disease is the finding of **hyalinized avascular villi** in segmental groupings reflecting the vascular territory of an upstream vessel.[77] A closely related pattern is **villous stromal karyorrhexis and hemorrhage (so-called "hemorrhagic endovasculitis")**.[81] The latter changes mimic changes seen in the placentas of stillborns and are probably due to vascular stasis.[82] They could indicate venous rather than arterial obstruction or might represent an early stage of either arterial or venous occlusion. Individual cases can show a mixture of both patterns. A diagnosis of **fetal thrombotic vasculopathy** is made when an average of 15 or more villi per parenchymal section show either pattern and this diagnosis has been shown to be an independent predictor of *cerebral palsy* in term infants.[95] Fetal thrombotic vasculopathy is usually characterized by large clusters of 20 or more avascular villi, but on occasion smaller clusters of 2–5 villi predominate suggesting smaller vessel disease. One third of cases with fetal thrombotic vasculopathy have demonstrable chorionic plate or stem villous thrombi in random histologic sections. Careful gross pathologic inspection can increase sensitivity by identifying chorionic plate thrombi prior to histologic examination. Other changes suggestive of fetal thromboocclusive disease include **fibromuscular sclerosis of stem vessels** and **intimal fibrin cushions**. Fibromuscular sclerosis is the concentric narrowing and obliteration of vascular lumina within stem villi lying between the actual site of obstruction and the avascular terminal villi.[83] Intimal fibrin cushions are collections of laminated fibrin within the walls of large fetal veins.[84] They may result from either increased venous pressure leading to intramural insudation of fibrin or incorporation of nonocclusive mural thrombi into the vascular wall. Calcification of intimal fibrin cushion reflects chronicity.

Disturbances of fetal vascular integrity

Hemorrhagic lesions occur at all levels of the fetal circulation. Etiologically they can be separated into degenerative lesions secondary to ischemia or viral infection and traumatic lesions related to turbulence in the intervillous space, tearing of fetal vessels at the time of labor and delivery, or iatrogenic complications of invasive procedures in utero.

Ischemic fetal capillary hemorrhages can occur following interruption of either maternal or fetal blood flow, as discussed above. **Acute villous stromal hemorrhage** is a secondary effect of abruptio placenta, especially in premature gestations. **Villous stromal karyorrhexis and hemorrhage ("hemorrhagic endovasculitis")** develops distal to thromboocclusive lesions of large fetal vessels and is most commonly seen in term pregnancies.

Some *congenital viral infections* in the so-called TORCH group can infect and lyse villous capillary endothelial cells leading to **villous stromal hemosiderosis**. Presently the most common viruses causing this pattern belong to the Herpesvirus group and include cytomegalovirus, herpes simplex virus, and varicella-zoster virus.[85] Historically, the most notorious vasculotropic virus affecting the placenta was rubella virus.[86]

Intervillous thrombi are spherical expansile hemorrhages in the intervillous space that are surrounded by compressed villous tissue. These lesions have been shown to contain fetal red blood cells.[87] Since the intervillous space is a maternal circulatory compartment, these lesions are by definition sites of fetomaternal hemorrhage. They most likely represent traumatic disruption of the terminal villous tree due to turbulent intervillous blood flow. They are more frequent in preterm placentas with increased syncytial knots and in hydropic placentas at term. Intervillous thrombi are very common and the degree of fetomaternal hemorrhage is usually not physiologically significant. Significance is increased when intervillous thrombi are large and/or multiple. Definitive diagnosis of significant or *massive fetomaternal hemorrhage* depends on other accompanying features such as low fetal hematocrit, positive maternal Kleihauer Betke testing, and/or the concomitant presence of secondary changes such as increased circulating nucleated red blood cells and fetal hydrops.

Massive subchorial thrombosis (subchorionic hematoma) is an idiopathic lesion defined by a large collection of clotted blood which distorts and elevates the chorionic plate.[88] This lesion was at one time believed to be a consequence of fetal death in that there were no surviving fetuses. Occasional survivors have since been reported. Because of the strong association with fetal demise and occasional cases where a direct tear in a fetal vessel has been identified, I believe that these are fetal hemorrhages arising from tears in major stem villous vessels. Other authors consider them to be accumulations of maternal blood. Several cases have been described in association with maternal thrombophilia.[89] It is possible that similar lesions may be pathogenically distinct, but it seems more likely that although the majority of blood in these lesions is maternal in origin they originate as fetal hemorrhages.

Traumatic tears in umbilical vessels near the insertion site or in the placental membranes have been discussed above. Most of these lesions occur either at the time of membrane rupture or in the process of fetal descent during parturition. Membranous vessels are often artifactually torn during placental removal after delivery of the fetus. Clinically significant tears are usually accompanied by a significant amount of adjacent hemorrhage, often displace neighboring tissues, and are generally associated with serious fetal distress.

Finally, **iatrogenic fetal hemorrhage** can occur as a consequence of diagnostic or therapeutic procedures performed in the antenatal period. Amniocentesis and percutaneous umbilical blood sampling are the most common procedures associated with hemorrhage. As with other traumatic injuries local spread and organization of the blood clot are key to the diagnosis. Only rarely can the actual site of injury be identified on the placenta after delivery.

Thrombophilia and placental pathology

A voluminous literature has arisen over the last 10 years debating the association of maternal thrombophilic states with severe preeclampsia, IUGR, abruptio placenta, and recurrent abortion. A considerable number of papers have also addressed the relationship of fetal thrombophilia to cerebral palsy, fetal stroke, and other fetal thromboembolic complications. This literature is reviewed elsewhere in this volume. Whether thrombophilia directly causes thrombotic and hemorrhagic lesions of the placenta or the lesions develop as a consequence of the clinical syndromes associated with thrombophilia is not clear. Reported associations of thrombophilia with specific placental lesions are summarized in Tables 8.1 and 8.2. A couple of studies and our own unpublished data and suggest that maternal thrombophilia has little impact on the prevalence of placental lesions in already complicated pregnancies (Table 8.4).[90,91] However, preliminary evidence suggests that anticoagulation in patients with thrombophilia not only decreases clinical disease but also the severity of placental lesions.[92] Although patients with severe fetal thromboocclusive lesions of the placenta probably have an increased prevalence of fetal thrombophilia (Table 8.3), the majority of such placentas are not associated with thrombophilia. An underlying caveat in any discussion of this topic is that it is highly likely that many more causes of underlying and acquired thrombophilia will be discovered in coming years.[93] For the present, the most important role of placental pathology is to document the pattern and extent of

Table 8.4 Maternal vascular obstructive lesions in pregnancies complicated by severe preeclampsia, abruptio placenta, or IUGR with and without maternal thrombophilia.

Maternal thrombophilia*	Cases tested	Mean placental weight (Z-score)¶	Increased syncytial knots	Villous infarcts	Intervillous fibrin
Positive	22	-0.66 ± 1.12	4 (18)	9 (41)	6 (27)
Negative	42	-0.64 ± 1.14	13 (31)	9 (21)	10 (24)

*Maternal thrombophilia = one or more of the following: Factor V Leiden, prothrombin 20210A, MTHFR (homozygous), evaluated by polymerase chain reaction using DNA extracted from maternal peripheral blood.
¶Z-score = standard deviations from the mean for gestational age.
Unpublished data, I. Ariel and R. Redline, Hadassah University Hospital, Jerusalem, Israel.

thrombosis and hemorrhage. When lesions recur in consecutive pregnancies or present in unusual circumstances (e.g., acute atherosis in a multiparous patient), a workup for underlying thrombophilia should be considered.

REFERENCES

1 Burrow, G., Ferris, T. *Medical Complications During Pregnancy.* Philadelphia, PA: W. B. Saunders Co., 1995.

2 Konje, J. C., Kaufmann, P., Bell, S. C., *et al.* A longitudinal study of quantitative uterine blood flow with the use of color power angiography in appropriate gestational age pregnancies. *Am. J. Obstet. Gynecol.*, 2001; **185**: 608–13.

3 Ramsey, E. M., Donner, M. W. *Placental Vasculature and Circulation.* Philadelphia, PA: W. B. Saunders Co., 1980.

4 Matijevic, R., Meekins, J. W., Walkinshaw, S. A., *et al.* Spiral artery blood flow in the central and peripheral areas of the placental bed in the second trimester. *Obstet. Gynecol.*, 1995; **86**: 289–92.

5 Craven, C. M., Zhao, L., Ward, K. Lateral placental growth occurs by trophoblast cell invasion of decidual veins. *Placenta*, 2000; **21**: 160–9.

6 Nanaev, A. K., Kosanke, G., Kemp, B., *et al.* The human placenta is encircled by a ring of smooth muscle cells. *Placenta*, 2000; **21**: 122–5.

7 Lanir, N., Aharon, A., Brenner, B. Procoagulant and anticoagulant mechanisms in human placenta. *Semin. Thromb. Hemost.*, 2003; **29**: 175–84.

8 Udagawa, K., Yasumitsu, H., Esaki, M., *et al.* Subcellular localization of PP5/TFPI-2 in human placenta: a possible role of PP5/TFPI-2 as an anti-coagulant on the surface of syncytiotrophoblasts. *Placenta*, 2002; **23**: 145–53.

9 Castellucci, M., Scheper, M., Scheffen, I., *et al.* The development of the human placental villous tree. *Anat. Embryol.*, 1990; **181**: 117–28.

10 Karimu, A. L., Burton, G. J. Human term placental capillary endothelial cell specialization: a morphometric study. *Placenta*, 1995; **16**: 93–9.

11 Pijnenborg, R., Bland, J. M., Robertson, W. B., *et al.* The pattern of interstitial trophoblastic invasion of the myometrium in early human pregnancy. *Placenta*, 1981; **2**: 303–16.

12 Brosens, I. A., Robertson, W. B., Dixon, H. G. The role of the spiral arteries in the pathogenesis of preeclampsia. *Obstet. Gynecol. Annu.*, 1972; **1**: 177–91.

13 De Wolf, F., Brosens, I., Ranger, M. Fetal growth retardation and the maternal arterial supply of the human placenta in the absence of sustained hypertension. *Br. J. Obstet. Gynaecol.*, 1980; **87**: 678–84.

14 De Wolf, F., Carreras, L. O., Moerman, P., *et al.* Decidual vasculopathy and extensive placental infarction in a patient with repeated thromboembolic accidents, recurrent fetal loss, and a lupus anticoagulant. *Br. J. Obstet. Gynaecol.*, 1982; **142**: 829–34.

15 Khong, T. Y., Hague, W. M. The placenta in maternal hyperhomocysteinaemia. *Br. J. Obstet. Gynaecol.*, 1999; **106**: 273–8.

16 Dommisse, J., Tiltman, A. J. Placental bed biopsies in placental abruption. *Br. J. Obstet. Gynaecol.*, 1992; **99**: 651–4.

17 Sebire, N. J., Fox, H., Backos, M., *et al.* Defective endovascular trophoblast invasion in primary antiphospholipid antibody syndrome-associated early pregnancy failure. *Hum. Reprod.*, 2002; **17**: 1067–71.

18 Caniggia, I., Winter, J., Lye, S. J., *et al.* Oxygen and placental development during the first trimester: implications for the pathophysiology of pre-eclampsia. *Placenta*, 2000; **21** (Suppl A): S25–30.

19 Xia, Y., Wen, H. Y., Kellems, R. E. Angiotensin II inhibits human trophoblast invasion through AT1 receptor activation. *J. Biol. Chem.*, 2002; **277**: 24601–8.

20 Trupin, L. S., Simon, L. P., Eskenazi, B. Change in paternity: a risk factor for preeclampsia in multiparas. *Epidemiology*, 1996; **7**: 240–4.

21 Zhou, Y., Damsky, C. H., Chiu, K., *et al.* Preeclampsia is associated with abnormal expression of adhesion molecules by invasive cytotrophoblasts. *J. Clin. Invest.* 1993; **91**: 950–60.

22 Khong, T. Y., De Wolf, F., Robertson, W. B., *et al.* Inadequate maternal vascular response to placentation in pregnancies complicated by pre-eclampsia and by small-for-gestational age infants. *Br. J. Obstet. Gynaecol.*, 1986; **93**: 1049–59.

23 Redline, R. W., Patterson, P. Preeclampsia is associated with an excess of proliferative immature intermediate trophoblast. *Hum. Pathol.*, 1995; **26**: 594–600.

24 Kaplan, C., Lowell, D. M., Salafia, C. College of American Pathologists Conference XIX on The Examination of the Placenta: Report of the Working Group on the Definition of Structural Changes Associated with Abnormal Function in the Matenal/Fetal/Placental Unit in the Second and Third Trimesters. 1991; 115.

25 Morgan, T., Craven, C., Lalouel, J. M., *et al.* Angiotensinogen Thr235 variant is associated with abnormal physiologic change of the uterine spiral arteries in first-trimester decidua. *Am. J. Obstet. Gynecol.*, 1999; **180**: 95–102.

26 Kitzmiller, J. L., Watt, N., Driscoll, S. G. Decidual arteriopathy in hypertension and diabetes in pregnancy: immunofluorescent studies. *Am. J. Obstet. Gynecol.*, 1981; **141**: 773–9.

27 Abramowsky, C. R., Vegas, M. E., Swinehart, G., *et al.* Decidual vasculopathy of the placenta in lupus erythematosus. *N. Engl. J. Med.*, 1980; **303**: 668–72.

28 Wallukat, G., Homuth, V., Fischer, T., *et al.* Patients with preeclampsia develop agonistic autoantibodies against the angiotensin AT1 receptor. *J. Clin. Invest.*, 1999; **103**: 945–52.

29 Matsumoto, T., Sagawa, N., Ihara, Y., *et al.* Relationship between lupus anticoagulant (LAC) and pregnancy-induced hypertension. *Reprod. Fertil. Dev.*, 1995; **7**: 1569–71.

30 Jackson, M. R., Walsh, A. J., Morrow, R. J., *et al.* Reduced placental villous tree elaboration in small-for-gestational-age pregnancies: relationship with umbilical artery Doppler waveforms. *Am. J. Obstet. Gynecol.*, 1995; **172**: 518–25.

31 Karsdorp, V. H., Dirks, B. K., van der Linden, J. C., *et al.* Placenta morphology and absent or reversed end diastolic flow velocities in the umbilical artery: a clinical and morphometrical study. *Placenta*, 1996; **17**: 393–9.

32 Macara, L., Kingdom, J. C., Kohnen, G., *et al.* Elaboration of stem villous vessels in growth restricted pregnancies with abnormal umbilical artery Doppler waveforms. *Br. J. Obstet. Gynaecol.*, 1995; **102**: 807–12.

33 Krebs, C., Macara, L. M., Leiser, R., *et al.* Intrauterine growth restriction with absent end-diastolic flow velocity in the umbilical artery is associated with maldevelopment of the placental terminal villous tree. *Am. J. Obstet. Gynecol.*, 1996; **175**: 1534–42.
34 Madazli, R., Somunkiran, A., Calay, Z., *et al.* Histomorphology of the placenta and the placental bed of growth restricted foetuses and correlation with the Doppler velocimetries of the uterine and umbilical arteries. *Placenta*, 2003; **24**: 510–6.
35 Mayhew, T. M., Barker, B. L. Villous trophoblast: Morphometric perspectives on growth, differentiation, turnover and deposition of fibrin-type fibrinoid during gestation. *Placenta*, 2001; **22**: 628–38.
36 Tominaga, T., Page, E. W. Accommodation of the human placenta to hypoxia. *Am. J. Obstet. Gynecol.*, 1966; **94**: 679–91.
37 MacLennan, A. H., Page, E. W. Accommodation of the human placenta to hypoxia. *Am. J. Obstet. Gynecol.*, 1966; **94**: 679–91.
38 Nelson, D. M., Crouch, E. C., Curran, E. M., *et al.* Trophoblast interaction with fibrin matrix. Epithelialization of perivillous fibrin deposits as a mechanism for villous repair in the human placenta. *Am. J. Pathol.*, 1990; **136**: 855–65.
39 Mayhew, T. M., Barker, B. L. Villous trophoblast: morphometric perspectives on growth, differentiation, turnover and deposition of fibrin-type fibrinoid during gestation. *Placenta*, 2001; **22**: 628–38.
40 Andres, R. L., Kuyper, W., Resnik, R., *et al.* The association of maternal floor infarction of the placenta with adverse perinatal outcome. *Am. J. Obstet. Gynecol.*, 1990; **163**: 935–38.
41 Mandsager, N. T., Bendon, R. W., Mostello, D., *et al.* Maternal floor infarction of placenta: prenatal diagnosis and clinical significance. *Obstet. Gynecol.*, 1994; **83**: 750–4.
42 Katzman, P. J., Genest, D. R. Maternal floor infarction and massive perivillous fibrin deposition: histological definitions, association with intrauterine fetal growth restriction, and risk of recurrence. *Pediatr. Dev. Pathol.*, 2002; **5**: 159–64.
43 Frank, H. G., Malekzadeh, F., Kertschanska, S., *et al.* Immunohistochemistry of two different types of placental fibrinoid. *Acta Anat.*, 1994; **150**: 55.
44 Katz, V. L., DiTomasso, J., Farmer, R., *et al.* Activated protein C resistance associated with maternal floor infarction treated with low-molecular-weight heparin. *Am. J. Perinatol.*, 2002; **19**: 273–7.
45 Sebire, N. J., Backos, M., Goldin, R. D., *et al.* Placental massive perivillous fibrin deposition associated with antiphospholipid antibody syndrome. *Br. J. Obstet. Gynaecol.*, 2002; **109**: 570–3.
46 Matern, D., Schehata, B. M., Shekhawa, P., *et al.* Placental floor infarction complicating the pregnancy of a fetus with long-chain 3-hydroxyacyl-CoA dehydrogenase (LCHAD) deficiency. *Mol. Genet. Metab.*, 2001; **72**: 265–8.
47 Wallenburg, H. C. S., Stolte, L. A. M., Jannsens, J. The pathogenesis of placental infarction. I. A morphologic study in the human placenta. *Am. J. Obstet. Gynecol.*, 1973; **116**: 835–46.
48 Naeye, R. L. Functionally important disorders of the placenta, umbilical cord, and fetal membranes. *Hum. Pathol.*, 1987; **18**: 680–91.
49 Dizon-Townson, D. S., Meline, L., Nelson, L. M., *et al.* Fetal carriers of the factor V Leiden mutation are prone to miscarriage and placental infarction. *Am. J. Obstet. Gynecol.*, 1997; **177**: 402–5.

50 Baergen, R., Chacko, S., Edersheim, T., *et al.* The placenta in thrombophilias (TH): A clinicopathologic study. *Mod. Pathol.*, 2001; **14**: 213A.

51 Fort, A., Morrison, J., Berreras, L., *et al.* Counseling the patient with sickle cell disease: Pregnancy outcome does not justify the maternal risk! *Am. J. Obstet. Gynecol.*, 1971; **111**: 324–7.

52 Morrison, J., Schneider, J., Whybrew, W., *et al.* Prophylactic transfusions in pregnant patients with sickle hemoglobinopathies: benefit versus risk. *Obstet. Gynecol.*, 1980; **56**: 274–80.

53 Fujikura, T., Froehlich, L. Diagnosis of sickling by placental examination. *Am. J. Obstet. Gynecol.*, 1968; **100**: 1122–4.

54 Pritchard, J. A., Mason, R., Corley, M., *et al.* Genesis of severe placental abruption. *Am. J. Obstet. Gynecol.*, 1970; **108**: 22–7.

55 Harris, B. A. Peripheral placental separation: A review. *Obstet. Gynecol. Surv.*, 1988; **43**: 577–81.

56 Naftolin, F., Khudr, G., Benirschke, K., *et al.* The syndrome of chronic abruptio placentae, hydrorrhea, and circumvallate placenta. *Am. J. Obstet. Gynecol.*, 1973; **116**: 347–50.

57 Elliott, J. P., Gilpin, B., Strong, T. H., Jr., *et al.* Chronic abruption-oligohydramnios sequence. *J. Reprod. Med.*, 1998; **43**: 418–22.

58 Odegard, R. A., Vatten, L. J., Nilsen, S. T., *et al.* Risk factors and clinical manifestations of pre-eclampsia. *Br. J. Obstet. Gynaecol.*, 2000; **107**: 1410–16.

59 Wiener-Megnagi, Z., Ben-Shlomo, I., Goldberg, Y., *et al.* Resistance to activated protein C and the Leiden mutation: high prevalence in patients with abruptio placentae. *Am. J. Obstet. Gynecol.*, 1998; **179**: 1565–7.

60 Acker, D., Sachs, B. P., Tracey, K. J., *et al.* Abruptio placentae associated with cocaine use. *Am. J. Obstet. Gynecol.*, 1983; **146**: 218–19.

61 Naeye, R. L., Harkness, W. L., Utls, J. Abruptio placentae and perinatal death. A prospective study. *Am. J. Obstet. Gynecol.*, 1977; **128**: 740–8.

62 Ananth, C. V., Smulian, J. C., Vintzileos, A. M. Incidence of placental abruption in relation to cigarette smoking and hypertensive disorders during pregnancy: a meta-analysis of observational studies. *Obstet. Gynecol.*, 1999; **93**: 622–8.

63 Torpin, R. Evolution of a placenta circumvallata. *Obstet. Gynecol.*, 1966; **27**: 98–101.

64 Major, C. A., de Veciana, M., Lewis, D. F., *et al.* Preterm premature rupture of membranes and abruptio placentae: is there an association between these pregnancy complications? *Am. J. Obstet. Gynecol.*, 1995; **172**: 672–6.

65 Kumar, M., Mehta, P. Congenital coagulopathies and pregnancy: report of four pregnancies in a factor X-deficient woman. *Am. J. Hematol.*, 1994; **46**: 241–4.

66 Inbal, A., Muszbek, L. Coagulation factor deficiencies and pregnancy loss. *Semin. Thromb. Hemost.*, 2003; **29**: 171–4.

67 Gruenwald, P., Levin, H., Yousem, H. Abruption and premature separation of the placenta. The clinical and pathologic entity. *Am. J. Obstet. Gynecol.*, 1968; **102**: 604–10.

68 Mooney, E. E., al Shunnar, A., O'Regan, M., *et al.* Chorionic villous haemorrhage is associated with retroplacental haemorrhage. *Br. J. Obstet. Gynaecol.*, 1994; **101**: 965–9.

69 Redline, R. W., Wilson-Costello, D. Chronic peripheral separation of placenta: The significance of diffuse chorioamnionic hemosiderosis. *Am. J. Clin. Pathol.*, 1999; **111**: 804–10.

70 Ogino, S., Redline, R. W. Villous capillary lesions of the placenta: Distinctions between chorangioma, chorangiomatosis, and chorangiosis. *Hum. Pathol.*, 2000; **31**: 945–54.
71 Yavner, D. L., Redline, R. W. Angiomyxoma of the umbilical cord with massive cystic degeneration of Wharton's jelly. *Arch. Pathol. Lab. Med.*, 1989; **113**: 935–7.
72 Jones, E. E. M., Rivers, R. P. A., Taghizadeh, A. Disseminated intravascular coagulation and fetal hydrops in a newborn infant in association with a chorangioma of placenta. *Pediatrics*, 1972; **50**: 901–5.
73 Tonkin, I. L., Setzer, E. S., Ermocilla, R. Placental chorangioma: a rare cause of congestive heart failure and hydrops fetalis in the newborn. *Am. J. Roentgenol.*, 1980; **134**: 181–3.
74 Kraus, F. T., Acheen, V. I. Fetal thrombotic vasculopathy in the placenta: cerebral thrombi and infarcts, coagulopathies, and cerebral palsy. *Hum. Pathol.*, 1999; **30**: 759–69.
75 Vern, T. Z., Alles, A. J., KowalVern, A., *et al.* Frequency of factor V-Leiden and prothrombin G20210A in placentas and their relationship with placental lesions. *Hum. Pathol.*, 2000; **31**: 1036–43.
76 Mooney, E., Vaughan, J., Ryan, F., *et al.* Placental thrombotic vasculopathy is not associated with thrombophilic mutations. *Lab. Invest.*, 2003; **83**: 303A.
77 Redline, R. W., Pappin, A. Fetal thrombotic vasculopathy: The clinical significance of extensive avascular villi. *Hum. Pathol.*, 1995; **26**: 80–5.
78 Fritz, M. A., Christopher, C. R. Umbilical vein thrombosis and maternal diabetes mellitus. *J. Reprod. Med.*, 1981; **26**: 320–4.
79 Redline, R. W., Wilson-Costello, D., Borawski, E., *et al.* Placental lesions associated with neurologic impairment and cerebral palsy in very low birth weight infants. *Arch. Pathol. Lab. Med.*, 1998; **122**: 1091–8.
80 DeSa, D. J. Rupture of fetal vessels on placental surface. *Arch. Dis. Child.*, 1971; **46**: 495–501.
81 Sander, C. H. Hemorrhagic endovasculitis and hemorrhagic villitis of the placenta. *Arch. Pathol. Lab. Med.*, 1980; **104**: 371–3.
82 Genest, D. R. Estimating the time of death in stillborn fetuses. 2. Histologic evaluation of the placenta – a study of 71 stillborns. *Obstet. Gynecol.*, 1992; **80**: 585–92.
83 Fox, H. *Pathology of the Placenta. Major Problems in Pathology.* Vol. 7. London, UK: Saunders, 1997.
84 DeSa, D. J. Intimal cushions in foetal placental veins. *J. Pathol.*, 1973; **110**: 347–52.
85 Mostoufi-zadeh, M., Driscoll, S. G., Biano, S. A., *et al.* Placental evidence of cytomegalovirus infection of the fetus and neonate. *Arch. Pathol. Lab. Med.*, 1984; **108**: 403–6.
86 Driscoll, S. G. Histopathology of gestational rubella. *Am. J. Dis. Child.*, 1969; **118**: 49–53.
87 Kaplan, C., Blanc, W. A., Elias, J. Identification of erythrocytes in intervillous thrombi: a study using immunoperoxidase identification of hemoglobins. *Hum. Pathol.*, 1982; **13**: 554–7.
88 Shanklin, D. R., Scott, J. S. Massive subchorial thrombohaematoma (Breus' mole). *Br. J. Obstet. Gynaecol.*, 1975; **82**: 476–87.
89 Heller, D. S., Rush, D., Baergen, R. N. Subchorionic hematoma associated with thrombophilia: report of three cases. *Pediatr. Dev. Pathol.*, 2003; **6**: 261–4.

90 Sikkema, J. M., Franx, A., Bruinse, H. W., *et al.* Placental pathology in early onset pre-eclampsia and intra-uterine growth restriction in women with and without thrombophilia. *Placenta*, 2002; **23**: 337–42.

91 Esposito, M., Pinar, H., Singer, D. B., *et al.* Does placental apthology reflect antiphospholipid test results independent of perinatal outcome? *Am. J. Obstet. Gynecol.*, 2001; **185**: S184.

92 Chacko, S., Edersheim, T., Etingen, O., *et al.* Thrombophilias in pregnancy: Does treatment improve outcome? *Pediatr. Dev. Pathol.*, 2001; **4**: 413–14.

93 Miletich, J. P., Prescott, S. M., White, R., *et al.* Inherited predisposition to thrombosis. *Cell*, 1993; **72**: 477–80.

94 Ariel, I., Anteby, E., Hamani, Y., *et al.* Placental pathology in fetal thrombophilia. *Hum. Pathol.*, 2004; **35**: 729–33.

95 Redline, R. W., O'Riordan, M. A. Placental lesions associated with cerebral palsy and neurologic impairment following term birth. *Arch. Pathol. Lab. Med.*, 2000; **124**: 1785–91.

9

Iron deficiency, folate, and vitamin B_{12} deficiency in pregnancy, obstetrics, and gynecology

William F. Baker Jr., M.D., F.A.C.P.[1] and Ray Lee, M.D.[2]

[1]Associate Clinical Professor of Medicine, Center for Health Sciences, David Geffen School of Medicine at University of California-Los Angeles, Los Angeles, CA, USA Thrombosis, Hemostasis, and Special Hematology Clinic, Kern Medical Center, Bakersfield; California Clinical Thrombosis Center, Bakersfield, California, USA
[2]Associate Professor of Internal Medicine, University of Texas Southwestern School of Medicine, Dallas, Texas, USA

Anemia is the single most common hematological problem faced by women. The most common anemia are iron deficiency anemia and folate deficiency megaloblastic anemia.[1] Iron deficiency alone affects nearly 20% of the world's population. Approximately 51% of pregnant women are anemic. This includes a prevalence of 56% in developing countries and 18% in developed countries.[2] Among these, 43% of women from developing countries and 12% of women from developed countries were already anemic, preconception.[3] The WHO has estimated that considering all forms of anemia, from 16,800 to 28,000 women of reproductive age die annually from anemia, with the greatest risk in younger women.[4] Of all anemias diagnosed during pregnancy, 75% are due to iron deficiency.[1]

The systemic effects of anemia of any cause may result in significant morbidity. Deficiencies of iron, folate and vitamin B_{12} result in unique clinical consequences. These are manifested throughout life. The underlying etiologies of each deficiency state may be somewhat different pre-puberty, during the child bearing years and post menopause. During pregnancy, the adverse effects of iron, folate and vitamin B_{12} deficiency extend beyond the health of the mother to the developing fetus. This chapter is divided into two sections. The first reviews the most common type of anemia, iron deficiency. The second section examines the deficiencies of folate and vitamin B_{12}. Because of the close interrelationship between folate, vitamin B_{12} and homocysteine in the methionine synthesis pathway, hyperhomocysteinemia is also discussed.

Hematological Complications in Obstetrics, Pregnancy, and Gynecology, ed. R. L. Bick *et al.* Published by Cambridge University Press.

Iron deficiency anemia

Introduction

Iron deficiency is the most prevalent single nutritional deficiency,[5] affecting as many as 200 million of the world's population.[6] Of the individuals with iron deficiency, 50% progress to iron deficiency anemia.[7] While iron deficiency might be expected in developing countries with widespread social and economic deprivation,[8,9,10,11] it also remains a significant problem in western nations as well.[12,13,14] In developed countries, the risk of iron deficiency appears to be greatest among low-income women during and after pregnancy.[15] When all ages of women are considered, iron deficiency remains the most frequently encountered health problem worldwide.[12]

It is clear that the prevalence of iron deficiency varies widely with geography, socioeconomic status and age.[16,17,18,19,20,21] A summary of prevalence is presented in Table 9.1.[12] In spite of the documented increases in the iron intake of infants and children,[22,23] the prevalence of iron deficiency anemia in low-income and pregnant women in the United States has not improved.[24] This apparent failure of

Table 9.1[2] Prevalence of iron deficiency.

NHANES III (United States of America)	
Iron deficiency	
Women ages 20–49	11%
Women ages 50–69	5%
Women ages ≥70	7%
Men 20–49	<1%
Men 50–69	2%
Men ≥70	4%
Iron deficiency anemia	
Women ages 20–49, nonpregnant	5%
Women ≥50	2%
Men 20–49	<1%
Men ≥50	≤2%
Pregnancy	
First trimester	9%
Second trimester	14%
Third trimester	37%
United Nations study of developing countries (estimates)[113]	
Iron deficiency anemia	
Adult women	18%
Adult men	10%
Pregnant women	18%–38%

United States efforts to identify and treat iron deficiency led the Centers for Disease Control and Prevention (CDC), in 1998, to publish new guidelines for the prevention and control of iron deficiency.[12]

The highest risk of iron deficiency occurs in women who are pre-menopausal and/or pregnant.[25,26] The etiologic origins and the consequences of iron deficiency are different in these younger women from those who are post-menopausal. Although menstrual loss, puerperal blood loss and nutritional insufficiency present an obvious source of iron deficiency in pre-menopausal women, iron loss frequently results from gastrointestinal blood loss in women of all ages.[27] Iron deficiency in post-menopausal women may be of gynecologic origin but may also result from any of the multiple sources of blood loss also seen in men.[28]

The basic pathophysiology, clinical and laboratory findings and approach to diagnosis of iron deficiency and iron deficiency anemia are identical in women and men of all ages.[17,29,30] Pregnancy, however, increases the need for maternal iron to supply fetal iron needs and to withstand the physiologic challenge of puerperal blood loss. Iron deficient premenstrual women are at increased risk for iron deficiency anemia during pregnancy.[31] Pregnancy also induces physiologic changes which may influence the results of laboratory studies.

Iron homeostasis

Iron homeostasis is achieved when iron absorption meets the physiologic needs for the formation of normal red blood cells and for normal cell physiology. Any increase in the utilization of iron or pathologic loss of iron-laden red blood cells results in an imbalance, which will ultimately lead to measurable deficiencies of iron and, finally iron deficiency anemia. Understanding basic iron homeostasis is essential to diagnosing and treating iron deficiency and iron deficiency anemia.

Functional iron is present in red blood cells as hemoglobin, available for oxygen storage in the tissues as myoglobin and for cellular aerobic metabolism in cytochromes. After circulating for 3–4 months, hemoglobin-containing red blood cells are removed from the circulation by the liver and spleen. Iron is extracted and stored in the spleen and bone marrow. Iron is primarily stored in tissue as ferritin or hemosiderin and transported by the protein transferrin. Iron deficiency results from an imbalance between intake, loss and tissue stores. (Table 9.2)[32] Once iron stores are depleted, with an iron intake of $\leq$70% of requirement, approximately 4 months of iron deficient erythropoiesis results in a 1.0 g/dl decrease in Hgb.[7] As defined by the WHO, anemia is present when the hemoglobin decreases to less than 12 mg/dl for premenopausal women and prepubertal patients and a hemoglobin of less than 13 g/dl for men and postmenopausal women.[33] Anemia in pregnancy is defined according to the trimester (as discussed below) but is generally described as hemoglobin below 11 g/dl.[1,34]

Table 9.2[22] Body iron distribution.

Storage (liver > marrow > spleen)
Men 1000 mg
Women 500 mg
Plasma 3 mg
Red cells 2000 mg
Other cells 1000 mg
Recirculation 20 mg
(Red cells to spleen to plasma or plasma to marrow to red cells)

The development of iron deficiency is a sequential four phase process, as shown in Figure 9.1 and summarized as follows:[32,35]

1. Decrease in storage iron
   a. Decrease in tissue iron
   b. Decreased marrow iron
   c. Decreased serum ferritin level
   d. Increased transferrin level
2. Decrease in iron for erythropoiesis
   a. Decreased mean corpuscular volume (MCV)
   b. Decreased mean corpuscular hemoglobin (MCHC)
   c. Decreased transferrin saturation
   d. Increased free erythrocyte protoporphyrin
3. Decrease in peripheral blood hemoglobin
   a. Decreased hemoglobin
   b. Decreased hematocrit
4. Decrease in peripheral tissue oxygen delivery
   a. Clinical signs
   b. Clinical symptoms

The World Health Organization dietary allowance for iron, based upon current knowledge of normal iron homeostasis, is 5 to 10 mg/day.[36,37] The amount of iron absorbed from the diet (<1% to >80%) is regulated by the gastrointestinal tract and depends upon the adequacy of iron stores.[38] Absorption is about 6% for men and 18% for nonpregnant women during childbearing years (reflecting lower iron stores resulting from menstruation and pregnancy). Dietary bioavailability is determined by the iron content and the presence of inhibitors of absorption such as phytates in bran, tannins in tea and polyphenols in certain vegetables versus enhancers such as heme iron in red meat, fish and poultry and vitamin C.[39] Average daily absorption of iron from the western diet is 4 to 5 mg/day. Iron stores vary from 1.0 to 1.4 grams of body iron in men to 0.4 grams in women.[40]

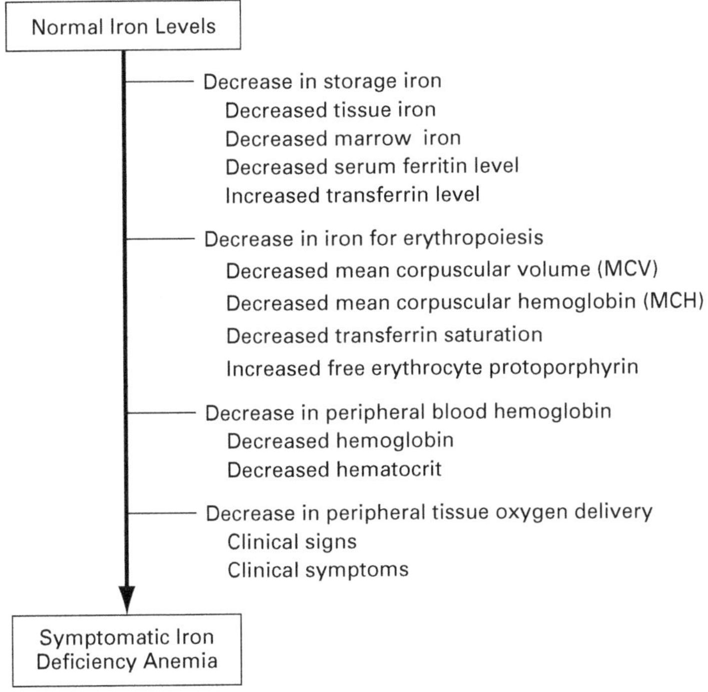

Figure 9.1 Phases of iron deficiency anemia.

Obligatory iron loss from skin cell desquamation, mucosal cell turnover and physiologic gastrointestinal loss amounts to 1 mg/day.[41] Iron deficiency may be expected with blood losses of 5 to 10 ml/day, the equivalent of 2.5 to 5 mg/day of iron. Iron loss during the childbearing years amounts to 0.3 to 0.5 mg/day.[39] To this is added the loss due to pregnancy and delivery of about 3 mg/day for a 280 day gestation (840 mg of iron).[42] Up to 2 years of normal dietary intake is required to replace the loss of iron incurred with each pregnancy. Over 500 mg of storage iron are required to avoid iron deficiency during pregnancy. These levels are present in only 20% of women; 40% of women have stores of 100–500 mg and 40% have no storage iron. Demand for iron increases from 0.8 mg/day early in pregnancy to 7.5 mg/day in late pregnancy. In spite of increased iron absorption during pregnancy, at least 20% of women not taking supplements have iron deficiency anemia.[43] In Scandinavian pregnant women, iron intake is as high as 9 mg/day, yet well below the recommended dietary allowance of 12 to 18 mg/day.[43] Multiple pregnancies progressively add to the iron deficit. Lactation places an added burden on maternal iron stores, with a loss of 0.5 to 1.0 mg/day.[44]

Table 9.3[22] Iron homeostasis.

IRON BALANCE Total body iron 4 grams	
INTAKE	LOSS
Western diet contains 10 to 20 mg/day	Obligatory loss (skin, lungs, renal, intestine)
Normal absorption	Men 1 mg/day
Men 1 mg/day	Women, non-menstruating 1 mg/day
Women, non-menstruating 1 mg/day	Women, menstruating 2 mg/day
Women, menstruating 2 mg/day	Blood loss 1 mg iron/1 gram red cells
During pregnancy or after blood loss 5 mg/day	

In premenopausal women, pathological blood loss leading to iron deficiency anemia may be due to excessive uterine bleeding (37%) but is also frequently the result of gastrointestinal bleeding (86% of women, including those with a concomitant gynecological cause).[27] Gastrointestinal pathology is the primary etiology of iron deficiency in postmenopausal women.[28]

Iron homeostasis may be altered by numerous environmental influences which include: an iron deficient diet, alcohol, medications, parasites and other factors predisposing to gastrointestinal hemorrhage (Table 9.3). Strict vegetarians require iron supplementation to avoid deficiency.[45] Grains, cereals and corn possess phytates and neutral detergent fibers which form insoluble complexes with iron, inhibiting absorption. Inadequate dietary vitamin C may reduce absorption of iron.[37,46] In underdeveloped countries, combined deficiencies of multiple nutrients including iron, vitamin C, riboflavin and thiamine may cause functional impairment without the specific features of any single deficiency.[46] Zinc[47–49] and vitamin A[50] deficiency also predispose to iron deficiency.

Alcohol may cause gastrointestinal hemorrhage but a traditional beer consumed by African women contains such substantial amounts of iron and folate that it may actually be protective against anemia.[51] Tannin-containing beverage consumption such as tea, in association with a largely vegetarian diet, impairs iron absorption.[52] Cigarette smoking, increasing in American women, raises mean hemoglobin levels[53] but is also a major risk factor for peptic ulcer disease and cancer; both associated with the development of iron deficiency anemia.[54]

A major problem in undeveloped countries is infestation with *Necatur americanus* (hookworm) and *Ancylostoma duodenale* (roundworm) which also cause iron deficiency from gastrointestinal blood loss.[55,56] Visceral leishmaniasis (*Leishmania donovani*) infestation may also result in gastrointestinal hemorrhage.[53,57]

Iron homeostasis during pregnancy

Changes in iron homeostasis during pregnancy reflect maternal physiologic changes and fetal demand for iron. Maternal plasma volume begins to increase starting at about 6 weeks gestation. The expansion of plasma volume, which peaks at about 1,250 ml (approximately 42% above the pre-pregnant state) is disproportionately greater than the corresponding increase in red cell mass. This results in a physiologic fall in the hemoglobin concentration. An initial rapid rise slows after 30 weeks gestation. Evidence of a positive correlation between the neonatal birth weight and the plasma volume expansion indicate that this is an important index of normal pregnancy. The red cell mass expands but at a slower rate, with a total increase of about 24% (250 ml) at term. Iron supplementation may produce an increase of up to 30%. Just as with the plasma volume, there seems to be a direct correlation between fetal growth and increased red cell mass.[1]

A marked decrease in the serum ferritin is observed between the 12th and 25th week of gestation as iron is utilized for the obligatory expansion of maternal red cell mass. During pregnancy, the placenta regulates iron transfer from the mother to fetus. Increased maternal iron absorption supports this process. Maternal iron absorption reaches peak efficiency after 30 weeks gestation. This corresponds to the period of greatest transfer of iron from the mother to fetus. Iron is carried by maternal transferrin, to transferrin receptors located on the apical surface of the placental syncytiotrophoblast. Endocytosis incorporates holotransferrin into the placental cell, iron is released and apotransferrin is returned to the maternal circulation. The free iron binds to ferritin in the placental cells, is transferred to apotransferrin entering from the fetal side of the placenta and is released as holotransferrin into the fetal circulation. Transport of iron from the maternal to fetal circulation is regulated by this placental iron transfer system. A decrease in maternal iron results in an increase in the number of placental transferrin receptors. More iron is then extracted from the maternal circulation by the placenta. The placental synthesis of ferritin inhibits further uptake of iron. When the mother is iron deficient, it appears that the capacity of the system is inadequate to maintain iron transfer to the fetus.[3]

In response to the net loss of maternal iron to the developing fetus, there is an increase in iron absorption from the gastrointestinal tract. A decrease of the maternal serum ferritin below 12 ug/l, stimulates absorption.[58] Absorption may triple from the first to third trimester. The molecular mechanisms whereby this occurs appear to involve the HFE gene and protein but are poorly understood.[59] Fetal iron needs in the first trimester are about 1 to 2 mg per day; 4 mg per day in the second trimester and 6 mg per day in the third trimester. Of approximately 1245 mg of iron to meet the demands of pregnancy, labor and delivery, basal maternal needs are 240 mg, 450 mg augments maternal blood volume, 80 mg deposits in the placenta, 225 mg is required for fetal needs and 250 mg is lost during a normal vaginal delivery.[14] The needs are met first by maternal tissue stores and then by increased absorption.

Clinical manifestations

Mild anemia, with the hemoglobin greater than 10 g/dl, is usually asymptomatic except during heavy physical exertion or in the presence of cardiovascular compromise.[60,61,62,63] Mild, nonspecific symptoms, frequently attributed to anemia and iron deficiency, require an alternative explanation.[64] Iron deficient adults involved in heavy labor may experience diminished work capacity and measurable cognitive deficiencies.[17,65] Severe anemia of any etiology (<5 g/dl) may cause a high cardiac output, high output failure and even tissue ischemia.[66]

Highly trained female athletes develop iron deficiency from dietary inadequacy, uncompensated menstrual losses, excessive losses from hemolysis, gastrointestinal bleeding and in sweat.[67,68,69,70] As many as 82% of female and 29% of male elite Canadian distance runners have been identified with low serum ferritin (less than 25 μg/l),[71,72] however, overt iron deficiency is found in only 3% to 7% of endurance runners.[73] The impact of iron deficiency with or without anemia is uncertain,[74] however, some studies do suggest significant impairment of performance.[75]

Neonatal iron stores are dependent upon those of the mother. Iron deficiency during the first two trimesters of pregnancy doubles the risk of pre-term delivery, triples the risk of neonatal low birth weight[76] and results in the delivery of iron deficient neonates.[3,14,77] In one study from India, severe maternal anemia (hemoglobin less than 7 g/dl) was associated with the greatest risk for intrauterine growth retardation and low birth weight. With a hemoglobin of less than 8.9 g/dl, there is a 4 to 6 times greater risk of prolonged labor and with the hemoglobin below 7.5 g/dl there is a 4.8 times greater risk of requiring cesarean section or operative vaginal delivery.[78] It appears that the greatest risk of low birth weight is associated with anemia during the first but not the second or third trimester.[79] Iron deficient children may experience delayed development and disturbed behavior, persisting until full repletion of iron stores.[80,81,82,83] Infants and children of iron deficient mothers are also at increased risk of developing iron deficiency anemia, undetected at birth.[83] In addition, maternal iron deficiency anemia has been correlated with increased fetoplacental angiogenesis during the first trimester leading to an increase in cardiovascular morbidity and mortality during adult life.[84] A trial of prophylactic oral iron supplementation has revealed that whereas neither the prevalence of anemia nor risk of preterm birth was not increased, the incidence of preterm low birth weight was reduced.[85]

Diagnosis

History and physical examination

Specific symptoms and signs may suggest iron deficiency anemia or chronic genitourinary or gastrointestinal blood loss. Pica is an uncommonly reported but not infrequent (as many as 50% of patients) symptom of severe iron deficiency,[86,87] and may include craving for earth or clay (geophagia), starch (amylophagia), ice (pagophagia), or even nuts.[88]

The pale green skin of chlorosis that is seen with severe iron deficiency appearing during the adolescent growth surge of maturing girls was first reported in the medical literature of the 1800s and disappeared during the first decade of the twentieth century.[89] Although chlorosis was once sine qua non for iron deficiency, pallor is the physical finding most often observed in patients with iron deficiency anemia.[90–92] Pruritis is occasionally due to iron deficiency and koilonychia is observed only in patients with severe, longstanding illness.[90] Blue sclera may be observed in teenage girls[93] and adults[94] with iron deficiency but has not been verified as a valuable diagnostic finding in children.[95]

Menorrhagia, metrorrhagia, or metromenorrhagia may be important clinical corollaries to the finding of iron deficiency. The average dietary consumption of iron may not be adequate to replace the loss consequent to menstrual blood loss and multiple or complicated pregnancies. Women of any age may present with chronic iron deficiency and no apparent gynecological explanation. A number of clinical studies have clearly demonstrated that gastrointestinal hemorrhage is the probable source of blood loss.[27,28,96]

Contraceptive method has also been identified as a factor in iron deficiency. Millman and colleagues have determined from a Danish study that women using oral contraception had a much shorter duration of menses than those using intrauterine devices (IUD) and other methods, resulting in a lower incidence of iron deficiency. Further, the recommendation is made that screening and preventive efforts be focused primarily in women with menses of greater than 5 days duration, with particularly heavy bleeding, those using an IUD and regular blood donors.[97]

Postmenopausal bleeding, particularly in women with a history of postmenopausal estrogen use or obesity, should be evaluated promptly for the presence of endometrial cancer.[98] Hematuria, a common gynecologic disorder usually resulting from acute hemorrhagic cystitis or incidental menstrual contamination may be overlooked as a sign of a primary genitourinary malignancy contributing to iron deficiency.[99]

Gastrointestinal symptoms of significant blood loss are easily recognized, however, even mild indigestion may be a symptom of a gastroesophageal source of hemorrhage. Many patients with occult gastrointestinal bleeding are asymptomatic.[27,28,96]

Abdominal and bimanual examination in women may reveal a gynecologic etiology of hemorrhage. Accompanying the bimanual pelvic examination with a rectal exam is also essential to diagnosis, as up to 12% of colon cancer is detected by the digital rectal examination. Stool specimens should be examined for the presence of occult blood, since gastrointestinal cancer or polyps will be found in 28% of patients with occult positive stools.[100]

Laboratory studies

The definition of both iron deficiency and iron deficiency anemia are primarily quantitative. Laboratory analysis includes hemoglobin, red cell indices, red cell dispersion width, serum iron, transferrin saturation and serum ferritin. To this may be added the serum transferrin receptors, free erythrocyte protoporphyrin, and bone marrow iron.

Anemia is diagnosed when there is a reduction of the hemoglobin in grams per 100 ml to at least two standard deviations below the mean, adjusted for age, sex, and altitude of residence.[101,102] Normal values increase in proportion to elevation of residence above sea level and in cigarette smokers. The mean normal hemoglobin for women is 14 g/dl, with a range of 12–16 g/dl. For men, normal hemoglobin is 16 g/dl, with a range of 14–18 g/dl. While increases in iron stores and in ineffective erythropoiesis occur in elderly women and men, these changes do not warrant the establishment of new geriatric norms.[103,104,105,106]

Twenty to 60% of pregnant women are found to have a hemoglobin level below 11.0 g/dl, defined by the WHO and others as anemia.[34,107] Table 9.4 summarizes the lower limit of normal hemoglobin during each stage of gestation.[34] Laboratory

Table 9.4[34,45] Normal hemoglobin values during pregnancy: pregnant women 5th percentile values.

Gestation in weeks	Hemoglobin
12	11.0
16	10.6
20	10.5
24	10.5
28	10.7
32	11.0
36	11.4
40	11.9

studies for the evaluation of anemia and iron deficiency during pregnancy may be influenced by inherent physiologic changes. During the first and second trimesters hemoglobin and hematocrit decrease as the maternal blood volume expands.[25,108] Women who have adequate iron intake experience a rise in both hemoglobin and hematocrit during the third trimester to levels noted pre-pregnancy.[34,109,110] A reduced hemoglobin from pre-pregnancy levels usually indicates iron deficiency, whereas, an increased hemoglobin (especially in the second trimester) indicates poor maternal blood volume expansion and is associated with hypertension, fetal growth retardation, death, premature delivery and low birth weight.[111–114] A hematocrit of >43% (normal 33% to 36%) has been associated with a four-times increased risk of fetal growth retardation.[112]

The diagnosis of iron deficiency anemia may also be reached by observing an increase in the hemoglobin in response to a therapeutic trial of iron supplementation. This clinical practice is appropriate during pregnancy, in premenopausal women with a history of heavy menstrual loss, those from underdeveloped countries, and women with a history of multiple pregnancies or a socioeconomic background at risk of dietary inadequacy. A trial of oral iron should be prohibited in most postmenopausal women from western countries, owing to the high likelihood of underlying occult gastrointestinal bleeding, including that from gastrointestinal malignancy.[27,28,115]

Iron deficiency is diagnosed when the serum ferritin, the most specific blood test, is ≤12 μg/l and excluded when >12 μg/l.[116,117] Correlation between low serum ferritin and absent bone marrow stainable iron is about 75%. The specificity of low serum ferritin for absent marrow iron is 98%. Indicating the importance of determination of the serum ferritin cut-off, it has been noted that when the lower limit for serum ferritin is set at <12 μg/l the sensitivity is 61% and specificity 98%.[118] In screening for iron deficiency in pregnant women from underdeveloped countries it has been recommended that the lower limit for ferritin be set at 30 μg/l.[8] Measurement of the ferritin during the first and second trimester may fail to predict the adequacy of iron stores during the third trimester.[119] Since ferritin is an acute phase reactant, acute or chronic inflammatory disorders may raise the levels, obscuring the diagnosis of iron deficiency.[120]

Serum iron, transferrin and percent saturation have significant limitations which may be accentuated during pregnancy and other states as seen in Table 9.5.[65,118] Recently, the protoporphyrin/heme ratio has been observed to rise in response to iron supplementation more dramatically than any other measurement of iron status in pregnant women.[121] For screening, van den Broek and colleagues have recommended a sequential evaluation including both the serum ferritin, as the most sensitive test and the transferrin ratio as the most specific.[8] Akesson[12] and others[122] have identified the serum transferrin receptor

Table 9.5[21,50] Misleading laboratory values in measurement of iron.

Increased serum iron
premenstrual state
ingestion of iron supplements
pregnancy
progesterone-based oral contraceptives
iron dextran injection
hepatitis
hemochromatosis
Decreased serum iron
diurnal variation with low values in mid-afternoon and very low near midnight during menstruation
acute or chronic inflammation
infection
malignancy
Increased total iron-binding capacity
progesterone-based oral contraceptives
Increased transferrin saturation
ingestion of iron supplements
progesterone-based oral contraceptives
iron dextran/sucrose injection
hemochromatosis
Decreased transferrin saturation
acute or chronic infection
inflammation
malignancy (transferrin saturation may be low or normal)

(soluble transferrin receptor) as 100% specific in identifying iron deficiency during pregnancy. This may be superior to both ferritin and transferrin saturation. As the serum ferritin is not only an iron storage protein but also an acute phase reactant, elevation is expected in the patient with an active inflammatory process. Assessment of the C-reactive protein is a useful method of determining the validity of an elevated serum ferritin as a marker of iron deficiency. Elevation of the C-reactive protein suggests that an elevated serum ferritin cannot be used for the diagnosis of iron deficiency. In this circumstance, the soluble transferrin assay is a very useful study, since it is unaffected by the presence of inflammation.[123]

Stainable marrow iron is the reference standard for iron deficiency. Although the absence of iron is not absolute proof of iron deficiency, the presence of stainable marrow iron (haemosiderin) reliably excludes iron deficiency.[65]

Table 9.6[32] Screening for iron deficiency and iron deficiency anemia.

Population	Frequency	Method
Adolescent nonpregnant girls ages 12 to <18	Every 5–10 yrs	Hemoglobin If low – 4-week trial of oral iron MCV, RDW, Ferritin if no response
Adult women	Annually if high risk	Hemoglobin If low – MCV, RDW, Ferritin
Pregnant women	First prenatal visit	Hemoglobin If low – MCV, RDW, Ferritin if <9.0, or if no response to oral iron refer for consultation

Screening for iron deficiency anemia

Screening for anemia is indicated for all adolescent girls (ages 12 to <18 years) and nonpregnant women of childbearing age every 5 to 10 years. Annual screening is indicated for women with risk factors for iron deficiency such as a history of heavy menstrual blood loss, menses >5 days duration, IUD use for contraception, gastrointestinal disease, low dietary iron intake, regular blood donors or previously diagnosed iron deficiency anemia.[97,124] Although it is recommended that all pregnant women receive low dose iron supplementation, screening for anemia remains an essential part of the first prenatal visit.[124] Screening for anemia and iron deficiency in postmenopausal women without major risk factors is not routinely recommended. A summary of the approach to screening is presented in Table 9.6.[32]

Diagnostic evaluation

Evaluation of the iron deficient patient must proceed to a determination of the specific etiology of poor iron absorption or of blood loss.[27] The diagnosis of anemia at the time of screening is based upon the finding of a hemoglobin <11.8 g/dl in girls from age 12 to 15 and <12.0 g/dl for adolescent girls over 15 and adult women. The normal values cited in Table 9.5 are used for the diagnosis during pregnancy. Table 9.7 outlines a basic categorization of anemia based on the MCV. Once the diagnosis of microcytic anemia has been reached, the evaluation must proceed to determine etiology. If iron deficiency is found, a precise cause must be determined. During pregnancy, unless the history and physical examination suggest an alternative source of iron depletion, therapy may proceed. If the initial hemoglobin is <9.0 g/dl, more intensive evaluation and referral for

Table 9.7 Classification of anemia (Hemoglobin <12.0 g/dl).

MCV (mm^3)	Category
80–100 mm^3	Normocytic
<80 mm^3	Microcytic
>100 mm^3	Macrocytic

Table 9.8 Etiologies of microcytic anemia.

Iron deficiency
Dietary deficiency
Blood loss
Thalassemia minor
B-Thalassemia intermedia and major
Sideroblastic (hereditary)
Anemia of chronic disease
Hemoglobinopathies (H or E)
Lead poisoning

consultation may be required. Clearly, failure to respond to oral iron with an elevation in hemoglobin (increase by 1 g/dl or hematocrit by 3%) within 4 weeks should prompt a more intensive investigation. Other possible etiologies of microcytic anemia are listed in Table 9.8.

In premenopausal women, pathological blood loss leading to iron deficiency anemia may be due to excessive uterine bleeding (37%) but is also frequently the result of gastrointestinal bleeding (86% of women).[27] Gastrointestinal pathology is the primary etiology of iron deficiency in postmenopausal women.[28] Nonpregnant, premenopausal women who fail to respond to a trial of oral iron or who have upper gastrointestinal symptoms should be considered for esophogastroduodenoscopy. Endoscopic evaluation of the colon is indicated in presence of lower intestinal symptoms or signs along with normal upper endoscopy.[27,28] Radiographic evaluation of the small bowel is indicated only if other studies fail to reveal a source of bleeding.[27,28,125,126] All iron deficient, postmenopausal women require a complete gastrointestinal evaluation to a certain diagnosis.

Treatment

All pregnant women should receive a daily oral dose of at least 27 mg of elemental iron to provide for the needs of pregnancy, labor and delivery and as prophylaxis against depletion of iron stores.[9,124,127–130] An iron supplement with a heme

Table 9.9[22,234] Treatment of iron deficiency.

Population	Therapy
Nonpregnant adolescent girls and women	Oral iron 60–120 mg/day
Pregnant women	Oral iron 60–120 mg/day
All groups	Counseling regarding a diet high in iron and correct all other dietary deficiencies
All groups	Monitor hemoglobin at 4 weeks and if hemoglobin rises by $\geq$1 g/dl diagnosis is confirmed and treat for 2 months, re-evaluate at 6 months. Re-evaluate if anemia persists
Refractory patients	Ferric gluconate complex in iron sucrose – approximately 1.0 gram total dose of elemental iron infused in 6 sessions; Erythropoietin – 150 IU/kg three times per week, combined with 100 mg/day parenteral elemental iron

component is preferred and is superior to an equivalent dose of pure organic iron.[127] The dose for treatment is 60 to 120 mg/day of elemental iron. Patients intolerant to oral iron or those with specific disorders which limit iron absorption may require parenteral iron therapy. Treatment is outlined in Table 9.9.

Therapy must continue throughout pregnancy. When the expected level of hemoglobin is achieved, the dose of oral iron may be reduced to 30 mg/day. Treatment is the same for iron deficiency in nonpregnant premenopausal, postpartum and postmenopausal women. For both primary prevention in premenopausal, pregnant and nonpregnant women, enhancement of the diet with foods high in iron is essential.[131] Women from underdeveloped countries, adolescent girls from developed countries and women with iron deficient diets, all require careful attention to correct dietary deficiencies. Counseling should be provided to all adolescent girls and women of childbearing age regarding the specifics of a diet high in available iron.[128,131]

Refractory iron deficiency anemia is a not uncommon problem during pregnancy. For treatment of iron deficiency, relatively large doses of iron are frequently administered. Side effects include gastrointestinal intolerance and oxidative damage. Delayed release preparations are somewhat better tolerated, however, many patients continue intolerant or unresponsive.[132] Concomitant with pharmacologic therapy, increased intake of dietary iron should continue. It has been recognized for many years that vitamin C is important for the absorption of iron from the gastrointestinal tract. It has now been demonstrated that the addition of folate to iron results in an improved response, with a greater elevation of hemoglobin in those treated with both compared to patients treated with iron alone. These results are independent of the underlying presence of folate deficiency.[133] The addition of riboflavin but not vitamin A may also help to enhance the effect of iron in iron deficient pregnant women.[134]

Patients who fail to respond to oral iron or who have severe intolerance, may be candidates for parenteral iron therapy. Intravenous iron sucrose has been extensively studied and determined to be safe and quite effective for the treatment of refractory iron deficiency anemia.[135–137] Studies have demonstrated a high success rate accompanied by a substantially decreased transfusion requirement.[138] In most refractory cases, and once the iron deficit has been fully reversed by parenteral iron, the addition of erythropoietin has proven quite successful.[138,139] A decreased post partum transfusion requirement has also been confirmed with the routine administration of 20,000 U recombinant erythropoietin immediately after delivery, given irrespective of the concomitant hemoglobin level.[140]

Conclusion

Iron deficiency remains a major health risk in the United States, in spite of the apparent availability of a high-quality diet. In the United States at least 7.8 million adolescent girls and premenopausal women are deficient.[5] World-wide, the challenge of identifying and treating iron deficiency is enormous.[7] Physicians involved in the primary care and in the obstetrical and gynecologic care of women of all ages must be aware of the nature of the problem and the correct approach to screening, diagnosis and treatment. The potential benefit to newborns and infants and to their mothers is substantial. Furthermore, a thorough diagnostic evaluation has considerable potential for uncovering a potentially lethal disease such as gastrointestinal malignancy in a curable phase.

Folate and vitamin B_{12} deficiency and hyperhomocysteinemia in obstetrics and gynecology

Introduction

Among the many metabolic changes that occur during pregnancy, the metabolism and maternal requirements of vitamins B_{12} and folate have received much attention due to the spectrum of clinical diseases associated with their deficiencies. In discussing these vitamins and their roles in health and disease, it is also necessary to discuss homocysteine, a molecule that shares biochemical pathways with folate and B_{12} and is itself an important marker for vascular disease as well as pregnancy complications. From the recognition many years ago that folate deficiency was associated with neural tube defects, research now indicates that folate, vitamin B_{12}, and homocysteine play roles in maternal and fetal health and may affect the health of older adult women.

The interrelationship between vitamin B_{12}, folate, and homocysteine

Vitamin B_{12}, or cobalamin, is found in a variety of animal-derived foods such as meats, eggs, and milk. After ingestion, vitamin B_{12} binds to its specific receptor, intrinsic factor, and this complex is absorbed in the terminal ileum. Average intake of cobalamin averages 5–7 mcg per day,[141] which exceeds the recommended daily allowance of 2 mcg per day. Vitamin B_{12} is required for only two enzymatic reactions in humans. The first reaction generates activated methyl groups in the methionine synthesis pathway that is discussed below. The second reaction, which converts methylmalonyl-CoA to succinyl-CoA, is important in the diagnosis of cobalamin deficiency.

Folate is a broad term encompassing the many different forms of naturally occurring and synthetic variants of folate. Folic acid refers to one synthetic form of folate found in many multivitamin supplements as well as fortified food products. Folate cannot be synthesized by man but is fortunately available from a wide variety of food sources including organ meats, leafy green vegetables, citrus fruit, bread, and dairy products. Cooking and ultraviolet radiation destroy many food sources of folate. After ingestion, folate is absorbed primarily in the jejunum and is taken up by the liver which processes and releases folate into the systemic circulation. Cells require folate for single-carbon transfer reactions: the catabolism of histidine, the interconversion of glycine and serine, the synthesis of thymidylate and purines, and the synthesis of methionine. The biochemical features of folic acid have recently been reviewed in detail.[142]

The interrelationship of vitamin B_{12}, folate, and homocysteine is best illustrated in the methionine synthesis pathway (Figure 9.2). Homocysteine is a central molecule in this process and can undergo remethylation or transsulfuration. In the remethylation cycle, methyltetrahydrofolate serves as the methyl donor to homocysteine in a vitamin B_{12} cofactor dependent reaction catalyzed by methionine synthase. Both folate and B_{12} are important in the normal processing of homocysteine since these two vitamins are required for remethylation. Inadequate stores of these vitamins place an individual at risk for hyperhomocysteinemia because homocysteine will accumulate if the reaction catalyzed by methionine synthase cannot continue at a normal rate. Methyltetrahydrofolate consumed in the methionine synthase-catalyzed reaction must be regenerated, and the final step of this process is catalyzed by 5,10-methylenetetrahydrofolate reductase (MTHFR). This enzyme is important because mutations of MTHFR cause hyperhomocysteinemia in adults. A cystathionine β-synthase mutation is the chief cause of homocystinuria, a rare childhood disease characterized by increased incidence

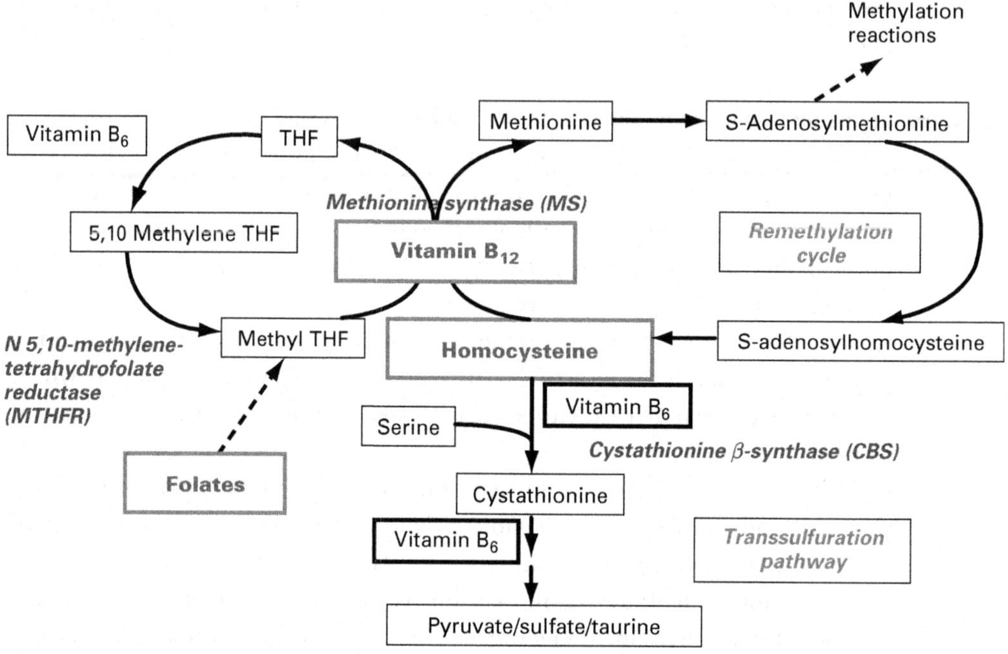

Figure 9.2 The methionine synthesis pathway. THF = tetrahydrofolate.

of thromboembolic disease.[143] Methionine synthase mutations are also known but have unclear clinical consequence. Hyperhomocysteinemia in adults has been associated with increased cardiovascular disease, and its role in the pathogenesis of disease is still under investigation.

Hyperhomocysteinemia

Elevated homocysteine levels are an important marker for folate and B_{12} deficiency in adults and will be discussed below. Hyperhomocysteinemia itself has received attention as a potential cause for a variety of clinical conditions, especially increased risk of vascular events in adults. Homocystinuria, the rare autosomal recessive condition causing markedly elevated homocysteine levels in the blood and urine, is usually diagnosed at a young age and is associated with a significant risk of thromboembolic complications that is a chief cause of early mortality.[143] Milder forms of hyperhomocysteinemia are common in adults and have also been linked to vascular disease; additional interest was generated when a common variant of MTHFR was discovered that caused hyperhomocysteinemia.[144] Later identified as a Cys677Thr mutation, this variant MTHFR showed reduced activity by approximately 50%.[144] In heterozygous (CT) MTHFR carriers, the mutation does not cause hyperhomocysteinemia, but homozygotes for the mutation (TT) show elevated homocysteine levels in the blood that are up to 25% above normal.[145] This Cys677Thr MTHFR mutation is common in the United States but shows ethnic variations; TT homozygotes are found in approximately 1% of African-Americans, 10% of Caucasian-Americans, and 20% of Hispanic-Americans.[146] Because the TT genotype is so common in the general population, it is better described as a polymorphism rather than a mutation and has been found in up to 50% of hyperhomocysteinemic adults.[145] The effects of the mutation appear to be 'treatable' in that increased folate intake lowers the homocysteine levels in TT homozygotes.[147–149] The U.S. folic acid fortification program, which started in 1998, will likely have an impact on the definition of 'normal' homocysteine levels because much of the hyperhomocysteinemic effect of the MTHFR TT genotype will likely be nullified. Other factors that may modestly increase homocysteine levels include impaired renal function, smoking, increased age, and male gender.[150] Thus, elevated homocysteine levels can also be due to environmental or genetic factors independent from adequate folate status.

The diagnosis of folate and B_{12} deficiency

The diagnosis of folate and vitamin B_{12} deficiency has been complicated by the discovery that mild forms of deficiency without overt clinical symptoms may be missed on basic screening tests using direct measurements of these vitamins. Common to both folate and B_{12} deficiency is the presence of a megaloblastic/macrocytic anemia, often accompanied by hypersegmentation of granulocytes. It is important to note that iron deficiency can occur simultaneously with B_{12} or folate deficiency with a resulting 'normocytic' anemia as measured by a Coulter counter. A high red cell distribution width (RDW) is a clue that more than one deficiency may exist, and can be confirmed by examination of the peripheral blood smear revealing both macrocytes and microcytes.

Laboratory measurement of folate and B_{12} include both direct and indirect measurements. Direct measurement of serum folate and B_{12} levels are commonly ordered when deficiency is suspected, but neither test is very sensitive or specific. For example, serum folate levels are affected by recent dietary changes and may not reflect tissue stores of folate, and even mild hemolysis will falsely elevate serum levels.[151] Erythrocyte folate levels are not as affected by dietary changes and offer theoretical advantages over serum folate, but clinical studies have shown that it does not have good sensitivity or specificity,[152] particularly in alcoholics and in pregnancy.[141] Similarly, serum B_{12} levels have been found to be in a low-normal range for a high percentage of patients who subsequently respond to B_{12} therapy[153] and conversely B_{12} levels may be suppressed due to folate deficiency that resolves with folate treatment.[141] Other causes of falsely raised or lowered B_{12} levels are listed in Table 9.10.

Table 9.10 Causes of falsely raised or depressed B_{12} levels.

Falsely depressed B_{12} levels
- Folate deficiency
- Myeloma
- High-dose vitamin C intake

Falsely raised B_{12} levels
- Liver disease
- Autoimmune diseases
- Myeloproliferative states

Indirect measurements assist in the diagnosis of folate and B_{12} deficiency. Rather than direct vitamin assays, indirect measurements of folate and B_{12} stores rely on detecting elevated levels of precursor molecules that accumulate when folate and/or B_{12} dependent reactions are blocked. Homocysteine, the precursor to methionine in the remethylation cycle, is expected to increase if either B_{12} or folate is deficient since both are required cofactors. Methylmalonic acid (MMA), the precursor for the conversion of methylmalonyl-CoA to succinyl-CoA, is expected to increase if a cobalamin deficiency exists but is not affected by folate stores. Based on clinical studies, homocysteine and MMA are now recognized as more sensitive and specific indicators of folate and cobalamin stores than the direct measurements of the vitamins themselves.[154] High homocysteine and MMA levels have been found to be more reliable markers of B_{12} deficiency, even in the absence of anemia, macrocytosis or subnormal serum B_{12} levels.[155,156] Likewise, high homocysteine is a sensitive marker for folate deficiency,[157] although it is not specific since it shares the same enzyme pathway with cobalamin. Two additional points should be emphasized. First, in addition to being useful diagnostically when levels are elevated, the indirect measurements have excellent negative predictive value in 'ruling-out' the presence of either folate or B_{12} deficiency when the levels are normal. In the study by Savage, only 1 out of 406 patients with documented cobalamin deficiency had normal levels of both homocysteine and methylmalonic acid.[157] Second, high homocysteine and/or MMA may be caused by other factors, notably renal insufficiency, hypovolemia, and as discussed above, the MTHFR TT genotype. That said, homocysteine and MMA have significantly improved our ability to diagnose or exclude folate and cobalamin deficiency. An approach to the diagnosis of B_{12} and folate deficiency using the above laboratory tests is shown in Figure 9.3.

Fluctuations in the blood levels of vitamins are known to occur in pregnancy though it is difficult to differentiate those changes that are physiological and not detrimental to fetal development from those which are pathological and potentially

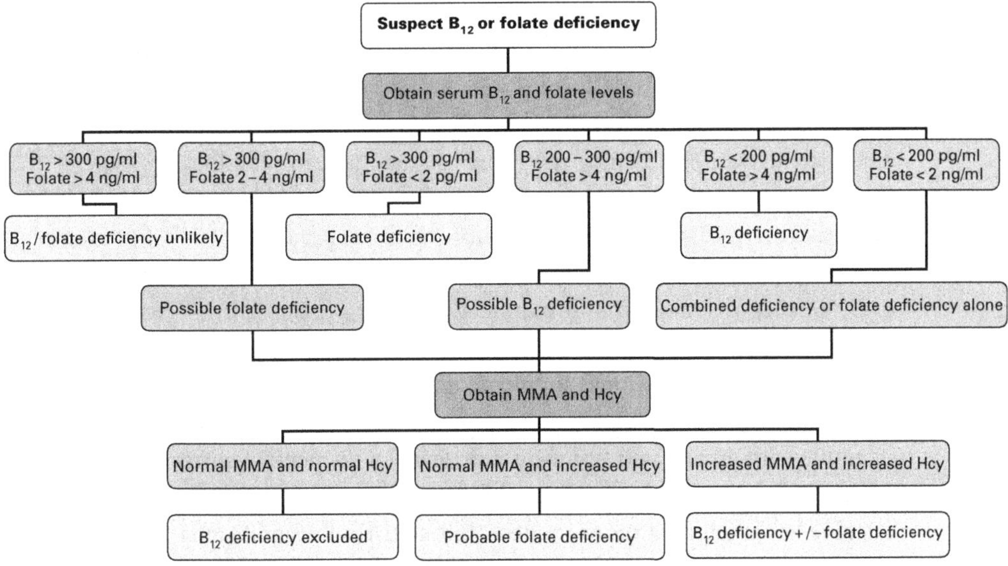

Figure 9.3 Proposed algorithm for evaluating patients with suspected vitamin B_{12} or folate deficiency. MMA = methylmalonic acid; Hcy = homocysteine.

harmful to the fetus. Vitamin B_{12} levels fall,[158–161] serum folate levels remain stable or fall slightly,[158,161,162] and homocysteine levels remain stable but may climb slightly during the third trimester,[159,161–163] in pregnant women. How these levels relate to each other, to changes in hormones, plasma volume and binding proteins, or to renal function is not well defined. Given this myriad of factors, interpreting results of serum folate, B_{12}, and homocysteine during pregnancy is a complicated task because reference norms have not been determined and standard adult reference ranges may not apply in pregnancy. Macrocytosis and other hematological changes are consistently seen in true folate and B_{12} deficiency and are as useful in pregnant women as they are in other adults.

Folate and vitamin B_{12} requirements in adults and during pregnancy

Folate

The actual and recommended daily intake of folate for adults and pregnant women continues to be a subject of much study, but one fact is emerging – the gap between the average and recommended folate consumption for Americans has narrowed over the past 5 years. In the past, the estimated folate intake for adult men and women has been 280 mcg and 210 mcg per day, respectively.[151] The current recommended daily folate intake for adults is 400 mcg daily.[128] In an attempt to narrow the gap between recommended and observed intake of folate and to prevent neural tube defects the Food and Drug Administration issued a regulation requiring that all enriched flour, rice, pasta, cornmeal, and other grain products contain 140 mcg of folic acid per 100 grams starting January 1998.[124] Because folic acid is a more bioavailable form of folate than most dietary forms of folate, this degree of fortification was thought to enhance the daily intake of folate by approximately 100–150 mcg per day of women in childbearing age.[124,164] Somewhat surprisingly, post-fortification studies have consistently revealed that the actual increase in dietary folate is more than was predicted.[165–168] For example, a recent study indicated that the actual increase in folate intake among adults is over 300 mcg per day, to approximately 650 mcg folate daily.[165] Jacques, *et al.* found that plasma folate levels doubled (from 4.6 to 10 ng/ml) in adults (mean age 55) not taking additional supplements since the start of the food fortification program.[168] Additionally, this study showed that the post-fortification percentage of adults with an elevated homocysteine level (>13 mcg/l) fell from 19% to 10% in those adults not taking additional folic acid supplements, while overall homocysteine levels fell by a more modest (but statistically significant) 7%.[168] Taking additional vitamin B supplements helped raise folate and B_{12} levels further while lowering homocysteine levels in this study. Thus it appears that the government's folic acid fortification program has exposed adults to increased folate from diet, perhaps even more than was originally envisioned.

The beneficial effects of folic acid supplementation for the general population are fortunately mirrored in the subpopulation of women in their childbearing years in preliminary studies. Caudill, *et al.*[169] examined the folate status of women between the ages of 18–45 in Southern California after folic acid fortification and found high serum and red cell folate levels along with low homocysteine levels in these women regardless of socioeconomic status. In a much larger study, the Centers for Disease Control showed an increase in serum folate since fortification from 6.3 to 16.2 ng/ml and a parallel rise in RBC folate from 181 to 315 ng/ml in women of childbearing age.[128,164]

Vitamin B_{12}

Vitamin B_{12} deficiency is uncommon in pregnancy, and unlike folate stores that can be depleted in months, normal cobalamin stores can last for years. The B_{12} needs of a pregnant woman are not thought to differ much from an average adult, and there is only a modest increase in recommended daily intake of vitamin B_{12} from 2.2 mcg daily to 2.4 mcg daily during pregnancy.[128,129]

Disorders related to folate and B_{12} deficiency and disorders related to hyperhomocysteinemia

Hematological sequelae of folate and B_{12} deficiency

Classically, folate and B_{12} deficiency in a non-pregnant adult is manifested by a megaloblastic/macrocytic anemia. Megaloblastosis refers to the changes in the

Table 9.11 Causes of macrocytosis.

Artifactual
- Markedly elevated blood sugar
- Cold agglutinins

Vitamin deficiency
- B_{12} deficiency
- Folate deficiency

Induced DNA defects
- Drug-induced altered DNA synthesis (folate antagonists, antiviral and anticonvulsant drugs)
- Inborn errors of metabolism (Lesch-Nyhan syndrome, orotic aciduria)

Metabolic derangements
- Myelodysplastic syndromes
- Liver disease
- Alcohol use
- Reticulocytosis
- Hypoxemia

bone marrow and macrocytosis in the peripheral blood; a deficiency of either will cause identical bone marrow features. It should also be remembered that macrocytosis does not specifically indicate that megaloblastic changes are occurring in the bone marrow. Other causes of macrocytosis are listed in Table 9.11. Two specific signs of megaloblastic changes are helpful: (1) hypersegmentation of neutrophils and (2) presence of macroovalocytes in the peripheral blood. As nuclear maturation is progressively delayed, megaloblastic erythroblasts in the bone marrow begin to lyse, causing an elevation of serum lactate dehydrogenase, indirect bilirubin, uric acid, as well as ferritin and iron.

Neuropsychiatric symptoms in B_{12} deficiency

One of the main clinical features that differentiate B_{12} deficiency from folate deficiency is the presence of neuropsychiatric symptoms. These can include posterolateral spinal column demyelinating symptoms, peripheral neuropathies, mood changes, and dementia-like memory loss (Table 9.12). Of these symptoms, peripheral neuropathy appears to be the most frequent clinical feature. Some of these changes are reversible with repletion of B_{12}, thus improvement can occur in days to weeks. The underlying pathophysiology remains unclear. Folate deficiency does not have neurological sequelae, so macrocytosis with neuropsychiatric symptoms should strongly suggest B_{12} deficiency.

Table 9.12 Neuropsychiatric manifestations of B_{12} deficiency.

Spinal Cord Changes

- Posterior column symptoms
  - Paresthesias in fingers and toes
  - Uncoordination of legs
  - Diminished vibratory sense/proprioception
- Lateral column symptoms
  - Weakness of legs > arms
  - Spasticity of legs > arms
  - Positive Babinski's sign

Central Nervous System Changes

- Dementia
- Personality changes
- Psychiatric disturbances

Obstetrical complications relating to a deficiency of vitamins, B_{12} or folate, or to elevated levels of homocysteine

Neural tube defects

One of the most well known problems related to folate deficiency in pregnancy is the group of disorders known as neural tube defects (NTDs). Spina bifida and anencephaly, the most common of the NTDs, occurred in approximately 2.5 out of 10,000 births in the United States in the early 1990s.[170] Although the association of maternal folate deficiency with fetal NTDs has been known for over forty years, the mechanism of this interaction remains unclear. Theories include a direct effect of low folate levels on impaired DNA synthesis[171] to an indirect effect of homocysteine toxicity on the fetus. Definitive evidence that treatment with folate can reduce the incidence of neural tube defects was shown in a randomized clinical trial carried out by the British Medical Research Council. In this study, women with a prior pregnancy affected by NTD were randomized to folate (4 mg), multivitamin (not a complete multivitamin – it did not include vitamin B_{12}, for example), or no intervention in a 2×2 factorial design. NTD-affected births decreased by 72% in women treated with folate.[144] The Institute of Medicine now recommends that pregnant women receive 600 mcg of folate daily, and women with prior NTD-associated pregnancy receive 4 mg of folate daily.[128,164]

Implementing an effective intervention has been difficult because neural tube closure is complete four weeks after conception, a time when many women are not aware that they are pregnant and may not be taking folate supplements. Folic acid fortification of food was clearly an attractive option that could eliminate or reduce the need for women to actively take folic acid supplements, but the U.S. program itself was controversial. Some have felt that the level of fortification was not enough,[172] others felt that it might be too much because B_{12} deficiency might be masked by folate repletion (which can reverse the anemia and hyperhomocysteinemia associated with a combined folate and B_{12} deficiency).[150] Thus far, folate fortification appears to have reduced the incidence of NTDs by approximately 20%.[173] Using birth certificate records, the prevalence of NTDs has decreased from 37.8 per 100,000 live births to 30.5 per 100,000 live births in the United States since 1998. Thus it appears that folate fortification has made an impact in reducing NTDs, though the ultimate degree of reduction remains to be seen.

Whether or not vitamin B_{12} status affects NTDs is not known. There are several key points to consider regarding vitamin B_{12} in pregnant women. First, true B_{12} deficiency is rare in pregnancy and is associated with a megaloblastic state.[151] Second, vitamin B_{12} levels fall throughout pregnancy, often to levels considered 'low' by adult reference standards, but are not associated with hyperhomocysteinemia or anemia.[159] Third, although most studies addressing a possible link between B_{12} and NTDs have used serum B_{12} levels and in aggregate have suggested a possible association,[174] methodological differences among the studies make such a conclusion difficult. Only a few studies have looked at methylmalonic acid levels during pregnancy,[148,175] but their small numbers also do not allow for clear conclusions to be drawn.

Miscarriage

Miscarriage occurs commonly in women with homocystinuria, who have fetal loss rates of almost 50%.[143] Studies of hyperhomocysteinemic women, with less elevated homocysteine values, have generally shown a positive association of high homocysteine levels with miscarriage. A meta-analysis of 10 case-control studies gave an odds ratio of 2.7 (95% CI 1.4 to 5.2) for women with recurrent early pregnancy loss (two or more spontaneous miscarriages before 16 weeks menstrual age) and elevated fasting levels of homocysteine.[176] A smaller link (odds ratio = 1.4, 95% CI 1.0 to 2.0) was found between the TT genotype of the MTHFR gene and recurrent miscarriages. Whether folate supplementation might be beneficial is not known, but a small trial using 15 mg of folic acid daily along with vitamin B_6 helped to normalize homocysteine levels in 25 hyperhomocysteinemic women, all with the TT MTHFR genotype, who had recurrent miscarriages.[177] Twenty of the 25 women subsequently carried a fetus to term without complications. Turning attention towards fetal characteristics, other studies suggest that spontaneously aborted fetuses carry certain combinations of genes more frequently, including the TT MTHFR genotype, which lowers fetal viability.[178,179] Thus, while elevated homocysteine may be found in a small subset of women with recurrent miscarriages, there is some hope that treatment with vitamins may allow these women to complete their pregnancies.

Preeclampsia

Preeclampsia occurs in up to 7% of nulliparas and 5% of multiparas during pregnancy[180] and while the etiology remains unclear, placental vasculopathy is seen pathologically and endothelial dysfunction has been postulated to play a significant role.[181] Homocysteine interferes with nitric oxide synthesis and homocysteine impairs endothelium dependent vasodilation.[182–184] Homocysteine has been associated with the development of pre-eclampsia in numerous case-control studies,[185–194] although an association with the MTHFR TT genotype has generally not been found.[189,194–198] Additionally, low serum folate and B_{12} levels generally do not correlate with preeclampsia.[185,189,190,193] In theory, if homocysteine can be lowered by increased folate intake and hyperhomocysteinemia plays a role in preeclampsia, then increased dietary folate should lessen the occurrence of preeclampsia. Although prospective clinical trial data are lacking, a retrospective analysis of the incidence of preeclampsia and eclampsia before and after folic acid supplementation in Canada did not show a decline following supplementation (3.8% before vs. 3.7% after).[199] Certainly more clinical trials are warranted in this area, but at the present, the roles of folate, B_{12}, and homocysteine in the diagnosis and treatment of preeclampsia are not well defined.

Other problems in pregnancy

The relationship of intrauterine growth retardation (IUGR) to homocysteine initially gave conflicting results with some positive correlations[187,200] and some negative correlations.[201,202] These studies were relatively small, but a recent large study[203] involving several hundred parents and children with and without IUGR failed to show any association to IUGR to elevated homocysteine values; in fact, most homocysteine values were in the normal range and relatively higher homocysteine levels in the mother and newborn were protective against IUGR. It is not clear why hyperhomocysteinemia might be protective or reflect a protective mechanism against IUGR, but it appears that hyperhomocysteinemia and IUGR are unlikely to be related events. Other studies have suggested a link between homocysteine and Down's syndrome[204] as well as congenital heart defects[205] and placental abruption.[206]

Folate and cancer

There are several putative mechanisms whereby folate deficiency may play a role in carcinogenesis.[207] First, deficiency of folate can cause a relative deficiency of the methyl donor S-adenosyl methionine leading to DNA and RNA hypomethylation. Hypomethylation of DNA may lead to activation of proto-oncogenes.[207] Additionally, folate is required for synthesis of purines and thymidylate, and folate deficiency may cause improper base pair incorporation into DNA leading to mutations. Several large case-control studies suggest that folate deficiency may increase risk for cancer, though the data with the MTHFR TT genotype is not as clear and even paradoxical.

Breast cancer

Many studies have attempted to find a link between breast cancer and folate intake; the majority of studies have not found a link except in women who have low folate intake and high alcohol intake. Large cohort studies including tens of thousands of women[208–211] and smaller case-control studies[212–216] provide the bulk of the evidence; folate intake was acquired via self-reporting of dietary habits by the study participants. Most studies show either no effect of folate on breast cancer risk in pre- or post-menopausal women,[210,213–215] or an association only with increasing alcohol intake,[208,211] itself a risk factor for breast cancer. Studies assessing the link between the MTHFR TT genotype and breast cancer have suggested a possible increased risk in TT genotype patients in premenopausal women only.[217,218] The only large trial measuring homocysteine in a cohort of women found no link between homocysteine levels and breast cancer.[219]

Other cancers

The data with regard to colon cancer and folate status provides an interesting parallel comparison with the data in breast cancer. Cohort and case-control studies provide most of the data, with the majority showing an inverse association of folate intake with colorectal carcinoma risk.[220–224] In contrast to the data in breast cancer, however, the TT MTHFR genotype appears to be protective against colon cancer.[223,225] A low folate status or increased alcohol intake negates the protective effect of the TT polymorphism in colon cancer. The mechanism of protection is not clear, but illustrates that gene-environment interactions are complex. In breast cancer, low intake of folate and the TT MTHFR genotype both appear to be risk factors, while in colon cancer, low intake of folate is a risk factor while the TT MTHFR genotype is a protective factor and the presence of both has a neutral effect. Studies on the effect of folate and cervical cancer have been recently reviewed,[226] with no clear link between low folate intake and the development of cervical carcinoma. Likewise, there is no clear link between folate status and development of lung cancer.[227–230]

Treatment

Folate and B_{12} deficiency

The approach to the treatment of folate and B_{12} deficiency depends on the clinical situation in which the diagnosis is suspected. When a megaloblastic anemia is the initial presenting problem, the anemia itself may be the most important symptom and transfusion of packed red blood cells may be indicated. Transfusion of one or two units should be enough to avert hemodynamic compromise and if possible, serum B_{12} and folate levels should be drawn before the transfusion to aid in diagnosis. If the patient is stable, workup can begin by checking serum B_{12} and folate levels, followed by homocysteine or methylmalonic acid levels to aid in diagnosis when the values are equivocal. Once the problem has been identified, treatment can be started with the appropriate vitamin, and if no etiology has been found, a search can commence for the cause of the deficiency.

Folate deficiency is most often related to inadequate dietary intake; pregnancy increases the metabolic demand for folate further as the placenta actively captures folate from the maternal circulation and releases it to the rapidly growing fetus. Folate demands may be heightened by multiparity and folate intake lessened by hyperemesis gravidarum. Fortunately, folate deficiency is effectively treated with folic acid supplements between 1–5 mg daily. Unlike food-derived folates, folic acid is very well absorbed and high doses can even overcome malabsorption problems. In non-pregnant adults, an appropriate response includes a reticulocytosis and drop in serum potassium levels in the first several days, resolution of hyperhomocysteinemia and hypersegmented neutrophils in a few weeks, and a normalization of the hemoglobin values in several months.[141]

B_{12} deficiency is a less common clinical condition than folate deficiency since intake and absorption of vitamin B_{12} (4 mcg) greatly exceeds the daily requirement of B_{12} (1 mcg) in most diets, and the body stores of B_{12} (2000–5000 mcg) are extensive enough to last for years. Because most mechanisms of B_{12} deficiency are related to absorptive problems, treatment is usually given by daily intramuscular injections of vitamin B_{12} for one week, followed by weekly injections for a month. Once the body stores have been repleted, oral B_{12} supplementation (1 mg daily) may be appropriate for some patients with ongoing malabsorption, though monthly 1 mg injections bypasses any absorption problems and ensures adequate levels. Repletion of B_{12} should result in normalization of the hematological abnormalities in a parallel manner to the treatment of folate deficiency. Recovery of neurological abnormalities is slower, requiring up to 6 months, and may be incomplete depending on the duration and degree of impairment at the time of diagnosis.

Hyperhomocysteinemia

Whether hyperhomocysteinemia arises from folate or vitamin B_{12} deficiency or from polymorphisms of enzymes involved in folate and B_{12} metabolism such as the MTHFR G677T mutation, treatment relies on increasing folate and B_{12} intake. While individual vitamin supplementation can lower homocysteine levels, multivitamins containing B_{12}, folate and vitamin B_6 are often used. Folate supplementation appears to have the most homocysteine lowering effect,[128,231] and addition of B_{12} lowers homocysteine values further. Effective doses used in homocysteine lowering trials are similar to doses used in folate and B_{12} deficiency: 1 to 5 mg of folic acid and 0.4 to 1 mg of vitamin B_{12}. Those who carry the TT MTHFR genotype can also be effectively treated with folic acid and vitamin B_{12}.[147,149,232,233]

Summary

Folate, vitamin B_{12}, and homocysteine are now seen as increasingly important mediators in the complex interaction of diet, genetics, health, and disease. For the obstetrician and gynecologist, the discoveries in this field have implications beyond caring for the pregnant woman; vascular disease and cancer are among the most important contributors of morbidity and mortality for the adult, post-menopausal woman. Although much of the clinical data is observational, well-designed clinical intervention trials have begun,[150] which should help guide clinicians on the appropriateness of offering vitamins in disease prevention for their patients.

REFERENCES

1 Sifakis, S. and G. Pharmakides, Anemia in pregnancy. *Ann. N. Y. Acad. Sci.*, 2000. **900**: 125–36.

2 Bergmann, R. L., *et al.*, Iron deficiency is prevalent in a sample of pregnant women at delivery in Germany. *Eur. J. Obstet. Gynecol. Reprod. Biol.*, 2002. **102**(2): 155–60.

3 Allen, L. H., Anemia and iron deficiency: effects on pregnancy outcome. *Am. J. Clin. Nutr.*, 2000. **71**(5 Suppl): 1280–4S.

4 Brabin, B. J., M. Hakimi, and D. Pelletier, An analysis of anemia and pregnancy-related maternal mortality. *J. Nutr.*, 2001. **131**(2S-2): 604–14S; discussion 614–15S.

5 Looker, A. C., *et al.*, Prevalence of iron deficiency in the United States. *Jama*, 1997. **277**(12): 973–6.

6 Schumann, K., B. Elsenhans, and A. Maurer, Iron supplementation. *J. Trace. Elem. Med. Biol.*, 1998. **12**(3): 129–40.

7 Viteri, F. E., A new concept in the control of iron deficiency: community-based preventive supplementation of at-risk groups by the weekly intake of iron supplements. *Biomed. Environ. Sci.*, 1998. **11**(1): 46–60.

8 van den Broek, N. R., *et al.*, Iron status in pregnant women: which measurements are valid? *Br. J. Haematol.*, 1998. **103**(3): 817–24.

9 Singh, K., Y. F. Fong, and S. Arulkumaran, The role of prophylactic iron supplementation in pregnancy. *Int. J. Food. Sci. Nutr.*, 1998. **49**(5): 383–9.

10 Adish, A. A., *et al.*, Risk factors for iron deficiency anaemia in preschool children in northern Ethiopia. *Public Health Nutr.*, 1999. **2**(3): 243–52.

11 Verhoeff, F. H., *et al.*, An analysis of the determinants of anaemia in pregnant women in rural Malawi–a basis for action. *Ann. Trop. Med. Parasitol.*, 1999. **93**(2): 119–33.

12 Akesson, A., *et al.*, Serum transferrin receptor: a specific marker of iron deficiency in pregnancy. *Am. J. Clin. Nutr.*, 1998. **68**(6): 1241–6.

13 Niederau, C., *et al.*, Screening for hemochromatosis and iron deficiency in employees and primary care patients in Western Germany. *Ann. Intern. Med.*, 1998. **128**(5): 337–45.

14 Blot, I., D. Diallo, and G. Tchernia, Iron deficiency in pregnancy: effects on the newborn. *Curr. Opin. Hematol.*, 1999. **6**(2): 65–70.

15 Bodnar, L. M., M. E. Cogswell, and K. S. Scanlon, Low income postpartum women are at risk of iron deficiency. *J. Nutr.*, 2002. **132**(8): 2298–302.

16 Kuizon, M. D., *et al.*, Assessment of iron status of Filipino pregnant women. *Southeast Asian J. Trop. Med. Public Health*, 1989. **20**(3): 461–70.

17 Baynes, R. D., Iron deficiency, In *Iron Metabolism in Health and Disease*, ed. J. H. Brock, 1994, W. B. Saunders: London, UK. p. 189–225.

18 Fleming, A. F., The aetiology of severe anaemia in pregnancy in Ndola, Zambia. *Ann. Trop. Med. Parasitol.*, 1989. **83**(1): 37–49.

19 Freire, W. B., Hemoglobin as a predictor of response to iron therapy and its use in screening and prevalence estimates. *Am. J. Clin. Nutr.*, 1989. **50**(6): 1442–9.

20 Strain, J. J., *et al.*, Iron sufficiency in the population of Northern Ireland: estimates from blood measurements. *Br. J. Nutr.*, 1990. **64**(1): 219–24.

21 Usanga, E. A., Iron stores of Nigerian blood donors as assessed by serum ferritin concentration. *Cent. Afr. J. Med.*, 1990. **36**(7): 170–3.

22 Yip, R., Iron deficiency: contemporary scientific issues and international programmatic approaches. *J. Nutr.*, 1994. **124**(8 Suppl): 1479–90S.

23 Yip, R., *et al.*, Declining prevalence of anemia among low-income children in the United States. *Jama*, 1987. **258**(12): 1619–23.

24 Perry, G. S., R. Yip, and C. Zyrkowski, Nutritional risk factors among low-income pregnant US women: the Centers for Disease Control and Prevention (CDC) Pregnancy Nutrition Surveillance System, 1979 through 1993. *Semin. Perinatol.*, 1995. **19**(3): 211–21.

25 Taylor, D. J., *et al.*, Effect of iron supplementation on serum ferritin levels during and after pregnancy. *Br. J. Obstet. Gynaecol.*, 1982. **89**(12): 1011–17.

26 Puolakka, J., *et al.*, Serum ferritin in the diagnosis of anemia during pregnancy. *Acta. Obstet. Gynecol. Scand. Suppl.*, 1980. **95**: 57–63.

27 Kepczyk, T., *et al.*, A prospective, multidisciplinary evaluation of premenopausal women with iron-deficiency anemia. *Am. J. Gastroenterol.*, 1999. **94**(1): 109–15.

28 Rockey, D. C., Gastrointestinal tract evaluation in patients with iron deficiency anemia. *Semin. Gastrointest. Dis.*, 1999. **10**(2): 53–64.

29 Bothwell, T. H., In *Iron Metabolism in Man*, ed. R. W. Charlton, 1979, Blackwell Scientific Publications: Oxford, UK.

30 Brittenham, G. M., Disorders or iron metabolism: iron deficiency and overload. 2nd edn. Hematology: Basic Principles and Practice, 1995, New York, NY: Churchill Livingstone. pp. 492–523.

31 Viteri, F. E., Effective iron supplementation does not happen in isolation. *Am. J. Clin. Nutr.*, 1997. **65**: 889–90.

32 Crosby, W. H., Physiology and pathophysiology of iron metabolism. *Hosp. Pract.*, (Off. Edn.)., 1991. **26** (Suppl 3): 7–10.

33 Groopman, J. E. and L. M. Itri, Chemotherapy-induced anemia in adults: incidence and treatment. *J. Natl. Cancer Inst.*, 1999. **91**: 1616–34.

34 Goodman, R. A., Current Trends-CDC criteria for anemia in children and child-bearing aged women. *MMWR Morb. Mortal Weekly Rep.*, 1989. **38**(22): 400–4.

35 Green, R., Disorders of inadequate iron. *Hosp. Pract.*, (Off. Edn)., 1991. **26** (Suppl 3): 25–9.

36 Bothwell, T. H., *et al.*, Nutritional iron requirements and food iron absorption. *J. Intern. Med.*, 1989. **226**(5): 357–65.

37 Woods, S., T. DeMarco, and M. Friedland, Iron metabolism. *Am. J. Gastroenterol.*, 1990. **85**(1): 1–8.

38 Hallberg, L., Bioavailability of dietary iron in man. *Annu. Rev. Nutr.*, 1981. **1**: 123–47.

39 Bothwell, T. H., Overview and mechanisms of iron regulation. *Nutr. Rev.*, 1995. **53**(9): 237–45.

40 Dallman, P. R., *et al.*, Influence of age on laboratory criteria in the diagnosis of iron deficiency anemia and iron deficiency in infants and children. In *Iron Nutrition in Health and Disease*, 1996: London John Libby and Co., pp. 156–170.

41 Green, R., *et al.*, Body iron excretion in man: a collaborative study. *Am. J. Med.*, 1968. **45**(3): 336–53.

42 Hallberg, L., Iron balance in pregnancy. In *Vitamins and Minerals in Pregnancy and Lactation*, ed. H. Berger, 1988, New York, NY: Raven Press, pp. 115–27.

43 Milman, N., *et al.*, Iron status and iron balance during pregnancy. A critical reappraisal of iron supplementation. *Acta Obstet. Gynecol. Scand.*, 1999. **78**(9): 749–57.

44 Kelton, J. G. and M. Cruikshank, Hematologic disorders of pregnancy. In Medical Complications During Pregnancy, 3rd edn, ed. J. Burrow. 1988, Philadelphia, PA: W. B. Saunders, pp. 65–85.

45 Lowik, M. R., *et al.*, Long-term effects of a vegetarian diet on the nutritional status of elderly people (Dutch Nutrition Surveillance System). *J. Am. Coll. Nutr.*, 1990. **9**(6): 600–9.

46 Bates, C. J., H. J. Powers, and D. I. Thurnham, Vitamins, iron, and physical work. *Lancet*, 1989. **2**(8658): 313–14.

47 Prasad, A. S., *et al.*, Zinc metabolism in patients with the syndrome of iron deficiency anemia, hepatosplenomegaly, dwarfism, and hypognadism. *J. Lab. Clin. Med.*, 1963. **61**(668): 537–49.

48 Arcasoy, A., *et al.*, Ultrastructural changes in the mucosa of the small intestine in patients with geophagia (Prasad's syndrome). *J. Pediatr. Gastroenterol. Nutr.*, 1990. **11**(2): 279–82.

49 Nishiyama, S., *et al.*, Zinc and IGF-I concentrations in pregnant women with anemia before and after supplementation with iron and/or zinc. *J. Am. Coll. Nutr.*, 1999. **18**(3): 261–7.

50 Rosenberg, E. H., Vitamin A and iron deficiency. *Nutr. Rev.* 1989. **47**(4): 119–21.

51 Mandishona, E. M., *et al.*, A traditional beverage prevents iron deficiency in African women of child bearing age. *Eur. J. Clin. Nutr.*, 1999. **53**(9): 722–5.

52 Disler, P. B., *et al.*, The effect of tea on iron absorption. *Gut*, 1975. **16**(3): 193–200.

53 Nordenberg, D., R. Yip, and N. J. Binkin, The effect of cigarette smoking on hemoglobin levels and anemia screening. *Jama*, 1990. **264**(12): 1556–9.

54 Fielding, J. E., Smoking: health effects and control (2). *N. Engl. J. Med.*, 1985. **313**(9): 555–61.

55 Stoltzfus, R. J., *et al.*, Epidemiology of iron deficiency anemia in Zanzibari schoolchildren: the importance of hookworms. *Am. J. Clin. Nutr.*, 1997. **65**(1): 153–9.

56 Kappus, K. D., *et al.*, Intestinal parasitism in the United States: update on a continuing problem. *Am. J. Trop. Med. Hyg.*, 1994. **50**(6): 705–13.

57 Steuchler, D., *Endemic Regions of Tropical Infections*, 1988, Toronto: M. H. Huber.

58 Barrett, J. F. R., P. G. Whittaker, and J. G. Williams, Absorption of non-haem iron from food during normal pregnancy. *Br. Med. J.*, 1994. **309**: 79–82.

59 Blot, I., D. Diallo, and G. Tchernia, Iron deficiency in pregnancy: effects on the newborn. *Curr. Opin. Hematol.*, 1999. **6**(2): 65–70.

60 Elwood, P. C., Evaluation of the clinical importance of anemia. *Am. J. Clin. Nutr.*, 1973. **26**(9): 958–64.

61 Gardner, G. W., *et al.*, Physical work capacity and metabolic stress in subjects with iron deficiency anemia. *Am. J. Clin. Nutr.*, 1977. **30**(6): 910–17.

62 Dallman, P. R., Iron deficiency: does it matter? *J. Intern. Med.*, 1989. **226**(5): 367–72.

63 Ohira, Y., *et al.*, Work capacity, heart rate and blood lactate responses to iron treatment. *Br. J. Haematol.*, 1979. **41**(3): 365–72.

64 Rangan, A. M., G. D. Blight, and C. W. Binns, Iron status and non-specific symptoms of female students. *J. Am. Coll. Nutr.*, 1998. **17**(4): 351–5.

65 Cook, J. D., Iron-deficiency anaemia. *Baillieres Clin. Haematol.*, 1994. **7**(4): 787–804.

66 Fowler, N. O., High cardiac output states, 5th edn. In *The Heart,* ed. J. Hurst. 1982, New York, NY: McGraw-Hill, pp. 477–90.

67 Steinkamp, I., Marathon running fails to influence RBC survival rates in iron-replete women. *Phys. Sportsmed.*, 1986. **14**: 89–92.

68 Rowland, T. W., Iron deficiency in the young athlete. *Pediatr. Clin. North Am.*, 1990. **37**(5): 1153–63.

69 Wishnitzer, R., Decreased cellularity and hemosiderin of the bone marrow in healthy and overtrained competitive distance runners. *Harefuah*, 1986. **14**: 86–92.

70 Balaban, E. P., *et al.*, The frequency of anemia and iron deficiency in the runner. *Med. Sci. Sports Exerc.*, 1989. **21**(6): 643–8.

71 de Wijn, J. F., *et al.*, Haemoglobin, packed cell volume, serum iron and iron binding capacity of selected athletes during training. *J. Sports Med. Phys. Fitness*, 1971. **11**(1): 42–51.

72 Clement, D. B. and R. C. Amundson, Nutritional intake and hematological parameters in endurance runners. *Phys. Sportsmed.*, 1982. **10**: 37–45.

73 Risser, W. L., *et al.*, Iron deficiency in female athletes: its prevalence and impact on performance. *Med. Sci. Sports Exerc.*, 1988. **20**(2): 116–21.

74 Selby, G. B., When does an athlete need iron? *Phys. Sportsmed.*, 1991. **19**: 96–105.

75 Risser, W. L., Iron deficiency in adolescents and young adults. *Phys. Sportsmed.*, 1990. **18**: 87–93.

76 Scholl, T. O., *et al.*, Anemia vs. iron deficiency: increased risk of preterm delivery in a prospective study. *Am. J. Clin. Nutr.*, 1992. **55**(5): 985–8.

77 Preziosi, P., *et al.*, Effect of iron supplementation on the iron status of pregnant women: consequences for newborns. *Am. J. Clin. Nutr.*, 1997. **66**(5): 1178–82.

78 Malhotra, M., *et al.*, Maternal and perinatal outcome in varying degrees of anemia. *Int. J. Gynaecol. Obstet.*, 2002. **79**(2): 93–100.
79 Hamalainen, H., K. Hakkarainen, and S. Heinonen, Anaemia in the first but not in the second or third trimester is a risk factor for low birth weight. *Clin. Nutr.*, 2003. **22**(3): 271–5.
80 Lozoff, B., E. Jimenez, and A. W. Wolf, Long-term developmental outcome of infants with iron deficiency. *N. Engl. J. Med.*, 1991. **325**(10): 687–94.
81 Pollitt, E., Iron deficiency and cognitive function. *Annu. Rev. Nutr.*, 1993. **13**: 521–37.
82 Idjradinata, P. and E. Pollitt, Reversal of developmental delays in iron-deficient anaemic infants treated with iron. *Lancet*, 1993. **341**(8836): 1–4.
83 Kilbride, J., *et al.*, Anaemia during pregnancy as a risk factor for iron-deficiency anaemia in infancy: a case-control study in Jordan. *Int. J. Epidemiol.*, 1999. **28**(3): 461–8.
84 Kadyrov, M., *et al.*, Increased fetoplacental angiogenesis during first trimester in anaemic women. *Lancet*, 1998. **352**(9142): 1747–9.
85 Cogswell, M. E., *et al.*, Iron supplementation during pregnancy, anemia, and birth weight: a randomized controlled trial. *Am. J. Clin. Nutr.*, 2003. **78**(4): 773–81.
86 Crosby, W. H., Pica: a compulsion caused by iron deficiency. *Br. J. Haematol.*, 1976. **34**(2): 341–2.
87 Farley, P. C. and J. Foland, Iron deficiency anemia. How to diagnose and correct. *Postgrad. Med.*, 1990. **87**(2): 89–93, 96, 101.
88 Pennington, G. R., Nuts and iron deficiency. *Med. J. Aust.* 1990. **153**: 571–2.
89 Crosby, W. H., Whatever became of chlorosis? *Jama*, 1987. **257**(20): 2799–800.
90 Dawson, A. A., *et al.*, Evaluation of diagnostic significance of certain symptoms and physical signs in anaemic patients. *Br. Med. J.*, 1969. **3**(668): 436–9.
91 Elwood, P. C., Anaemia. *Lancet*, 1974. **2**(7893): 1364–5.
92 Strobach, R. S., *et al.*, The value of the physical examination in the diagnosis of anemia. Correlation of the physical findings and the hemoglobin concentration. *Arch. Intern. Med.*, 1988. **148**(4): 831–2.
93 Osler, W., *Primary or Essential Anemia. The Principles and Practice of Medicine*, ed. W. Osler. 1908, East Norwalk, CT: Appleton and Lange, pp. 721–35.
94 Kalra, L., A. N. Hamlyn, and B. J. Jones, Blue sclerae: a common sign of iron deficiency? *Lancet*, 1986. **2**(8518): 1267–9.
95 Barton, L. L. and A. D. Friedman, Blue sclerae and iron deficiency. *Am. J. Dis. Child.*, 1990. **144**(11): 1180–1.
96 Bini, E. J., P. L. Micale, and E. H. Weinshel, Gastrointestinal endoscopy in premenopausal women with iron deficiency anemia: determination of the best diagnostic approach. *Am. J. Gastroenterol.*, 1999. **94**(6): 1715.
97 Milman, N., J. Clausen, and K. E. Byg, Iron status in 268 Danish women aged 18–30 years: influence of menstruation, contraceptive method, and iron supplementation. *Ann. Hematol.*, 1998. **77**(1–2): 13–9.
98 Geisinger, K. R., *et al.*, Endometrial adenocarcinoma. A multiparameter clinicopathologic analysis including the DNA profile and the sex steroid hormone receptors. *Cancer*, 1986. **58**(7): 1518–25.

99 Mohr, D. N., *et al.*, Asymptomatic microhematuria and urologic disease. A population-based study. *Jama*, 1986. **256**(2): 224–9.
100 Jones, R. S. and M. H. Sleisinger, Cancer of colon and rectum. In *Gastrointestinal Disease*, 2nd edn, ed. M. H. Sleisinger. 1978, Philadelphia, PA: W. B. Saunders, pp. 1785–801.
101 McPhee, S. J., The evaluation of anemia. *West J. Med.*, 1982. **137**(3): 253–7.
102 Dallman, P. R., R. Yip, and C. Johnson, Prevalence and causes of anemia in the United States, 1976 to 1980. *Am. J. Clin. Nutr.*, 1984. **39**(3): 437–45.
103 Freedman, M. L., Anemias in the elderly: physiologic or pathologic? *Hosp. Pract* (Hosp Ed)., 1982. **17**(5): 121–9, 133–6.
104 Htoo, S. H. and R. L. Koghoff, Erythrocyte parameters in the elderly: argument against new geriatric normal values. *J. Am. Gerialr. Soc.*, 1979. **27**: 547–52.
105 Lipschitz, D. A., C. O. Mitchell, and C. Thompson, The anemia of senescence. *Am. J. Hematol.*, 1981. **11**(1): 47–54.
106 Marx, J. J., Normal iron absorption and decreased red cell iron uptake in the aged. *Blood*, 1979. **53**(2): 204–11.
107 CDC, CDC criteria for anemia in chldren and childbearing -aged women. *MMWR Recomm. Rep.*, 1989. **38**: 400–04.
108 Bothwell, T. H., Iron Deficiency in Women, R. W. Charlton, ed. 1981, Washington, D.C.: The Nutrition Foundation.
109 Svanberg, B., *et al.*, Absorption of supplemental iron during pregnancy – a longitudinal study with repeated bone-marrow studies and absorption measurements. *Acta Obstet. Gynecol. Scand. Suppl.*, 1975(48): 87–108.
110 Sjostedt, J. E., *et al.*, Oral iron prophylaxis during pregnancy: a comparative study on different dosage regimens. *Acta. Obstet. Gynecol. Scand.*, 1977. **60**(Suppl.): 3–9.
111 Steer, P., *et al.*, Relation between maternal haemoglobin concentration and birth weight in different ethnic groups. *BMJ*, 1995. **310**(6978): 489–91.
112 Lu, Z. M., *et al.*, The relationship between maternal hematocrit and pregnancy outcome. *Obstet. Gynecol.*, 1991. **77**(2): 190–4.
113 Garn, S. M., *et al.*, Maternal hematologic levels and pregnancy outcomes. *Semin. Perinatol.*, 1981. **5**(2): 155–62.
114 Murphy, J. F., *et al.*, Relation of haemoglobin levels in first and second trimesters to outcome of pregnancy. *Lancet*, 1986. **1**(8488): 992–5.
115 Harris, G. J. and J. N. Simson, Causes of late diagnosis in cases of colorectal cancer seen in a district general hospital over a 2-year period. *Ann. R. Coll. Surg. Engl.*, 1998. **80**(4): 246–8.
116 Alper, B. S., R. Kimber, and A. K. Reddy, Using ferritin levels to determine iron-deficiency anemia in pregnancy. *J. Fam. Pract.*, 2000. **49**(9): 829–32.
117 Guyatt, G. H., *et al.*, Laboratory diagnosis of iron-deficiency anemia: an overview. *J. Gen. Intern. Med.*, 1992. **7**: 145–53.
118 Hallberg, L., *et al.*, Screening for iron deficiency: an analysis based on bone-marrow examinations and serum ferritin determinations in a population sample of women. *Br. J. Haematol.*, 1993. **85**(4): 787–98.
119 Allen, L. H., Pregnancy and iron deficiency: unresolved issues. *Nutr. Rev.*, 1997. **55**(4): 91–101.

120 Lipschitz, D. A., J. D. Cook, and C. A. Finch, A clinical evaluation of serum ferritin as an index of iron stores. *N. Engl. J. Med.*, 1974. **290**(22): 1213–16.

121 Madan, N., *et al.*, Monitoring oral iron therapy with protoporphyrin/heme ratios in pregnant women. *Ann. Hematol.*, 1999. **78**(6): 279–83.

122 Suominen, P., *et al.*, Serum transferrin receptor and transferrin receptor-ferritin index identify healthy subjects with subclinical iron deficits. *Blood*, 1998. **92**(8): 2934–9.

123 Breymann, C., Iron deficiency and anaemia in pregnancy: modern aspects of diagnosis and therapy. *Blood Cells Mol. Dis.*, 2002. **29**(3): 506–16.

124 Food and Nutrition Board, Folate. *Dietary reference intakes for thiamine, riboflavin, niacin, vitamin B6, folate, vitamin B12, pantothenic acid, biotin and choline/a report of the Standing Committee on the Scientific Evaluation of Dietary Reference Intakes and its Panel on Folate, Other B Vitamins, and Choline and Subcommittee on Upper Reference Levels of Nutrients, Food and Nutrition Board, Institute of Medicine*, 1998, Washington, D.C: National Academy Press, pp. 196–305.

125 Rockey, D. C., Gastrointestinal evaluation for premenopausal women with iron deficiency anemia: what is appropriate? *Am. J. Med.*, 1998. **105**(4): 356–7.

126 Bini, E. J., P. L. Micale, and E. H. Weinshel, Evaluation of the gastrointestinal tract in premenopausal women with iron deficiency anemia. *Am. J. Med.*, 1998. **105**(4): 281–6.

127 Eskeland, B., *et al.*, Iron supplementation in pregnancy: is less enough? A randomized, placebo controlled trial of low dose iron supplementation with and without heme iron. *Acta Obstet. Gynecol. Scand.*, 1997. **76**(9): 822–8.

128 Recommendations to prevent and control iron deficiency in the United States. Centers for Disease Control and Prevention. 1998. **47**: 1–29.

129 *Public Health Service: Caring for Our Future: The Content of Prenatal Care. A Report of the Public Health Expert Panel on the Content of Prenatal Care*, 1989, Washington D.C.: U.S. Department of Agriculture and U.S. Department of Health and Human Services.

130 Makrides, M., *et al.*, Efficacy and tolerability of low-dose iron supplements during pregnancy: a randomized controlled trial. *Am. J. Clin. Nutr.*, 2003. **78**(1): 145–53.

131 Anderson, S. A., *Guidelines for the Assessment and Management of Iron Deficiency in Women of Childbearing Age*, 1991, Bethesda, MD: U.S. Department of Health and Human Services, Food and Drug Administration, Center for Food Safety and Applied Nutrition.

132 Beard, J. L., Effectiveness and strategies of iron supplementation during pregnancy. *Am. J. Clin. Nutr.*, 2000. **71**(5 Suppl): 1288–94S.

133 Juarez-Vazquez, J., E. Bonizzoni, and A. Scotti, Iron plus folate is more effective than iron alone in the treatment of iron deficiency anaemia in pregnancy: a randomised, double blind clinical trial. *Bjog*, 2002. **109**(9): 1009–14.

134 Suprapto, B., Widardo, and Suhanantyo, Effect of low-dosage vitamin A and riboflavin on iron-folate supplementation in anaemic pregnant women. *Asia Pac. J. Clin. Nutr.*, 2002. **11**(4): 263–7.

135 Bashiri, A., *et al.*, Anemia during pregnancy and treatment with intravenous iron: review of the literature. *Eur. J. Obstet. Gynecol. Reprod. Biol.*, 2003. **110**(1): 2–7.

136 Bayoumeu, F., *et al.*, Iron therapy in iron deficiency anemia in pregnancy: intravenous route versus oral route. *Am. J. Obstet. Gynecol.*, 2002. **186**(3): 518–22.

137 Breymann, C., *et al.*, Efficacy and safety of intravenously administered iron sucrose with and without adjuvant recombinant human erythropoietin for the treatment of resistant iron-deficiency anemia during pregnancy. *Am. J. Obstet. Gynecol.*, 2001. **184**(4): 662–7.
138 Perewusnyk, G., *et al.*, Parenteral iron therapy in obstetrics: 8 years experience with iron-sucrose complex. *Br. J. Nutr.*, 2002. **88**(1): 3–10.
139 Sifakis, S., *et al.*, Erythropoietin in the treatment of iron deficiency anemia during pregnancy. *Gynecol. Obstet. Invest.*, 2001. **51**(3): 150–6.
140 Hatzis, T., *et al.*, The effects of recombinant human erythropoietin given immediately after delivery to women with anaemia. *Curr. Med. Res. Opin.*, 2003. **19**(4): 346–9.
141 Hoffman, A. A., *Hematology: Basic Principles and Practice*, ed. R. Hoffman. Philadelphia, PA: Elsevier Churchill Livingstone, 2000, pp. 446–85.
142 Lucock, M., Folic acid: nutritional biochemistry, molecular biology, and role in disease processes. *Mol. Genet. Metab.*, 2000. **71**(1–2): 121–38.
143 Mudd, S. H., *et al.*, The natural history of homocystinuria due to cystathionine beta-synthase deficiency. *Am. J. Hum. Genet.*, 1985. **37**(1): 1–31.
144 Kang, S. S., *et al.*, Thermolabile methylenetetrahydrofolate reductase in patients with coronary artery disease. *Metabolism*, 1988. **37**(7): 611–3.
145 Brattstrom, L., *et al.*, Common methylenetetrahydrofolate reductase gene mutation leads to hyperhomocysteinemia but not to vascular disease: the result of a meta-analysis. *Circulation*, 1998. **98**(23): 2520–6.
146 Botto, L. D. and Q. Yang, 5,10-Methylenetetrahydrofolate reductase gene variants and congenital anomalies: a HUGE review. *Am. J. Epidemiol.*, 2000. **151**(9): 862–77.
147 Guinotte, C. L., *et al.*, Methylenetetrahydrofolate reductase 677C→T variant modulates folate status response to controlled folate intakes in young women. *J. Nutr.*, 2003. **133**(5): 1272–80.
148 Silaste, M. L., *et al.*, Polymorphisms of key enzymes in homocysteine metabolism affect diet responsiveness of plasma homocysteine in healthy women. *J. Nutr.*, 2001. **131**(10): 2643–7.
149 Pullin, C. H., *et al.*, Optimization of dietary folate or low-dose folic acid supplements lower homocysteine but do not enhance endothelial function in healthy adults, irrespective of the methylenetetrahydrofolate reductase (C677T) genotype. *J. Am. Coll. Cardiol.*, 2001. **38**(7): 1799–805.
150 Lee, R. and E. P. Frenkel, Hyperhomocysteinemia and thrombosis. *Hematol. Oncol. Clin. North Am.*, 2003. **17**(1): 85–102.
151 Frenkel, E. P. and D. A. Yardley, Clinical and laboratory features and sequelae of deficiency of folic acid (folate) and vitamin B12 (cobalamin) in pregnancy and gynecology. *Hematol. Oncol. Clin. North Am.*, 2000. **14**(5): 1079–100, viii.
152 Snow, C. F., Laboratory diagnosis of vitamin B12 and folate deficiency: a guide for the primary care physician. *Arch. Intern. Med.*, 1999. **159**(12): 1289–98.
153 Pennypacker, L. C., *et al.*, High prevalence of cobalamin deficiency in elderly outpatients. *J. Am. Geriatr. Soc.*, 1992. **40**(12): 1197–204.
154 Klee, G. G., Cobalamin and folate evaluation: measurement of methylmalonic acid and homocysteine vs. vitamin B(12) and folate. *Clin. Chem.*, 2000. **46**(8 Pt 2): 1277–83.

155 Lindenbaum, J., *et al.*, Diagnosis of cobalamin deficiency: II. Relative sensitivities of serum cobalamin, methylmalonic acid, and total homocysteine concentrations. *Am. J. Hematol.*, 1990. **34**(2): 99–107.

156 Lindenbaum, J., *et al.*, Neuropsychiatric disorders caused by cobalamin deficiency in the absence of anemia or macrocytosis. *N. Engl. J. Med.*, 1988. **318**(26): 1720–8.

157 Savage, D. G., *et al.*, Sensitivity of serum methylmalonic acid and total homocysteine determinations for diagnosing cobalamin and folate deficiencies. *Am. J. Med.*, 1994. **96**(3): 239–46.

158 Baker, H., *et al.*, Vitamin profile of 563 gravidas during trimesters of pregnancy. *J. Am. Coll. Nutr.*, 2002. **21**(1): 33–7.

159 Koebnick, C., *et al.*, Longitudinal concentrations of vitamin B(12) and vitamin B(12)-binding proteins during uncomplicated pregnancy. *Clin. Chem.*, 2002. **48**(6 Pt 1): 928–33.

160 Chery, C., *et al.*, Hyperhomocysteinemia is related to a decreased blood level of vitamin B12 in the second and third trimester of normal pregnancy. *Clin. Chem. Lab. Med.*, 2002. **40**(11): 1105–8.

161 Cikot, R. J., *et al.*, Longitudinal vitamin and homocysteine levels in normal pregnancy. *Br. J. Nutr.*, 2001. **85**(1): 49–58.

162 Walker, M. C., *et al.*, Changes in homocysteine levels during normal pregnancy. *Am. J. Obstet. Gynecol.*, 1999. **180**(3 Pt 1): 660–4.

163 Murphy, M. M., *et al.*, The pregnancy-related decrease in fasting plasma homocysteine is not explained by folic acid supplementation, hemodilution, or a decrease in albumin in a longitudinal study. *Am. J. Clin. Nutr.*, 2002. **76**(3): 614–9.

164 *U.S. Department of Agriculture and U.S. Department of Health and Human Services: Nutrition and Your Health: Dietary Guidelines for Americans*, 1995, Washington, D.C.: U.S. Department of Agriculture and U.S. Department of Health and Human Services.

165 Choumenkovitch, S. F., *et al.*, Folic acid intake from fortification in United States exceeds predictions. *J. Nutr.*, 2002. **132**(9): 2792–8.

166 Quinlivan, E. P. and J. F. Gregory, 3rd, Effect of food fortification on folic acid intake in the United States. *Am. J. Clin. Nutr.*, 2003. **77**(1): 221–5.

167 Lawrence, J. M., *et al.*, Trends in serum folate after food fortification. *Lancet*, 1999. **354**(9182): 915–16.

168 Jacques, P. F., *et al.*, The effect of folic acid fortification on plasma folate and total homocysteine concentrations. *N. Engl. J. Med.*, 1999. **340**(19): 1449–54.

169 Caudill, M. A., *et al.*, Folate status in women of childbearing age residing in Southern California after folic acid fortification. *J. Am. Coll. Nutr.*, 2001. **20**(2 Suppl): 129–34.

170 Mathews, T. J., M. A. Honein, and J. D. Erickson, Spina bifida and anencephaly prevalence – United States 1991–2001. *MMWR Recomm. Rep.*, 2002. **51**(RR-13): 9–11.

171 Friso, S., *et al.*, A common mutation in the 5,10-methylenetetrahydrofolate reductase gene affects genomic DNA methylation through an interaction with folate status. *Proc. Natl. Acad. Sci. USA*, 2002. **99**(8): 5606–11.

172 Wald, N. J., *et al.*, Quantifying the effect of folic acid. *Lancet*, 2001. **358**(9298): 2069–73.

173 Honein, M. A., *et al.*, Impact of folic acid fortification of the US food supply on the occurrence of neural tube defects. *Jama*, 2001. **285**(23): 2981–6.

174 Ray, J. G. and H. J. Blom, Vitamin B12 insufficiency and the risk of fetal neural tube defects. *Qjm*, 2003. **96**(4): 289–95.

175 McMullin, M. F., *et al.*, Homocysteine and methylmalonic acid as indicators of folate and vitamin B12 deficiency in pregnancy. *Clin. Lab. Haematol.*, 2001. **23**(3): 161–5.

176 Nelen, W. L., *et al.*, Hyperhomocysteinemia and recurrent early pregnancy loss: a meta-analysis. *Fertil. Steril.*, 2000. **74**(6): 1196–9.

177 Quere, I., *et al.*, Vitamin supplementation and pregnancy outcome in women with recurrent early pregnancy loss and hyperhomocysteinemia. *Fertil. Steril.*, 2001. **75**(4): 823–5.

178 Zetterberg, H., *et al.*, Increased frequency of combined methylenetetrahydrofolate reductase C677 T and A1298 C mutated alleles in spontaneously aborted embryos. *Eur. J. Hum. Genet.*, 2002. **10**(2): 113–18.

179 Isotalo, P. A., G. A. Wells, and J. G. Donnelly, Neonatal and fetal methylenetetrahydrofolate reductase genetic polymorphisms: an examination of C677 T and A1298 C mutations. *Am. J. Hum. Genet.*, 2000. **67**(4): 986–90.

180 Gabbe, S. B., *Obstetrics – Normal and Problem Pregnancies*, S. Gabbe, ed. 2002, Philadelphia, PA: Churchill Livingstone. pp. 947–74.

181 Roberts, J. M. and D. W. Cooper, Pathogenesis and genetics of pre-eclampsia. *Lancet*, 2001. **357**(9249): 53–6.

182 Stuhlinger, M. C., *et al.*, Homocysteine impairs the nitric oxide synthase pathway: role of asymmetric dimethylarginine. *Circulation*, 2001. **104**(21): 2569–75.

183 Schlaich, M. P., *et al.*, Mildly elevated homocysteine concentrations impair endothelium dependent vasodilation in hypercholesterolemic patients. *Atherosclerosis*, 2000. **153**(2): 383–9.

184 Tawakol, A., *et al.*, Hyperhomocyst(e)inemia is associated with impaired endothelium-dependent vasodilation in humans. *Circulation*, 1997. **95**(5): 1119–21.

185 Rajkovic, A., P. M. Catalano, and M. R. Malinow, Elevated homocyst(e)ine levels with preeclampsia. *Obstet. Gynecol.*, 1997. **90**(2): 168–71.

186 Raijmakers, M. T., *et al.*, Plasma thiol status in preeclampsia. *Obstet. Gynecol.*, 2000. **95**(2): 180–4.

187 Leeda, M., *et al.*, Effects of folic acid and vitamin B6 supplementation on women with hyperhomocysteinemia and a history of preeclampsia or fetal growth restriction. *Am. J. Obstet. Gynecol.*, 1998. **179**(1): 135–9.

188 Sorensen, T. K., *et al.*, Elevated second-trimester serum homocyst(e)ine levels and subsequent risk of preeclampsia. *Gynecol. Obstet. Invest.*, 1999. **48**(2): 98–103.

189 Lachmeijer, A. M., *et al.*, Mutations in the gene for methylenetetrahydrofolate reductase, homocysteine levels, and vitamin status in women with a history of preeclampsia. *Am. J. Obstet. Gynecol.*, 2001. **184**(3): 394–402.

190 Cotter, A. M., *et al.*, Elevated plasma homocysteine in early pregnancy: a risk factor for the development of severe preeclampsia. *Am. J. Obstet. Gynecol.*, 2001. **185**(4): 781–5.

191 Cotter, A. M., *et al.*, Elevated plasma homocysteine in early pregnancy: a risk factor for the development of nonsevere preeclampsia. *Am. J. Obstet. Gynecol.*, 2003. **189**(2): 391–4; discussion 394–6.

192 Lopez-Quesada, E., M. A. Vilaseca, and J. M. Lailla, Plasma total homocysteine in uncomplicated pregnancy and in preeclampsia. *Eur. J. Obstet. Gynecol. Reprod. Biol.*, 2003. **108**(1): 45–9.

193 Sanchez, S. E., *et al.*, Plasma folate, vitamin B(12), and homocyst(e)ine concentrations in preeclamptic and normotensive Peruvian women. *Am. J. Epidemiol.*, 2001. **153**(5): 474–80.
194 Powers, R. W., *et al.*, The 677 C-T methylenetetrahydrofolate reductase mutation does not predict increased maternal homocysteine during pregnancy. *Obstet. Gynecol.*, 2003. **101**(4): 762–6.
195 Prasmusinto, D., *et al.*, The methylenetetrahydrofolate reductase 677 C→T polymorphism and preeclampsia in two populations. *Obstet. Gynecol.*, 2002. **99**(6): 1085–92.
196 O'Shaughnessy, K. M., *et al.*, Factor V Leiden and thermolabile methylenetetrahydrofolate reductase gene variants in an East Anglian preeclampsia cohort. *Hypertension*, 1999. **33**(6): 1338–41.
197 Kobashi, G., *et al.*, Absence of association between a common mutation in the methylenetetrahydrofolate reductase gene and preeclampsia in Japanese women. *Am. J. Med. Genet.*, 2000. **93**(2): 122–5.
198 Murphy, R. P., *et al.*, Prospective evaluation of the risk conferred by factor V Leiden and thermolabile methylenetetrahydrofolate reductase polymorphisms in pregnancy. *Arterioscler. Thromb. Vasc. Biol.*, 2000. **20**(1): 266–70.
199 Ray, J. G. and M. M. Mamdani, Association between folic acid food fortification and hypertension or preeclampsia in pregnancy. *Arch. Intern. Med.*, 2002. **162**(15): 1776–7.
200 de Vries, J. I., *et al.*, Hyperhomocysteinaemia and protein S deficiency in complicated pregnancies. *Br. J. Obstet. Gynaecol.*, 1997. **104**(11): 1248–54.
201 Hogg, B. B., *et al.*, Second-trimester plasma homocysteine levels and pregnancy-induced hypertension, preeclampsia, and intrauterine growth restriction. *Am. J. Obstet. Gynecol.*, 2000. **183**(4): 805–9.
202 Burke, G., *et al.*, Intrauterine growth retardation, perinatal death, and maternal homocysteine levels. *N. Engl. J. Med.*, 1992. **326**(1): 69–70.
203 Infante-Rivard, C., *et al.*, Unexpected relationship between plasma homocysteine and intrauterine growth restriction. *Clin. Chem.*, 2003. **49**(9): 1476–82.
204 O'Leary, V. B., *et al.*, MTRR and MTHFR polymorphism: link to Down syndrome? *Am. J. Med. Genet.*, 2002. **107**(2): 151–5.
205 Wenstrom, K. D., *et al.*, Association of the C677T methylenetetrahydrofolate reductase mutation and elevated homocysteine levels with congenital cardiac malformations. *Am. J. Obstet. Gynecol.*, 2001. **184**(5): 806–12; discussion 812–17.
206 Eskes, T. K., Clotting disorders and placental abruption: homocysteine – a new risk factor. *Eur. J. Obstet. Gynecol. Reprod. Biol.*, 2001. **95**(2): 206–12.
207 Lamprecht, S. A. and M. Lipkin, Chemoprevention of colon cancer by calcium, vitamin D and folate: molecular mechanisms. *Nat. Rev. Cancer*, 2003. **3**(8): 601–14.
208 Zhang, S., *et al.*, A prospective study of folate intake and the risk of breast cancer. *Jama*, 1999. **281**(17): 1632–7.
209 Rohan, T. E., *et al.*, Dietary folate consumption and breast cancer risk. *J. Natl. Cancer Inst.*, 2000. **92**(3): 266–9.
210 Feigelson, H. S., *et al.*, Alcohol, folate, methionine, and risk of incident breast cancer in the American Cancer Society Cancer Prevention Study II Nutrition Cohort. *Cancer Epidemiol. Biomarkers Prev.*, 2003. **12**(2): 161–4.

211 Sellers, T. A., *et al.*, Interaction of dietary folate intake, alcohol, and risk of hormone receptor-defined breast cancer in a prospective study of postmenopausal women. *Cancer Epidemiol. Biomarkers Prev.*, 2002. **11**(10 Pt 1): 1104–7.

212 Graham, S., *et al.*, Nutritional epidemiology of postmenopausal breast cancer in western New York. *Am. J. Epidemiol.*, 1991. **134**(6): 552–66.

213 Freudenheim, J. L., *et al.*, Premenopausal breast cancer risk and intake of vegetables, fruits, and related nutrients. *J. Natl. Cancer Inst.*, 1996. **88**(6): 340–8.

214 Potischman, N., *et al.*, Intake of food groups and associated micronutrients in relation to risk of early-stage breast cancer. *Int. J. Cancer*, 1999. **82**(3): 315–21.

215 Shrubsole, M. J., *et al.*, Dietary folate intake and breast cancer risk: results from the Shanghai Breast Cancer Study. *Cancer Res.*, 2001. **61**(19): 7136–41.

216 Sharp, L., *et al.*, Folate and breast cancer: the role of polymorphisms in methylenetetrahydrofolate reductase (MTHFR). *Cancer Lett.*, 2002. **181**(1): 65–71.

217 Semenza, J. C., *et al.*, Breast cancer risk and methylenetetrahydrofolate reductase polymorphism. *Breast Cancer Res. Treat.*, 2003. **77**(3): 217–23.

218 Langsenlehner, U., *et al.*, The common 677C>T gene polymorphism of methylenetetrahydrofolate reductase gene is not associated with breast cancer risk. *Breast Cancer Res. Treat.*, 2003. **81**(2): 169–72.

219 Zhang, S. M., *et al.*, Plasma folate, vitamin B6, vitamin B12, homocysteine, and risk of breast cancer. *J. Natl. Cancer Inst.*, 2003. **95**(5): 373–80.

220 Giovannucci, E., *et al.*, Alcohol, low-methionine–low-folate diets, and risk of colon cancer in men. *J. Natl. Cancer Inst.*, 1995. **87**(4): 265–73.

221 Giovannucci, E., *et al.*, Multivitamin use, folate, and colon cancer in women in the Nurses' Health Study. *Ann. Intern. Med.*, 1998. **129**(7): 517–24.

222 Su, L. J. and L. Arab, Nutritional status of folate and colon cancer risk: evidence from NHANES I epidemiologic follow-up study. *Ann. Epidemiol.*, 2001. **11**(1): 65–72.

223 Ma, J., *et al.*, Methylenetetrahydrofolate reductase polymorphism, dietary interactions, and risk of colorectal cancer. *Cancer Res.*, 1997. **57**(6): 1098–102.

224 Slattery, M. L., *et al.*, Methylenetetrahydrofolate reductase, diet, and risk of colon cancer. *Cancer Epidemiol. Biomarkers Prev.*, 1999. **8**(6): 513–18.

225 Chen, J., *et al.*, A methylenetetrahydrofolate reductase polymorphism and the risk of colorectal cancer. *Cancer Res.*, 1996. **56**(21): 4862–4.

226 Eichholzer, M., *et al.*, Folate and the risk of colorectal, breast and cervix cancer: the epidemiological evidence. *Swiss Med. Wkly*, 2001. **131**(37–38): 539–49.

227 Shen, H., *et al.*, Dietary folate intake and lung cancer risk in former smokers: a case-control analysis. *Cancer Epidemiol. Biomarkers Prev.*, 2003. **12**(10): 980–6.

228 Heijmans, B. T., *et al.*, A common variant of the methylenetetrahydrofolate reductase gene (1p36) is associated with an increased risk of cancer. *Cancer Res.*, 2003. **63**(6): 1249–53.

229 Jatoi, A., *et al.*, Folate status among patients with non-small cell lung cancer: a case-control study. *J. Surg. Oncol.*, 2001. **77**(4): 247–52.

230 Bandera, E. V., *et al.*, Diet and alcohol consumption and lung cancer risk in the New York State Cohort (United States). *Cancer Causes Control*, 1997. **8**(6): 828–40.

231 Erickson, J. D., Mulinare, J., Yang, Q. n., CDC. Folate status in women of childbearing age-United States. *MMWR*, 2000; **49**, 962–5.

232 Malinow, M. R., *et al.*, The effects of folic acid supplementation on plasma total homocysteine are modulated by multivitamin use and methylenetetrahydrofolate reductase genotypes. *Arterioscler. Thromb. Vasc. Biol.*, 1997. **17**(6): 1157–62.

233 Woodside, J. V., *et al.*, Effect of B-group vitamins and antioxidant vitamins on hyperhomocysteinemia: a double-blind, randomized, factorial-design, controlled trial. *Am. J. Clin. Nutr.*, 1998. **67**(5): 858–66.

234 Sifakis, S., *et al.*, Erythropoietin in the treatment of iron deficiency anemia during pregnancy. *Gynecol. Obstet. Invest.*, 2001; **51**: 150–6.

10

Thrombosis prophylaxis and risk factors for thrombosis in gynecologic oncology

Georg-Friedrich von Tempelhoff, M.D., F.A.C.T.H.

Specialist in Gynecology and Obstetrics, Department of Obstetrics and Gynecology, GP Rüsselsheim, Teaching Hospital of the Johannes Gutenberg-University Main 2, Rüsselsheim, Germany

Introduction

Malignancy is an independent risk factor for the development of venous thrombosis (VT)[1] and the latter belongs to the most common and life-threatening complications in patients with gynecological malignancy. Most thrombotic complications are recognized while patients undergo cancer treatment. Breast cancer patients under observation were found to experience VT in 0 to 3% compared to an overall incidence per year of about 0.3% in women. Incidence of VT does not exceed 1.5% following surgery for breast cancer, irrespectively of whether patients had radical or breast conserving surgery.[2,3] VT occurs in about 1 out of 5 patients after Wertheim – Meigs surgery for cervical and endometrial cancer despite receiving thrombosis prophylaxis[2,4,5] and every 4th patient with ovarian malignancy is confronted with VT during the time of primary treatment (surgery and first-line chemotherapy).[6,7,8] According to a statement by the *Subcommittee Thrombosis and Haemostasis in Malignancy* of the *International Society on Thrombosis and Haemostasis (ISTH)* a 5% incidence of VT can be expected in the course of adjuvant chemotherapy for breast cancer,[9] which is of concern since most breast cancer patients will receive adjuvant chemotherapy. According to the *American Cancer Society (ACS)*[10] estimates for 2004, 217,000 new cases of invasive breast cancer, 50,840 cases of uterine cancer and 25,580 cases of ovarian cancer will be diagnosed in the United States. Thus some 13,000 patients (6%) with breast cancer, 10,000 patients with uterine malignancy, and 6,300 women with ovarian cancer will develop thrombosis within the first year after diagnosis of cancer. Despite the widespread acceptance of the increased risk for VT in cancer patients, among physicians, a lack of confidence exist when, how, and how long a cancer patient should receive prophylaxis during the course of cancer disease. This discrepancy may be in part explained by the lack of uniform – or to be precise – adequate and negotiable guidelines/

Hematological Complications in Obstetrics, Pregnancy, and Gynecology, ed. R. L. Bick *et al.* Published by Cambridge University Press.

recommendations for VT prophylaxis apart from surgical interventions. Moreover, valid data on the incidence of VT within a particular type of cancer and apart from the surgical period are rare or even absent. Symptomatic VT is an infrequent event, even in thrombosis prophylaxis or prevention trials thus the overall VT rate is low as long as screening procedures are not applied.[11] In a Pan-European trial of the *European Organisation for Research and Treatment of Cancer* (EORTC –55962) a 3% rate of symptomatic VT was recently reported after radical hysterectomy for uterine cancer.[12] In a meta-analysis the incidence after uterine cancer surgery was more than 6 times higher (118/600; 19.6%) when VT screening was performed.[13] Early discharge from hospital after surgery and the increasing outpatient management, e.g. during adjuvant and second-line chemotherapy, reduces patients' surveillance, thus clinical manifestation of VT often is misinterpreted or remains unrecognized. As a result the true incidence of thrombotic complications likewise is dramatically underestimated in the course of malignant disease, which is supported by the high rate of previously undiagnosed thrombotic events in cancer patients that are found in autopsy studies.[14]

The clinical importance of asymptomatic thrombosis has been a matter of discussion for many years but such interpretations are interrogative and should always consider the potential risk of thrombus embolization and of post thrombotic syndrome that further confines life-quality in a cancer patient.

Risk factors for VT in gynecologic malignancy

Development of thrombosis in malignancy is the result of multiple conditions that commonly coincide in a cancer patient. Apart from the surgery, systemic cancer treatment is an independent risk factor for VT in patients.[3] For individual risk assessment, predisposing and temporary risk factors must be defined and their cumulative appearance should guide the decision for VT prophylaxis also apart from the surgical period. A risk-assessed model (RAM) with defined risk categories has been designed in an international collaboration of experts[15] (Table 10.1). Although such RAM seems useful, especially in hospitalized patients, during clinical workaday in many patients it is difficult or even impossible to assign them to an equivocal risk category. Predisposing factors, which include the patient's history, e.g. previous VT, known hereditary or acquired thrombophilia, co morbidity, or higher age of patient, can be obtained relatively easily. The number of temporary risk factors is extensive and – most important – dynamic, which often necessitates reevaluation of the overall risk in a cancer patient. Metastatic disease in particular is a predisposing factor for VT since co morbidity rises and according to RAM in such patients prophylaxis is indicated.

Table 10.1 Experts' recommendation for indication of thrombosis prophylaxis application in non-surgical patients according to a risk-assessed model (RAM) introduced at the VTE meeting in Lisbon, November 2003.

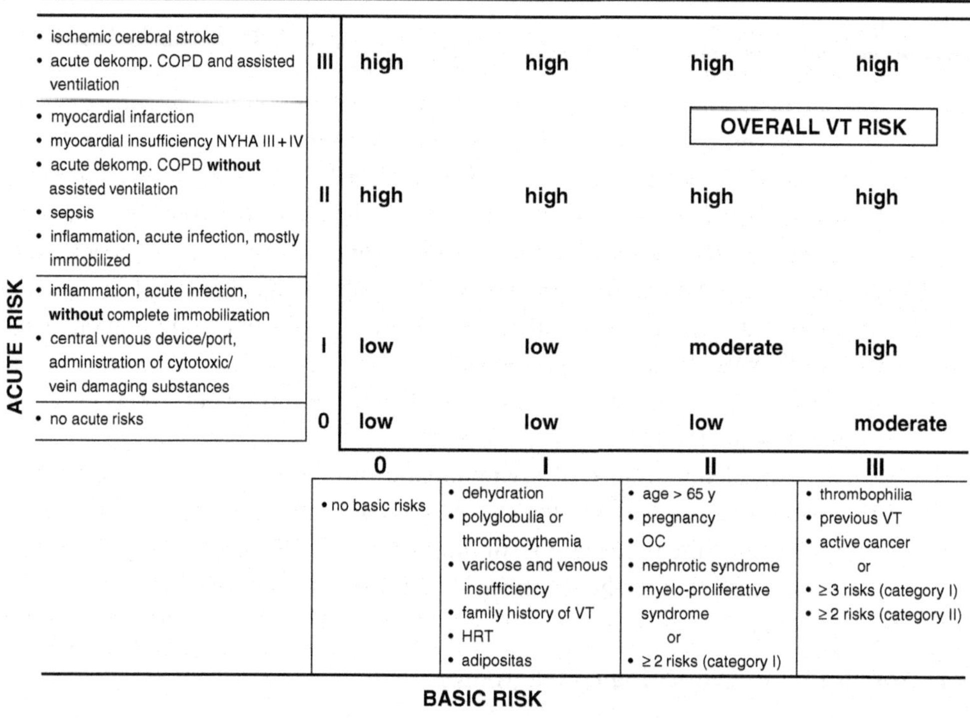

OVERALL VT RISK

ACUTE RISK		BASIC RISK 0	BASIC RISK I	BASIC RISK II	BASIC RISK III
• ischemic cerebral stroke • acute dekomp. COPD and assisted ventilation	III	high	high	high	high
• myocardial infarction • myocardial insufficiency NYHA III + IV • acute dekomp. COPD **without** assisted ventilation • sepsis • inflammation, acute infection, mostly immobilized	II	high	high	high	high
• inflammation, acute infection, **without** complete immobilization • central venous device/port, administration of cytotoxic/ vein damaging substances	I	low	low	moderate	high
• no acute risks	0	low	low	low	moderate
		0	I	II	III
BASIC RISK		• no basic risks	• dehydration • polyglobulia or thrombocythemia • varicose and venous insufficiency • family history of VT • HRT • adipositas	• age > 65 y • pregnancy • OC • nephrotic syndrome • myelo-proliferative syndrome or • ≥ 2 risks (category I)	• thrombophilia • previous VT • active cancer or • ≥ 3 risks (category I) • ≥ 2 risks (category II)

Source: Venous Thrombosis Experts meeting (VTE), Lisbon, November 2nd–4th 2003.

There is a significant correlation between a rising age of patient and the risk of VT after surgery.[16] The relative risk for postoperative VT, when compared with an age below, is 4-fold higher over an age of 19 years, is 12 fold increased at the age over 39 years and 35-fold increased when the age is more than 60 years.[17] In healthy individuals, an age over 60 years represents a permanent risk factor for post-operative VT through accumulation of physiological changes in the elderly. These include low-grade coagulation activation accompanied by reduced fibrinolytic activity and a higher prevalence of atheriosclerotic changes with impaired endothelial anticoagulant properties, as well as insufficient venous valve function that is associated with reduced blood flow.[18] The latter is further negatively influenced by a set of rheological changes triggered by an increase in fibrinogen turn over, higher plasma viscosity, and an increased erythrocyte rigidity and – aggregation.[19] Thus impairment of all three cornerstones of the Virchow – Trias

Table 10.2 Risk categories for VT in surgical patients.[20]

Risk	Low	Moderate	High	Very high
Localization of VT	uncomplicated surgery, age <40 y, no additional risk factors	abdominal and vaginal surgery age >40 y, no additional risk factors	abdominal and vaginal surgery age >40 y, additional risk factors	abdominal and vaginal cancer surgery, age >60 y
Distal VT (%)	2	10–20	20–40	40–80
Proximal VT (%)	0.4	2–4	4–8	10–20
Symptomatic PE (%)	0.2	1–2	2–4	4–10

tend to the worse with an increasing age. Accordingly the patient's age is a major stratifying determinant within the risk categories, that have been developed by the *European Consensus Conference*[20] in surgical patients that also apply to gynecologic/surgical patients (Table 10.2).

Immobilization, e.g. bed-rest prior to surgery predisposes to venous stasis and thus to VT. The role of an increased BMI (>24 kg/m^2) for the development of VT is a point at issue. Hormonal replacement therapy in a postmenopausal woman may not increase the risk for thrombosis during surgery.[21] While hormonal replacement therapy (HRT) in a postmenopausal woman may not increase the risk for thrombosis during surgery[21] the Women's Health Initiative trial[109] found a two- to three-fold higher rate of VT in patients receiving HRT continuous and daily as compared to women that were given placebo (HR 2.11; 95% CI: 1.58–2.82) during an average follow up of 5.6 years. Moreover the presence of factor V Leiden mutation nearly six-fold increased the risk for VT during HRT.[110] However, a history of primary thrombosis, e.g. one that occurred during hormonal contraception, is associated with a higher risk of recurrence. During surgery the duration of anesthesia and the extend of surgical intervention are important determinants for the risk of postoperative VT, whereas general anesthesia particularly for more than 5 h carries a higher risk as compared to segmental spine anesthesia. Extent of pelvic lymphadenectomy at surgical staging for uterine cancer is an independent risk factor for the occurrence of postoperative complications including VT. In a recent study, according to multiple logistic regression, removal of more than 14 nodes was the only condition associated with at least one postoperative complication ($OR = 2.56$, $P < 0.01$), while removal of more than 19 nodes ($OR = 9.7$, $P < 0.01$) was the only variable significantly associated with the development of two postoperative complications.[22] A time-interval of less than 30 days between two surgical interventions further increases the risk for VT.[23]

In malignancy the presence of hemostaseological and hemorheological defects in addition to cancer induced hypercoagulability predisposed to thrombosis. Acquired defects include inhibitor deficiency[24] and hypofibrinolysis[25] that occur during chemotherapy, functional resistance to activated Protein C (APC),[26,27] and high antiphospholipid antibody titres[28] that may not develop for the course of cancer disease.[29] Genetically determined hemostaseologic risk-factors of VT include gene-mutation of factor V (Leiden), factor II (prothrombin G20210A), thrombomodulin, methyl-tetrahydrofolate-reductase (MTHFR), or 4G5G polymorphism of the plasminogen activator inhibitor-1 (PAI-1) gene, whereas factor V mutation is present in about 11 to 20% of all patients with VT[30] and factor II mutation, that is found in about 5 to 10% of patients with VT[31], has been shown to increases the risk of VT 3.8-fold.[32] However, their contribution to the pathogenesis of VT in malignancy apart from catheter-related thrombosis is less studied and may be of secondary importance.[27,33,34] Finally, the common presence of hyper viscosity – a syndrome, that is caused by high cellular concentrations in myelo-proliferative malignancy, e.g. polycythemia Vera, and hematocrit independent with high plasma viscosity in patients with solid tumors,[35] is a risk-factor for VT.[36,37,38]

VT during gynecologic cancer surgery

Surgery for malignant compared to benign gynecologic diseases is associated with a three-fold higher VT incidence. In a set of ten trials without prophylaxis and a comparable study design, VT incidence postoperatively was assessed in patients who had surgery for benign and malignant gynecologic diseases (Table 10.3). The rate was 13.4% (n = 78) in 579 patients confirmed by fibrinogen up-take test after

Table 10.3 VT in patients undergoing gynecologic surgery without prophylaxis.

	Number of patients (N)	Incidence of VT%	Incidence of PE%
Bonnar & Walsh, *Lancet ii, 1972*	140	15	0.7
Ballard *et al., Obstet. Gynecol. Brit. Cwlth., 1973*	55	29	0
Walsh *et al., Obstet. Gynecol. Brit. Cwlth., 1974*	262	14	2.7
Taberner *et al., BMJ, 1988*	49	23	0
Adolf *et al., Gynäkol. Geb. Frauenhlk., 1978*	75	29	0
Clarke-Pearson *et al., Am. J. Obstet. Gynecol., 1983*	97	12.4	1
Clarke-Pearson *et al., Gynecol. Oncol., 1984*	382	12.4	1.3
Clarke-Pearson *et al., Obstet. Gynecol., 1984*	12	34.6	1.9
Turner and Brookes, *Brit. J. Obstet. Gynec., 1984*	92	4.3	0
Clarke-Pearson *et al., Obstet. Gynecol., 1990*	103	18.4	0

Table 10.4 VT incidence after different prophylactic methods in patients undergoing general surgery.

	Trials (n)	Absolute VT incidence postoperatively (n)	Relative VT incidence postoperatively (%)	95% CI
Without prophylaxis	54	1,084/4,310	25	24–27
Aspirin	5	372/76	20	16–25
Elastic stockings	3	196/28	14	10–20
UFH*	47	10,339/784	8	7–8
NMH	21	9,364/595	6	6–7
IPC	2	132/4	3	1–8

*UFH: unfractionated heparin; LMWH: low molecular weight heparin; IPC: intermit. pneumat. compression.

Source: Pooled data from randomized trials (published at the *VIth ACCP Consensus Conference on Antithrombotic Therapy*).[96]

vaginal and abdominal hysterectomy for benign pathology and was 20.3% (n = 78) in 384 patients after cancer surgery. In an early trial by Walsh and colleagues from 1974,[39] 26% of patients after the Wertheim-Meigs operation and 45% after ovarian and vulva cancer surgery developed VT postoperatively. In 1987, Clarke-Pearson and colleagues reported a mean incidence of 12% after abdominal hysterectomy for non-malignant indication and after ovarian cancer surgery, while 16% of patients undergoing Wertheim surgery, 23% after surgery for endometrial cancer, 32% after radical vulvectomy, and 88% of patients who had exenterating surgery, had VT postoperatively.[40]

In general surgery the use of aspirin for thrombosis prophylaxis had little effect on the incidence of VT when compared to that of patients without prophylaxis (Table 10.4). In 1980 the use of Dextran for thrombosis prophylaxis in a small study of gynecologic cancer patients was rather disappointing since 28.0% of patients developed VT postoperatively.[41] A review of studies in which different prophylactic methods were randomly tested against placebo or no prophylaxis in gynecologic patients undergoing cancer surgery (**UFH**: unfractionated heparin, **LMWH**: low molecular weight heparin, **IPC**: intermittent pneumatic compression or **EC**: graduated elastic compression), the rate was between 4.9% (LMWH) and 11.5% (ICE) postoperatively and thus significantly lower as compared to a rate of 20.0% in patients who randomly received no prophylaxis (Figure 10.1). In 1,225 patients who had vaginal and abdominal operations for non-oncologic indication VT incidence was 5.4% (n = 66) postoperatively, whereas thrombosis screening in 966 women revealed a mean incidence of 14.6% (n = 141) after surgery for genital cancer. Most of detected VT were located in the calf veins (~17.0%), while ~2.0%

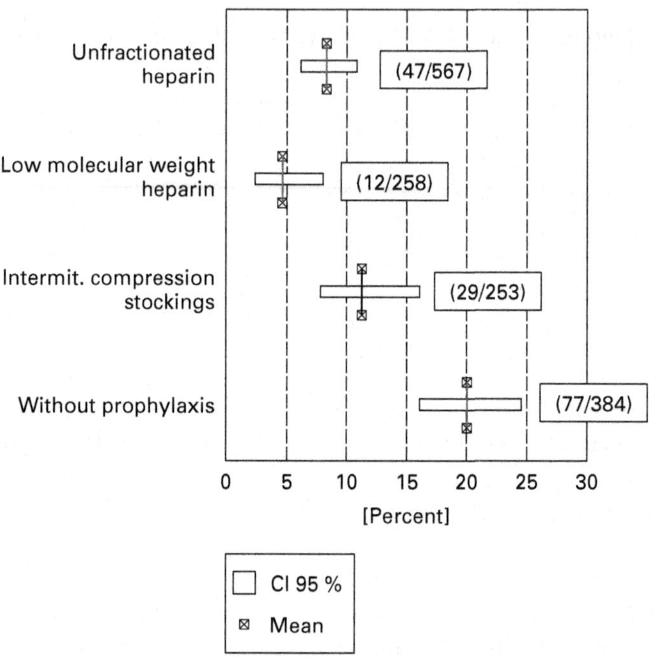

Figure 10.1 Thrombosis incidences (95 confidence interval) after different prophylactic methods in gynecologic patients undergoing cancer surgery.

were found in the proximal veins. Among these, earlier trials used fibrinogen up-take test for screening and diagnosing VT, which offers a lower sensitivity for the detection of thrombi in the femoral and pelvic veins. Thus the estimated rate of proximal VT likely is underestimated. This is supported by trials that used phlebography for VT screening and found more proximal VT than calf vein thrombosis.[42,43] Ovarian cancer patients had the lowest incidence of VT (6.3%) after standard abdominal surgery, while the "Wertheim" operation (radical hysterectomy plus extended retroperitoneal lymphadenectomy) for cervix or uterine cancer was followed by a VT rate of 19.5% and 19.9% respectively (Figure 10.2).[13] In these trials thrombosis prophylaxis was given up to day 7–10 postoperatively which might be too short since 8.3% of ovarian cancer patients developed late thrombotic complications thereafter while no prophylaxis was given.[6] White and colleagues retrospectively investigated the early and late incidence of symptomatic VT after surgery in patients that were recorded in the *California Patient Discharge Data Set* from 1992–96. ICD-9-CM (*International Classification of Disease, 9th Revision Clinical Modification*) numbers associated with thrombosis were identified and the incidence of VT during stay in hospital as well as after discharge until day 91 postoperatively was calculated in 1,653,275 patients with and without cancer that previously had surgery (Table 10.5). VT incidence was 1.28% (n = 244)

Table 10.5 Incidence of symptomatic VT within 91 days of surgery before and after discharge from hospital in patients with and without cancer. The numbers of patients with thrombosis are shown and the rate (%) is calculated accordingly.[44]

	Patients without cancer		Cancer patients	
	VT incidence upto day 91 postoperatively [N (%)]	VT incidence **after discharge** upto day 91 postoperatively [N (%)]	VT incidence upto day 91 postoperatively [N (%)]	VT incidence **after discharge** upto day 91 postoperatively [N (%)]
Neurosurgery	395/0.83	0.51	215/3.21	2.47
Head/neck surgery	25/0.10	0.06	144/0.83	0.43
Thoracic surgery	1,806/0.68	0.39	654/1.00	0.61
Gastrointestinal surgery	1,177/0.38	0.20	988/1.77	0.81
Urologic surgery	319/0.34	0.23	814/1.30	0.76
Gynecologic surgery	402/0.25	0.19	244/1.28	0.74
Orthopedic surgery	4,689/1.30	0.96	324/2.49	1.38

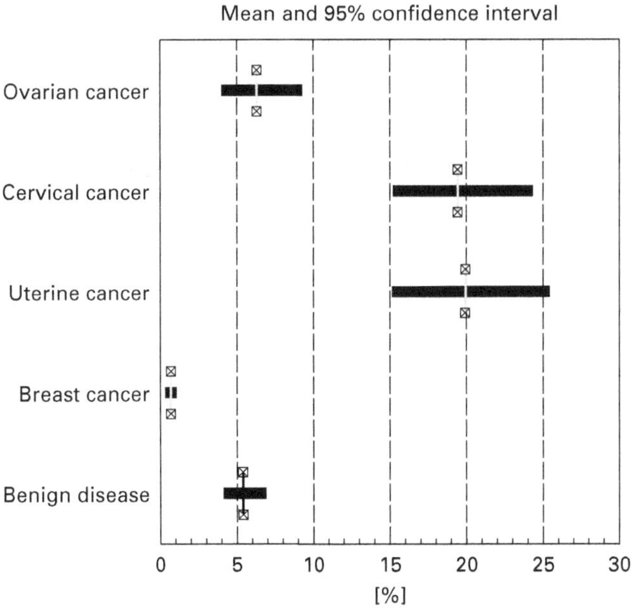

Figure 10.2 Postoperative VT in gynecologic cancer patients who received prophylaxis (ovarian cancer: 23/366; cervical cancer: 64/329; uterine cancer: 54/271; breast cancer: 12/1,717) and in patients with benign gynecologic disease (66/1,225). Meta-analysis including 13 trials.

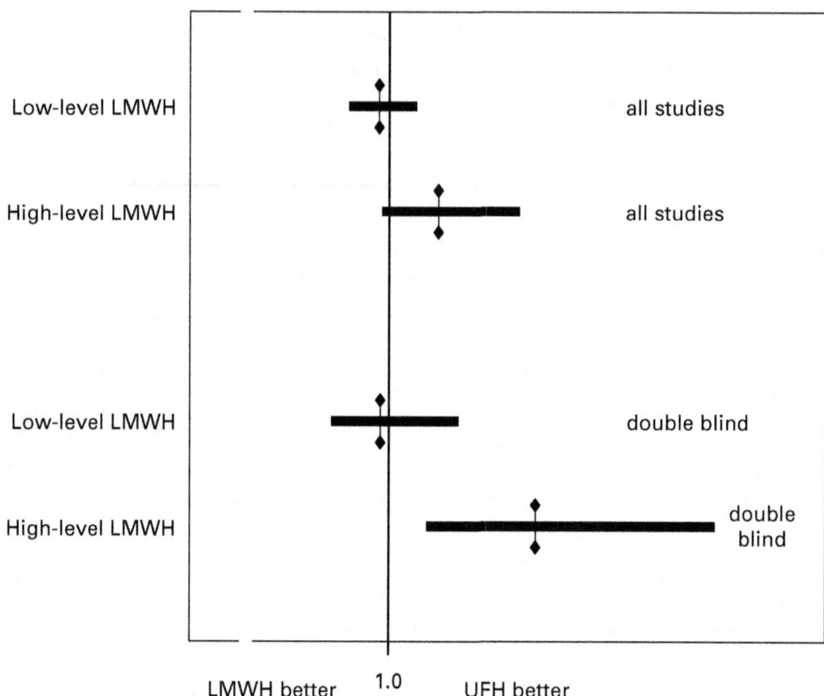

Figure 10.3 Odds-Ratio (95 CI) of wound hematoma after low and high doses of LMWH and after low-dose heparin (UFH). Meta-analysis by Kakkar.[50]

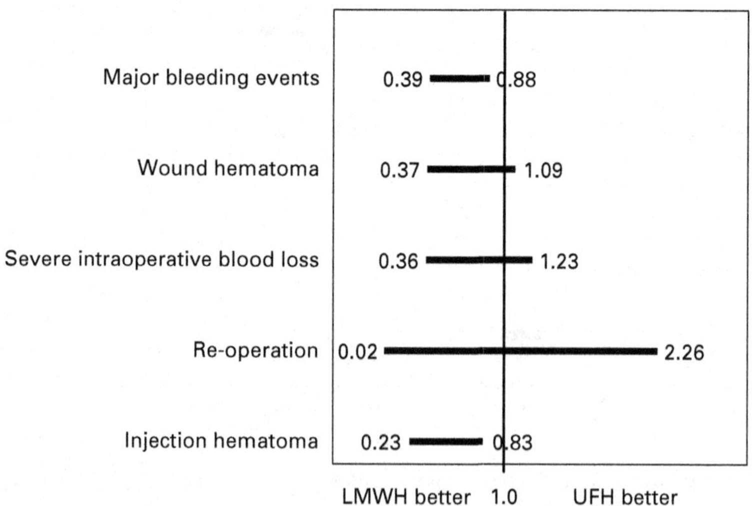

Figure 10.4 Odds-Ratio (95% CI) of major bleeding complications after gynecologic cancer surgery.

within 3 months after surgery in a total of 19,006 women with gynecologic cancer, whereas more than half of these events (n = 141; 57.8%) occurred after discharge from hospital.[44] Extending the time of postoperative heparin prophylaxis may reduce the high rate of late VT in gynecologic cancer patients, which is supported by the results of the Enoxacan II trial. Continuation of VT prophylaxis (Enoxaparin 40 mg/d s.c.) after cancer surgery for a total of 4 weeks (n = 165) was associated with a 60% risk reduction for the development of VT within 28 days after surgery, whereas the incidence of phlebographically confirmed VT (n = 9; 5.5%) was significantly lower as compared to cancer patients receiving placebo (23/167; 13.3%; $p = 0.01$).[11]

In women undergoing radical pelvic surgery of the highly vascularized retroperitonal area for treatment of genital cancer the risk of severe bleeding complications may be higher as compared to that during general surgery.[45] However, the introduction of *low-dose heparin* prophylaxis during gynecologic cancer surgery seemed not to potentiate the risk for hemorrhagic diathesis in patients.[46] Changes in homeostasis that trigger the risk for VT in the elderly may also admit responsibility for a lower risk of bleeding associated with the use of anticoagulants for VT prophylaxis. After thrombosis prophylaxis with Nadroparin (once 0.3 ml/d) during general surgery including gynecologic cancer surgery a patient's age > 60 y was associated with a 67% risk reduction for the development of wound hematoma (n = 9; 2.0%) as compared to younger patients (n = 27; 5.8%; $p < 0.01$).[45] Studies comparing LMWH and UFH prophylaxis during cancer surgery including gynecologic patients found similar or better safety after LMWH prophylaxis while efficacy was comparable.[47,48,49] In 1995 a meta-analysis performed by Kakkar and colleagues found a lower risk of bleeding after LMWH compared to UFH prophylaxis postoperatively.[50] However, higher doses of LMWH in randomized trials had significantly higher rate of wound hematoma as compared to low-dose heparin prophylaxis (UFH) (Figure 10.3). The lower rate of minor hemorrhagic complications after LMWH prophylaxis as compared to UFH may be due to reduced inhibition of platelet aggregation. In a double blind randomized trial in patients undergoing gynecologic cancer surgery,[2] incidence of major bleeding events and the number of necessary blood transfusions were statistically significantly lower after Certoparin prophylaxis (Novartis AG – once daily 3,000 anti Xa Units) as shown in Figure 10.4.

VT during radiotherapy

Reviewing the charts of one gynecologic institution, 81 women with genital cancer and an episode of VT were identified within a 10 year period (1984–95) by Morgan and colleagues.[51] Most thrombotic complications were diagnosed within 3 months of radiation (43% 32/81), while 38% (n = 28) occurred postoperatively and

24% (n = 25) during chemotherapy. Although no conclusion on the incidence of VT during radiotherapy can be drawn from these data, the distribution of their occurrence is surprising. Prior to the introduction of HDR-AL techniques (high dose rate after loading) using ^{192}IR, VT was a substantial complication during intra vaginal/uterine radium therapy, which needs several hours to days. In 1962 an incidence of symptomatic VT of 2.5% within 48 h after 2,540 intra vaginal/uterine radium applications without prophylaxis was found, whereas PE occurred in 0.6% and 0.1% had lethal PE.[52] In 347 gynecologic cancer patients the risk for postoperative VT was significantly increased when radiotherapy had preceded surgery (RR = 1.108; $p < 0.05$).[5] In the recent literature there is little information on the role of VT in gynecologic cancer patients undergoing radiotherapy. Among 132 gynecologic patients with endometrial cancer who received oral anticoagulation (Cumarin INR: 2.0–3.5) during pre- or postoperative radiotherapy Graf and colleagues[53] found a VT incidence of 6.8% and an incidence of non-lethal PE of 3.8%, while in 5.3% bleeding complications occurred. In a subsequent study,[54] 136 uterine cancer patients either received low molecular weight heparin (LMWH; once 5,000 anti Xa/die s.c. Fragmin), or an oral anticoagulant (acenocoumarol, Sintron INR: 2.0–3.5) during primary or post surgery radiotherapy. The incidence of non-lethal PE was 5.9% in the LMWH group vs. 5.8% in the oral anticoagulant prophylaxis group. Bleeding complications occurred in 1.5% in the LMWH group and in 2.9% while receiving oral anticoagulants. In a study by Kemkes-Matthes from 1995[55] a 10 to 30 minute HDR-AL therapy was not associated with an increase in coagulation activation after 6 or 24 h as indicated by normal and – compared to the pre-treatment values – unchanged levels of thrombin–antithrombin complexes, d-dimer, and prothrombin 1 + 2. Symptoms of VT were observed in none of the patients and the authors concluded that prophylaxis is not recommended during HDR-AL therapy. In a recent trial 37 women with uterine cancer received 4 cycles of postoperative HDR-AL therapy that was given weekly. No routine VT prophylaxis was applied. Tests performed before each radiation session neither revealed coagulation activation nor reduced fibrinolytic response or changes in blood rheology in the course of treatment. Non-invasive VT screening took place at the same times but revealed no episodes of VT.[56]

VT during chemotherapy

In literature the reported incidences of clinical VT in breast cancer patients undergoing adjuvant chemotherapy excluding catheter-related VT is about 5%[9] and was twice as high upon screening for VT.[25] A systematic review[57] found 6 studies in which a total of 3,101 patients received adjuvant non-hormonal chemotherapy for breast cancer whereas the incidence of VT in these trials was between 1.3% and 10% (mean 4.5%). Most of them used CMF therapy (cyclophosphamide, methotrexate, 5-fluorouacil) and the average mean VT incidence was 4.2% compared to 4.8% when anthracycline regimens were given. In 4 studies chemotherapy for advanced stage disease in 444 breast cancer patients was associated with an average mean VT incidence of 9.8%.

During adjuvant tamoxifen/chemotherapy for breast cancer in 4 trials ($n = 1{,}102$) an average mean VT incidence of 4.8% (range of means: 3.1% to 9.3%) was recorded, which is more than twice as high as compared to the average mean rate of 1.7% (range of means: 0 to 5.6%) found in 8 studies during adjuvant tamoxifen mono therapy based on a total of 3,184 patients. Tamoxifen or toremifen mono therapy for metastatic breast cancer in 3,370 patients from 5 studies revealed comparable rate for VT (average mean VT incidence 2.1%; range of means: 0.8% to 3.2%) as seen after adjuvant tamoxifen mono therapy. Data from the *International Breast Cancer Intervention Study (IBIS-I) trial* revealed significantly higher risk for VT in those who received tamoxifen in a chemopreventive setting as compared to women from a matched control group not receiving tamoxifen (OR, 4.7; 95% CI, 2.2 to 10.1).[58] Interestingly, a trial by the *Stockholm Breast Cancer Study Group*[59] found no significant differences in the incidence of hospital admissions due to VT in 2,365 postmenopausal breast cancer patients who were randomly assigned to either adjuvant tamoxifen treatment (49/1,188; 4.1%) or no hormonal therapy (45/1,177; 3.8%; HR: 1.06; CI 95%: 0.71–1.6; $p > 0.05$). During MPA (medroxy-progesterone acetate) mono therapy at a dose of 500–1,200 mg/d in 6 studies including 1,225 patients with advanced stage breast cancer, the reported VT incidence was between 0.9% to 14.5% (mean: 4.1%) compared to 4.1% (range of means: 3.5% to 4.7%) in 407 patients from 4 studies receiving megestrol acetate (MA). Treatment regimens with Taxane, which is a new antineoplastic substance obtained from extracts of yew tree, have become the standard in advanced breast cancer, whereas an 11% incidence of clinical VT occurred during 6 cycles of docetaxel and estramustine phosphate combination therapy in 36 women.[60] In 2 trials of 130 ovarian cancer patients receiving platinum based chemotherapy VT incidence was 10.6% and 12.0% respectively (Table 10.6).[7,61]

A search for hemostaseological and hemorheological changes associated with different antineoplastic substances was performed in a number of trials among which CMF-regimens were best studied in breast cancer. Patients receiving CMF chemotherapy show a temporary reduction in protein C and S activity/antigen levels soon after the 1st cycle,[62,24] which possibly is caused by methotrexate induced inhibition of tetrahydrofolate-dependent protein synthesis, e.g. nucleic acids, pyrimidine, and purine. The reduction of coagulation inhibitors is

Table 10.6 Systematic review – trials on the incidence of chemo/hormonal therapy related VT in breast cancer patients.[57]

Cytostatika regimens	Authors	TNM	Patients (n)	Arterial thrombosis n (%)	VT n (%)
Cyclophosphamide	R. Weiss *Cancer Treat. Rep., 1981*; ***65:*** *677–9*	$T_{1–4}\,N_{0–2}\,M_0$	433	–	22 (5.1%)
Methotrexate	T. Saphner *J. Clin. Oncol., 1991*; ***9:*** *286–94*	$T_{1–4}\,N_{0–2}\,M_0$	603	0	9 (1.5%)
Fluorouacil (CMF) without hormonal substances	M. N. Levine *N. Engl. J. Med., 1988*; ***318:*** *404–7*	$T_{1–2}\,N_{0–1}\,M_0$	102	–	9 (8.8%)
	S. E. Rifkin *J. Clin. Oncol., 1994*; ***12:*** *2078–85*	$T_{1–3}\,N_{0–2}\,M_0$	300	0	4 (1.3%)
	M. N. Levine *Lancet, 1994*; ***343:*** *886–9*	$T_{1–4}\,N_{0–2}\,M_1$	159	0	7 (4.4%)
	A. Falanga *Thromb. Haemost., 1998*; ***79:*** *23–7*	$T_{1–4}\,N_{0–2}\,M_1$	16	0	2 (12.5%)
	L. Goodnough *Cancer, 1984*; ***54:*** *1264–8*	$T_{1–4}\,N_{0–2}\,M_1$	159	4 (2.5%)	20 (12.6%)
	A. Manni *Cancer Treat. Rep., 1980*; ***64:*** *111–16*	$T_{1–4}\,N_{0–2}\,M_1$	110	–	11 (10.0%)
Anthracycline	J. G. Wall *Am. J. Med., 1989*; ***87:*** *501–4*	$T_{1–2}\,N_{0–1}\,M_0$	901	7 (0.8%)	–
Adriamycin	J. G. Wall *Am. J. Med., 1989*; ***87:*** *501–4*	$T_{1–4}\,N_{0–2}\,M_0$	113	6 (5.3%)	–
Epirubicin	P. C. Clahsen *J. Clin. Oncol., 1994*; ***12:*** *1266–71*	$T_{1–4}\,N_{0–2}\,M_0$	1,292	0	27 (2.1%)

Cyclophosphamide	v.Tempelhoff *J. Clin. Oncol.*, *1996*; ***14:*** *2560–8*	T_{1-4} N_{0-2} M_0	50	0	5 (10.0%)
(AC, EC)	T. Saphner *J. Clin. Oncol.*, *1991*; ***9:*** *286–94*	T_{1-4} N_{0-2} M_0	321	1 (0.3%)	8 (2.4%)
Taxane regimens docetaxel	S. E. Soule *Ann. Oncol.*, *2002*; ***13:*** *1612–5*	T_{1-4} N_{0-2} M_1	36	–	4 (11.1)
Combination regimens	K. I. Pritchard *J. Clin. Oncol.*, *1996*; ***14:*** *2731–7*	T_{1-3} N_{0-2} M_0	353	3 (0.9%)	33 (9.3%)
	M. N. Levine *N. Engl. J. Med.*, *1988*; ***318:*** *404–7*	T_{1-3} N_{0-2} M_0	103	1 (1.0%)	4 (3.9%)
Tamoxifen CMF with and without anthracycline	B. Fisher *J. Clin. Oncol.*, *1990*; ***8:*** *1005–18*	T_{1-3} N_{0-2} M_0	383	–	12 (3.1%)
	S. E. Rifkin *J. Clin. Oncol.*, *1994*; ***12:*** *2078–85*	T_{1-3} N_0 M_0	303	–	11 (3.6%)
	K. Bober-Sorcinelli *Proc. Asco.*, *1986*; ***5:*** *64**	T_{1-4} N_{0-2} M_{0-1}	52	–	7 (13.5%)
Tamoxifen	K. D. Pemberton *Blood Coag. Fibrin.*, *1993*; ***4:*** *935–42*	T_{1-4} N_{0-2} M_0	89	–	5 (5.6%)
	K. I. Pritchard *J. Clin. Oncol.*, *1996*; ***14:*** *2731–7*	T_{1-3} N_{0-2} M_0	352	4 (1.1%)	5 (1.4%)
	B. Fisher *J. Clin. Oncol.*, *1990*; ***8:*** *1005–18*	T_{1-3} N_{0-2} M_0	367	–	6 (1.6%)
	S. E. Rifkin *J. Clin. Oncol.*, *1994*; ***12:*** *2078–85*	T_{1-3} N_{0-2} M_0	295	0	0
	B. Fisher *N. Eng. J. Med.*, *1989*; ***320:*** *479–84*	T_{1-3} N_0 M_0	1,318	–	12 (0.9%)
	R. R. Love *Arch. Int. Med.*, *1992*; ***152:*** *317–20*	T_{1-4} N_{0-2} M_0	70	–	1 (1.2%)

Table 10.6 (*cont.*)

Cytostatika regimens	Authors	TNM	Patients (n)	Arterial thrombosis n (%)	VT n (%)
	C. C. Mamby *Cancer Res. Treat., 1994;* ***30:*** *311–4*	$T_{1–4}$ $N_{0–2}$ M_0	32	–	0
	C. C. McDonald *BMJ, 1995;* ***311:*** *977–80*	$T_{1–4}$ $N_{0–2}$ M_0	661	39 (5.9%)	15 (2.8%)
	D. F. Hayes *J. Clin. Oncol., 1995;* ***13:*** *2556–66*	$T_{1–4}$ $N_{0–2}$ M_1	215	4 (1.8%)	5 (2.3%)
	L. Beex *Cancer Treat. Rep., 1981;* ***65:*** *179–85*	$T_{1–4}$ $N_{0–2}$ M_1	1975	–	15 (0.8%)
	A. Lipton *Cancer Treat. Rep., 1984;* ***68:*** *887–8*	$T_{1–4}$ $N_{0–2}$ M_1	220	0	7 (3.2%)
	M. Castigl-Gertsch *Ann. Oncol., 1993;* ***4:*** *735–40*	$T_{1–4}$ $N_{0–2}$ M_1	64	0	2 (3.1%)
	M. Gershanovich *Br. Can. Res. Treat., 1997;* ***75:*** *251–62*	$T_{1–4}$ $N_{0–2}$ M_1	149	3 (2.0%)	2 (1.3%)
Toremifen	D. F. Hayes *J. Clin. Oncol., 1995;* ***13:*** *2556–66*	$T_{1–4}$ $N_{0–2}$ M_1	433	6 (1.38%)	12 (2.8%)
	M. Gershanovich *Br. Can. Res. Treat., 1997;* ***75:*** *251–62*	$T_{1–4}$ $N_{0–2}$ M_1	314	2 (0.6%)	4 (1.3%)

MPA (medroxy-progesterone acetate high dose) *combination regimens with chemotherapy	F. Pannuti *Eur. J. Cancer. Clin. Oncol.*, *1988*; ***24:*** *423–9*	T_{1-3} N_{0-2} M_0	62	–	1 (1.6%)
	M. Castigl-Gertsch *Ann. Oncol.*, *1993*; ***4:*** *735–40*	T_{1-4} N_{0-2} M_1	55	–	8 (14.5%)
	G. Bastert *Med. Welt.*, *1984*; ***34:*** *61–9*	T_{1-4} N_{0-2} M_1	94	–	2 (2.1%)
	K. Pollow *Tumordiag. Ther.*, *1993*; ***14:*** *49–55*	T_{1-4} N_{0-2} M_1	846	–	13 (1.5%)
	G. R. Della Cuna *Tumori.*, *1978*; ***64:*** *143–51*	T_{1-4} N_{0-2} M_1	101	–	1 (0.9%)
	G. Samonis *Oncology 1994*; ***51:*** *411–5*	T_{1-4} N_{0-2} M_1	29	–	1 (3.4%)
	JABCS group *Jp. J. Cancer Res.*, *1993*; ***84:*** *455–61**	T_{1-4} N_{0-2} M_1	44	–	1 (2.3%)
MA (megestrol-acetate)	J. S. Abrams *Oncology*, *1992*; ***49*** *Suppl 2: 12–17*	T_{1-4} N_{0-2} M_1	50	–	2 (4.0%)
	A. Buzdar *J. Clin. Oncol.*, *1996*; ***14:*** *2000–11*	T_{1-4} N_{0-2} M_1	253	–	12 (4.7%)
	H. L. Parnes *Blood Coag. Fibrin.*, *1993*; ***4:*** *935–42*	T_{1-4} N_{0-2} M_1	57	–	2 (3.5%)
	S. Tchekmedyian *Sem. Oncol.*, *1988*; ***15*** *Suppl 1: 44–9*	T_{1-4} N_{0-2} M_1	47	–	2 (4.3%)

*combination regimens with chemotherapy

accompanied by increasing PAI-1 levels (Plasminogen activator inhibitor type 1) that may signal a cytotoxic reaction of the vascular endothelium.[63] CMF treated patients had less deformable erythrocyte, which could be a result of lipid-oxidation, induced by cyclophosphamide metabolites Acrolein and Phosphoramide mustard.[64] During adjuvant anthracyclin based chemotherapy coagulation inhibitors in addition to anti thrombin activity were unchanged while PAI activity increased and remained high throughout chemotherapy.[25] During both, chemotherapy in the adjuvant setting for breast cancer using EC (Epirubicine, Cyclophosphamide) as well as first-line PEC chemotherapy for ovarian cancer (Cisplatinum, Epirubicine Cyclophosphamide), levels of the d-dimer and fibrinogen in addition to rheological variables, e.g. plasma viscosity and erythrocyte aggregation markedly reduced. Thus there was no evidence of chemotherapy induced coagulation activation.[25,65,66] Moreover, none of the markers studied in these trials was able to predict the development of VT in patients. Upon reevaluation of all patients with a previous diagnosis of VT during adjuvant EC and first line PEC chemotherapy ($n = 10$) in half of them hereditary thrombophilia defect, i.e. heterozygous gene mutation of the factor V Leiden and/or Factor II was present (unpublished data). The increasing use of antibody treatment for breast cancer, e.g. Trastuzumab so far has not been associated with the development of VT. However, during antiangiogenic therapy using a potent inhibitor of vascular endothelial growth factor (VEGF) receptor-1 and -2 (SU5416), 3 of 17 patients with miscellaneous cancer types developed VT whereas levels of the von Willebrand antigen, soluble tissue factor, and soluble E-selectin significantly increased during therapy signaling an activation of endogenous thrombin formation and endothelial cell activation that was most pronounced in the presence of VT.[67]

Findings in studies on Tamoxifen induced changes of blood coagulation are widely inconsistent and predominantly revealed a moderate reduction of anti thrombin levels/activity which however was not associated with the development of VT in these trials.[57] In the *IBIS-I trial*[58] from 53 women who had VT while receiving tamoxifen in chemopreventive setting, blood samples were available and all were negative for the Factor V Leiden and prothrombin mutations compared to a prevalence of 5.0% and 1.9% respectively in 159 control women.

In 1990 Edwards and colleagues[68] showed that heparin could abolish chemotherapy induced coagulation activation. In 8 of 16 patients receiving different regimens of chemotherapy for various advanced malignancies, a single injection of 5,000 IU of UFH heparin immediately after blood collection and before chemotherapy resulted in significantly lower FPA levels 45 minutes after chemotherapy ($p < 0.02$) as compared to patients that received no heparin. Levine and colleagues[69] performed a double blind randomized trial of very-low-dose warfarin for prevention of VT in stage IV breast cancer. A total of 152 patients with advanced stage breast cancer daily received dose-adjusted warfarin (international normalized ratio: 1.3 to 1.9) throughout different chemotherapy regimens until one week thereafter. During chemotherapy 4.4% of patients without concurrent warfarin prophylaxis developed VT (7/159) – one of which complicated by non-fatal PE – and one patient of the warfarin treated group had PE. Warfarin recipients had an 85% lower risk for VT as compared to patients not receiving prophylaxis ($p = 0.03$), which was not shouldered by an increase in major bleeding complication. In another small prospective randomized trial by Falanga *et al.*,[70] during 9 cycles of CMF chemotherapy in advanced stage breast cancer the same daily dosage of warfarin resulted in significantly lower mean levels of the d-dimer, thrombin–antithrombin (TAT), and prothrombin fragment 1+2 (F1+2) between the 4th and 6th cycle as compared to patients who did not receive warfarin prophylaxis. VT occurred in 2 women of the placebo group ($n = 16$) and in none of the warfarin treated patients (0/9). Recently, a prospective randomized trial (FAMOUS) found comparable rates of symptomatic VT in a total of 385 patients who either received a LMWH (Dalteparin 5,000 IU) once-daily s.c. (2.4%) or placebo (3.3%), with bleeding rates of 4.7% and 2.7%, respectively.[71] The use of LMWH once daily s.c. (3,000 anti Xa Certoparin, Novartis) during PEC chemotherapy in patients with a previous diagnosis of VT after ovarian cancer surgery ($n = 6$) successfully prevented re thrombosis, while 6 of 41 patients without prophylaxis VT were diagnosed upon non-invasive screening.[61]

VT in cancer patients with central venous catheters

In the course of cancer disease, placement of a central venous catheter (CVC) often remains the last resort to access the venous system in a patient. However, their use potentially bears the risk of acute and late complications one of which is VT. Short-term CVC (1–14 days) include percutaneous internal jugular, subclavian, and femoral lines in addition to the peripherally inserted central catheters (PICCs). Long-term catheters such as surgically tunneled devices or CVCs that are connected to a totally implanted port-system may remain *in situ* for months or even years. Apart from intraluminal clot formation, which is a common event[72], the development of partially or completely occluding thrombi in the blood vessel may involve up to 66% of all CVC.[70] Most of these thrombi were found non-occlusive and in a trial by Balestreri *et al.*[74] only 10.5% of 26 oncologic patients with catheter-related VT (cr-VT) had complete thrombosis and all were clinically silent. Less than a quarter of patients with cr-VT present symptoms such as local venous distention and numbness, a painful shoulder, or a swollen arm, and neck or head that will guide to a diagnosis of cr-VT. Meanwhile a number of studies have been published in which the incidence of symptomatic cr-VT ranged between 0.3%[75] and 28.3%.[76] When venography was used for screening of cr-VT the incidence is somewhat higher and ranges between 27%[77] and 66%,[73] whereas most of these are asymptomatic. The risk for upper limb cr-VT (UL-cr-VT) in cancer patients seems highest within the first weeks of CVC insertion.[78,79] In a prospective study by De Cicco *et al.* serial venography revealed that 64% of all UL-cr-VTs were diagnosed on day 8, 34% on day 30, and 2% on day 105 after insertion of CVCs.[73] A review by Ruesch and colleagues[80] found that the rate of cr-VT was not dependant on whether the subclavian or jugular veins were access points. After insertion of a peripherally implanted central catheter in the basilic, brachial, or cephalic veins most trials found a lower overall incidence of cr-VT compared to CVC in non-oncologic patients,[81] whereas venographic screening revealed a high rate of 23% – that were predominantly located in the cephalic veins.[82] The risk of PE coming from catheter related upper extremity VT has been estimated low in earlier reports. Recently some smaller trials that included cancer patients reported a lung-scan proven incidence of 16.5[83] to 23.6%.[84] In 4 studies reviewed by Kuter,[85] incidence of PE was 11% in patients with UL-VT, which is comparable with the rate of asymptomatic PE seen in patients with symptomatic lower extremity VT.

After catheter insertion, a fibrin sheath forms around the catheter,[86] which is almost always colonized by cocci[87] but does not seem to predict subsequent cr-VT of the vessel in which the catheter is placed.[88] Few studies have recorded the prevalence of inherited thrombophilia (F V Leiden mutation, F II 20210A gene mutation) in cancer patients with cr-VT. In 252 consecutive cancer patients the cumulative incidence of cr-VT was 30% (clinically manifested thrombosis: 7%). The relative risk of factor V Leiden or prothrombin G20210A mutation for thrombosis was 2.7 (CI 95% 1.9 to 3.8).[89] In women with locally advanced or metastatic breast cancer who received fluorouracil-based chemotherapy through a totally implanted access port another trial found a 60% risk-increase for cr-VT in heterozygous carriers of factor V mutation ($P = 0.04$).[90] In contrast, Leebeek and colleagues[34] found significantly higher prevalence of high antiphospholipid antibody titers and reduced levels of antithrombin (also seen by de Cicco[91]) in patients with vs. without cr-VT while factor V Leiden or prothrombin G20210A mutation was equally distributed in all patients. Incorrect positioning of the distal catheter tip is an independent risk factor for cr-VT.[92] Only five of 87 patients with a correctly positioned distal catheter tip (i.e. either in the superior vena cava or at the junction between the right atrium and the superior vena cava) developed thrombosis, compared with 12 of 26 patients with a misplaced catheter ($P < 0.001$).

In a number of trials prophylaxis was given to cancer patients with CVC and the rate of cr-VT was assessed clinically or using objective methods (Table 10.7). After very low-dose warfarin prophylaxis an incidence of symptomatic cr-VT between

Table 10.7 VT incidence during different prophylactic regimens in patients with CVC.

	Prophylaxis regimens	Screening procedure	Type of CVC	Cr-VT (total)	Cr-VT UFH prophylaxis [n/n (%)]	Cr-VT LMWH prophylaxis [n/n (%)]	Cr-VT warfarin prophylaxis [n/n (%)]	Cr-VT without prophylaxis [n/n (%)]	Duration [(days)]	p value
Mismetti, P.[97] *prospective, randomized*	Warfarin 1 mg/d LMWH 2,850 IU	venography	CICC		–	6/21 (28.6)	4/24 (16.7)	–	90	$p = 0.48$
Bern, M. M.[98] *prospective, randomized*	Warfarin 1 mg/d	venography	Port	37.5%	–	–	4/42 (9.5)	15/40 (37.5)	90	$p < 0.001$
Boraks, P.[99] *retrospective*	Warfarin 1 mg/d	clinically	CICC	9.0%	–	–	5/108 (4.6)	15/115 (13.0)	diff.	$p = 0.03$
Nightingale, C. E.[100] *prospective*	Warfarin 1 mg/d	clinically	CICC				(5.1)		diff.	
Heaton, D. C.[101] *prospective, randomized*	Warfarin 1 mg/d	clinically	CICC	14.8%	–	–	8/45 (17.7)	5/43 (11.6)	90	n.s.
Couban, S.[102] *prospective, randomized*	Warfarin 1 mg/d	clinically	CICC	4.3%	–	–	6/130 (4.6)	5/125 (4.0)	diff.	n.s.
Minassian, V. A.[103] *retrospective*	UFH low dose	clinically	PICC CICC Port		(4.0)	–	–	(11.0)	5–16 months	$p = 0.004$
Harter, C.[104] *prospective*	UFH low dose	clinically	CICC	1.5%	4/233 (1.5)	–	–	–	diff.	

Table 10.7 *(cont.)*

	Prophylaxis regimens	Screening procedure	Type of CVC	Cr-VT (total)	Cr-VT UFH prophylaxis [n/n (%)]	Cr-VT LMWH prophylaxis [n/n (%)]	Cr-VT warfarin prophylaxis [n/n (%)]	Cr-VT without prophylaxis [n/n (%)]	Duration [(days)]	p value
Cortelezzia, A.[105] *retrospectively*	UFH, 2,500 IU/d 24 h. cont. infus. LMWH 3,800 IU/d s.c. *Nadoparin*	clinically	PICC CICC	15.5%	28/169 (16.6)	1/21 (4.7)	1	–	19	
Monreal,[106] *prospective, randomized*	LMWH 2,500 IU/d s.c. *Fragmin*	venography	Port	31.0%	–	1/16 (6.3)	–	8/13 (61.5)	90	p = 0.002
Pucheu, A.[107]	LMWH 2,500 anti-Xa U/d s.c. *Dalteparin*	duplex	CICC	11.9%	–	3/46 (6.5)	–	11/72 (15.3)	diff.	p = 0.2
Reichardt, P.[108]		clinically	CICC	5.5%	–	17/294 (5.8)	–	10/194 (5.3)	114	n.s.

4.6 and 17.7% was found compared to a rate of 11.6 and 13.0% in those patients who had no prophylaxis. In a prospective analysis of 949 insertion of CVC that were needed for ambulatory chemotherapy the incidence of symptomatic cr-VT was 5.1% in patients who received very low-dose warfarin.[100] Heaton *et al.*[101] found no differences in the incidences of cr-VT in hematological cancer patients with and without warfarin 1 mg/d. Another trial by Eastman and colleagues[93] used the same dose of warfarin for prophylaxis in patients with metastatic melanoma or renal cell carcinoma in whom a surgically implanted central venous device was placed before starting IL-2 therapy, but found no reduced incidence of cr-VT compared to patients without prophylaxis. These results are in accordance with that of a recent trial in which 255 cancer patients had similar cr-VT incidences despite prophylaxis with very low-dose warfarin in about half of the patients.[102] Mismetti and colleagues found a non-significant higher incidence of cr-VT in 57 cancer patients who received a fixed dose LMWH (Nadroparin) (6/21) as compared to patients who had very low-dose warfarin for VT prophylaxis.[97] In 382 consecutive patients receiving a stem cell transplantation (SCT) two consecutive regimens with Nadroparin were used for cr-VT prophylaxis (7 days 2,850 IE Nadroparin and 10 days 5,700 IE Nadroparin). While the overall incidence of cr-VT was 6.9% in 382 patients with 390 catheters, 8% of patients receiving one of the prophylactic Nadroparin regimens developed VT compared to 6% in a comparable control group without prophylaxis.[94] In a prospective open randomized trial long-term administration of 2,500 IU Fragmin once daily or nothing was given to cancer patients who underwent placement of a long-term port subclavian venous catheter. As the incidence of VT reached 62% (8/13) in the group without prophylaxis compared to 6% (1/16) during LMWH treatment this study was terminated earlier than planned.[106] Reichard *et al.*[108] performed a large double blind placebo controlled trial in cancer patients using Dalteparin for prevention of cr-VT but found similar VT rates in the verum and placebo treated arm.

Recommendations for thrombosis prophylaxis in gynecologic patients

Thrombosis prophylaxis in patients undergoing gynecologic cancer surgery

There are sufficient data from randomized double-blind trials available that have demonstrated a significant reduction of venous thromboembolic complications in association with different prophylactic regimens in patients undergoing pelvic and abdominal cancer surgery. According to the European and American risk stratifications of VT during surgery (Table 10.2) women undergoing genital cancer surgery belong to the "very high risk" category and pharmacological methods in addition to physical strategies (IPC, ES) are indicated. Low molecular

Table 10.8 Thrombosis prophylaxis during surgery in gynecologic cancer patients. Recommendation according to the ACCP.[96]

	Heparin*	Dose	Duration
UFH	low dose	5,000 U	8–12 h, starting 1–2 h before surgery
LMWH	Dalteparin	5,000 U 10–12 h	before surgery and once daily after surgery
	Enoxaparin	4,000 U 10–12 h	10–12 h before surgery and once daily after surgery
Heparinoids	Danaparoid	750 U 1–2 h	before surgery and twice daily after surgery

*approved by the FDA for use in the United States

weight heparin regimens represent the first choice as they have widely replaced the use of low-dose heparin prophylaxis in most countries (Table 10.8). Although the risk of VT during breast cancer surgery is comparably low, VT prophylaxis in patients should be considered. Prolongation of prophylaxis for at least 4 weeks seems beneficial in terms of a further reduction of late VT. In the presence of HIT II (heparin-induced thrombocytopenia) or other rare conditions of contraindications to heparin, heparinoids (Table 10.8), Dextrane or adjusted-dose warfarin may be an alternative but should be avoided as a routine procedure for prophylaxis in gynecologic surgery.

Thrombosis prophylaxis during cytoreductive therapy

So far, thrombosis prophylaxis is not routinely applied during conventional chemotherapy for gynecologic malignancy, either in the adjuvant setting or in patients with advanced-stage malignancy. Apart from high costs and – in terms of oral anticoagulation – the need of laboratory monitoring, general prophylaxis is not indicated in most patients. The incidence of thrombosis during MPA or tamoxifen treatment compared to chemotherapy is low and therefore hormonal anticancer treatment alone does not justify thrombosis prophylaxis. Following the RAM shown in Table 10.1, chemotherapy (acute risk I) for treatment of metastatic or active cancer (basic risk III) represents a high risk of VT in patients, thus pharmacological prophylaxis is indicated. Treatment of occult micro metastasis or supposed tumor residuals after surgery in the adjuvant setting in an otherwise healthy individual carries a low risk of VT according to RAM and prophylaxis is not recommended. Most breast cancer patients with a history of VT during adjuvant treatment are postmenopausal and previously had mastectomy.[9] A more recent trial found a 5.5% incidence of VT upon screening in 348 patients with breast cancer during the first 9 months of adjuvant chemotherapy.[95] None of the premenopausal women (n = 69) developed VT but more often it was diagnosed in the presence of a tumor greater than 5 cm, in nodal positive women having more than 9 positive axillary lymph nodes and in women with a history of VT. Therefore such a constellation may guide the decision for thrombosis prophylaxis during chemotherapy. The role of congenital thrombophilia (factor V Leiden mutation, prothrombin mutation) in the pathogenesis of VT associated with systemic cancer treatment is still to be determined. Since one out of four patients with ovarian cancer develops VT during primary cancer treatment concomitant thrombosis prophylaxis throughout therapy should be considered.

Thrombosis prophylaxis can either be given orally, e.g. very-low-dose warfarin or using heparin, whereas LMWH is a particularly suitable drug for this indication. Prophylaxis should be started 3 to 4 days before the beginning of chemotherapy and continued throughout chemotherapy at a prophylactic dose using self-injecting systems. The platelet count should be monitored 2 to 3 times in the first month to exclude heparin-induced thrombocytopenia.

Apart from high-risk patients (Table 10.1) and those who have intra vaginal/uterine radium therapy, prophylaxis is not recommended while undergoing radiotherapy, e.g. HDR-AL.

Recommendations for VT prophylaxis in cancer patients with central venous catheters

According to the RAM shown in Table 10.1, insertion of a CVC alone is a weak risk factor for VT and routine prophylaxis is not needed. Central venous catheter installation in a cancer patient is often required for application of second line chemotherapy, parenteral nutrition or for patients' surveillance (a.o.). Thus, most of these reasons are likely associated with advanced stage (active) malignancy and therefore prophylaxis is recommended. According to the recommendation of the *VIth ACCP (American College of Chest Physicians) Consensus Conference on Antithrombotic Therapy*[96] cancer patients with long-term CVC for chemotherapy should also receive prophylaxis with either warfarin 1 mg/d or LMWH s.c. to prevent axillary-subclavian VT. At the 1997 meeting of the *Subcommittee Thrombosis and Haemostasis in Malignancy* of the *ISTH* low-dose warfarin prophylaxis (1 mg/d) is the drug of first choice in patients with CVC during chemotherapy. In the case of clot development LMWH was suggested as an alternative.[9] In order to minimize the risk of cr-VT the smallest acceptable catheter diameter should be used.

Synopsis

According to the American and European Consensus Conferences patients undergoing major cancer surgery are at very high risk for the development of VT and therefore require appropriate prophylaxis. LMWH has become the drug of first choice and should be combined with physical methods, e.g. ES, ICP. In the medical patients malignancy itself is an independent risk factor for VT. Nonetheless it is the responsibility of the physician to individually assess the risk profile in a cancer patient prior to commencement of cancer treatment, and a RAM may be useful. Insertion of a CVC in cancer patients receiving chemotherapy does not require VT prophylaxis as long as additional risk-factors do not coincide. Duration of VT prophylaxis after surgery is still a matter of debate but an increasing number of studies found significant reduction of late VT which is of particular concern in ovarian cancer patients. Hencc, VT is a frequent complication in gynecologic malignancy that one should be aware of when planning therapeutic management of patients.

REFERENCES

1 Alikhan, R., Cohen, A. T., Combe, S., *et al.* Prevention of venous thromboembolism in medical patients with enoxaparin: a subgroup analysis of the MEDINOX study. *Blood Coag. Fibrinolysis*, 2003; **14**: 341–6.

2 Heilman, L., Tempelhoff, von G.-F., Kirkpatrick, J. P., *et al.* Comparison of unfractionated versus low molecular weight heparin for deep vein thrombosis prophylaxis during breast and pelvic cancer surgery: Efficacy, safety and follow-up. *Clin. Appl. Thromb. Hemost.*, 1998; **4**: 268–73.

3 Clahsen, P. C., Cornelis, J. H., van der Velde, J. P. J., *et al.* Thromboembolic complications after perioperative chemotherapy in women with early breast cancer: A European Organization for Research and Treatment of Cancer Breast Cooperative Group Study. *J. Clin. Oncol.*, 1994; **12**: 1266–71.

4 Clarke-Pearson, D. L., Jelovsek, F. R., Creasman, W. T. Thromboembolism complicating surgery for cervical and uterine malignancy: Incidence, risk factors and prophylaxis. *Obstet. Gyn.*, 1983; **61**: 87–94.

5 Clarke-Pearson, D. L., Colemann, R. E., Synan, I. S., *et al.* Venous thromboembolism prophylaxis in gynecologic oncology: A prospective controlled trial of low dose heparin. *Am. J. Obstet. Gynecol.*, 1983; **145**: 606–13.

6 Tempelhoff, von G.-F., Dietrich, M., Niemann, F., *et al.* Blood coagulation and thrombosis in patients with ovarian malignancy. *Thromb. Haemost.*, 1997; **77**: 456–61.

7 Canney, P. A., Wilkinson, P. M. Pulmonary embolism in patients receiving chemotherapy for advanced ovarian cancer. *Eur. J. Cancer. Clin. Oncol.*, 1985; **21**: 585–7.

8 Henderson, P. H., Jr. Multiple migratory thrombophlebitis associated with ovarian carcinoma. *Am. J. Obstet. Gynecol.*, 1955; **70**: 452–5.

9 Levine, M. N. Prevention of thrombotic disorders in cancer patients undergoing chemotherapy. *Thromb. Haemost.*, 1997; **78**: 133–6.

10 American Cancer Society. Cancer Facts & Figures 2004. National Cancer Institute Surveillance, Epidemiology, and End Results program. American Cancer Society No. 5008.04.

11 Bergqvist, D., Agnelli, G., Cohen, A. T., *et al.* ENOXACAN II Investigators. Duration of prophylaxis against venous thromboembolism with enoxaparin after surgery for cancer. *N. Engl. J. Med.*, 2002: **346**: 975–80.

12 Trimbos, J. B., Franchi, M., Zanaboni, F., *et al.* "State of the art" of radical hysterectomy; current practice in European oncology centres. *Eur. J. Cancer*, 2004; **40**: 375–8.
13 Heilmann, L., Tempelhoff, von G.-F., Schneider, D. Prevention of thrombosis in gynecological malignancy. *Clin. Appl. Thromb. Hemost.*, 1998; **4**: 153–9.
14 Saeger, W., Genzkow, M. Venous thromboses and pulmonary embolisms in post–mortem series: Probable causes by correlation of clinical data and basic diseases. *Path. Res. Pract.*, 1994; **190**: 394–9.
15 Venous Thrombosis Experts meeting (VTE), Lisbon, November 2nd–4th 2003.
16 Silverstein, M. D., Heit, J. A., Mohr, D. N., *et al.* 3rd Trends in the incidence of deep vein thrombosis and pulmonary embolism: a 25-year population-based study. *Arch. Intern. Med.*, 1998; **158**: 585–93.
17 Lowe, G. D. Venous and arterial thrombosis: epidemiology and risk factors at various ages. *Maturitas*, 2004; **47**: 259–63.
18 Fowkes, F. G. R., Pell, J. P., Donnan, P. T., *et al.* Sex differences in susceptibility to etiologic factors for peripheral athersiosclerosis. *Arterioscler. Thromb.*, 1994; **14**: 862–8.
19 Heilmann L. Blutrheologie und Thrombose. In Gerinnungsstörung in Gynäkologie und Geburtshilfe. Thieme stuttgart, New York, NY: Rath, W. und Heilmann, L. Thieme, 1999, pp. 10–6.
20 European Consensus Statement on the prevention of venous thromboembolism. *Int. Angiol.*, 1992; **11**: 151–6.
21 Shackelford, D. P., Lalikos, J. F. Estrogen replacement therapy and the surgeon. *Am. J. Surg.*, 2000; **179**: 333–6.
22 Franchi, M., Ghezzi, F., Riva, C., *et al.* Postoperative complications after pelvic lymphadenectomy for the surgical staging of endometrial cancer. *J. Surg. Oncol.*, 2001; **78**: 232–7.
23 Bergqvist, D., Lindblad, B. Incidence of venous thromboembolism in medical and surgical patients. In Bergqvist, A. J., Comerosa. A. N., Nicolaides (eds.), *Prevention of Venous Thromboembolism.* London, Med-Orion. 1994, pp. 175–80.
24 Rogers, J. S., Murgo, A. J., Fontana, J. A., *et al.* Chemotherapy for breast cancer decreases plasma protein C and protein S. *J. Clin. Oncol.*, 1988; **6**: 276–81.
25 Tempelhoff, von G.-F., Dietrich, M., Hommel, G., *et al.* Blood coagulation during adjuvant Epirubicin/Cyclophosphamide chemotherapy in patients with primary operable breast cancer. *J. Clin. Oncol.*, 1996; **14**: 2560–8.
26 Nijziel, M. R., van Oerle, R., Christella, M., *et al.* Acquired resistance to activated protein C in breast cancer patients. *Br. J. Haematol.*, 2003; **120**: 117–22.
27 Haim, N., Lanir, N., Hoffman, R., *et al.* Acquired activated protein C resistance is common in cancer patients and is associated with venous thromboembolism. *Am. J. Med.*, 2001; **110**: 91–6.
28 Ozguroglu, M., Arun, B., Erzin, Y., *et al.* Serum cardiolipin antibodies in cancer patients with thromboembolic events. *Clin. Appl. Thromb. Hemost.*, 1999; **5**: 181–4.
29 Zuckerman, E., Toubi, E., Golan, T. D., *et al.* Increased thromboembolic incidence in anti-cardiolipin-positive patients with malignancy. *Br. J. Cancer* 1995; **72**: 447–51.
30 De Stefano, V., Chiusolo, P., Paciaroni, K., *et al.* Epidemiology of factor V Leiden: clinical implications. *Semin. Thromb. Hemost.*, 1998; **24**: 367–79.

31 Crowther, M. A., Kelton, G. K. Congenital thrombophilic states associated with venous thrombosis: A qualitative overview and proposed classification system. *Ann. Intern. Med.*, 2003; **138**: 128–4.

32 Hillarp, A., Zoller, B., Svensson, P. J., *et al.* The 20210 A allele of the prothrombin gene is a common risk factor among Swedish outpatients with verified deep venous thrombosis. *Thromb. Haemost.*, 1997; **78**: 990–2.

33 Ramacciotti, E., Wolosker, N., Puech-Leao, P., *et al.* Prevalence of factor V Leiden, FII G20210A, FXIII Val34Leu and MTHFR C677T polymorphisms in cancer patients with and without venous thrombosis. *Thromb. Res.*, 2003; **109**: 171–4.

34 Leebeek, F. W., Stadhouders, N. A., van Stein, D., *et al.* Hypercoagulability states in upper-extremity deep venous thrombosis. *Am. J. Hematol.*, 2001; **67**: 15–19.

35 Tempelhoff, von G.-F., Pollow, K., Heilmann, L., *et al.* Impact of rheological variables in cancer. *Seminars Thromb. Hemost*, 2003; **29**: 499–513.

36 Patterson, W. P., Caldwell, C. W., Doll, D. C. Hyperviscosity syndromes and coagulopathies. *Sem. Oncol.*, 1990; **17**: 210–6.

37 Humphreys, W. V., Walker, A., Charlesworth, D. Altered viscosity and yield stress in patients with abdominal malignancy: Relationship to deep venous thrombosis. *Br. J. Surg.*, 1976; **63**: 559–61.

38 Tempelhoff, von G.-F., Heilmann, L., Hommel, G., *et al.* Hyperviscosity Syndrome in ovarian malignancy. *Cancer*, 1998; **82**: 1104–11.

39 Walsh, J. J., Bonnar, J., Wright, F. W. A study of pulmonary embolism and deep leg vein thrombosis after major gynecological surgery using labelled fibrinogen – phlebography and lung scanning. *J. Obstet. Gynecol. Brit. Cwlth.*, 1974; **81**: 311–16.

40 Clarke-Pearson, D. L., deLong, E. R., Synan, J. S., *et al.* Variables associated with postoperative deep venous thrombosis. A prospective study of 411 gynecologic patients and creation of a prognostic model. *Obstet. Gynecol.*, 1987; **69**: 146–50.

41 Hohl, M. K., Lüscher, K. P., Tichy, J., *et al.* Prevention of postoperative thromboembolism by Dextran 70 or low dose heparin. *Obstet. Gynecol.*, 1980; **55**: 497–500.

42 Heilmann, L., Kruck, A., Schindler, E. Thromboseprophylaxe in der Gynäkologie: Doppelblindvergleich zwischen niedermolekularen (LMWH) und unfraktionierten (UFH) Heparin. *Geburtsh Frauenheilk*, 1989; **48**: 803–7.

43 Heilmann, L., Tempelhoff, von G.-F., Herrle, B., *et al.* Low dose heparin versus niedermolekulares Heparin zur Thromboseprophylaxe in der operativen gynäkologischen Onkologie. *Geburtsh Frauenheilk*, 1997; **57**: 1–6.

44 White, R. H., Zhou, H., Romano, S. Incidence of symptomatic venous thromboembolism after different elective or urgent surgical procedures. *Thromb. Haemost.*, 2003; **90**: 446–55.

45 Kakkar, V. V., Murray, W. J. G. Efficacy and safety of low molecular weight heparin (CY216) in preventing postoperative venous thromboembolism: a co-operative study. *Br. J. Surg.*, 1985; **72**: 786–91.

46 Clarke-Pearson, D. L., DeLong, E., Synan, I. S., *et al.* A controlled trial of two low-dose-heparin regimens for the prevention of postoperative deep vein thrombosis. *Obstet. Gynecol.*, 1990; **75**: 683–9.

47 Nurmohamed, M. T., Verhaeghe, R., Haas, S., *et al.* A comparative trial of a low molecular weight heparin (enoxaparin) versus standard heparin for the prophylaxis of postoperative deep vein thrombosis in general surgery. *Am. J. Surg.*, 1995; **169**: 567–71.

48 Fricker, J-P., Vergnes, Y., Schach, R., *et al.* Low dose heparin versus low molecular weight heparin (Kabi 2165, Fragmin) in the prophylaxis of thromboembolic complications of abdominal oncological surgery. *Eur. J. Clin. Invest.*, 1988; **18**: 561–7.

49 Kakkar, V. V., Cohen, A. T., Edmonson, R. A., *et al.* Low molecular weight versus standard heparin for prevention of venous thromboembolism after major abdominal surgery. *Lancet*, 1993; **341**: 251–65.

50 Kakkar, V. V. Effectiveness and safety of low molecular weight heparins (LMWH) in the prevention of venous thrombembolism (VTE). *Thromb. Haemostas.*, 1995; **74**: 364–8.

51 Morgan, M. M., Iyengar, T. D., Napiorkowski, B. E., *et al.* The clinical course of deep vein thrombosis in patients with gynecological cancer. *Gynecol. Oncol.*, 2002; **84**: 67–71.

52 Ludwig, H. Klinisch – experimentelle Untersuchungen zur thromobotischen Diathese bei der gynäkologischen Radiumbehandlung. *Geburtsh Frauenhlk*, 1962; **22**: 1121–3.

53 Graf, A. H., Graf, B., Brandis, M. G., *et al.* Oral anticoagulation in patients with gynecological cancer and radiotherapy: a retrospective analysis of 132 patients. *Anticancer Res.*, 1998; **18**: 2047–51.

54 Graf, A. H., Graf, B., Traun, H., *et al.* Risiko und Prophylaxe thromboembolischer Komplikationen bei gynäkologischen Malignomen. *Gynäkol Geburtshilf Rundsch*, 1996; **36**: 37–45.

55 Kemkes-Matthes, B., Münstedt, K., Matthes, K. J., *et al.* Blood coagulation activation markers during iridium HDR – AL therapy in patients with uterine cancer. *Ann. Haemat.*, 1995; **70**(Suppl.1): A 61 (Abstract).

56 Tempelhoff, von G.-F., Heilmann, L., Pollow, K., *et al.* Monitoring of rheological variables during postoperative high-dose brachytherapy for uterine cancer. *Clin. Appl. Thrombosis/Hemostasis*, 2004; **10**: 239–48.

57 Tempelhoff, von G.-F., Pollow, K., Schneider, D., *et al.* Chemotherapy and thrombosis in gynecological malignancy. *Clin. Appl. Thrombosis/Hemostasis*, 1999; **5**: 92–104.

58 Duggan, C., Marriott, K., Edwards, R., *et al.* Inherited and acquired risk factors for venous thromboembolic disease among women taking tamoxifen to prevent breast cancer. *J. Clin. Oncol.*, 2003; **21**: 3588–93.

59 Rutqvist, E., A, Mattson for the Stockholm Breast Cancer Study Group. Cardiac and thromboembolic morbidity among postmenopausal women with early stage breast cancer in a randomized trial of adjuvant tamoxifen. *J. Natl. Cancer Inst.*, 1993; **85**: 1298–306.

60 Soule, S. E., Miller, K. D., Porcu, P., *et al.* Combined anti-microtubule therapy: a phase II study of weekly docetaxel plus estramustine in patients with metastatic breast cancer. *Ann. Oncol.*, 2002; **13**: 1612–5.

61 Tempelhoff, von G.-F., Niemann, F., Schneider, D., *et al.* Blood rheology during chemotherapy in patients with ovarian cancer. *Thromb. Res.*, 1998; **90**: 73–82.

62 Feffer, S. E., Carmasino, L. S., Fox, R. L. Acquired protein C deficiency in patients with breast cancer receiving cyclophosphamide, methotrexate and 5 floururacil. *Cancer*, 1989; **63**: 1303–7.

63 Rella, C., Coviello, M., Giotta, F., *et al.* A prethrombotic state in breast cancer patients treated with adjuvant chemotherapy. *Breast Cancer Res. Treat.*, 1996; **40**: 151–9.
64 Vasigara-Singh, W., Subramaniam, S., Shyama, S., *et al.* Changes in erythrocyte membrane lipids in breast cancer patients after radiotherapy and chemotherapy. *Chemotherapy*, 1996; **42**: 65–70.
65 Tempelhoff, von G.-F., Niemann, F., Schneider, D., *et al.* Gerinnungsuntersuchungen und Thromboseinzidenz während der Cisplatin/Epirubicin/Cyclophosphamid Chemotherapy beim Ovarialkarzinom. *Geburtsh Frauenhlk*, 1997; **57**: 595–601.
66 Tempelhoff, von G.-F., L., Heilmann. Thrombosis and hemorheology in patients with breast cancer and adjuvant chemotherapy. *Clin. Hemorheology*, 1995; **15**: 311–23.
67 Kuenen, B. C., Levi, M., Meijers, J. C. M., *et al.* Analysis of coagulation cascade and endothelial cell activation during inhibition of vascular endothelial growth factor/vascular endothelial growth factor receptor in cancer patients. *Arterioscler. Thromb. Vasc. Biol.*, 2002; **22**: 1500–5.
68 Edwards, R. L., Klaus, M., Mathews, E., *et al.* Heparin abolishes the chemotherapy induced increase in plasma fibrinopeptid A levels. *Am. J. Med.*, 1990; **89**: 25–8.
69 Levine, M., Hirsh, J., Gent, M., *et al.* Double-blind randomised trial of very-low-dose warfarin for prevention of thromboembolism in stage IV breast cancer. *Lancet*, 1994; **343**: 886–9.
70 Falanga, A., Levine, M. N., Consonni, R., *et al.* The effect of very-low-dose warfarin on markers of hypercoagulation in metastatic breast cancer: Results from a randomized trial. *Thromb. Haemost.*, 1998; **79**: 23–7.
71 Kakkar, A. K., Levine, M. N., Kadziola, Z., *et al.* Low molecular weight heparin, therapy with dalteparin, and survival in advanced cancer: the fragmin advanced malignancy outcome study (FAMOUS). *J. Clin. Oncol.*, 2004; **22**: 1944–8.
72 Ray, S., Stacey, R., Imrie, M., *et al.* A review of 560 Hickman catheter insertions. *Anaesthesia*, 1996; **51**: 981–5.
73 De Cicco, M., Balestieri, L. Central venous thrombosis: An early and frequent complication in cancer patients bearing a long term silastic catheter – A prospective study. *Thromb. Res.*, 1997; **86**: 101–13.
74 Balestreri, L., De Cicco, M., Matovic, M., *et al.* Central venous catheter-related thrombosis in clinically asymptomatic oncologic patients: a phlebographic study. *Eur. J. Radiol.*, 1995; **20**: 108–11.
75 Smith, V. C., Hellett, J. W. Subclavian vein thrombosis during prolonged catheterisation for parenteral nutrition: Early management and long-term follow-up. *South Med. J.*, 1983; **76**: 606–13.
76 Lokich, J. J., Becker, B. Subclavian vein thrombosis in patients treated with infusion chemotherapy for advanced malignancy. *Cancer*, 1983; **52**: 1586–9.
77 Ladefoged, K., Jarnum, S. Long term parenteral nutrition. *BMJ*, 1978; **2**: 262–78.
78 Tolar, B., Gould, J. R. The timing and sequence of multiple device-related complications in patients with long-term indwelling Groshong catheters. *Cancer*, 1996; **78**: 1308–13.
79 Luciani, A., Clement, O., Halimi, P., *et al.* Catheter-related upper extremity deep venous thrombosis in cancer patients: a prospective study based on Doppler US. *Radiology*, 2001; **220**: 655–60.

80 Ruesch, S., Walder, B., Trammer, M. R. Complications of central venous catheters: Internal jugular veins VS. subclavian vein access – A systematic review. *Crit. Care Med.*, 2002; **30**: 454–60.
81 Grove, J. R., Pevec, W. C. Venous thrombosis related to peripherally inserted central catheters. *J. Vasc. Interv. Radiol.*, 2000; **11**: 837–40.
82 Allen, A. W., Megargell, J. L., Brown, D. B., *et al.* Venous thrombosis associated with the placement of peripherally inserted central catheters. *Vasc. Interv. Radiol.*, 2000; **11**: 1309–14.
83 Monreal, M., Raventos, A., Lerma, R., *et al.* Pulmonary embolism in patients with upper extremity DVT associated to venous central lines – a prospective study. *Thromb. Haemost.*, 1994; **72**: 548–50.
84 Monreal, M., Lafoz, E., Ruiz, J., *et al.* Upper-extremity deep venous thrombosis and pulmonary embolism. A prospective study. *Chest*, 1991; **99**: 280–3.
85 Kuter, D. J. Thrombotic complications of central venous catheters in cancer patients. *Oncologist*, 2004; **9**: 207–16.
86 Hoshal, V. L. Jr., Ause, R. G., Hoskins, P. A. Fibrin sleeve formation on indwelling subclavian central venous catheters. *Arch. Surg.*, 1971; **102**: 253–8.
87 Raad, I., Costerton, W., Sabharwal, U., *et al.* Ultrastructural analysis of indwelling vascular catheters: a quantitative relationship between luminal colonization and duration of placement. *J. Infect. Dis.*, 1993; **168**: 400–7.
88 Starkhammar, H., Bengtsson, M., Morales, O. Fibrin sleeve formation after long term brachial catheterisation with an implantable port device. A prospective venographic study. *Eur. J. Surg.*, 1992; **158**: 481–4.
89 Van Rooden, C. J., Rosendaal, F. R., Meinders, A. E., *et al.* The contribution of factor V Leiden and prothrombin G20210A mutation to the risk of central venous catheter-related thrombosis. *Haematologica*, 2004; **89**: 201–6.
90 Mandala, M., Curigliano, G., Bucciarelli, P., *et al.* Factor V Leiden and G20210A prothrombin mutation and the risk of subclavian vein thrombosis in patients with breast cancer and a central venous catheter. *Ann. Oncol.*, 2004; **15**: 590–3.
91 De Cicco, M., Matovic, M., Balestreri, L., *et al.* Antithrombin III deficiency as a risk factor for catheter-related central vein thrombosis in cancer patients. *Thromb. Res.*, 1995; **78**: 127–37.
92 Schwarz, R. E., Coit, D. G., Groeger, J. S. Transcutaneously tunneled central venous lines in cancer patients: an analysis of device-related morbidity factors based on prospective data collection. *Ann. Surg. Oncol.*, 2000; **7**: 441–9.
93 Eastman, M. E., Khorsand, M., Maki, D. G., *et al.* Central venous device-related infection and thrombosis in patients treated with moderate dose continuous-infusion interleukin-2. *Cancer*, 2001; **91**: 806–14.
94 Lagro, S. W., Verdonck, L. F., Borel, Rinkes, I. H., *et al.* No effect of nadroparin prophylaxis in the prevention of central venous catheter (CVC)-associated thrombosis in bone marrow transplant recipients. *Bone Marrow Transplant*, 2000; **26**: 1103–6.
95 Tempelhoff, von G.-F., Heilmann, L. Thrombosis – a clue of poor prognosis in primary non-metastatic breast cancer? *Breast Cancer Res. Treat.*, 2002; **73**: 275–7.
96 Geerts, W. H., Heit, J. A., Clagett, G. P., *et al.* Prevention of venous thromboembolism. *Chest*, 2001; **119**(1 Suppl.): 132–75S.

97 Mismetti, P., Mille, D., Laporte, S., *et al.* CIP Study Group. Low-molecular-weight heparin (nadroparin) and very low doses of warfarin in the prevention of upper extremity thrombosis in cancer patients with indwelling long-term central venous catheters: a pilot randomized trial. *Haematologica*, 2003; **88**: 67–73.

98 Bern, M. M., Lokich, J. J., Wallach, S. R. Very low doses of warfarin can prevent thrombosis in central vein catheters: a randomized prospective trial. *Ann. Intern. Med.*, 1990; **112**, 4428–32.

99 Boraks, P., Seale, J., Price, J., *et al.* Prevention of central venous catheter associated thrombosis using minidose warfarin in patients with haematological malignancies. *Br. J. Haematol.*, 1998; **101**: 483–6.

100 Nightingale, C. E., Norman, A., Cunningham, D., *et al.* A prospective analysis of 949 long-term central venous access catheters for ambulatory chemotherapy in patients with gastro-intestinal malignancy. *Eur. J. Cancer*, 1997; **33**: 398–403.

101 Heaton, D. C., Han, D. Y., Inder, A. Minidose (1 mg) warfarin as prophylaxis for central vein catheter thrombosis. *Intern. Med. J.*, 2002; **32**: 84–8.

102 Couban, S., Goodyear, M., Burnell, M. A randomized double-blind placebo-controlled study of low-dose warfarin for the prevention of symptomatic central venous catheter-associated thrombosis in patients with cancer. *Blood*, 2002; **100**(suppl.): 703a [abstract].

103 Minassian, V. A., Sood, A. K., Lowe, P., *et al.* Longterm central venous access in gynecologic cancer patients. *J. Am. Coll. Surg.*, 2000; **191**: 403–9.

104 Harter, C., Salwender, H. J., Bach, A., *et al.* Catheter-related infection and thrombosis of the internal jugular vein in hematologic-oncologic patients undergoing chemotherapy: a prospective comparison of silver-coated and uncoated catheters. *Cancer*, 2002; **94**: 245–51.

105 Cortelezzia, A., Fracchiolla, N. S., Maisonneuve, P., *et al.* Central venous catheter-related complications in patients with hematological malignancies: a retrospective analysis of risk factors and prophylactic measures. *Leuk. Lymphoma*, 2003; **44**: 1495–501.

106 Monreal, M., Alastrue, A., Rull, M., *et al.* Upper extremity deep venous thrombosis in cancer patients with venous access devices – prophylaxis with a low molecular weight heparin (Fragmin). *Thromb. Haemost.*, 1996; **75**: 251–3.

107 Pucheu, A., Leduc, B., Sillet-Bach, I., *et al.* Experimental prevention of deep venous thrombosis with low-molecular-weight heparin using implantable infusion devices. *Ann. Cardiol. Angeiol. (Paris)*, 1996; **45**: 59–63.

108 Reichardt, P., Kretzschmar, A., Biakhov, M. A phase III randomized, double-blind, placebo-controlled study evaluating the efficacy and safety of daily low-molecular-weight heparin (dalteparin sodium, fragmin) in preventing catheter-related complications (CRCs) in cancer patients with central venous catheters (CVCs). *Proc. Am. Soc. Clin. Oncol.*, 2002; **21**: 369a.

109 Anderson, G. L., Judd, H. L., Kaunitz, A. M., *et al.* Women's Health Initiative Investigators. Effects of estrogen plus progestin on gynecologic cancers and associated diagnostic procedures: the Women's Health Initiative randomized trial. *JAMA*, 2003; **290**: 1739–48.

110 Herrington, D. M., Vittinghoff, E., Howard, T. D., Factor V Leiden, hormone replacement therapy, and risk of venous thromboembolic events in women with coronary disease. *Arterioscler. Thromb. Vasc. Biol.*, 2002; **22**: 1012–17.

11

Low molecular weight heparins in pregnancy

Debra A. Hoppensteadt, Ph.D., Jawed Fareed, Ph.D.,[1] Harry L. Messmore, M.D.,[2] Omer Iqbal, M.D.,[3] William Wehrmacher, M.D.,[4] and Rodger L. Bick M.D., Ph.D.[5]

[1]Professor of Pathology and Pharmacology, Loyola University Chicago, Maywood, Illinois, USA, email: dhoppen@lumc.edu
[2]Professor Emeritus, Department of Medicine, Loyola University Chicago, Maywood, Illinois, USA
[3]Research Assistant Professor, Department of Pathology, Loyola University Chicago, Maywood, Illinois, USA
[4]Professor Emeritus, Department of Physiology, Loyola Univeristy Chicago, Maywood, Illinois, USA
[5]Clinical Professor of Medicine and Pathology, University of Texas Southwestern Medical Center; Director: Dallas Thrombosis Hemostasis and Vascular Medicine Clinical Center, Dallas, Texas, USA

The pathophysiology of the thrombotic process is multicomponent and involves blood, vascular system, humoral mediators and target sites. Furthermore, the intiating event and the site of thrombogenesis play a key role in the overall pathogenesis. The process of thrombogenesis is depicted in Figure 11.1. Initially, vascular injury results in the localized alterations of the vessels, generation of tissue factor, and subsequent activation of platelets. Activated cells mediate several direct or signal transduction induced processes resulting in the activation of platelets. Cellular activation also results in the release of various mediators which amplify vascular spasm and the coagulation process. Adhesion molecules, cytokines, oxidative stress and flow conditions signficantly contribute to the ischemic and occlusive outcome. Drugs that target various sites of the activation process have been developed to control thrombotic events. Because of the coupled pathophysiology, a drug that targets a single site may not be able to produce the desired therapeutic effects. Furthermore, many of these mediators produce localized actions at cellular and subcellular levels. Feedback amplification processes also play an important role in the pathology of these disorders and interruption of these pathways can be a therapeutic goal. This understanding has led to the concept of polytherapy in the management of thrombotic disorders.

Pregnancy and thrombosis

Pregnancy is associated with a hypercoagulable state that can lead to thrombosis and thromboembolism.[1,2] The risk of venous thromboembolism (VTE) in

Hematological Complications in Obstetrics, Pregnancy, and Gynecology, ed. R. L. Bick *et al.* Published by Cambridge University Press.

Mechanism of thrombogenesis

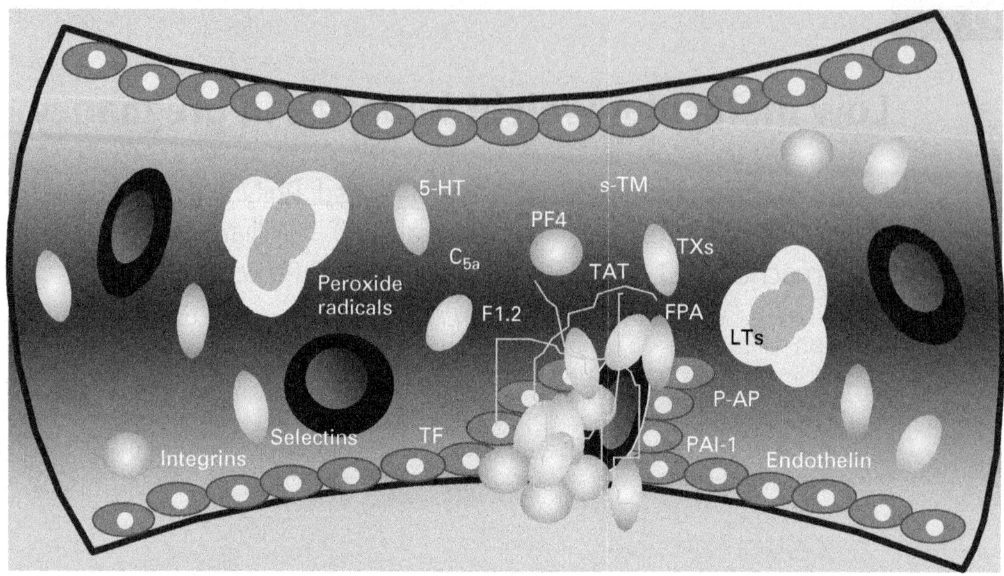

Figure 11.1 Diagrammatic representation of the mechanisms of thrombogenesis. Both the cellular and humoral components of the vascular system contribute to the formation of thrombus. Endothelial dysfunction and damage result in the formation of platelet thrombi which are able to trigger activation of coagulation. Cellular adhesion molecules and other mediators further augment this process. The composition of plasma proteins also play a key role in the eventual clot formation.

pregnancy is approximately six times higher than in non-pregnant women.[3] Pulmonary embolism occurs in 16% of pregnant women with untreated deep vein thrombosis.[3] This in turn can lead to both morbidity and mortality during pregnancy. Many factors contribute to the risk of thrombosis during pregnancy. These include age, cesarean delivery, prolonged immobilization, prior thrombosis, and obesity (Table 11.1). The coexistence of thrombophilia compounds this risk. The puerperium, the six week period following delivery, is associated with a higher rate of thrombosis than pregnancy itself.[4]

Thrombosis during pregnancy can be attributed to alteration in hemostasis as shown in Table 11.2. Several physiologic changes during pregnancy can predispose women to thrombosis. Release of tissue thromboplastin occurs at the time of placental separation causing alteration in the coagulation system.[5] In addition, increased levels of markers of coagulation activation can be detected in the circulation by the end of the first trimester.[6] The levels of most coagulation proteins increase during pregnancy with fibrinogen and factor VIII levels increasing to 2–3 times normal.[7] There is also a significant decrease in free and total

Table 11.1 Risk factors for VTE in pregnancy.

- Age
- Obsesity
- Immobilization
- Thrombophilia
- Protein C deficiency
- Protein S deficiency
- Factor V Leiden mutation
- Prothrombin 20210 mutation
- Antiphospholipid syndrome

Table 11.2 VTE in pregnancy: Etiology.

Mechanical	Hemostatic
• enlarged uterus obstructs venous return	• ↑ factors II, V, VII, VIII, and X activity
• venous atonia caused by hormonal effects	• ↑ von Willebrand factor
	• ↑ fibrinogen
	• ↓ fibrinolysis
	• ↓ free protein S
	• acquired resistance to protein C
	• platelet activation

protein S in the second trimester.[8] Simultaneously, a decrease in fibrinolytic activity occurs during the third trimester, and in the early stages of labor, due to the generation of plasminogen activator-2 by the placenta.[5,9] Platelet activation and increased platelet turnover also occurs leading to an increased risk of thrombosis.[10] Mild thrombocytopenia occurs in approximately 8.3% of healthy women at term.[11] The causes of this are multifactorial.

In pregnancy local pressure of the gravid uterus causes stasis of the venous return from the lower limbs.[12] Trauma to the pelvic veins during vaginal delivery or tissue injury during cesarean section also contribute to a hypercoagulable state.[13] Compression of the left iliac vein by the crossing right iliac artery is a local, mechanical factor that is believed to cause a 3-fold higher incidence of DVT in the left leg compared to the right leg. If there are obstetric complications such as abruptio placenta, preeclampsia, threatened abortion, prolonged labor, etc., the risk of thrombosis is even higher.[14] The association of right ovarian vein thrombosis with late stage pregnancy and early puerperium can be a cause of right lower abdominal and flank pain, fever, and embolization in the lung.[15]

Thrombophilia is common in approximately 20% of pregnant women having some type of genetic predisposition to thrombosis.[1,2] Several genetic mutations associated with an increased risk of thrombosis include Factor V Leiden, Prothrombin 20210 and methyltetrahydrofolate reductase deficiency (MTHFR). Other causes of thrombophilias include antithrombin, protein C, protein S deficiency, and heparin cofactor II deficiency, and antiphospholipid antibodies.

There is convincing evidence that women who are positive for the antiphospholipid antibodies (APAs) are also at increased risk for developing thrombosis and pregnancy loss.[16] Women with recurrent pregnancy loss should be screened for the APAs during the early part of the pregnancy. The clincial manifestations of APAs include DVT, PE, coronary or peripheral artery thrombosis, cerbrovascular or retinal thrombosis, and pregnancy mobidity. Most of the miscarriages (94%) in women with APAs occur in the first trimester. There is a correlation between the titer of APAs and the risk of recurrent thrombosis and spontaneous abortions. A summary of the literature reports that 5.3% of normal women, 20% of women with recurrent pregnancy loss, and 37% women with systemic lupus have APAs. The management of women with APAs is tricky due to the fact that only limited clinical trials evaluating therapy have been performed.[17]

Taking a detailed family history on pregnant patients, genetic testing and population studies of thrombophilia have led to improved risk assessments and early intervention for thrombosis in pregnancy. Other groups of women who may need prophylaxis during pregnancy include those with a history of past thrombosis, prosthetic heart valves, native valvular heart disease, and patients with antiphospholipid syndrome.[18] Pregnant women with thrombophilia require prolonged anticoagulant therapy such as coumadin, which cross the placenta and has adverse effects on the fetus.[19,20] Some of the newer agents such as the low molecular weight heparins (LMWHs) (see below) may be useful in these cases. LMWHs do not bind to endothelium and have a lower affinity to plasma proteins, which results in more predictable bioavailability and elimination kinetics.[19] This suggests that LMWHs may have several advantages of UFH for use in pregnancy. The management of thrombosis and thrombophilia during pregnancy has been refined over the past 5 years due to the better understanding of the pathophysiology of thrombosis during pregnancy and the development of newer anticoagulants for the treatment of thrombosis. The prevention and management of venous thrombosis in pregnancy is a controversial area, due to the fact that there are no major clinical studies to support evidence based practice.[20]

Low molecular weight heparins

While heparin has been used as the sole anticoagulant for nearly half a century, its use has been associated with several adverse effects, in particular the white clot syndrome, alternately known as heparin-induced thrombocytopenia and heparin-associated thrombosis (HIT/HITTS). The need for an alternate anticoagulant prompted the development of several newer anticoagulant agents which are obtained from either natural or synthetic/biosynthetic techniques. Currently, several of the newer drugs are being tested in various antithrombotic and cardiovascular indications. The LMWHs represent deploymerized heparin derivatives with better safety and efficacy profiles. Both heparin and LMWHs release an endogenous inhibitor, namely tissue factor pathway.

From the earlier studies it became evident that low-dose subcutaneous heparin produced prophylactic antithrombotic effects in surgical patients. This is due to the absorption of the low molecular weight components of heparin which exhibit mostly anti-Xa activity and produce a long-lasting effect. At the same time the bioavailability of smaller molecular weight components is markedly high. This observation led to the development of depolymerized heparin derivatives which exhibit similar properties to LMW components of heparin. In addition, these agents show decreased toxicity profiles in terms of lesser bleeding, osteoporosis, and HIT/HITTS potential.

LMWHs are now widely accepted as drugs of choice for post-surgical prophylaxis and treatment of DVT and the management of acute coronary syndromes. Currently these agents are also being developed for several additional indications. Because of manufacturing differences, each of the LMWHs exhibit distinct pharmacologic and biochemical profiles. The specific activity of these agents in the anticoagulant assays ranges from 35–45 anti-IIa U/mg whereas the specific activity in terms of anti-Xa units is designated as 80–120 anti-Xa U/mg. LMWHs are capable of producing product specific dose and time dependent antithrombotic and bleeding effects in animal models of thrombosis. While the ex vivo effects are initially present at dosages that are antithrombotic, these agents have been found to produce sustained antithrombotic effects without any detectable ex vivo anticoagulant actions.

All of the LMWHs are prepared by depolymerization of porcine mucosal heparin preparations. LMWHs are either prepared by chemical or enzymatic digestion methods as shown in Figure 11.2. Most LMWHs exhibit approximately one-third of the molecular weight of regular heparin. Initially, the clinical batches of LMWHs were prepared by fractionation of heparin. However, because of cost the limited availability of heparin for the sizeable isolation of these agents, chemical and enzymatic depolymerization procedures were developed. Physical methods such as irradiation have also been employed in the preparation of these agents. All of the currently available LMWHs are usually manufactured by chemical depolymerization. Controlled depolymerization processes are widely used to produce products with similar molecular weights, however, marked differences in the chemical composition of each of these products were inflicted during depolymerization process.

Table 11.3 Low molecular weight heparin (LMWH).

	Median molecular weight	Anti-Xa IU/mg	Anti-IIa IU/mg	Xa/IIa
Enoxaparin	4800	104	32	3.3
Dalteparin	5000	122	60	2.0
Nadroparin	4500	94	31	3.0
Tinzaparin	4500	90	50	1.8
Clivarine	3900	130	40	3.3

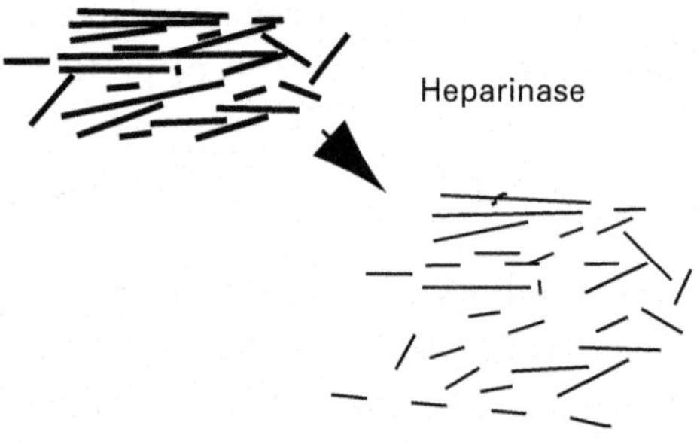

Figure 11.2 Heparin represents a polycomponent drug composed of high and low molecular weight fractions. Heparin can be depolymerized to produce low molecular weight heparins. Unfractionated heparin represents a molecular weight of 15,000 daltons, whereas the low molecular weight heparins represent one-third the molecular weight of heparin. The anticoagulant properties of low molecular weight heparin are weaker and these agents have a better safety and efficacy index.

Although the depolymerization process results in lower molecular weight heparin products (MW 4–8 kDa) as shown on Table 11.3, these products exhibit differences in their molecular, structural, and functional properties. Optimized methods are currently employed to prepare LMWHs which exhibit a similar molecular profile. However, due to the significant differences in the chemical or enzymatic procedures, structural variations are found in all of these agents. These differences, therefore, exert significant influence on the biologic action of these products.[21,22] Safety and efficacy comparison of these agents in well-designed clinical trials to demonstrate clinical differences in each of the individual products have only become available recently. Initial attempts to standardize LMWHs on the basis of their biologic actions, such as anti-Xa potency, have failed. A potency designation on the basis of the anti-Xa actions only represents one of the several properties of these agents. Furthermore, this assay only measures the AT based actions of some of the components of these agents. Many of the pharmacologic actions of LMWHs are based on the non-AT affinity components of the drugs. The non-AT III affinity components of LMWHs are also capable of producing several biologic effects such as the coagulation inhibitor, tissue factor pathway inhibitor (TFPI) release, HC II activation, and platelet selectin modulation.

Despite the clinical effectiveness of the LMWHs in various thrombotic conditions, the mechanism of action of these agents is not completely understood. More recently, it has been suggested that endogenous release of a Kunitz-type inhibitor, TFPI, may be a contributing factor to the mediation of the antithrombotic actions of these agents.[23,24] This inhibitor is also known as lipoprotein associated coagulation inhibitor, which is released from vascular sites. It is interesting to note that most of the studies on LMWH have eluded to the relevance of the anti-Xa effect with the antithrombotic action of these agents. However, after subcutaneous administration of these agents, circulating anti-Xa activity is not detectable in samples collected 12 hours after the administration of prophylactic dosages. Despite this, the patients remain in an antithrombotic state. Thus, additional mechanisms such as the release of TFPI may contribute to the overall action of these agents. LMWHs are also known to produce endothelial modulation and may release fibrinolytic activators such as t-PA and antiplatelet substances such as prostacyclin. Thus, LMWHs are effective in the control of thrombogenesis which itself is a complicated process. Endothelial dysfunction, platelet activation, white cell activation, and plasmatic process contribute to this process. Since LMWHs are polycomponent drugs with multiple sites of action, these agents are capable of controlling the process of thrombogenesis at several target sites. Unfortunately, most of the clinical trials have been designed to determine the clinical outcome with these drugs and very little is known on the pharmacologic mechanisms involved in the mediation of their action. The pharmacologic profiles of individual LMWHs has been extensively studied by various investigators. However, only limited data on the comparison of all of the available LMWHs is available at this time. Pharmacologic differentiation and inequivalence of these agents has been reported previously.[25–29]

It is now widely accepted that unlike unfractionated heparin, LMWHs exhibit both structural and functional heterogeneity and each of these agents, therefore, represents a distinct drug entity. From the clinical trials for the prophylaxis of DVT, it is evident that most of the commercially available LMWHs at optimized dosage can be used for this indication. These dosages, however, vary and are product specific. In these indications, relatively lower dosages (20–40 mg either once a day or twice a day) are used in the subcutaneous regimen. While the amidolytic anti-Xa activity can be assigned to a given LMWH, a product equivalence can not be claimed for any two products at either gravimetric or biologic potency adjusted/assigned units. Based on various discussions each of the LMWH preparations is now considered to be a distinct drug requiring individual optimization for different prophylactic and therapeutic indications.

LMWHs are also developed for therapeutic, cardiovascular, and long-term home therapy at high dosages for various indications (3–5 times higher). When these agents are used intravenously at higher dosages, the observed differences in their pharmacologic characteristics will be proportionately modified. These differences, therefore, determine the individual product profile in terms of safety and efficacy. It is, therefore, necessary to perform preclinical studies for a given indication measuring the dosage to be used for human trials. While it may not be possible to compare all products, any claims for product equivalence for a given indication must be supported by both preclinical and clinical applications. In vitro potency adjustment and equivalence claims for a product are not predictive of its in vivo behavior. Most of the clinical trials carried out on LMWHs are carried out in anti-Xa units and individualized dosages, thus these trials can not be compared.

LMWHs have been developed for several clinical indications. Several preclinical and clinical studies have been carried out on these agents or are in the process of being completed.[25,30–34] These agents have been tested for the management of post-PTCA restenosis where a high dosage of these agents is used. At higher total dosages of 100–200 mg total dosage in various regimens, LMWHs are proposed for use in various interventional cardiovascular procedures. In both the preclinical and clinical studies, LMWHs have been observed to produce beneficial effects.[34,35] In these conditions, tissue factor is released after interventional procedures. Thus, TFPI may play a key role in the mediation of the actions of LMWHs. Thus, additional studies on the relevance of TFPI to the clinical outcome with these agents may be useful.

The impressive clinical performance of LMWHs is primarily due to their polypharmacologic actions. In post-surgical states, the role of these agents as drugs of choice is well documented. Surgical trauma produces a sizeable release of tissue factor from various sites. This mediator is a potent thrombogenic agent and is capable of activating both the plasmatic and cellular sites. LMWHs are capable of releasing an endogenous inhibitor to tissue factor, namely TFPI. The subcutaneously administered LMWH produces a sustained release of this mediator. Thus, it effectively inhibits the action of tissue factor and helps in the control of thrombogenesis.

The pharmacologic differences among LMWHs can only be demonstrated by comparing these agents in valid and properly designed studies. Such studies are currently lacking and warrant further investigation. For example, in some of the newer indications, such as thrombotic stroke, large dosages of LMWHs will be used for therapeutic purposes and for the management of cardiovascular disorders. To validate the safety of these agents, Phase I studies should be carried out prior to giving the patients these agents at such higher dosages. It must be emphasized that in many of these indications, patients already received several other drugs depending upon the clinical conditions. To date, a systematic study on drug interactions is also not available. Such studies should also be carefully designed to elucidate the interactions of LMWHs with such agents as antiplatelet, thrombolytic, and vascular modulatory drugs. It is also desirable to obtain information on additional interactions of these agents with drugs that are commonly used.

Recognizing the clinical usefulness of LMWHs, the American College of Chest Physicians, 2004 Consensus conference has unequivocally endorsed the use of LMWHs in high risk major surgery, hip replacement, knee replacement, and high risk multiple trauma.[36] The consensus statement also includes favorable comments for LMWHs in contrast to the oral anticoagulant drugs for knee surgery. Needless to say, these recommendations are based on well-designed clinical trials and were objectively developed by a panel of experts. It is also important that such recommendations have taken into account the product specific clinical outcome. Besides the prophylaxis of post surgical and medical DVT/PE, guidelines for the treatment have also been endorsed. In addition on the LMWHs, namely enoxaparin is now approved for the management of acute coronary syndromes. Thus, the ACCP consensus statement has also endorsed the use of this agent.

There are several newer clinical trials in progress using different products in indication specific protocols. These trials are designed to investigate the effects of LMWHs in the treatment of DVT/PE, cancer associated thrombosis, stroke, and several cardiovascular indications. Each of these trials was designed either empirically or by considering results of pilot trials on a given product. The dosages used are product specific. Some of these trials employ relatively high dosage for long periods of time. In these situations, each product will have its own clinical profile. The results of these trials will certainly validate the notion that all LMWHs are not the same. The future consensus conferences will also consider the product based differences and a collective statement based on the performance of LMWHs as a group must be based on valid meta-analysis.

In some of the clinical trials and preclinical studies LMWHs have been reported to exhibit reduced morbidity and mortality associated with thrombosis during pregnancy suggesting that these drugs may also have therapeutic value in pregnancy.[37] Once again suggestions have been made that some of these LMWHs may be better in producing their effects than others.

In the United States there are three LMWHs currently approved for the prophylaxis and treatment of DVT. One of these LMWHs is also approved for an additional indication for the management of unstable angina and non-Q wave myocardial infarction. In addition to the approved uses LMWHs are currently tested for the management of thrombotic and ischemic stroke, malignancy associated thrombosis and transplantation associated vasculopathies. Being a polypharmacologic agent these drugs are expected to find usages in several other clinical indications. Well-designed clinical trials in which various pharmacokinetic and pharmacodynamic parameters are also studied will provide additional evidence on the clinical individuality of each of these drugs. Additional studies on the pharmacologic and biochemical profiles of each of the individual drugs will provide useful information on the mechanism and site of action of these drugs.

Anticoagulant therapy during pregnancy

The indications for anticoagulation in pregnancy include prophylaxis and/or treatment of DVT, history of chronic anticoagulation for prior conditions, and risk of pregnancy loss. Studies to support the use of anticoagulation therapy in preeclampsia and the hemolysis elevated liver enzymes low platelet (HELLP) syndrome have recently been reported.[38,39] Historically, UFH was the anticoagulant used during pregnancy, because unlike warfarin it does not cross the placental barrier and cause teratogenic effects.[2] However, UFH can be difficult to dose during pregnancy and requires monitoring using the activated partial thromboplastin time (APTT). Side effects with prolonged treatment of UFH, include osteoporotic fractures and loss of bone mass. Greer has estimated that in pregnancy, UFH treatment results in 30% of women losing at least 10% of their bone mass and 2% experience fractures.[2] LMWHs offer an alternative to UFH since they have better bioavailability, do not cross the placenta, are easy to use, and reportedly have a lower incidence for osteoporosis.[2]

There are several studies on the administration of LMWHs during pregnancy.[40–50] In one study enoxaparin 40 mg was administered to 13 pregnant women during early pregnancy (12–15 weeks), late pregnancy (30–33 weeks), and in the postpartum period (6–8 weeks after delivery). During pregnancy, the maximum concentration and last measurable anti-Xa levels were considerably lower than in the postpartum period ($p = 0.05$).[42] This difference is probably due to the increased renal clearance of the LMWH during pregnancy.[42] An adjustment in the dosage of LMWH may therefore be required to maintain anti-Xa activity in pregnancy. Enoxaparin has also been studied in women requiring thromboprophylaxis after delivery by cesarean section. Two dosages on enoxaparin, 20 and 40 mg once a day, were compared with UFH 7,500 IU twice a day.[43] Although the study was small, 17 women, no thrombotic or bleeding events were observed.[43] Another study in women undergoing abortion due to fetal malformation confirmed that enoxaparin does not pass the placental barrier.[44] This suggests that enoxaparin may be without risk to the fetus if taken during pregnancy. However, since the level of enoxaparin was measured using a functional method, the presence of other non-anticoagulant effects of this drug cannot be ruled out.

A small randomized controlled trial in 107 women compared dalteparin to UFH. No thrombotic events were report in either group however, the bleeding complications were higher in the UFH treated group.[45] Two larger trials have conformed the safety and efficacy of enoxaparin during pregnancy.[46,47] In a total of 111 woman treated with 40 mg of enoxaparin, no thrombotic or hemorrhagic events were reported. Several larger studies also confirmed the safety and efficacy of enoxaparin during pregnancy.[48,49] One of these studies reported a congenital abnormality rate of 2.5%, which is consistent with the literature.[48]

A comprehensive literature summarized the findings of 40 published studies involving women treated with LMWHs.[50] Among these patients, 47% received dalteparin, 26% enoxaparin, and 27% other LMWHs. Highly variable dosing regimens and treatment regimens were reported. The major outcomes included 9 thromboembolic events, 8 cases of DVT, 4 pulmonary embolisms, 4 cases of thrombophlebitis, 1 placental abruption, 12 cases of preeclampsia, 27 bleeding episodes, and 2 fractures due to osteoporosis. Local skin reactions were observed in 18 patients. Overall these studies showed that LMWHs are safe and effective, although additional studies are warranted.[51]

A placebo controlled randomized study in 202 women, showed no benefit to using aspirin and prednisone in pregnant women with prior pregnancy loss and APAs.[52] Additional trials with UFH comparing aspirin and UFH to aspirin alone, showed improved fetal survival with the combination.[52,53] Results of published trials using LMWHs suggest that LMWHs are efficacious in women with APAs and fetal loss. The available data suggests that aspirin and heparin therapy are the treatment of choice for prevention of pregnancy loss in women with APAs. It is very likely that LMWHs will also prove to be effective in this indication.

Pregnant women with high titer APAs and no pregnancy losses, but previous DVT should be considered for prophylaxis with UFH or LMWH. Women with APAs who have no previous history of thrombosis or pregnancy loss should still be considered for prophylaxis with UFH or LMWHs.

A recent study of pregnant patients with elevated titers of anticardiolipin β_2-glycoprotein I antibody may be at increased risk for fetal–maternal complications.[54]

Recommendation from the ACCP Consensus

The Consensus Conference on Antithrombotic Therapy of the American College of Chest Physicians (ACCP) has developed guidelines to help clinicians make treatment decisions for patients. These recommendations along with the physicians' clinical judgement need to be considered prior to treatment. These experts in the field, have developed a systematic approach to grading the strength of the treatment recommendations to minimize bias and aid in the interpretation. In this grading system the 1A-1C recommendations are strong recommendations that can apply to most patients. The 2A grading is a intermediate-strength recommendation depending on circumstances or the patient. A 2B recommendation is weak where alternative approaches may be better in some patients. The 2C grading is a very-weak recommendation where other alternative therapy may be as good. These are only recommendations and it is up to the individual physician to assess the patient and determine what is the best treatment under the given circumstances for each patient.

Management of pregnant patients at increased risk for VTE

For a single episode of previous VTE associate with a transient risk factor, surveillance and postpartum anticoagulation is recommended. For a single incidence of idiopathic VTE in patients not already on long-term anticoagulation surveillance of mini-dose UFH, moderate dose UFH or prophylaxis with LMWH, plus postpartum anticoagulation is recommended. For a single episode of VTE and confirmed thrombophilia in patients not already receiving long-term anticoagulant therapy mini-dose UFH, moderate dose UFH or prophylaxis with LMWH, plus postpartum anticoagulation is recommended. The indication for active prophylaxis is stronger in women with antithrombin deficiency. For no prior VTE and confirmed thrombophilia mini-dose UFH, moderate dose UFH or prophylaxis with LMWH, plus postpartum anticoagulation is recommended. For multiple episodes of VTE and/or women receiving long-term anticoagulation (single episode of VTE, either idiopathic or associated with thrombophilia), adjusted-dose UFH, or prophylaxis or adjusted-dose LMWH, followed by resuming long-term anticogulation postpartum is recommended. These are all grade 1C recommendations.

Treatment of VTE of pregnancy

Adjusted-dose LMWH throughout pregnancy or UFH IV bolus, followed by a continuous infusion (to maintain APTT in therapeutic range) for at least 5 days, followed by adjusted-dose UFH for the remainder of the pregnancy. Therapy should be stopped 24 hours prior to delivery. If the woman is at high risk to develop recurrent VTE, defined as proximal DVT within 2 weeks, therapeutic UFH should be initiated and stopped 4–6 hours before expected delivery. Postpartum therapy should be administered for at least 6 weeks. This is a grade 1C recommendation.

Unexpected pregnancy or planned pregnancy in patients already receiving long-term anticoagulation

These patients should be told about the risks before pregnancy. Frequent pregnancy tests should be performed and adjusted-dose LMWH or UFH should be substituted for warfarin when pregnancy is achieved. Alternately, UFH or LMWH can replace warfarin before conception. Both of these treatments have limitations. The first treatment assumes warfarin is safe during the first 4–6 weeks of gestation. The second treatment approach extends the use of UFH or LMWH. The recommendations are for the first treatment approach. However, the first option has an increased risk of serious osteoporosis in the mother, particularly if she is not a primipara or older patient. The patient should be so advised. This is a 1C recommendation.

Prophylaxis in patients with mechanical heart valves

Three treatment modalities have been recommended. The first is aggressive adjusted-dose UFH (s.c. every 12 hours in a dose to keep APTT at least twice control) throughout pregnancy. The second is adjusted-dose LMWH throughout pregnancy, adjusted according to weight or to keep 4 hour post administration anti-Xa level at 1.0 U/ml. The third approach is UFH or LMWH as given in the first two approaches, until the 13th week, change to warfarin until the middle of the third trimester, then restart UFH or LMWH until delivery.

These are all grade 2C recommendations.

Management of pregnant women at increased risk for pregnancy loss

Women with three or more miscarriages should be screened for APAs. If one of the losses occurred in the second trimester, screening for thrombophilia should be performed. In addition, women with prior severe or recurrent preeclampsia, IUGR, abruption, or other unexplained complications should be screened for congenital thrombophilia and APAs. Pregnant women with APAs and a history of multiple pregnancy losses or preeclampsia, IUGR, or abruption should be treated with antepartum aspirin plus mini-dose or moderate dose UFH or prophylaxis with LMWH. This is a grade 1B recommendation.

Women who are homozygous for the methylenetetrahydrofolate reductase (MTHFR) variant (C677T) should be treated with folic acid supplements prior to conception or if already pregnant, as soon as possible. This is a 2C recommendation. Women with a thrombophilic deficiency who have experienced recurrent miscarriages, a second triemster or later loss or preeclampsia, IUGR or abruption should also be considered for low-dose aspirin plus mini-dose UFH or prophylaxis with LMWH. These women should also receive postpartum anticoagulation. This is a grade 2C recommendation.

Patients positive for APAs and a history of venous thrombosis, who are receiving long-term therapy, during pregnancy should be treated with adjusted-dose UFH or LMWH throughout the pregnancy and return to oral anticoagulants postpartum. This is a grade 2C recommendation. In addition, women positive for APAs and no history of VTE or pregnancy loss should be considered at risk for the development of DVT and pregnancy loss. Four treatment approaches have been recommended. These treatments are surveillance, mini-dose UFH, prophylactic LMWH or low-dose aspirin (80–325 mg qd). This is also a 2C recommendation.

A statement from the American College of Obstetricians and Gynecologists also supports the use of enoxaparin in pregnancy with two precautions.[55] LMWHs are not recommended in pregnant women with prosthetic heart valves. This warning came after reports of frequent valvular thrombosis in pregnant women treated with LMWH.[56] The second precaution is that LMWHs should not be administered 24–48 hours prior to the administration of epidural analgesics during labor. This stems from the warning issued on increased risk of hematomas, that may lead to permanent paralysis when LMWHs are used with spinal/epidural analgesics.[57] In addition, use of non-steroidal anti-inflammatory agents or other drugs that alter hemostasis may increase this risk.

In view of the fact that a study showed that the use of LMWHs in non-pregnant subjects with mechanical heart valve replacement was successful, it encourages us to evaluate this therapy in pregnant patients.[58]

In a 1999 article, Messmore *et al.* suggested that a study such as the one cited above would provide encouragement to start a trial of LMWH in pregnant patients with mechanical heart valves.[59] There are some successful anecdotal reports which should provide some guidance as to dosages that might be safe and effective.[59–61] Monitoring with anti-Xa levels should be a part of such a study, assuring a dosage to provide a blood level of at least 1.0 AXa U/ml. Monitoring for osteoporosis is advisable as well inspite of reports that it should be less than with heparin therapy.

Another special problem encountered uncommonly in pregnancy is heparin-induced thrombocytopenia (HIT). A number of anecdotal reports have supported the use of danaparoid (ORG 10172-Orgaran) in pregnant patients with the HIT syndrome. None of these were patients with prosthetic heart valves. This drug has a low probability of interaction with the HIT antibody, but testing with platelet aggegation or serotonin release assay has been reported to be positive in some cases. Thus, it is important to test for the HIT antibody and avoid its use if the test is positive. Platelet counts during use are advisable. A thorough review of the use of danaparoid in HIT patients has been published by Chong and Magnani.[62,63] This drug is no longer marketed in the United States, but it is available in Canada and Europe. It is marketed by the Organon Corporation and inquiries should be directed to them.

It is obvious that the pregnant patient is underserved by the pharmaceutical industry and the medical community in the area of hypercoagulable syndromes and thromboembolism. Dedicated research in this area is vitally needed.

Newer antithrombotic and anticoagulant drugs

Several newer anticoagulant and antithrombotic drugs have been introduced recently (Figure 11.3). These drugs represent a wide array of agents with molecular and functional diversity, however with the exception of heparins most of these drugs are monotheraputic and target specific sites in hemostatic process.[43,44] Of these agents the synthetic pentasaccharide is noteworthy. While this agent is not developed for specific indications in pregnancy, it has been clinically validated in various thrombotic disorders. Pentasaccharide primarily produces its anticoagulant actions by interacting with endogenous antithrombin and inhibits thrombin generation. Pentasaccharide is a relatively small molecule (MW <2,000 daltons) and in its free form it is expected to pass the placental barrier. However, when complexed with antithrombin it does not pass through the placental barrier. Since pentasaccharide exists in an equilibrium, it is likely that it may pass through the placental barrier. However, no data are available in clinical setting on this issue. While pentasaccharide may be useful in pregnancy associated thrombosis, the questions related to its effect on fetal growth and hemostatic process are not known. Regardless of this issue, pentasaccharide and its analogues should be considered for this indication. However, some preclinical studies are needed prior to the initiation of the clinical trial in this area.

The recognition of HIT syndrome has led to the development of various antithrombin agents such as hirudin, hirulog, angiomax, and argatroban. All of these agents are currently used as potential anticoagulants in heparin compromised patients. All agents are capable of passing through the placental barrier. Therefore, their utilization in pregnancy associated thrombotic indications may be inhibited. Currently, several new anti-Xa and anti-IIa drugs are being developed. Of these exanta or ximelagatran is in advanced clinical development. This drug is approved in France for post orthopedic surgical thrombosis. However, in the US this agent is under consideration by the US FDA. Ximelagatran has been clearly validated in post-surgical thrombosis and atrial fibrillation. However, ximelagatran has a relatively small molecular weight (<500 daltons) and is capable of passing through the placental barrier. Furthermore, it has been shown to produce an increase in liver enzymes. Thus, this drug and similar antithrombin agents may not be useful in pregnancy.

Both the parenteral and oral forms of anti-Xa agents are also currently being developed. These agents also represent small molecular weight (<500 daltons)

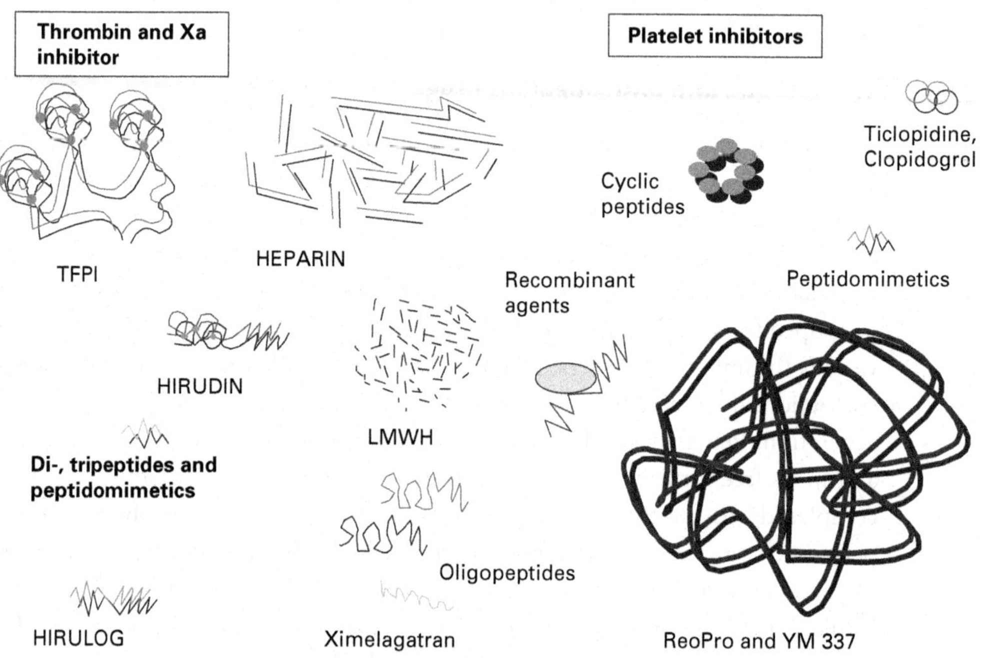

Figure 11.3 A composite illustration for the newly developed anticoagulant and antithrombotic drugs. These agents include a wide array of drugs with both the molecular and functional heterogeneity. These include synthetic peptides and peptidomimetics, natural and recombinant proteins, natural glycosaminoglycans and synthetic and biotechnology produced glycomimetics. Most of the newer drugs are monotherapeutic agents and target a single site such as thrombin or factor Xa. Heparins are the only drugs with polytherapeutic effects.

synthetic agents which are capable of passing through the placental barrier. There are no studies available on the relatively safety and efficacy of these agents in pregnancy at the clinical and preclinical level. However, the relative safety of the anti-Xa drugs may be higher than the anti-IIa drugs. Thus, additional studies are warranted on these agents for their potential usefulness in pregnancy.

While the newly developed antithrombotic drugs may be of value for the acute and extended management of thrombosis, their relative usefulness in the pregnant patient is questionable. The most unmet need in this area is to replace long-term use of heparin and LMWHs. Since the extended use of heparin may result in osteoporosis, the LMWHs represent an optimal approach to manage pregnancy associated thrombosis. Despite several clinical trials with different LMWHs, a recommendation on the use of these agents is primarily not endorsed. Additional large scale trials to validate the safety and efficacy of various LMWHs are needed. The coming years will witness the introduction of several newer antithrombotic agents in the management of thrombosis, whose efficacy in pregnancy-related thrombosis will require clinical validation.

REFERENCES

1 Toglia, M. R., Weg, J. G. Current concepts. VTE during pregnancy. *N. Engl. J. Med.*, 1996; **335**: 108–14.

2 Greer, I. A. Exploring the role of low-molecular-weight heparins in pregnancy. *Semin. Thromb. Hemost.*, 2002; **28**(Suppl. 3): 25–31S.

3 Eldor, A. Management of thrombophilia and antiphospholipid syndrome during pregnancy In *Consultative Hemostasis and Thrombosis*, ed. Kitchens, C., Alving, B., Kessler, C. Philadelphia, PA: W. B. Saunders Co. Elsevier Science, 2002, pp. 449–60.

4 Howard, P. A. Low molecular weight heparin in special populations. *J. Infus. Nurs.*, 2003; **26**(5): 304–10.

5 Bonnar, J., Prentice, C. R., McNicol, G. P., *et al.* Haemostatic mechanisms in the uterine circulation during placental seperation. *Br. Med. J.*, 1970; **1**: 564–70.

6 Greer, I. A. In *Haemostasis and Thrombosis in Pregnancy*, ed. Bloom, A. L., Forbes, C. D., Thomas, D. P., *et al.* Edinburgh: Churchill Livingstone, 1994, p. 987.

7 Greer, I. A. Thrombosis in pregnancy: maternal and fetal issues. *Lancet*, 1999; **353**: 1258–65.

8 Leduc, L., Wheeler, J. M., Kirshon, B., *et al.* Coagulation profile in severe preeclampsia. *Obstet. Gynecol.*, 1992; **79**: 14.

9 Astedt, B., Lecander, I., Ny, T. Placental type plasminogen activator inhibitor: PAI-2. *Fibrinolysis*, 1987; **1**: 203–9.

10 Redman, C. W. Platelets and the beginning of preeclampsia. *N. Engl. J. Med.*, 1990; **323**: 478.

11 Burrows, R. F., Hunter, D. J., Andrew, M., *et al.* A prospective study investigating the mechanism of thrombocytopenia in preeclampsia. *Obstet. Gynecol.*, 1987; **70**: 334.

12 Greer, I. A. Epidemiology, risk factors and prophylaxis of venous thrombo-embolism in obstetrics and gynaecology. *Baillieres Clin. Obstet. Gynaecol.*, 1997; **11**: 403–30.

13 Macklon, N. S., Greer, I. A., Bowman, A. W. An ultrasound study of gestational and postural changes in the deep venous system of the leg in pregnancy. *Br. J. Obstet. Gynaecol.*, 1997; **104**: 191–7.

14 Rutherford, S. E., Phelan, J. P. Thromboembolic disease in pregnancy. *Clin. Perinatol.*, 1986; **13**: 719.

15 Brown, T. K., Munsick, R. A. Puerperal ovarian vein thrombophlebitis: A syndrome. *Am. J. Obstet. Gynecol.*, 1971; **109**: 263–73.

16 Lockshin, M. D. Pregnancy loss in the antiphospholipid syndrome. *Thromb. Haemost.*, 1999; **82**: 641–8.

17 Greaves, M. Antiphospholipid antibodies and thrombosis (Letter; Comment). *Lancet*, 1999; **354**: 1031.

18 Long, A. A., Ginsberg, J. S., Brill-Edwards, P., *et al.* The relationship of antiphospholipid antibodies to thromboembolic disease in systemic lupus erythematosus: a cross-sectional study. *Thromb. Haemost.*, 1991; **66**: 520–4.

19 Ginsberg, J. S., Brill-Edwards, P., Johnston, M., *et al.* Relationship of antiphospholipid antibodies to pregnancy loss in patients with systemic lupus erythematosus: a cross-sectional study. *Blood*, 1992; **80**: 975–80.

20 Ginsberg, J. S., Greer, I., Hirsh, J. Use of antithrombotic agents during pregnancy. *Chest*, 2001; **119**: 1225–315.

21 Fareed, J., Walenga, J. M., Kumar, A., *et al.* A modified stasis thrombosis model to study the antithrombotic actions of heparin and its fractions. *Semin. Thromb. Hemost.*, 1985; **11**: 155.

22 Fareed, J., Hoppensteadt, D., Huan, X., *et al.* Comparative study on the in vitro and in vivo activities of seven low molecular weight heparins. *Hemostasis*, 1989; **18**(Suppl. 3): 3.

23 Abildgaard, U., Sandset, P., Lindahl, A. Tissue factor pathway inhibitor. In *Recent Advances in Blood Coagulation*, 6th edn, ed. Poller, L. Edinburgh: Churchill Livingstone, 1993, pp. 105–24.

24 Bronze, G. J. Tissue factor pathway inhibitor and the current concept of blood coagulation. *Blood Coag. Fibrinolysis*, 1995; **6**(1): 7–12S.

25 Fareed, J., Hoppensteadt, D., Jeske, W., *et al.* Low molecular weight heparins: pharmacologic profile and product differentiation. *Am. J. Cardiol.*, 1995; **82**(5B): 3–10L.

26 Fareed, J., Hoppensteadt, D., Jeske, W., *et al.* Low molecular weight heparins: are they different?. *Can. J. Cardiol.*, 1998; **14**(28): 28–34E.

27 Brieger, D., Dawes, J. Production method affects the pharmacokinetic and ex vivo biologic properties of low molecular weight heparins. *Thromb. Haemost.*, 1997; **77**(2): 317–22.

28 Fareed, J., Hoppensteadt, D., Jeske, W., *et al.* Low molecular weight heparins: a developmental perspective. *Exp. Opin. Invest. Drugs.*, 1997; **6**(6): 705–20.

29 Wolzt, M., Eder, M., Welterman, A., *et al.* Comparison of the effects of different low molecular weight heparins on the hemostatic system activation in vivo in man. *Thromb. Haemost.*, 1997; **78**(2): 876–9.

30 Hoppensteadt, D., Jeske, W., Fareed, J., *et al.* The role of tissue factor pathway inhibitor in the mediation of the antithrombotic actions of heparin and low molecular weight heparin. *Blood Coag. Fibrinolysis*, 1995; **6**: S57.

31 Bognacki, J., Hammelburger, J. Functional and immunologic methods for the measurement of human tissue factor pathway inhibitor. *Blood Coag. Fibrinolysis*, 1995; **6**: S65.

32 Hoppensteadt, D., Walenga, J. M., Fasanella, A., *et al.* TFPI antigen levels in normal human volunteers after intravenous and subcutaneous administration of unfractionated heparin and low molecular weight heparin. *Thromb. Res.*, 1995; **77**(2): 175.

33 Fareed, J. Basic and applied pharmacology of low molecular weight heparins. *Pharmacy and Therapeutics*, 1995; **46**: 16–24S.

34 Fareed, J., Callas, D., Hoppensteadt, D., *et al.* Recent developments in antithrombotic agents. *Invest. Exp. Opin. Drugs*, 1995; **4**: 389–412.

35 Fareed, J., Walenga, J. M., Pifarre, R. Newer approaches to the pharmacologic management of acute myocardial infarction. *Cardiac Surgery: State of the Art Reviews*, 1992; **6**: 101.

36 Hirsh, J., Guyatt, G., Albers, G., *et al.* The seventh ACCP conference on antithrombotic and thrombolytic therapy: evidence based medicine. *Chest*, 2004: **126**: 167–696S.

37 Hunt, B. J., Doughty, H. A., Majumdar, G., *et al.* Thromboprophylaxis with low-molecular-weight heparin in high risk pregnancies. *Thromb. Hemost.*, 1997; **77**: 39.

38 Kobayashi, T. K., Terao, T., Ikenoue, T., *et al.* Treatment of severe preeclampsia with antithrombin concentrate: results of a prospective feasibility study. *Semin. Ped. Thromb. Hemost.*, 2003; **29**(6): 645–53.

39 Ohta, K., Kobashi, G., Hata, A., *et al.* Association between a variant of the glutathione s-transferase p1 gene (GSTP1) and hypertension in pregnancy in Japanese: interaction with parity, age, and genetic factors. *Semin. Thromb. Hemost.*, 2003; **29**(6): 653–8.

40 Eldor, A. Thrombophilia, thrombosis and pregnancy. *Thromb. Haemost.*, 2001; **86**(1): 104–11.

41 Sanson, B. J., Lensing, A. W., Prins, M. H., *et al.* Safety of low-molecular-weight heparin in pregnancy: a systematic review. *Thromb. Haemost.*, 1999; **81**: 668–72.

42 Casele, H. L., Laifer, S. A., Woelkers, D. A., *et al.* Changes in the pharmacokinetics of the low-molecular-weight heparin enoxaparin sodium during pregnancy. *Am. J. Obstet. Gynecol.*, 1999; **181**: 1113–17.

43 Gibson, J. L., Ekevall, K., Walker, I., *et al.* Puerperal thromboprophylaxis: comparison of the anti-Xa activity of enoxaparin and unfractionated heparin. *Br. J. Obstet. Gynaecol.*, 1998; **105**: 795–7.

44 Forestier, F., Daffos, F., Capella-Pavlovsky, M. Low molecular weight heparin (PK 10169) does not cross the placenta during the second trimester of pregnancy: studied by direct fetal blood sampling ultrasound. *Thromb. Res.*, 1984; **34**: 557–60.

45 Pettila, V., Kaaja, R., Leinonem, P., *et al.* Thromboprophylaxis with low molecular weight heparin (dalteparin) in pregnancy. *Thromb. Res.*, 1999; **96**: 275–82.

46 Nelson-Piercy, C., Letsky, E. A., de Swiet, M. Low molecular weight heparin for obstetric thromboprophylaxis: experience of sixty-nine pregnancies in sixty-one women at high risk. *Am. J. Obstet. Gynecol.*, 1997; **176**: 1062–8.

47 Ellison, J., Walker, I. D., Greer, I. A. Antenatal use of enoxaparin for the prevention and treatment of thromboembolism in pregnancy. *Br. J. Obstet. Gynaecol.*, 2000; **107**: 1116–21.

48 Lepercq, J., Conard, J., Borel Derlon, A., *et al.* Venous thromboembolism during pregnancy: a systematic review. *Thromb. Haemost.*, 1999; **81**: 668–72.

49 Sanson, B. J., Lensing, A. W. A., Prins, M. H., *et al.* Safety of low-molecular weight heparin in pregnancy: a systematic review. *Thromb. Haemost.*, 1999; **81**: 668–72.

50 Enson, M. H. H., Stephenson, M. D. Low-molecular-weight heparins in pregnancy. *Pharmacotherapy*, 1999; **19**: 1013–25.

51 Ginsberg, J. S., Greer, I., Hirsh, J. Use of antithrombotic agents during pregnancy. In Dalen J. E., Hirsh, J., Guyatt G. H., eds. Sixth ACCP Consensus Conference on Antithrombotic Therapy. *Chest*, 2001; **119**(Suppl. 1): 122–31S.

52 Rai, R., Cohen, H., Dave, M., *et al.* Randomised controlled trial of aspirin and aspirin plus heparin in pregnant women with recurrent miscarriage associated with phospholipid antibodies (or antiphospholipid antibodies). *Br. Med. J.*, 1997; **314**: 253–7.

53 Kutteh, W. H. Antiphospholipid antibody-associated recurrent pregnancy loss: treatment with heparin and low dose aspirin is superior to low-dose aspirin alone. *Am. J. Obstet. Gynecol.*, 1996; **174**: 1584–89.

54 Yamada, H., Kato, E. H., Morikawa, M., *et al.* Anticardiolipin B2-glycoprotein I antibody: is a high titer related to unfavorable pregnancy outcome? *Semin. Thromb. Hemost.*, 2003; **29**(6): 639–43.

55 AGOC Committee Opinion: safety of Lovenox in pregnancy. *Obstet. Gynecol.*, 2002; **100**(4): 845–6.

56 Aggarwal, M. Use of low-molecular-weight heparin in pregnant women with mechanical heart valves. *Mayo Clin. Proc.*, 2002; **77**: 1133–4.

57 Wu, C. L. Regional anesthesia and anticoagulation *J. Clin. Anesth.*, 2001; **13**: 49–58.

58 Montalescot, G., Polle, V., Collet, J. P., *et al.* Low molecular weight heparin after mechanical heart valve replacement. *Circulation*, 2000, **20**: 1083–6.

59 Messmore, H. L., Kundur, R., Wehrmacher, W., *et al.* Anticoagulant therapy of pregnant patients with prosthetic heart valves: rationale for a clinical trial of low molecular weight heparin. *Clin. Appl. Thrombosis/Hemostasis*, 1999; **5**(2): 73–7.

60 Chan, W. S., Anand, S., Ginsberg, J. S. Anticoagulation of pregnant women with mechanical heart valves. *Arch. Intern. Med.*, 2000; **160**: 191–6.

61 Vitale, N., de Feo, M., de Santo, L. S., *et al.* Dose-dependent fetal complications of warfarin in pregnant women with mechanical heart valves. *J. Am. Coll. Cardiol.*, 1999; **33**: 1637–41.

62 Chong, B., Magnani, H. Danaparoid for the treatment of heparin induced thrombocytopenia. In *Heparin Induced Thrombocytopenia*, 2nd edn, ed. Warkentin, T. E., Greinacher, A. Basel, Switzerland: Marcel Dekker Inc., NY, 2001, pp. 323–47.

63 Magnani, H. N. Heparin-induced thrombocytopenia (HIT): an overview of 230 patients treated with orgaran (org 10172). *Thromb. Hemost.*, 1993; **70**(4), 554–61.

64 Hoppensteadt, D., Walenga, J. M., Fareed, J. Heparin, low-molecular-weight heparins, and heparin pentasaccharide. Basic and clinical differentiation. *Hematol. Oncol. Clin. N. Am.*, 2003; **17**: 313–41.

65 Fareed, J., Hoppensteadt, D. A., Bick, R. L. Management of thrombotic and cardiovascular disorders in the new millennium. *Clin. Appl. Thrombosis/Hemostasis*, 2003; **9**(2): 101–8.

12

Post partum hemorrhage: Prevention, diagnosis, and management

William F. Baker, Jr., M.D., F.A.C.P.,[1] Joseph Mansour, M.D.[2] and Arthur Fontaine, M.D.[3]

[1]Associate Clinical Professor of Medicine, Center for Health Sciences, David Geffen School of Medicine at University of California-Los Angeles, Los Angeles, CA, USA Thrombosis, Hemostasis, and Special Hematology Clinic, Kern Medical Center, Bakersfield, California; California Clinical Thrombosis Center, Bakersfield, California, USA
[2]Associate Professor, Department of Obstetrics and Gynecology, Kern Medical Center, Bakersfield, California, USA
[3]Chairman of Radiology, Mercy Hospital, Bakersfield, California, USA

Introduction

Although childbirth is a wonderful and enjoyable experience by most, it still is an anatomically traumatic event, associated with tissue injury, vascular disruption and the potential for blood loss. All deliveries are accompanied by physiologic hemorrhage from the genital tract, and the abdominal soft tissue in cesarean section (Table 12.1). Post partum hemorrhage (PPH) is an obstetrical complication, which can transform a normal physiologic process of labor and delivery into a life-threatening emergency within minutes. A routine cesarean section can be complicated by massive hemorrhage. The healthy mother may quickly become a patient in the critical care unit, requiring all of the available skill and resources of physicians, nurses, the medical laboratory and the blood bank for survival. A thorough knowledge of the risk factors, preventive strategies, approach to diagnosis and management of PPH are required to properly care for women presenting for delivery. Once PPH is diagnosed, hospital facilities and/or referral centers, laboratories and blood banks must be readily available to provide the optimal chance for a successful outcome. The availability of blood replacement and modern critical care are major determinants of survival in women who develop post partum hemorrhagic shock. Mortality from PPH is strongly correlated with substandard care.[1] Clearly, it is the problem of PPH that most vividly illustrates the difference, worldwide, between management of the puerperium in developed countries from that in underdeveloped countries.[2] Good prenatal care to detect and treat correctable risk factors and active management of the third stage of labor can usually prevent PPH. This chapter reviews the pathophysiology

Hematological Complications in Obstetrics, Pregnancy, and Gynecology, ed. R. L. Bick *et al.* Published by Cambridge University Press.

Table 12.1 Physiologic parturition hemorrhage.

Physiologic/normal vascular injury
Placental separation
Uterine vascular separation
Cervical laceration (minor)
Vaginal laceraton (minor)
Perineal laceration (minor)
Episiotomy
Cesarean section
Cutaneous and abdominal wall incision
Uterine incision

of PPH and the underlying risk factors for its occurrence, strategies to identify and properly treat high-risk patients (including those with hemorrhagic diatheses), as well as the approach to clinical, laboratory, and radiological diagnosis and management involving the use of pharmacologic agents, blood products, interventional radiology, and surgery.

Incidence

Post partum hemorrhage is a major cause of maternal morbidity and mortality, causing the death of 150,000 women per year, worldwide. Post partum hemorrhage is the underlying factor in 17% to 40% of the maternal mortality per year in underdeveloped countries.[3,4] This amounts to a risk of death from PPH in developing countries of 1 in 1,000.[4] By contrast, in the United Kingdom, the risk of mortality from PPH is 1 in 100,000.[5] Hemorrhage is the leading cause of maternal mortality and PPH accounts for the majority of it.[6,7]

The United States incidence of post partum hemorrhage (as defined by the American College of Obstetrics and Gynecology) is 3.9% for vaginal deliveries and 6.4% for cesarean sections.[8–10] The incidence of PPH may, however, be greatly influenced by the approach to the third phase of labor. When management of the third stage of labor is active and includes the routine use of an oxytocic agent after delivery, the risk of PPH is reduced by 40%.[11,12] Mortality and morbidity from PPH are related not only to hemorrhagic shock but also to other systemic consequences. In the absence of blood replacement (as occurs most often in underdeveloped countries), the mother may die of exsanguination.[2,13] Hemorrhagic shock may also lead to pathologic derangements triggering multiple organ dysfunction syndrome (MODS)[5,14] or, at the least, may result in significant post partum anemia. Post partum iron deficiency anemia may cause symptoms of malaise, fatigue and may impair effective breast-feeding. The true clinical impact of PPH is therefore, not easily quantified. It is estimated that morbidity from PPH affects 20 million women per year, worldwide.[15]

Definition of post partum hemorrhage

The World Health Organization (WHO) has defined PPH as the post partum loss of greater than 500 ml of blood after delivery.[16] While this definition may be considered arbitrary, it is a volume of hemorrhage that, untreated may be sufficient to cause hemorrhagic shock and death.[17,18] Post partum hemorrhage after cesarean section is defined as blood loss in excess of 1,000 ml.[10] This is also defined by the American College of Obstetrics and Gynecology as either a 10% change in hematocrit between admission and post partum or the need for a blood transfusion.[8] Primary PPH is defined as blood lost within the first 24 hours of delivery and secondary PPH as that which occurs from 24 hrs to 12 weeks post partum. Early hemorrhage is far more common than late.[10] Primary PPH may also be characterized as either placental or extra-placental hemorrhage.[19] While the widely accepted definition of PPH is more than 500 ml of blood lost, the diagnosis rests also on other clinical features. A more useful definition is any blood loss, which causes a physiological change threatening the woman's life.[20] In the severely anemic woman, for example, a mere 250 ml blood loss might result in the same adverse clinical outcomes as the loss of a larger volume in a woman with normal hemoglobin (Hgb).[19,21]

The definition of PPH has been further categorized by the addition of the terms major PPH and severe or massive PPH. These are cases in which the volume of blood lost is greater than 1,000 ml (major PPH) to 1,500 ml (severe or massive PPH). Severe PPH may be further defined as a Hgb drop of $\geq$4 g/dl and transfusion of $\geq$4 units of blood. Table 12.2 summarizes the accepted definitions of PPH. In a United Kingdom study, severe PPH was approximated to occur in 6.7 per 1,000 deliveries.[5,22] The source of blood loss may also greatly influence clinical consequences and management. Bleeding from the body and fundus of uterus usually responds to uterotonic agents, however, hemorrhage from the lower uterine segment may require more vigorous medical and/or surgical intervention.[19]

Massive (severe) post partum hemorrhage

While hemorrhagic shock may result from as little as 250 ml of blood loss in especially vulnerable patients, most lethal consequences of PPH occur when the

Table 12.2 Definitions of post partum hemorrhage.

Blood loss of >500 ml following vaginal delivery and >1,000 ml following a cesarean section
Early PPH
Blood lost within the first 24 hours of delivery
Late PPH
Blood lost from 24 hours to 12 weeks after delivery
Major PPH
Blood loss >1,000 ml
Massive/severe PPH
Blood loss >1,500 ml
PPH in severely anemic women
Blood loss >250 ml

volume and rate of blood loss is much greater. Massive (also termed severe) post partum hemorrhage has been variably defined.[14] In general, the definitions include reference both to the total volume of blood transfused and the overall clinical consequences. With blood loss of over 1,500 ml (about 25% of total blood volume), massive hemorrhage resulting in hemorrhagic shock should be anticipated. The usual definition includes blood loss requiring the replacement of the patient's total blood volume or transfusion of more than 10 units of blood within 24 hrs. Another definition includes the need for replacement of 50% of circulating blood volume in less than 3 hours or blood loss at the rate of more than 150 ml per minute. Unfortunately, in obstetrical emergencies the volume of blood lost may be difficult to estimate due to occult hemorrhage within the uterus, broad ligament or peritoneum.[14]

The pathologic consequences of hemorrhagic shock due to massive post partum hemorrhage are tissue hypoxia, acidosis, the release of pro-inflammatory cytokines and the precipitation of the systemic inflammatory response syndrome (SIRS),[23–26] the triggering of disseminated intravascular coagulation (DIC) with associated systemic microvascular thrombosis, and organ hypoperfusion (Table 12.3).[27–29] Clinically, patients may then progress to the multiple organ dysfunction syndrome (MODS), including renal failure,[30] hepatic failure, adult respiratory distress syndrome (ARDS),[31] hypoxic brain injury, Sheehan's syndrome (avascular necrosis of the anterior pituitary gland),[14,32] myocardial ischemia, myocardial infarction[33] and death (Table 12.4).[23–27,34–38] Further complicating the clinical picture are the consequences of resuscitation, including left ventricular failure due to fluid volume overload, intravascular hemolysis (further stimulating DIC) due to massive transfusions, dilutional coagulopathy, electrolyte disturbances and surgical complications such as injury to the ureters and bladder. The primary causes of preventable

Table 12.3[26,38,133,134,136] Pathologic consequence of hemorrhagic shock.

- Diagnosis of Systemic Inflammatory Response Syndrome (SIRS)
  - Clinical criteria: 2 or more for diagnosis
    - Abnormal body temperature (>38 °C or <36 °C)
    - Tachycardia (HR >90)
    - Tachypnea (RR >20 or PCO2 <32 mmHg)
    - Abnormal WBC count (WBC >12 K or <4 K)
  - Associated disease states
    - Systemic sepsis
    - Hemorrhagic shock
    - Massive transfusion
    - Cardiopulmonary bypass
    - Surgery
    - Trauma
    - CPR
    - Others
- Pathophysiology of SIRS
  - Release of cytokines and factors
    - IL-2, IL-6, IL-8, Tumor Necrosis Factor alpha and others
  - Endothelial dysfunction
    - Expression of E and P selectins
  - Stimulation of thrombosis and fibrinolysis
    - PAI-1 increased
    - Elevated VWF
    - Elevated thrombomodulin
    - Elevated t-PA
    - Elevated F1+2, TAT complexes and D-Dimer

HR = heart rate, RR = respiratory rate, WBC = white blood count, IL-2 = Interleukin-2, IL-6 = Interleukin-6, IL-8 = Interleukin-8, PAI-1 = plasminogen activator inhibitor type-1, VWF = von Willebrand factor, t-PA = tissue plasminogen activator, F1 + 2 = prothrombin factor 1 + 2, TAT = thrombin-antithrombin.

death in massive PPH are delayed fluid volume and blood replacement, delay in recognizing and appropriately treating DIC and delay in controlling surgical bleeding.[14]

Antepartum hemorrhage

While separate from PPH, antepartum hemorrhage is often the predictor of PPH. Antepartum hemorrhage complicates as many as 2–5% of pregnancies

Table 12.4 Clinical manifestations of MODS.

Cerebrovascular thrombosis
Cerebral infarction
Pituitary infarction (Sheehan's Syndrome)
Hypoxic brain injury
Hypoxic encephalopathy
Coronary thrombosis
Myocardial ischemia
Myocardial infarction
LV dysfunction
Microvascular thrombosis
Adult Respiratory Distress Syndrome (ARDS)
Acute renal failure
Acute hepatic failure
Skin necrosis
Mesenteric thrombosis
Acute adrenal failure

with etiologies ranging from potentially lethal placenta previa to genital infections. Generally, antepartum hemorrhage is defined as that occurring after the 20th week of gestation.[17] Table 12.5 summarizes etiologies of antepartum hemorrhage. The most common causes are placenta previa and placental abruption. Both may culminate in massive PPH. Other etiologies may have less severe consequences but, as in the case of genital infections, may still require careful diagnosis and effective treatment. Nearly 25% of women with antepartum hemorrhage are found to have placental abruption or placenta previa, with a fetal loss rate of 32%.[39] Adverse pregnancy outcomes are also noted in as many as a third of patients with antepartum hemorrhage from causes other than placenta previa or abruption.[40]

In order to exclude placenta previa and placental abruption, a thorough diagnostic investigation including pelvic ultrasound (US), is indicated when any pregnant patient presents with antepartum hemorrhage.[41–44] If assessment confirms the presence of a viable fetus, and bleeding stops, conservative management is appropriate. If hemorrhage is life threatening or if the fetus is nonviable, immediate delivery is indicated.[17] Identification of placenta previa, as well as other placental abnormalities allows for planning of appropriate management and offers potential life-saving benefits. Other placental abnormalities may also be identified and allow an appropriate approach to delivery.

Table 12.5 Etiology of antepartum hemorrhage.

Placenta previa
Placental abruption
Marginal bleeding
Bloody show during labor (cervical effacement)
Cervicitis
Vaginal and cervical trauma
Vulvovaginal varicosities
Genital neoplasm (benign and malignant)
Vulvovaginal infection
Hematuria
Vasa previa (hemorrhage from fetal blood vessels caused by abnormal cord insertion, if membranes are ruptured)

Pathophysiology of post partum hemorrhage

Risk factors for post partum hemorrhage

The majority of women who develop post partum hemorrhage have underlying risk factors, which are recognizable antepartum. For these, carefully managed pregnancy, labor, and delivery can dramatically reduce the likelihood of bleeding. Risk factors can be characterized as either clinical or hematological, obstetrical, anatomical or systemic and can be recognized antepartum or occurring unexpectedly during the puerperium. Predisposition to PPH may occur with (1) abnormal placentation, (2) birth trauma, (3) uterine atony, (4) maternal blood volume deficiency, (5) hemorrhagic diathesis, and (6) other factors (including uterine artery aneurysms and varices;[45,46] as outlined in Table 12.6.[41] Women who have previously had a cesarean section are also at increased risk of PPH due to placental accretism. The incidence of placenta previa with placental accretism correlates directly with the number of cesarean scars, and it is not surprising that the risk of a morbidly adherent placenta increases from 5% with no previous cesarean section; 10 to 24% with one; 38–49% with two; and 67% with three previous cesarean scars.[47] Hemorrhagic diatheses include von Willebrand disease, coagulation factor defects, platelet and vascular defects. Hemorrhagic diatheses predisposing to hemorrhage include not only inherited coagulation defects but also acquired deficiencies of coagulation factors in acute fatty liver of pregnancy, HELLP syndrome (hemolytic anemia, elevated liver enzymes, and low platelets), cholestasis of pregnancy, and factor VIII inhibitors.

Table 12.6[5,10,17,41] Risk factors for post partum hemorrhage.

- Abnormal placentation
  - Placenta previa
  - Placental abruption
  - Placenta accreta/increta/percreta
  - Bicornate uterus
  - Leiomyoma
  - Prior uterine surgery/cesarean section
  - Hydatidiform mole
  - Retained placental fragments
- Birth trauma
  - Episiotomy (medioloateral > midline)
  - Cesarean section
  - Cervical or vaginal tear
  - Low or mid forceps delivery
  - Uterine rupture
  - Uterine inversion
- Uterine atony
  - Multiple gestations
  - High parity
  - Over distended uterus
    - Large fetus
    - Multiple fetuses
    - Hydramnios
    - Distended with clots
  - Complications of anesthesia or analgesia
    - Halogenated agents
    - Conduction analgesia with hypotension
  - Myometrial dysfunction
    - Rapid labor
    - Prolonged labor
    - Oxytocin or prostaglandin augmented labor
    - Tocolytic agents
    - Chorioamnionitis
  - Previous uterine atony
- Maternal blood volume deficiency
  - Small maternal size
  - Submaximal maternal hypervolemia
  - Constricted maternal hypervolemia
    - Preeclampsia
    - Eclampsia

Table 12.6[5,10,17,41] *(cont.)*

Hemorrhagic diathesis
Inherited coagulopathy
Acquired coagulopathy
Disseminated intravascular coagulation (DIC)
Amniotic fluid embolism
Placental abruption
Retained dead fetus
Severe preeclampsia and eclampsia
Saline-induced abortion
Massive transfusion
Severe intravascular hemolysis
Systemic sepsis
Systemic inflammatory response syndrome
Therapeutic anticoagulation
Dilutional coagulopathy (massive volume resuscitation)
Thrombotic thrombocytopenic purpura
Other factors
Nulliparity
Obesity
Native American ancestry
Prior postpartum hemorrhage

Causes of post partum hemorrhage

The causes of post partum hemorrhage may be organized into three groups (Table 12.7). First, are those disorders in which hemorrhage originates primarily from pathologic vascular injury of the uteroplacental junction, uterus, cervix, vagina or perineum and uterine atony. The second group includes women in whom PPH results from the usual degree of uteroplacental vascular disruption or birth trauma concomitant with an underlying inherited or acquired hemorrhagic diathesis. Finally, are women who experience peripartum hypovolemic shock or other complications of pregnancy, which trigger DIC. Failure of normal physiologic contraction of uterine arteries may occur as the result of a morbidly adherent or retained placenta, uterine atony or uterine rupture. Pathologic injury to the birth canal may result in active vaginal bleeding or interstitial bleeding into a large vaginal hematoma. When abruptio placenta, amniotic fluid embolism, sepsis or hemorrhagic shock trigger DIC, massive vaginal and cesarean incision bleeding are associated with systemic hemorrhage.

Table 12.7 Causes of post partum hemorrhage.

Pathologic vascular injury
Abnormal placental separation
Placenta previa
Placenta abruption
Placenta accreta/increta/percreta
Ectopic pregnancy
Hyatidiform mole
Uterine vascular injury/dysfunction
Uterine rupture
Uterine atony
Uterine inversion
Cervical laceration (major)
Vaginal laceraton (major)
Perineal laceration (major)
Episiotomy (complicated)
Cesarean section/cesarean hysterectomy with surgical misadventure
Physiologic trauma complicated by underlying hemorrhagic diatheses
Fibrinogen deficiency (hypo or dysfibrinogenemia)
Factor II deficiency
Factor V deficiency
Factor VII deficiency
Factor VIII deficiency/inhibitors
Factor IX deficiency
Factor X deficiency
Factor XI deficiency
Factor XIII deficiency
Passovoy defect
Platelet defects
Von Willebrand disease
α-2-antiplasmin deficiency
α-2-macroglobulin deficiency
Disseminated intravascular coagulation (DIC)
Amniotic fluid embolism
Placental abruption
Hemorrhagic shock
Septicemia

Maternal physiology and parturition

In order to compensate for the vascular injury and physiologic blood loss associated with delivery, there are a number of compensatory changes in maternal physiology. By pregnancy term, uteroplacental blood flow is as brisk as 600 ml per minute.[19] As parturition involves the separation of the placenta from the uterine wall in the third stage of labor, physiologic adaptations have developed to prevent the otherwise inevitable exsanguination. In anticipation of blood loss, maternal plasma volume expands by 42% and the red cell mass expands by 24% by the third trimester[48] (Table 12.8). By late in pregnancy, the healthy mother has a total blood volume of 6–7 liters, compared to normal of approximately 5 liters (70 ml/kg).[14] In pre-eclamptic patients, plasma volume fails to expand normally and is as much as 9% lower than in patients without preeclampsia.[49,50] In addition to the increase in plasma volume and red cell mass, third trimester pregnancy is characterized by intensification of the intrinsically hypercoagulable state of normal pregnancy. Measurable increases occur in the levels of fibrinogen, factors VII, VIII, X, and von Willebrand factor[51] and with decreased levels of Protein S (associated with an increase in the level of C4 binding protein). Fibrinolytic activity is inhibited as the result of increased levels of plasminogen activator inhibitor (PAI-1).[52] This hyper-coagulable state of pregnancy not only predisposes to thrombotic complications but also may blunt the impact of underlying inherited hemorrhagic diatheses and alter coagulation tests, making the prediction of PPH more difficult. Typically, the prothrombin time (PT) and partial thromblastin time (PTT) shorten

Table 12.8[49] Physiological changes in pregnancy.

Third trimester
Maternal plasma volume expands 42%
Red cell mass expands 24%
Total blood volume of 6–7 liters
Increases in
Fibrinogen
Factor VII
Factor VIII
Factor X
Von Willebrand factor
Plasminogen Activator Inhibitor (PAI-1)
Decreases in Protein S
Fibrinolytic activity inhibited
Preeclampsia patients
Plasma volume expands 9% lower than normal patients (33%)

during the third trimester of pregnancy.[51] Markers of active thrombosis and fibrinolysis are noted with elevations of D-Dimer and thrombin-antithrombin complexes.

Prevention of post partum hemorrhage

Antepartum preparation

The recognition of clinical and obstetrical risk factors for PPH is an essential step in preventing post partum hemorrhage. Prenatal evaluation must include a thorough history and physical examination and screening laboratory studies. Required laboratory studies include a complete blood count (CBC), prothrombin time (PT) and activated partial thromblastin time (PTT). In the event there is a personal or family history of easy bruising, bleeding, excessive hemorrhage with minor injury, surgery, pregnancy or labor and delivery, a thorough investigation must be undertaken. Patients with a history of metromenorrhagia must be assessed, as 17% will be found to have a hemorrhagic diathesis.[53] A complete screening evaluation is required including the CBC, PT, PTT and also a template bleeding time (TBT) or alternative assay of platelet function (Table 12.9). Based upon the results of these screening studies, suspicion may be then directed to specific hemorrhagic diatheses, as outlined in Table 12.10. Follow-up laboratory studies of clotting factors, platelet function assays and other confirmatory studies may then be performed to define a specific diagnosis. From this is estimated the associated risk of PPH.

An often-overlooked issue in the pregnant woman is the willingness to receive blood transfusion. Religious beliefs may preclude transfusion and without fore knowledge the potential exists for catastrophic consequences. If it is evident from the prenatal history that this is the case, preparation is required to plan for potential PPH. This will include attention to prevent and treat anemia, careful management of identified risk factors and provision for a blood substitute to be used in an emergency.[54,55]

Preparation must also include planning for the physiologic hemorrhage associated with uncomplicated vaginal and cesarean delivery. Prevention, early identification and effective treatment of prenatal anemia (usually iron deficiency) is essential to preventing normal bleeding from becoming a serious medical complication.[56] Women who are anemic at the time of PPH are at increased risk of the complications of decreased oxygen carrying capacity, may require an increased number of units of packed red cells for resuscitation and are exposed to an increased risk of systemic complications.

Table 12.9 Prenatal laboratory screening evaluation.

CBC
PT (Prothrombin time)
PTT (Activated partial thromboplastin time)
TBT (Template bleeding time) (indicated if there is a personal or family history of hemorrhage)

Table 12.10 Screening tests for the laboratory differentiation of hemorrhagic diatheses.

Laboratory test	Vascular disorder	Platelet function	Platelet number	Blood proteins
Platelet count	Normal	Normal	Abnormal	Normal
Template bleeding time	Abnormal	Abnormal	Abnormal	Normal[a]
Prothrombin time	Normal	Normal	Normal	Abnormal or normal[b]
Partial thromboplastin time	Normal	Normal	Normal	Abnormal or normal[b]

[a] Except von Willebrand's syndrome.
[b] Prothrombin time and/or partial thromboplastin time will be prolonged depending on the factor involved; factor XIII deficiency and alpha-2-antiplasmin deficiency not detected by prothrombin time or partial thromboplastin time.

Antepartum hemorrhagic diatheses

The inherited coagulopathies are well-described risk factors for PPH. Disturbances in the antigenic or functional levels of most of the components of the coagulation or fibrinolytic systems have the potential for predisposing to hemorrhage. In normally functioning hemostasis, activation of the intrinsic pathway, involving factors VIII and IX, leads to activation of the common pathway. Stimulation of the extrinsic coagulation pathway (tissue factor pathway) by factor VII also results in activation of the common pathway. In the common pathway, activation of the prothrombinase complex of factor Xa with factor Va, calcium and phospholipid results in the conversion of prothrombin to thrombin which then converts fibrinogen to fibrin (cross-linked as the result of factor XIII) (Figure 12.1). Platelets function to provide primary hemostasis and stimulate the activation of the coagulation cascade. Abnormal function of any of the coagulation factors may impair normal hemostasis. Hyperfunction of the fibrinolytic system may rapidly degrade an otherwise normal clot. A simple schematic of the coagulation system is presented in Figure 12.1. The delicate balance between thrombosis and hemorrhage is illustrated in Figure 12.2.

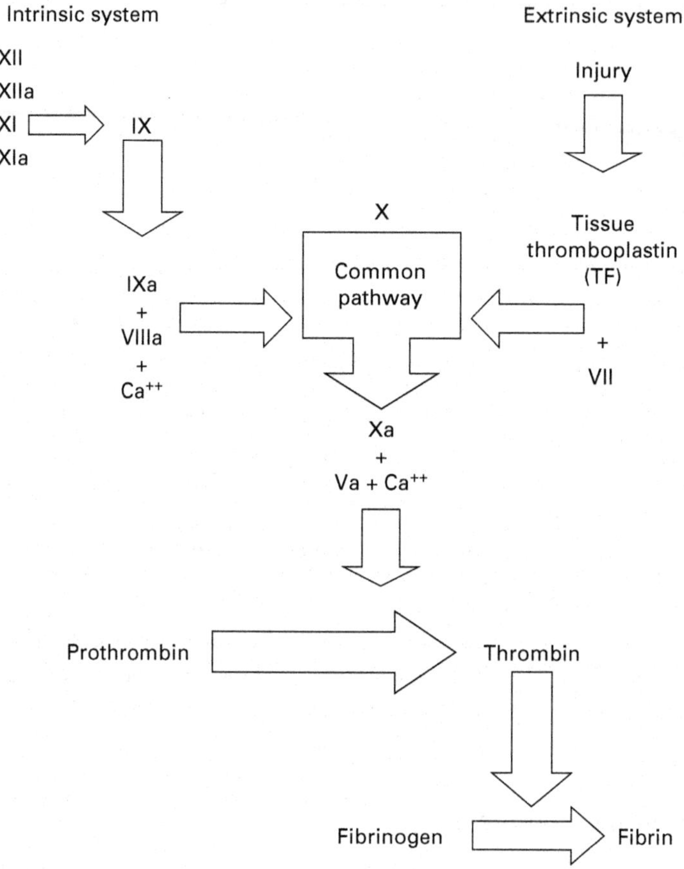

Figure 12.1 Coagulation pathway.

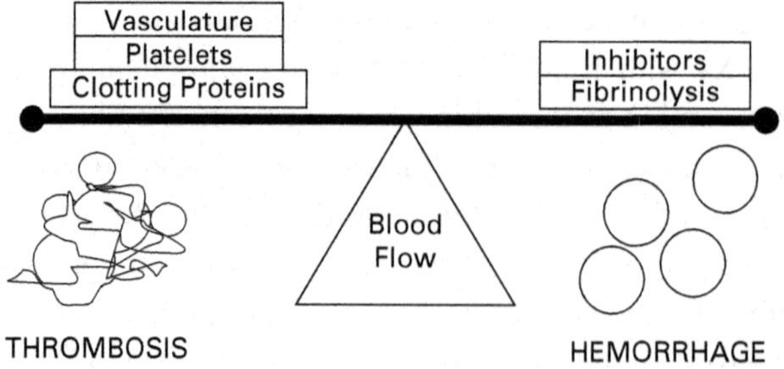

Figure 12.2 The balance of thrombosis and hemorrhage.

Table 12.11 Hemorrhagic diatheses.

Deficiency/Defects	PT	PTT	TBT	Platelets
Fibrinogen deficiency	↑	↑	↔	↔
Factor II deficiency	↑	↑	↔	↔
Factor V deficiency	↑	↑	↔	↔
Factor VII deficiency	↑	↔	↔	↔
Factor VIII deficiency/inhibitors	↔	↑	↔	↔
Factor IX deficiency	↔	↑	↔	↔
Factor X deficiency	↑	↑	↔	↔
Factor XI deficiency	↔	↑	↔	↔
Factor XIII deficiency	↔	↔	↔	↔
Prekallikrein deficiency	↔	↑	↔	↔
Passovoy defect	↔	↑	↑	↔
Von Willebrand disease	↔	↑	↑	↔
α-2-antiplasmin deficiency	↔	↔	↔	↔
α-2-macroglobulin deficiency	↔	↔	↔	↔
Platelet defects				
Thrombocytopenia	↔	↔	↑	↓
Thrombocytopathy	↔	↔	↑	↔
DIC	↑	↑	↑	↓

↑ = increase, ↔ = no change, ↓ = decrease

When local vascular injury in the uterus and lower genital tract occurs in patients with disorders of coagulation factors or of platelets, significant blood loss results from failure of primary and/or secondary hemostasis. Patients usually, but not always, will provide a history of easy bruising, gum bleeding, epistaxis, soft tissue bleeding with or without a history of trauma, post-operative or previous post partum hemorrhage or metromenorrhagia. The primary hemorrhagic disorders recognized to place women at risk for PPH are listed in Table 12.11 and include von Willebrand disease, deficiencies of factors (II, V, VII, VIII, IX, X, XI, XIII), deficiency or dysfunction of fibrinogen, deficiency of the plasmin inhibitors alpha-2-antiplasmin and alpha-2-macroglobulin, and disorders which decrease platelet numbers (immune thrombocytopenia) or impair platelet function.

When the diagnosis of a primary hemorrhagic diathesis is known, the problem becomes one of simply planning an appropriate management strategy (Table 12.12). Many patients with von Willebrand disease, thrombocytopenia or thrombocytopathy (platelet function defects) have no history of unusual bleeding and proceed into labor undiagnosed. It is in such patients who begin labor with a previously unsuspected hemorrhagic diathesis, that the risk of PPH is

Table 12.12 Management of hemorrhagic diatheses during pregnancy and puerperium.

Hemorrhagic diathesis	Hemostasis	Treatment
Fibrinogen defects	Fibrinogen level >60 to 100 mg/dl	Infusion of cryoprecipitate
Factor II defects	Elevation of factor II level to 50% of normal	Administration of PCC[a] or FFP[b]
Factor V defects	Factor V levels above 30%	Administration of FFP[b] or infusion of cryoprecipitate
Factor VII defects	Factor VII levels at 30% of normal	Factor VII replacement, administration of FFP[b] or PCC[a]
Factor VIII: C defects	Rise in factor VIII: C to at least 50% or 80–100% for severe and acute hemorrhage	Infusion of factor VIII most effective; for mild bleeding bed rest, topical thrombin or DDAVP
Factor IX defects	Factor IX level of 100% of normal	Replacement therapy with factor IX from FFP[b] or PCC[a]; may require surgery
Factor X defects	Factor X level of 15 to 20% of normal or 50% just before delivery	Administration of factor X from FFP[b]
Factor XI defects	Factor XI levels to 70% of normal	Administration of FFP,[b] factor XI concentrate (Europe) and/or antifibrinolytic agents
Prekallikrein deficiency	–	No therapy required
Kininogen defect	–	No therapy required
Passovoy defect	–	Administration of FFP[b]
Alpha-2-antiplasmin	–	Epsilon α-aminocaproic acid (EACA) or tranexamic acid
Factor XIII	Factor XIII level at 2% to 3% of normal	Infusion of FFP[b] or cryoprecipitate and prophylaxis for surgery, labor and delivery
Von Willebrand disease	Increase in VWF and factor VIII to the normal range	DDAVP, cryoprecipitate, and humate-P
Platelet defects	Platelet count of 50,000 at delivery	Platelet transfusion; administration of glucocorticoids, intravenous IgG, and splenectomy for ITP

[a] Prothrombin complex concentrate.
[b] Fresh frozen plasma.

greatest. In those patients with an established diagnosis, therapeutic approaches have been developed to reduce the risk of PPH and allow safe delivery. When PPH occurs, therapy must be directed to correct the primary defect, as well as the specific complications, such as blood loss, hypotension, or post partum anemia. The effective treatment options for the inherited and acquired hemorrhagic diatheses are summarized below.

Fibrinogen defects

While dysfibrinogenemias are the best recognized, both quantitative and qualitative defects of fibrinogen are identified. Afibrinogenemia and hypofibrinogenemia inheritance is usually autosomal recessive. Congenital hypodysfibrinogenemia is also reported as an autosomal dominant disorder characterized by both qualitative and quantitatively abnormal fibrinogen.[57] Since clinical manifestations of bleeding are usually only associated with the puerperium, surgery, trauma or menses, therapy may only be indicated in specific situations. Without treatment, congenital afibrinogenemia results in miscarriage at 6–8 weeks gestation due to hemorrhage.[58] Newborns with the disorder may present with umbilical stump bleeding at birth, intra-articular bleeding and occasionally intracranial hemorrhage.[59] The mother with dysfibrinogenemia, afibrinogenemia or hypodysfibrinogenemia, may bleed from the uterus, birth canal, gastrointestinal tract or other mucous membranes.

Treatment consists primarily of infusion of cryoprecipitate. In the pregnant patient, prevention of spontaneous abortion and genital hemorrhage requires the fibrinogen level be maintained at >60 to 100 mg/dl.[60,61] As the pregnancy progresses, fibrinogen clearance increases, thus the dose requirement increases. Continuous infusion of fibrinogen concentrate (not available in the United States) or cryoprecipitate is recommended during labor and delivery to maintain the fibrinogen level at a minimum of 150 to 200 mg/dl.[60] This approach has proven successful at allowing uneventful pregnancy, labor and delivery of a normal fetus. There is, however, a report of placental abruption, placental infarction and post partum deep vein thrombosis in a woman who was treated in a similar manner with cryoprecipitate.[58] Cryoprecipitate contains 80–120 U of factor VIII, 40–70% of the original plasma of von Willebrand factor and 150–250 mg of fibrinogen.[62] It is postulated that the increased factor VIII and von Willebrand factor levels may have contributed to thrombosis.[58]

Factor II defects

Factor II (prothrombin) deficiency is a very rare autosomal recessive disorder. Quantitative defects in factor II (prothrombin) may be either hypoprothrombinemia or aprothrombinemia. The deficiency may also be qualitative. Clinical manifestations primarily occur in the presence of a homozygous defect. These include spontaneous, severe bleeding with the formation of large hematomas, massive gastrointestinal or other mucosal membrane hemorrhage, as well as bleeding due to delivery, surgery or trauma. Heterozygous patients occasionally bleed spontaneously but usually only with surgery or trauma.[59] Therapy is indicated in the presence of hemorrhage or in anticipation of delivery, surgery or invasive procedures.[63]

Treatment consists of prothrombin complex concentrates[64] or fresh frozen plasma.[65] Elevation of the functional factor II level to about 50% of normal is adequate to prevent puerperal and post partum hemorrhage. Fresh frozen plasma has approximately 400 mg of fibrinogen and 200 U of other clotting factors (including prothrombin), in about 250 ml of plasma. Infusion begins with a loading dose of 15–20 ml/kg, followed by 5 ml/kg every 24 hours as needed to achieve hemostasis. Prothrombin complex concentrates (PCC) contain prothrombin, factor VII, IX and X and proteins C and S. PCC are highly thrombogenic (may lead to pathologic thrombi including DIC) and are not to be administered concomitantly with antifibrinolytic agents. Therapy is initiated with 20 U/kg as a loading dose followed by 10 U/kg daily.[66]

In addition to clinical assessment, therapy is monitored with the PT and PTT. The precise quantitative measurement of factor II may not be available in all clinical laboratories, however, is the most accurate method of documenting laboratory improvement with treatment. Resolution of clinical hemorrhage should accompany stabilization of functional factor II levels at about 50%.

Factor V defects

Factor V deficiency is autosomal recessive and, fortunately, very rare. Homozygous individuals may experience mucosal membrane and gastrointestinal hemorrhage, spontaneous hematomas, spontaneous intra-articular bleeding, intracranial bleeding, and large ecchymoses.[59] Severe bleeding may occur with delivery, surgery or trauma. Heterozygous patients rarely bleed. Therapy must consider not only the level of factor V, which correlates poorly with clinical manifestations, but the frequent presence of concomitant disorders of hemostasis. These include: combined congenital factor V and factor VIII deficiency, combined factor V deficiency with von Willebrand's syndrome and factor V Quebec (with moderately low levels of plasma factor V combined with low levels of platelet alpha granules).[63,64]

Treatment consists of administration of fresh frozen plasma at 10 ml/kg or cryoprecipitate. The goal of treatment is to keep the factor V levels above 30%.

As the half-life of factor V is about 24 hours, infusion is required only every 24 hours.[59] Therapy also includes clinical support until hemorrhage is controlled. Prophylaxis is indicated for homozygotes during labor and delivery, and for major surgery or interventional procedures. Monitoring of therapy requires following the PT and activated partial thromboplastin time (APTT). At least 30% of normal activity of the PT and APTT are desired.

Factor VII defects

Factor VII (proconvertin) deficiency is a rare autosomal recessive disorder, which may result from either complete absence of factor VII or the presence of a dysfunctional factor. Homozygotes have factor VII levels of less than 10% and heterozygotes have levels of about 50%.[67] Clinical manifestations include: mucosal membrane bleeding with severe epistaxis, intrapulmonary and gastrointestinal hemorrhage, intra-articular bleeding, umbilical stump bleeding and intracranial hemorrhage in the homozygotic newborn and severe hemorrhage with childbirth, surgery, invasive procedures or trauma. Heterozygous patients rarely bleed except at the time of delivery, surgery or trauma.[63] Normal pregnancy induces a fourfold rise in the factor VII levels during pregnancy but it is unclear to what degree this is due to increased factor production or to enhanced function. Furthermore, it is not known to what degree pregnancy induces an increase in the factor VII deficient woman.[68] As it is clear that deficiency confers an increased risk for hemorrhage and that any labor may potentially require cesarean delivery, it is acknowledged that prophylaxis should be provided to prevent puerperal and post partum hemorrhage.[67]

Primary treatment consists of factor VII replacement. Although fresh frozen plasma may be used, prothrombin complex concentrates (associated risk of blood born illness) containing a high concentration of factor VII promptly increase factor VII levels. A widely available recombinant factor VII (Novoseven®) is also rapidly effective without the usual risks associated with the administration of products of whole blood, and is now recommended. The required dose ranges from 15 to 30 mg/kg body weight, as monitored by the PT.[69] Treatment with both bolus[67] and constant infusion[70] methods have been demonstrated effective at preventing hemorrhage during and after cesarean delivery. A level of factor VII at 30% of normal should be achieved for effective therapy.[59] Since the factor VII half-life is only four to six hours, repeat boluses or continuous infusion is needed to maintain an adequate level. Therapy is indicated in the presence of clinical evidence of hemorrhage or in anticipation of and following vaginal or cesarean delivery, major surgery or invasive procedures. Monitoring of therapy is dependent upon bedside clinical evaluation and factor VII levels. While, as in diagnosis, a prolonged PT and normal PTT are helpful, they are not the optimal guides to therapy.

Factor VIII: C defects

In spite of the complexities of precise diagnosis and characterization, the presentation, clinical consequences, and treatment of all of the forms of factor VIII: C deficiency are similar. Patients with the sex-linked recessive absence of VIII: C (90%) (hemophilia A), with dysfunctional VIII: C (10%), and with anti-factor VIII antibodies (autoantibodies) all bleed. The severity of bleeding correlates with the absolute level of functional VIII: C. Patients with levels of 0 to 5% have severe and spontaneous bleeding, those with levels of 5 to 10% experience moderate bleeding, including some spontaneous hemorrhage, and patients with levels of 10 to 40% may experience only mild bleeding and rarely bleed spontaneously. Patients with the lowest levels of VIII: C bleed in infancy with hemorrhage at circumcision, spontaneously bleeding into large muscles and joints and intracranial. With growth and development intra-articular hemorrhage followed by joint fibrosis may be crippling. Hemorrhage may occur into closed muscle compartments resulting in peripheral nerve injury, which may be permanent if not identified and treated promptly. All patients with VIII: C deficits are, to a greater or lesser extent as determined by the level of VIII: C, prone to surgical bleeding. Similarly, there is a considerably increased risk of hemorrhage subsequent to childbirth, trauma or special procedures.[59,64,71]

Patients with factor VIII autoantibodies may not be identified antepartum. Factor VIII autoantibodies are present at a rate of 0.2 to 1 cases per million per year, of which 7–11% of the cases occur during pregnancy.[72] A large review of 215 non-hemophiliac patients with acquired factor VIII inhibitors identified 47% of patients with underlying illness such as autoimmune disease and malignancy, 46% with no underlying disorder, and 7% occurring in women post partum.[73] Presentation during pregnancy is uncommon. Post partum hemorrhage is usually late, presenting about a week after apparently uncomplicated delivery.[41] Post partum hemorrhage, whether early or late, is uncommon. More often, non-hemophiliac women with acquired factor VIII antibodies, develop soft tissue and joint bleeding from 1 month to over one year after delivery. Acute PPH with a fatal outcome due to uncontrolled hemorrhage is reported.[74]

Therapy with infusion of factor VIII remains the key element in successful treatment, both for hemophiliacs and patients with autoantibodies. Delivery must be carefully managed to decrease the risk of serious intracranial hemorrhage in the affected newborn, occurring most commonly with prolonged labor, vacuum extraction, and forceps delivery.[59] Patients with mild bleeding may be managed simply with bed rest, topical thrombin or 1-D-amino-8-D-Arginine Vassopressin (DDAVP). Hemophiliacs who demonstrate a baseline factor VIII: C level of >5 U/dl may respond to DDAVP. A trial of DDAVP must demonstrate rise in factor VIII: C levels to at least 30 U/dl, 30 to 60 minutes after the dose, before this approach may be relied upon for minor surgery.[64] Factor VIII replacement is required in anticipation of delivery by vaginal or cesarean route, in anticipation of neuraxial anesthesia, or as treatment for acute hemorrhage.[75] Spontaneous hemorrhage is unlikely with factor VIII levels below 20% of normal, however with severe hemorrhage, levels of 80% to 100% are required for hemostasis.[76] Since cryoprecipitates may include variable amounts of factor VIII, large amounts of fibrinogen, and carry some risk of viral transmission, therapy with recombinant factor VIII concentrates is preferred. For emergency treatment, an infusion of recombinant factor VIII concentrate at 30 units/kg may be expected to increase the circulating level by 50%. The treatment goal in the presence of acute severe hemorrhage is between 50% to 100% of normal factor VIII levels.[59,71] Control of hemorrhage should follow. Precise calculation of dose is primarily indicated in the antepartum whether delivery is expected by vaginal or cesarean route. The formula for administration of recombinant factor VIII concentrate is as follows: [59]

Units needed = desired level − initial level
Dose of factor VIII = units needed × 0.5 × body weight (kg)
Milliliters of concentrate needed = total units needed/units/ml concentrate

The biologic half-life of factor VIII is 12 hours. Treatment is guided by the clinical situation. Patients who present with hemorrhage are treated emergently. Postpartum hemorrhage requires adjusted dose infusions every 12 hours, until clinical and laboratory stabilization is achieved. After cesarean section delivery, therapy is also required until all wounds are healed.[76]

Spontaneous recovery from factor VIII autoantibodies is likely but may take years. Treatment with immunosuppression may hasten remission in as many as 40%,[74] but is of little use in the acute setting. The most rapid induction of remission in a post partum woman with acquired factor VIII inhibitors, with immunosuppression has been 15 days after therapy with the combination of methylprednisolone (3 mg/kg/day for 8 days then 1 mg/kg/day) and cyclosphamide (150 mg/day for 5 days then 100 mg/day).[77] Patients with factor VIII inhibitors usually fail to demonstrate the expected increase in factor VIII: C activity level following recombinant factor VIII infusion. In clinical situations when more serious bleeding is present or anticipated (as in labor and delivery), the level of the inhibitor should be quantified via the Bethesda assay[78] and a precise dose of recombinant factor VIII concentrate administered to exactly neutralize the inhibitor. The correct dose may be estimated by applying the formula above and assuming that the patient level of VIII:C is 0%. While plasma exchange and extracorporeal inhibitor absorption with protein A columns have been met with some success in clearing the antibodies, DDAVP has not been effective. In the past, treatment with factor VIII concentrates carried a significant risk of hepatitis and human immunodeficiency virus (HIV) infection. New recombinant products have eliminated this risk.[79,80] Unfortunately, however, the presence of autoantibodies which rapidly inactivate factor VIII may require the use of alternative therapy not needed in the hemophiliac without autoantibodies. This problem has led to the development and use of Porcine factor VIII (Hyate:C®), Factor VIII Inhibitor Bypassing Activity (FEIBA), Autoplex® and recombinant factor VIIa.[79,80] Treatment with these agents proceeds according to the formula presented above and is guided by the serial measurement of factor VIII: C levels and bedside clinical assessment. Occasionally, in severe deficiencies, a dysfunction of platelet aggregation develops requiring platelet transfusions. Thrombotic complications remain a concern with the use of prothrombin complex concentrates. A highly predictable and effective alternative to recombinant factor VIII therapy for inhibitor patients appears to be recombinant factor VIIa.[81] Therapy for patients with factor VIII inhibitors may be complex, but properly managed is expected to produce a successful outcome of pregnancy and the puerperium.

Monitoring of therapy requires careful bedside evaluation and measurement of quantitative factor VIII: C. While at the time of diagnosis, the PTT will be prolonged and the PT normal, normalization of these parameters is not an adequate indication of therapeutic efficacy.

Factor IX defects

Hemophilia B (Christmas disease) is a sex linked recessive disorder in which factor IX is absent in 70 to 90% of patients and dysfunctional in 10 to 30%. The clinical manifestations of hemophilia B are quite similar to those expressed in hemophilia A. Severity of hemorrhage correlates with the level of quantitative or qualitative deficiency. Deep muscle hemorrhage, intra-articular, intracranial and severe bleeding from mucosal membranes may occur. In severe deficiency (0 to 5% factor IX level) spontaneous hemorrhage is frequent, in moderate deficiency (5 to 10% factor IX level) spontaneous bleeding is occasional and in mild deficiency (10 to 40% factor IX level) spontaneous hemorrhage is rare.[82] Management involves not only replacement of the deficient factor but also local or interventional treatment of the complications.[59,71]

Replacement therapy with factor IX contained in fresh frozen plasma or prothrombin complex concentrates containing factor IX has been the hallmark of treatment.[59] The risk of viral infection and the risk of thrombosis posed by the presence of fibrinogen and other procoagulants, have prompted a change in preferred therapy to highly purified factor IX products. These include AlphaNine®, MonoNine® and the recombinant factor IX, Benefix®.[64,83] The dose of purified factor IX administered in anticipation of labor and delivery, surgery or in the presence of acute hemorrhage should achieve a factor IX level of 100% of normal. A calculated dose may be given as with factor VIII replacement, however, due to the wide extravascular presence of factor IX, the initial loading dose must be 1.5 to 2.0 times the calculated dose based on plasma volume.[83] Factor IX inhibitors have rarely been reported in nonhemophiliac post partum women.[84] Plasmaphoresis, immunoabsorption and immunosuppressives may also be effective.[85] Patients with hemophilia B not only require infusion therapy but also may require invasive procedures or surgery as well as considerable medical support during episodes of hemorrhage.

Monitoring requires frequent clinical follow-up and serial measurement of factor IX levels. In spite of the observed prolongation of the PTT in the presence of a normal PT, monitoring of these levels is of limited value in clinical management. In milder cases, both the PT and PTT may be normal.

Factor X

The autosomal recessive disorder of factor X deficiency is very rare. Clinical features are umbilical stump bleeding, subcutaneous hemorrhage and bleeding with childbirth, surgery, invasive procedures and trauma. Deep-tissue bleeding is not generally observed. Severe bleeding from mucosal membranes, including gastrointestinal, genitourinary and intrapulmonary sites primarily occurs in homozygotes. Menorrhagia is frequent and there is a significant risk for PPH.[83] Pregnancy is often complicated by recurrent miscarriage and preterm delivery in homozygotes. The risk for hemorrhage correlates with factor X levels below 15% to 30% of normal. The presentation is frequently with the observation of a prolonged PT and PTT, with mild prolongation in heterozygotes and marked prolongation in homozygotes. Heterozygotes are usually asymptomatic.[59,63]

Treatment includes administration of factor X contained in fresh frozen plasma at 15–20 ml/kg loading dose followed by 5 ml/kg daily maintenance dose or a calculated dose of prothrombin complex concentrates (associated risk of thrombosis). As no spontaneous or other hemorrhage will occur if the factor X level is 15% to 30% of normal, the target level for treatment is usually 15% to 20%. Factor replacement is indicated during pregnancy, labor and delivery.[59,64] The target level in anticipation of delivery is 50% of normal. Although only 13 pregnancies have been reported in the medical literature, it appears clear that prophylactic replacement therapy is effective at allowing uncomplicated delivery, both vaginal and cesarean.[86]

Monitoring includes clinical assessment and measurement of factor X levels. The prolonged PTT, PT and Russell's viper venom time (RVVT) are useful for diagnosis but not therapy.

Factor XI

The deficiency of factor XI is inherited as an incomplete autosomal recessive genotype and the clinical manifestations are quite variable. Patients present with an isolated prolongation of the PTT and normal PT. There may be no history of bleeding or severe bleeding and there may be variable degrees of hemorrhagic risk. Heterozygous patients are rarely symptomatic. Bleeding is most often associated with factor XI levels less than 10%, but there is no clear correlation between the risk of hemorrhage and the factor XI level. Mucosal bleeding, particularly from the oral mucosa and genitourinary tract is common. A prior familial or personal history of abnormal bleeding best correlates with future risk.[71] Factor XI deficiency has also been reported as first presenting with acute PPH.[87]

With or without a prior history of hemorrhage, it is advised that individuals with levels less than 20% be pretreated with FFP to raise the levels to 70% in anticipation of surgery, labor and delivery. Infusion of fresh frozen plasma may be used to increase factor XI levels, but the volume of infusion may be significant (15–20 ml/kg loading dose followed by 5 ml/kg/day). Available in Europe, factor XI concentrate is recommended in a dose calculated to raise the factor XI level to 70% of normal (0.7 U/ml). Treatment is recommended during labor to maintain this level for 3–4 days after vaginal delivery and 4–5 days after cesarean delivery. Antifibrinolytic agents (tranexamic acid and ε-aminocaproic acid, trasylol) may be added to replacement therapy for refractory PPH.[87] Although a prolonged PTT and normal PT are useful for diagnosis, they are not of value for therapy. Both a precise diagnosis and appropriate management require the measurement of factor XI levels.

Prekallikrein deficiency

The diagnosis of prekallikrein (Fletcher factor) deficiency is usually noted on routine evaluation of coagulation with a PTT. While the PTT is markedly prolonged and the PT normal, suggesting a number of other disorders, the important distinctive feature of Fletcher trait is the absence of clinical manifestations.[59,83] Since there is no hemorrhagic or thrombotic diathesis, no therapy or monitoring is required. Confusion between this and other much more serious disorders, however, may lead to life-threatening errors in management. Evaluation with a prekallikrein assay to confirm the diagnosis is critical.

Kininogen

Similarly to defects in prekallikrein, deficiency of kininogen is not associated with either hemorrhage or thrombosis. Diagnosis is important primarily due to the potential confusion between this and other disorders presenting with a prolonged PTT and a normal PT. In the appropriate setting, measurement of high-molecular weight kininogen may be indicated. No therapy is required.[83]

Passovoy defect

The Passovoy defect is a poorly delineated abnormality characterized by autosomal dominant inheritance and a moderate degree of hemorrhage. Mucosal bleeding, excessive menstrual bleeding, spontaneous bruising and severe bleeding with childbirth, trauma or surgery are observed. The administration of fresh frozen plasma will correct clinical bleeding and may be used in preparation for delivery or surgery. Monitoring is primarily clinical. Although the detection of a prolonged PTT and normal PT are useful for diagnosis, they are not useful for therapy.[59]

Alpha-2-antiplasmin

The rare autosomal recessive disorder of alpha-2-antiplasmin deficiency may result in severe hemorrhage in homozygous patients. Severe mucosal membrane bleeding (especially genitourinary), spontaneous bruising and subcutaneous hematoma formation, intra-articular bleeding, traumatic hemorrhage and surgical bleeding are characteristic.

Treatment primarily is indicated in the presence of major hemorrhage. Therapies of choice are either epsilon α-aminocaproic acid (EACA), 10 mg/kg three times daily or tranexamic acid, 500 mg two to three times daily, either orally or intravenously. Supportive and interventional therapy may also be required for severe bleeding. No prophylaxis is indicated.

Monitoring is primarily clinical, since all global clotting studies are normal and the only laboratory abnormality is a low level of alpha-2-antiplasmin. Low level elevations of fibrin degradation products (FDP) may be observed but these are also not useful as a guide to therapy.[59,64]

Factor XIII

The rare autosomal recessive disorder of deficiency of factor XIII may have severe clinical consequences. Since only 10% of normal levels of factor XIII are required for normal hemostasis, bleeding only occurs in homozygotes. At least 90% of patients present with delayed umbilical stump bleeding. Delayed hemorrhage is also typical in spontaneous and traumatic deep muscle hemorrhage and delayed post-traumatic or spontaneous intracranial bleeding (the most common cause of death). Deep-tissue bleeding may result in bone pseudotumor formation. Intra-articular hemorrhage is rare. Men are sterile and women experience spontaneous abortion. Postoperative hemorrhage and delayed wound healing are observed.[88] Therapy must address both the coagulopathy and the clinical consequences of bleeding.

Treatment is primarily indicated in the presence of major hemorrhage. Hemorrhage requires infusion of fresh frozen plasma (2–3 ml/kg) or cryoprecipitate (one bag/10 kg) every 4–6 weeks. The goal is to maintain the factor XIII level at 2% to 3% of normal.[59] Prophylaxis has been effective at sustaining pregnancy (prophylactic fresh frozen plasma every 14 days or factor XIII concentrate every 21 days).[83] Cryoprecipitate is also effective. Prophylaxis is indicated for surgery, labor and delivery and therapy must continue for 3–4 weeks to avoid complications.

Monitoring is primarily clinical, since the diagnosis is difficult to establish and readily available laboratory studies are non-existent. A specific assay for factor XIII cross-linking activity is required for diagnosis.

Von Willebrand disease

Von Willebrand disease (vWD) is of variable inheritance and characterized by easy and spontaneous bruising, petechiae and purpura, mucosal membrane hemorrhage and bilateral epistaxis in early childhood. Deep-tissue bleeding is rare but hemorrhage may be severe with surgery, trauma or labor and delivery. Table 12.13 characterizes the various types of von Willebrand disease. Table 12.14 summarizes the diagnostic evaluation for von Willebrand disease. Table 12.15 compares von Willebrand disease with factor VIII deficiency (and inhibitors).[59,89] During pregnancy, von Willebrand factor levels rise after the 11th week gestation. Early hemorrhage due to first trimester miscarriage and both early[90] and late PPH (when the levels again drop to pre-pregnancy levels) are reported.[89] Women with vWD may normalize the levels of von Willebrand factor (vWF) and factor VIII levels but do not normalize the template bleeding time (thus remain at risk of PPH).[91]

Treatment in preparation for delivery is advised for both vaginal and cesarean deliveries. As the defect in primary hemostasis due to platelet dysfunction can usually be well managed by meticulous surgical technique, PPH most closely correlates with the factor VIII: C level. Vaginal deliveries are deemed safe if the factor VIII: C level is >50 U/dl. Prophylactic therapy for delivery is recommended if the level is <30 U/dl. Available therapies for von Willebrand's are DDAVP, cryoprecipitate (contains abundant amounts of VWF) and Humate-P® (a stable,

Table 12.13[59] Von Willebrand disease.

Type I
Von Willebrand syndrome type IA
Autosomal dominant
Concordant decrease in factor VIII: C, factor VIII: CAg, VW factor, VW factor Ag
WF multimer analysis reveals decrease in normal structure and distribution
Von Willebrand syndrome type IB
Same as IA but disproportionate decrease in large VWF multimers
Type II
Von Willebrand syndrome type IIA
Autosomal dominant trait
Discordant decreases in factor VIII: C (reduced), factor VIII: CAg (reduced), VW factor (very reduced), VW factor Ag (reduced)
Depolymerization of VWF complex with many multimeric "fast" forms
Von Willebrand syndrome type IIB
Autosomal dominant trait
Discordant findings as in type IIA
Factor VIII: C near normal
VWF factor Ag moderately reduced
Enhanced platelet agglutination to ristocetin
Depolymerization of VWF complex but fewer monomeric forms than IIA
Type III
Von Willebrand syndrome type III/IV
Severe hemorrhage of many sites
High incidence of consanguinity
Very prolonged template bleeding time
Very reduced factor VIII: C
Very reduced VWF (ristocetin cofactor)
Very reduced VWF: Ag

Table 12.14 Diagnostic evaluation for suspected von Willebrand disease.

Template bleeding time
Activated partial thromboplastin time
Factor VIII: C assay
Von Willebrand's (ristocetin cofactor assay)
VWF factor: Ag (Factor VIII: RAg) assay
Agarose gel analysis of VWF multimers

Table 12.15 Comparison of von Willebrand disease with factor VIII: C deficiency.

	von Willebrand	Factor VIII: C deficiency
Inheritance	Autosomal dominant	Sex-linked recessive
Bleeding time	Prolonged	Normal
Factor VIII: C	Moderately decreased	Markedly decreased
VWF: Ag (VIII:RAg)	Decreased	Normal
VWF (ristocetin cofactor)	Decreased	Normal
Platelet adhesion	Abnormal	Normal
Clinical features	Mucosal bleeding, petechiae, purpura	Deep-tissue bleeding

purified, sterile, lyophilized concentrate of factor VIII, prepared from pooled human plasma containing higher concentrations of von Willebrand factor).

The choice of treatment depends upon the von Willebrand disease type and the specific setting. Patients diagnosed antenatally can be thoroughly evaluated and the type of VWD well characterized. In patients with all but Type 2 VWD, a trial of DDAVP may be administered as 0.3 μg/kg intravenously with peak von Willebrand factor (VWF) and factor VIII: C levels assessed 30 to 60 minutes later. An increase in VWF and factor VIII: C levels to the normal range indicates that DDAVP may be relied upon and administered in the late second stage of labor, immediately post partum and 12 hours later.[91,92] If there is no response to, or in the presence of severe deficiencies such as Type 2B VWD and Type 3 VWD, replacement therapy with cryoprecipitate or Humate-P® is required. Humate-P® therapy is individualized depending upon the risk or severity of hemorrhage. For acute hemorrhage, 15 U/kg (factor VIII units) is administered as a bolus followed by 8 U/kg every 8 hours for the first 24 hours and the same dose every 12 hours for 3–4 days. Prior to delivery (or surgery) doses of 20–26 U/kg are advised. Post partum or postoperatively, 15 U/kg every 8 hours for at least 10 days should be administered. Cryoprecipitate is generally administered as 1 to 3 bags of cryoprecipitate per day per 10 kg of body weight. If Humate-P or cryoprecipitate are not available, fresh frozen plasma may be used to raise the level of factor VIII: C to near 80% to 100% of normal or to normalize the template bleeding time (usually 10 to 15 ml/kg per day).[59,93]

Epidural anesthesia is possible with attention to maintain adequate factor VIII and VWD levels. Both vaginal and cesarean delivery are possible with proper planning and prophylactic therapy. Preventing both early and late PPH also requires continued therapy for 7–10 days for a vaginal delivery and 14 days for cesarean delivery.[92]

Platelet defects

Thrombocytopenia of pregnancy may occur as incidental thrombocytopenia of pregnancy or autoimmune thrombocytopenia. Incidental thrombocytopenia is not associated with hemorrhagic complications. The incidence in pregnancy is 7–8% and platelet counts usually range from 95,000 to 150,000, but may be as low as 40 to 80,000.[94] Autoimmune thrombocytopenia (idiopathic thrombocytopenic purpura, (ITP)) during pregnancy may result in PPH and the risk of PPH correlates with the platelet count less than 50,000. Treatment is indicated if the platelet count falls below 50,000. Therapeutic intervention includes the administration of glucocorticoids, intravenous IgG and splenectomy (preferred in the 2nd trimester). There is a risk of PPH and fetal thrombocytopenia, especially in vaginal deliveries. Vaginal delivery has been discouraged in favor of planned cesarean section, however, this remains at issue. Labor and delivery in a woman with ITP should anticipate PPH with platelet transfusion as needed to elevate the platelet count to 50,000 at the time of delivery.[94]

The occurrence of thrombocytopathy resulting from inherited and acquired platelet defects is well described. Clearly, the impact on pregnancy, labor and delivery varies, depending on the disorder. Typically, the clinical manifestations are easy bruising, soft tissue bleeding, mucosal hemorrhage and hypermenorrhea.[66] There is a risk for PPH. Treatment is expectant, with preparation for prompt administration of blood and platelets should PPH occur. Careful monitoring of the Hgb and clinical monitoring are required during the puerperium.

Management of labor

A major factor in the prevention of PPH is the active management of the third stage of labor. Treatment of the laboring patient is a "hands on" process, involving regular assessment and modification of therapy based upon the minute-to-minute physiologic changes experienced by the laboring mother and her fetus. During the first two stages of labor, prevention of PPH largely rests with early identification of placental abruption. Typical findings include vaginal bleeding, uterine tenderness or back pain, fetal distress, high frequency contractions, uterine hypertonus, idiopathic preterm labor, and dead fetus.[41]

The third stage of labor is the time from delivery of the baby to separation and expulsion of the placenta.[41] The third stage is perhaps the most important phase of labor from the standpoint of prevention of PPH.[41] It is during the third phase that placental separation and delivery occurs, the uterus contracts and uterine arteries constrict and clot.[41] The purpose of management in the third stage of labor is to decrease the duration of this stage since the incidence of PPH increases as the duration lengthens.[41] There are no uniform criteria for the length of normal third stage labor. However, it is commonly accepted that 30 minutes is the endpoint for intervention in the absence of hemorrhage.[41]

Management of the third stage of labor may be physiological or "active".[95,96] Physiological management involves gentle pressure with the hand on the abdomen over the uterine fundus to assist delivery of the separated placenta. This is contrasted with "active management" involving the use of pharmacologic agents to stimulate uterine contraction, assist delivery of the placenta, and reduce the risk of uterine atony.[95] The first hour after delivery has been characterized as the "fourth stage" of labor and it is during this time that PPH is most likely to appear. Careful monitoring of maternal blood pressure and pulse are advised immediately after delivery and every fifteen minutes for this critical first hour.[41]

The goal of active management of the third stage of labor is to assist uterine contraction, thus reducing the risk of uterine atony, accelerating the delivery of the placenta and reducing the risk of post partum hemorrhage.[96] It is during the third stage that life-threatening PPH is likely to occur, thus any maneuver that shortens this phase reduces the incidence of PPH. It has been well demonstrated that active management reduces the amount of blood lost at delivery and reduces the need for transfusion.[97] With active management, including the use of a uterotonic drug, the risk of PPH is decreased over 40%.[11,12,98] The key elements of active management include: (1) administration of uterotonic agents, (2) delivery of the placenta by controlled cord traction, (3) uterine massage.[12,96]

Uterine contraction during the 3rd phase appears to be influenced by endogenous prostaglandins and oxytocin. Prostaglandins gradually rise in the first stage and increase rapidly during the second stage, reaching a peak in the third stage immediately before and after delivery of the placenta.[21] Prostaglandin F levels are highest 5 minutes after placental separation and subsequently demonstrate a rapid decline.[99] Oxytocin levels also rise progressively during labor, peak within minutes of crowning of the fetal head and plateau until placental delivery, when they rapidly decline.[100] A close interaction between endogenous prostaglandins and oxytocin is evident but the precise mechanism has not been well established.[21] Understanding of the role of oxytocin and prostaglandins has led to their pharmacologic use to prevent and control PPH (Table 12.16).

The preferred uterotonic agent is oxytocin. Immediately after delivery of the newborn and subsequent to uterine palpation to verify the absence of a second fetus, 10 U of oxytocin is administered intravenously (IV) or intramuscularly (IM). This is effective within 2–3 minutes, stimulates uterine contraction and is well tolerated by most women.[96] There is no advantage to giving oxytocin prior to delivery of the placenta, however, such timing does not increase the risk of a retained placenta.[101] Oxytocin is the preferred oxytocic agent due to its rapid

Table 12.16[49,108] Uterotonic agents.

Agent	Indication	Dose
Oxytocin	Routine[a]/PPH[b]	10–20 mg
Ergometrine	PPH[b]	10–20 mg
Syntometrine	Routine[a]/PPH[b]	0.2 mg
Prostaglandin F_2	PPH[b]	0.2 mg
Prostaglandin E_2	PPH[b]	0.2 mg
Misoprostol	Routine[a]/PPH[b]	600 μg

[a] Routine = active management of the third stage of labor.
[b] PPH = post partum hemorrhage.

effectiveness, prompt onset of action, low risk of side effects and tolerance by most women. Administration is associated with approximately 22% reduction in post partum blood loss and 40% reduction in the frequency of PPH.[12,98] When administered by rapid IV bolus, oxytocin has been complicated by acute, life threatening hypotension.[102]

Alternative agents include the ergot alkaloids, ergometrine and syntometrine (a combination of 5 U of oxytocin and 0.5 mg of ergometrine)[103] and the prostaglandin misoprostol.[15,21,104–108] Ergometrine administration may be complicated by hypertension, intracerebral hemorrhage[109] and coronary artery spasm.[110] The ergot alkaloids are administered IM as 0.2 mg of ergometrine or 1 ampule of syntometrine. The ergots are contraindicated in women with pre-eclampsia, eclampsia or hypertension.

Misoprostol has the advantage of administration as a rectal suppository or oral tablet and may be stored at room temperature.[15,105–108,111] Misoprostol is effective at inducing uterine contraction but is associated with a significantly increased risk of shivering and post partum elevation of body temperature to greater than 38 degrees C. A large (9,264 women received misoprostol and 9,266 received oxytocin), multinational World Health Organization trial concluded that oxytocin 10 mg IM or IV is preferred over misoprostol 600 mcg, administered orally.[107]

The other two components of active management involve proper application of the techniques of controlled cord traction and uterine massage. These methods are well described and must be performed properly to avoid serious complications such as uterine atony, cord avulsion, uterine inversion and retained placental fragments. The essentials of controlled cord traction and placental delivery are as follows: (1) once cord pulsation stops in a healthy newborn, clamp the cord close to the perineum, (2) while holding the cord with one hand, place the other over the woman's pubic bone and exert gentle counter-pressure over the uterus, (3) await a strong uterine contraction with slight tension on the cord, (4) encourage the mother to push with uterine contraction and while continuing to exert counter-pressure on the uterus, very gently pull downward on the cord to deliver the placenta, (5) if the placenta fails to descend after 30–40 seconds of cord traction, hold the cord until the next contraction and repeat the process with the next contraction, (6) with delivery, hold the placenta in 2 hands and gently turn it until the membranes are twisted and complete placental delivery, (7) any tearing of membranes must be followed by careful inspection of the upper vagina and cervix with removal of any retained fragments, (8) the placenta must then be carefully inspected for missing fragments and if any are missing, immediate uterine examination and removal of retained tissue is then required.[96]

Uterine massage mechanically assists the contraction of the uterus and is effective at combating uterine atony. After delivery of the placenta, the uterus must be continuously massaged until it is well contracted. Palpation for contraction is then required every 15 minutes for the first 2 hours and massage is repeated as needed to assure continued uterine contraction. It is important to monitor carefully for uterine relaxation, even after apparent initial contraction.[96]

Diagnosis of post partum hemorrhage

The diagnosis of PPH primarily rests with bedside clinical evaluation (Table 12.17). A history of predisposition to PPH and knowledge of the patient's condition throughout labor assists the development of an index of suspicion for PPH that may influence the interpretation of changes in the post partum vital signs, physical examination and the post partum Hgb. Following the definition of PPH as blood loss in excess of 500 ml is a reasonable guide, however, as little as 250 ml of blood loss may be of clinical significance in a patient who is anemic at presentation for delivery. The volume of parturition blood loss may be difficult to quantify and is frequently underestimated, as a mixture of fluids (blood, amniotic fluid, urine, stool) may accompany delivery. After delivery, determination of the volume of blood lost vaginally can be made by quantifying blood collected in bedpans, from the weight of saturated pads and linens (1 ml of blood weighs 1 gm).[15] Frequently, however, the volume of blood loss is an estimation made by obstetrical nurses, midwives and obstetricians and is frequently only 50% of the actual loss.[18] Occasionally, as much as 1000 ml of blood may accumulate in a large uterus and not produce vaginal bleeding.[41] Bleeding may be sudden and massive, but also characterized by continuous hemorrhage, which does not produce hypotension until the volume of blood lost is substantial. At cesarean section, measurement of blood loss is usually much more precise, as blood is collected from the

Table 12.17 Diagnosis of PPH.

Diagnostic approach
History and physical examination
Clinical impression (accurate 90% of the time given a thorough Hx and PE)
Laboratory evaluation
Differential diagnosis
Secondary evaluation: laboratory, radiographic, examination under anesthesia/surgery
Differential diagnosis
Focal bleeding
Uterus
Birth canal
Cesarean wound
Systemic bleeding
DIC
Combined etiologies
Focal bleeding with DIC
Patients on antiplatelet therapy or anticoagulants
Patients with underlying disorders of hemostasis

surgical field via suction catheters. Typically, massive PPH is readily apparent from simple observation. Profuse bleeding may be seen from the vagina or surgical field. Rarely, however, normal pregnancy, pre-eclampsia[112] or HELLP[113] may lead to the formation of hepatic hematomae or cause frank hepatic rupture. Massive intra-abdominal hemorrhage presents as acute abdominal distention and hemorrhagic shock.[41,114,115]

Hemorrhagic shock

In massive PPH, features of hypovolemic shock may ensue, with hypoperfusion of vital organs resulting in changes in mental status, decreased urine output and acute cardiovascular collapse or cardiac arrest. Except in placental abruption and amniotic fluid embolism,[116,117] hemodynamic changes directly correlate with the volume of extravasated blood.[14] In the normal non-pregnant patient a loss of 500 ml (10% of total blood volume) may cause no symptoms or vasovagal syncope; 1000 ml loss (20% of total blood volume) orthostatic hypotension and exertional tachycardia; 1500 ml loss (30% of total blood volume) flat neck veins supine but normal blood pressure and pulse with orthostatic hypotension; 2000 ml (40% of total blood volume) reduced central venous pressure, cardiac output and systolic blood pressure, tachycardia, air hunger and cold clammy skin; 2500 ml

Table 12.18[14,289,290] Indices of severity in hemorrhagic shock.

Parameter	Compensated	Mild	Moderate	Severe
Blood loss (ml)	500–1,000	1,000–1,500	1,500–2,000	>2,000
Heart rate (bpm)	<100	>100	>120	>140
Systolic pressure (mm Hg)	Normal	Orthostatic drop	70–80	<70
Arterial pO2	Normal	Normal	Decreased	<59 torr (FiO2 >0.4)*
Arterial pCO2	Decreased	Decreased	Decreased	Decreased or normal
Arterial pH	Increased	Decreased	Decreased	Severe decrease
Cardiac index (l/min × M^2) (Nonsurvivors)	3.5–4.0	2.5–3.5	2.2–2.8	1.5–2.0
Urinary output	>30 cm^3/hr	20–30 cm^3/hr	5–20 cm^3/hr	Anuria
Mental status	Normal	Agitated	Confused	Coma
Fetal heart rate	Normal	Tachycardia	Bradycardia	Severe bradycardia

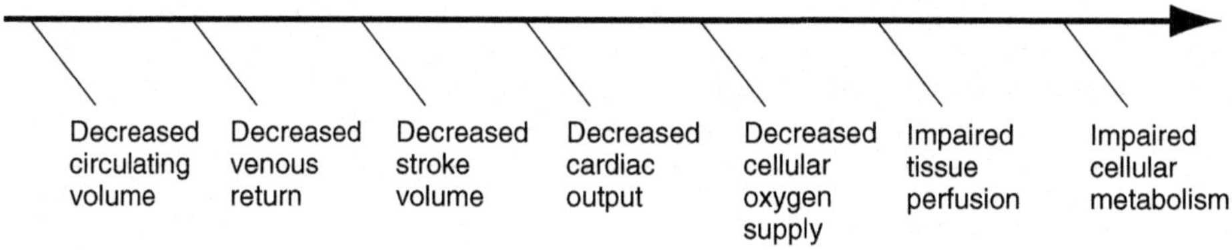

Decreased circulating volume → Decreased venous return → Decreased stroke volume → Decreased cardiac output → Decreased cellular oxygen supply → Impaired tissue perfusion → Impaired cellular metabolism

*Consistent with ARDS.

(50% of total blood volume) shock with reduced systolic and diastolic blood pressure, tachycardia, reduced urine output, changes in mental status or coma (Table 12.18).[62,118–120]

Physiologic and pathologic changes unique to pregnancy, however, may affect the response of the blood pressure and pulse.[14,121] Third trimester hypervolemia may prevent the expected degree of hypotension and tachycardia resulting from the loss of even large volumes of blood. Hemorrhage may actually induce initial hypertension, resulting in a confusing clinical picture.[41] Sympathetic compensation for acute PPH results in intense peripheral vasoconstriction, cardiac tachycardia, increased myocardial contractility (associated with increased myocardial oxygen consumption),[122] and decreased blood flow to the uterus and placenta.[121] Women with severe pre-eclampsia do not have the normal degree of hypervolemia and are thus predisposed to hypotension even with less than the normal post partum blood loss. Fetal distress related to uteroplacental hypoperfusion is usually evident by fetal monitoring and is an important indication of maternal systemic

Table 12.19 Clinical manifestations of hemorrhagic shock.

Organ system	Early shock	Late shock
Blood volume, normal – 5 l (70 ml/kg)	Loss of 25–30%	35–45%
CNS	Altered mentation	Coma
Cardiovascular	Orthostatic hypotension, tachycardia	Myocardial ischemia, arrythmias, LV failure, supine hypotension
Respiratory	Normal tachypnea	Tachypnea, cyanosis, respiratory failure (ARDS)
Renal	Oliguria	Anuria
Hepatic	No change	Elevated liver enzymes, hepatic failure
Gastrointestinal	No change	Gastrointestinal bleeding, bowel ischemia
Hematologic	Normocytic anemia	Thrombocytopenia, DIC
Metabolic	Respiratory alkalosis	Lactic acidosis, hypocalcemia, hypomagnesemia, hyponatremia

CNS (central nervous system); LV (left ventricle); ARDS (adult respiratory distress syndrome); DIC (disseminated intravascular coagulation).

perfusion.[14,121] Amniotic fluid embolism (AFE) is characterized by sudden cardiopulmonary decompensation followed by the development of acute hemorrhagic DIC.[117,123–127] Presenting symptoms of AFE are, typically, seizure-like activity (30%), dyspnea (27%), fetal bradycardia (17%) and hypotension (13%). This initial presentation is usually followed by hemorrhagic DIC.[126]

The clinical manifestations of hemorrhagic shock allow classification as "early" shock or "late" shock. These are summarized in Table 12.19.[118] Early shock is characterized by decreased mean arterial pressure, stroke volume, cardiac output, central venous pressure, and pulmonary capillary wedge pressure. Tissue oxygen extraction increases and overall oxygen consumption decreases as there is a measurable increase in arteriovenous oxygen levels.[128] The intense catecholamine release resulting from acute hemorrhage results in an intense increase in venular tone resulting, effectively, in an autotransfusion as the large volume (70% of total blood volume stored in the venules) in this reservoir enters the arterial circulation. Extracellular fluid and electrolyte shifts resulting from cellular dysfunction promotes the transport of water and sodium into muscles and potassium to the extracellular fluid.[129,130] Heart rate, myocardial contractility, and systemic and pulmonary vascular resistance increase and there is selective, centrally mediated arteriolar vasoconstriction. The result is decreased perfusion to the kidneys, splanchnic beds, skin and uterus in attempt to maintain perfusion to the heart, brain and adrenal glands.[130,131] Compensatory mechanisms begin to fail when the blood volume deficit exceeds 25%.[131] Subsequently, blood pressure and cardiac output decrease and any additional blood loss results in rapidly intensifying maldistribution of blood flow, focal tissue hypoxia, metabolic acidosis and organ dysfunction. Leukotrienes and cytokines are released, platelet aggregation is stimulated and vasoactive mediators are released.[132]

As shock progresses from mild to severe, the degree of systemic tissue hypoperfusion progressively worsens and organ system dysfunction intensifies. In early shock, prompt volume resuscitation reverses hemodynamic changes and may forestall the development of organ ischemia. Early shock may be separated into the shock phase followed by the post resuscitation phase. Inflammatory signaling pathways are activated early in the shock phase and key genes which control inflammatory mechanisms are rapidly upregulated at the time of resuscitation.[133] A systemic inflammatory response progresses to multiple organ dysfunction syndrome (MODS).[120,122,134–136] As hemorrhage continues and shock persists, anaerobic metabolism supervenes, multiple organ dysfunction syndrome intensifies and shock becomes irreversible, accompanied by a mortality of over 30% and substantial risk of permanent tissue injury in survivors, including anoxic brain injury.[119,137]

Management of post partum hemorrhage

Resuscitation

Clearly, the aspect of PPH treatment, which has the greatest influence on outcome is resuscitation from acute hypovolemia. Delay in initiating therapy is the major factor in maternal morbidity and mortality.[1,14] As much as any other factor, it is the prompt availability of intravenous fluids, blood and blood products, which is responsible for the difference in mortality between the developed and underdeveloped nations.[2,13] While the problem of PPH is one of acute blood loss, the primary effort of resuscitation is restoration of intravascular volume. A general guide to therapy during the critical first hour is the mnemonic ORDER: *O*xygenate, *R*estore circulating volume, *D*rug therapy, *E*valuate response to therapy, *R*emedy the underlying cause.[35,118,138] This has also been restated as: *O*rganization, *R*estoration of blood volume, *D*efective blood coagulation, *E*valuation of response, *R*emedy the cause of bleeding.[14] Critical to success is a clear plan of action, an organized approach to care involving physicians, nurses, intensive care facilities, medical laboratory and blood bank.[14,35] A failure in any one of the required components may doom the resuscitative efforts.

The initial step in resuscitation is to provide adequate oxygenation. Although initially not presenting with respiratory compromise (except in cases of amniotic fluid embolism), patients with acute PPH may quickly experience a profound decrease in oxygen carrying capacity and a decrease in effective respirations associated with cerebral hypoperfusion and obtundation.[118] Rapid volume infusion of crystalloid should be administered through large bore intravenous catheters. Two peripheral catheters of 14–16 gauge should be inserted and 1,000 to 2,000 ml administered rapidly.[5,14,118] In patients with severe PPH, central venous pressure catheters and multi-lumen pulmonary artery catheters should be strongly considered. These allow accurate measurement of intravascular volume and greatly facilitate the maintenance of normovolemia, which is an essential goal of therapy.[35,120,139] Although delayed volume resuscitation has been evaluated in patients with traumatic hemorrhagic shock,[140] it is generally accepted that the faster the intravascular volume deficit can be corrected and the more effective management is at maintaining normovolemia, the greater the possibility of avoiding hypovolemic shock.[118]

Comparative trials have demonstrated the superiority of crystalloid over colloid for acute intravenous volume resuscitation.[141] A 4% increase in mortality is noted in PPH patients resuscitated with colloid rather than crystalloid.[141] If colloid is used, it should not be given in pre-eclampsia patients who develop PPH, until 2,000 ml of crystalloid have been infused.[14] Albumin should also be avoided in critically ill patients, as there is a 6% increased rate of mortality used for volume expansion.[142] The disadvantage of crystalloid is the rapid movement from the intravascular to the extravascular space, necessitating three to four times greater volumes of fluid for replacement of intravascular volume deficits, contributing to severe tissue edema.[118,143]

The crystalloids of choice for resuscitation are Ringer's lactate, Hartmann's solution and 0.9% saline.[5,144] As the administration of 1000 ml of Ringer's lactate only increases intravascular volume by 200 ml (80% enters the extravascular space) large volumes of crystalloid are required to correct hypovolemia.[5,144] Dextrose solution is not indicated, as not only does a mere 10% of the infused volume remain in the intravascular space but dextrose may also impair platelet function and hinder blood compatibility testing.[118,145]

Immediately upon the diagnosis of PPH, type and cross-match for packed red blood cells should be requested on an emergency basis. While awaiting compatible blood, massive crystalloid infusion must be continued. When hemorrhage is truly massive and accompanied by signs of hypovolemic shock, type O negative (universal donor) blood should be administered.[14] Red cell transfusion is clearly indicated when acute volume depletion amounts to 2,000 to 3,000 ml (40% of total blood volume).[146] Universal donor blood is required if cross-matched blood is not available by the time 3.5 L of crystalloid has been infused.[5] Blood should be infused as rapidly as possible through large bore intravenous catheters.[35] In massive PPH, one or more units of red cells may be required per hour to keep up with the lost blood.[14] It is the maintenance of intravascular volume and red blood cell carrying capacity, which will most influence morbidity and mortality.[147]

Blood component therapy

Packed red blood cells

Although the infusion of whole blood is ideal for replacement of red cells and blood volume, it has numerous limitations and is rarely available. Component therapy is now preferred. Table 12.20 summarizes the available blood components for use in PPH. The primary method of increasing red blood cell mass is with the administration of packed red blood cells (PRBCs).[62,148,149] The use of PRBCs decreases the volume of infused white blood cells with the associated risk of sensitization due to white cell antigens. PRBCs are provided as 200 to 250 ml volume including preservative and anticoagulant.[62] An adequate oxygen carrying

Table 12.20[62] Blood products in the management of PPH.

Product	Volume	Components
PRBCs	CPD, CPDA-1, 250 ml AS 350 ml	CPD, CPDA-1, WB 200–250 ml plasma removed, Hct 70–80% WB with most plasma removed and 100 ml of AS added, Hct 50–60%
FFP	200–250 ml	150–250 mg per unit of fibrinogen, factors II, VII, IX, X, protein S and C, antithrombin
Platelets	50 ml	>5.5 × 10^{10} PLT plus plasma, 10^8 WBC, trace to 0.5 ml RBC
Cryoprecipitate	5–15 ml	80–120 U of factor VIII, 40 to 70% of original plasma of von Willebrand factor and 150–250 mg fibrinogen

FFP = fresh frozen plasma, AP = anticoagulant/preservative, AS = additive solution, CPD = citrate phosphate dextrose anticoagulant, CPDA-1 = citrate phosphate dextrose adenine anticoagulant, WB = whole blood, PLT = platelets, WBC = white blood cells, RBC = red blood cells.

capacity is maintained in most women with Hgb levels of 7 g/dl. Actively bleeding patients should be transfused with Hgb levels between 7 and 10 g/dl. The combination of PRBCs and crystalloid should be administered at a rate, which at least matches the rate of loss, compensates for deficits and maintains intravascular normovolemia.[150] Generally, each unit of PRBCs will increase the Hgb level by approximately 1 gm/dl and Hct by 3–4% (in the absence of active bleeding).[149] Another goal of transfusion is to maintain the packed cell volume (PCV) above 30, as below this level platelet function may deteriorate.[151]

As PRBCs include only small amounts of clotting factors and few platelets, when massive transfusions (replacement of one or more blood volumes within 24 hrs, which is approximately 10 units of blood in a 70 kg individual)[14,152] are required, clotting factors and platelets must be provided independently. As the blood lost includes plasma volume and red cells, the concomitant administration of crystalloid, plasma and platelets is required to not only maintain intravascular volume but also allow effective hemostasis and maintain electrolyte balance.[14,118,149] Blood must be transfused through intravenous lines with 0.9% saline rather than Ringer's lactate (which contains calcium and causes red cell agglutination) or 5% dextrose (which causes red cell hemolysis).[14,35,149] The citrate anticoagulant in banked blood may complex with serum calcium and dramatically reduce ionized calcium levels, predisposing to impaired myocardial contractility and cardiac arrhythmias. Calcium chloride (10 ml 10% calcium chloride, given intravenously) is, therefore, recommended after every fourth unit of blood.[150] Hypothermia is a significant risk in patients requiring massive transfusion and may cause hypocalcemia by interfering with hepatic metabolism of citrate, provoke cardiac arrhythmias, produce thrombocytopenia due to platelet sequestration and trigger DIC.[62,153–155] For this reason it is advised that blood be administered with the use of a blood warmer and the patient treated with warming blankets. Every effort should be made to maintain normothermia.[5,156] Blood should be infused through a 170–200 μm filter, but the use of micro-aggregate filters, leukocyte poor or irradiated units is not required in the setting of acute massive blood loss when large volumes of blood must be administered rapidly.[5,118]

Although estimations of volume of blood loss are possible from direct collection via drains, suctioned blood, and blood soaked dressings, this is not an adequate indication of the volume of PRBCs required. Frequent monitoring of the Hgb and Hct allows estimation of the deficit in red blood cell mass and provides a guide for red cell transfusion. Every effort should be made to cross-match blood well in anticipation of the patient's immediate needs, staying at least 3–4 units ahead, with blood available in the blood bank. During resuscitation from active hemorrhage, it is essential to remember that there is continued loss of red cells and plasma. Measurement of the Hgb does not directly reflect the loss of intravascular volume.

Measurement of the Hgb and Hct may not reflect the true degree of acute hemorrhagic anemia until 72 hours after bleeding has ceased.[62] Frequent measurement is required of not only Hgb and Hct but also of the platelet count (which may also be reduced by consumption), electrolytes (may be dramatically affected by crystalloid infusion) and coagulation parameters.[147,157]

Autotransfusion

In a variety of operative and postoperative settings, blood is collected and processed for re-infusion by a Cell Saver® device that permits continuous autotransfusion.[158–161] Blood collected is anti-coagulated, filtered and centrifuged, allowing the re-infusion of red blood cells. The process is not associated with an increased risk of infection or amniotic fluid embolism and is accompanied by the reduced risk of transfusion reaction, autoimmunization and infection from blood-born pathogens.[49]

Fresh frozen plasma

Since resuscitation with crystalloid and PRBCs does not include platelets or clotting factors, frequent monitoring of the platelet count, PT and PTT are necessary to anticipate the need for transfusion of platelets and clotting factors. In resuscitation from hemorrhagic shock, there is no clear indication for the prophylactic or "routine" administration of FFP or platelets.[118,143,145,162,163] Rather, therapy with both must be guided by the need to replace specific deficits.[149,164] A unit of FFP (250 ml) contains approximately 150–250 mg per unit of fibrinogen, factors II, VII, IX, X, protein C, protein S and antithrombin.[41,62] The primary indications for FFP are massive transfusion and the replacement of factors VIII and V.[62,165–168] During massive blood transfusion (>1 blood volume within a few hours), coagulation defects arise more from dilutional thrombocytopenia than depletion of clotting factors. A one blood volume hemorrhage is associated with a loss of about 60% of available clotting factors.[169,170] In the absence of DIC, the coagulopathy associated with massive transfusion is most associated with deficiency of fibrinogen (<50 mg/dl) and clotting factors less than 20% of normal.[171] Although the PT and PTT are frequently prolonged, the most useful predicators of hemorrhage are the platelet count <50,000, fibrinogen level <50 mg/dl and PT or PTT ratios (patient/control) of >1.8.[167,171]

The administration of FFP is guided by the necessity for clotting factor replacement as best measured by the PT and PTT. The PT and PTT are, however, of limited value as predictors of the degree of hemodilution or of the potential for bleeding.[170] Empiric therapy, pending the laboratory results is often required, although not preferred. When the PT and/or PTT are prolonged to greater than 1.5 times normal and diffuse hemorrhage is noted, an initial infusion of FFP is recommended at a starting dose of 12–15 ml/kg (4–5 units of FFP).[14] Subsequent FFP therapy should be guided by the need for factor replacement, as required to maintain the PT and PTT <1.5 times normal.[146] This will require approximately 4 units of FFP for every 6 units of PRBCs.[14] The use of FFP for clotting factor replacement must be carefully guided by repeat laboratory studies and clinical assessment. Correction of the PT and PTT to normal is not usually required to achieve hemostasis.

In the presence of DIC or other primary clotting factor deficiencies, much larger volumes of FFP or specific factor replacement may be required. The use of FFP in DIC must be integrated into an overall plan for treatment, as the use of FFP without inhibition of microvascular thrombosis is likely to further potentiate systemic thrombosis, factor consumption and fibrinolysis, thus worsening the prognosis for recovery.[172–175] For fibrinogen replacement (100 mg/dl levels required for normal hemostasis), large volumes of FFP may be required. A preferred alternative is cryoprecipitate, which contains much more fibrinogen (150–250 mg per 50 ml unit), as well as factor VIII and von Willebrand factor.[149] The complications of FFP therapy primarily result from rapid administration of large volumes and include hypothermia, citrate toxicity and hyperkalemia.[167]

Platelets

The administration of platelets must be guided by the clinical assessment, platelet count and estimated platelet function. Although, in the otherwise stable patient, spontaneous hemorrhage is unlikely unless the platelet count is less than 10,000, in the post partum patient and in the presence of PPH, the target level is a platelet count above 50,000.[5,146] In acute blood loss, thrombocytosis occurs promptly, with increases in platelet count to as high as $1{,}000 \times 10^9$/L.[176–178] Patients with PPH are expected to exhibit thrombocytosis, however, in massive PPH, resuscitation with crystalloid and PRBCS results in dilutional thrombocytopenia, usually observed with replacement of 1.5 to 2.0 times blood volume replacement.[14,170,179] Actively bleeding patients should be transfused to maintain the platelet count above 50,000.[14,149] Prophylactic administration of platelets is, however, not indicated.[118,162,180]

In DIC, fibrinogen degradation products profoundly inhibit platelet function,[172,181,182] principally through binding to the GPIIb/IIIa receptor.[66,172,175] In the actively hemorrhaging patient with continued bleeding in spite of adequate replacement of clotting factors and fibrinogen, platelets may be required due to platelet dysfunction, even if the platelet count is >50,000.[62,183]

The primary risk of platelet transfusion is the development of platelet alloantibodies and RBC alloantibodies. Platelet cross-matching by HLA typing is not readily available, nor appropriate, in the emergency setting. The use of ABO-matched platelets is preferred, but not required.[62] Since there remain small numbers of RBCs, even after careful platelet preparation, platelets infused which are not ABO and Rh matched to the patient may induce the development of anti-D (Rho) antibodies. This may be an important concern in the woman who intends future pregnancy and may be prevented by the administration of a single 300 μg dose of Rho immune globulin for every 15 ml of RBC (assume 2 ml of blood per each 6 unit platelet pack).[149]

Cryoprecipitate

The indication for infusion of cryoprecipitate is to rapidly replace fibrinogen, von Willebrand factor, fibronectin and the clotting factors VIII and XIII.[184] Cryoprecipitate contains 80–120 U of factor VIII, 40–70% of the original plasma of von Willebrand factor and 150–250 mg of fibrinogen.[62,167] Patients with PPH and DIC are usually profoundly hypofibrinogenemic. Infusion with FFP as a source of fibrinogen may require large volume FFP infusions, whereas the volume of cryoprecipitate required to increase the fibrinogen level to the same degree is 5 times lower.[184] PPH patients confirmed or suspected to also have DIC should be promptly evaluated for fibrinogen deficiency and transfused with cryoprecipitate at a rate necessary to keep the fibrinogen level above 100 mg/dl.[5,149] Prophylactic therapy is not indicated. In the patient with DIC, cryoprecipitate is only indicated as a component of an overall management plan and should not be administered without concomitant antithrombotic therapy, as doing so simply sustains systemic microvascular thrombosis and perpetuates MODS.[172,175]

Hemostatic agents

Factor VIIa

Factor VII is the clotting factor unique to the extrinsic clotting system. The tissue factor-factor VIIa complex triggers the conversion of factor X to Xa. Recombinant factor VIIa has been used effectively in refractory PPH to control hemorrhage.[185–187] Although, generally considered contraindicated, successful hemostasis and outcome have also been achieved in PPH patients with refractory hemorrhage and DIC.[186,188,189] Therapy has included the administration of one or more doses ranging from 60 U/kg to 120 U/kg. An initial dose has been usually followed by at least one additional dose and repeated infusion is guided by the initial response and clinical course.[185,186] As the mechanism of action involves stimulation of the common pathway of coagulation on the platelet surface, leading to local fibrin deposition, the effectiveness of this approach depends upon the presence of adequate levels of factors X, V, prothrombin and fibrinogen.

Pharmacologic therapy

Uterotonics

As the major cause of PPH is uterine atony and since the major source of blood lost is usually from the uterus, pharmacologic measures to stimulate uterine contraction and vascular constriction are first line therapy. Concomitant with fluid resuscitation, oxytocin is recommended by intravenous bolus of 10–20 U followed by 20 U in 500 ml of normal saline.[190] This is followed by methyl ergometrine 0.4 mg intravenously. Cases not responding to this regimen may be administered intramyometrial prostaglandin F 2α (15-methyl-PGF2; carboprost tromethamine) at a dose of 0.25 mg intramuscularly or intramyometrialy every 15 minutes to a maximum of 2 mg.[54] Therapeutic failures have also been treated quite successfully with a 600 to 800 mcg dose of rectal misoprostol (response within 30 s to 3 min).[21,108,191] In comparison to Syntometrine (ampoule with 5 U oxytocin and 500 mcg ergometrine maleate), misoprostol is more effective at controlling PPH.[103,106] Studies comparing intravenous versus intramyometrial administration of carboprost have demonstrated superiority of the intramyometrial route for control of PPH.[192,193] In refractory cases, this has been successful in controlling PPH, when administered as a vaginal suppository or by intrauterine irrigation.[49,193]

Side effects to prostaglandins are not uncommon, as PGF2 is associated with side effects in 20% of women, including provocation of bronchospasm (contraindicated in patients with a history of asthma), diarrhea, hypertension, vomiting, fever, flushing and tachycardia[49] and PGE2 may cause fever in 50% and transient diastolic hypotension in 10%.[49] Ergot derivatives and prostaglandin analogues are also identified as causative factors in acute myocardial infarction and cardiac arrest during initial treatment for PPH.[33,194,195]

Antifibrinolytic agents

The therapeutic use of the antifibrinolytic agents ε-aminocaproic acid (EACA), tranexamic acid (AMCA) and trasylol has been suggested in patients with PPH, DIC and refractory life-threatening hemorrhage.[196] Antifibrinolytic therapy is however, generally regarded as contraindicated in DIC, due to potentiation of microvascular thrombosis.[172,175] EACA has been used in primary fibrinolysis,[197,198] AMCA has been used to reduce blood loss at cesarean section[199] and for primary fibrinolysis[197,200,201] and trasylol to inhibit the initiation of SIRS associated with cardiopulmonary bypass.[197,202] Tranexamic acid has been used successfully for refractory PPH as 1 g intravenously every 4 hours for 12 hours.[203] In the setting of massive PPH with DIC, fibrinolytic agents must only be considered as a component of a comprehensive approach to management. Since the primary pathology of DIC is microvascular thrombosis, concomitant antithrombotic therapy is required.[196]

Vasopressors

Other pharmacologic agents of use in the patient with PPH, primarily assist control of hemodynamic instability and treatment of DIC. Although the primary insult in PPH is hypovolemia, as volume and blood deficits are treated, cardiotonic and vasoconstrictor agents may be required temporarily to maintain an adequate mean blood pressure. These agents include the inotropic agents dopamine, dobutamine, and isoproterenol and the vasopressor agents epinephrine, norepinephrine, vasopressin, metaraminol bitartrate, inamrinone, milrinone acetate, and phenylephrine. Vasopressin, by action on unique receptors, causes intense vasospasm. In addition to use as a systemic vasoconstrictor, vasopressin has been used successfully in a dilute solution for intrauterine injection for intractable uterine hemorrhage resulting from placenta accreta.[54,204] Initiation of therapy with the agent of first choice, dopamine is indicated if the mean arterial pressure is less than 60 mm Hg. The goal for blood pressure maintenance should be a mean of 90 mm Hg.[37,118,205]

Patients who present with acute PPH are hypotensive and tachycardic as the result of acute blood loss resulting in intravascular hypovolemia. The logical and appropriate therapy is to replace volume. Unfortunately, patients with massive PPH frequently present with acute, severe hypotension and active acute hemorrhage. Although crystalloid may be available for rapid infusion, blood may not be and the patient may either suffer frank cardiac arrest or appear near arrest with very low or undetectable blood pressure. As a therapy of last resort, the prompt administration of vasopressor agents may stimulate heart rate, increase myocardial contractility and intensify peripheral vasoconstriction to assist central vital organ perfusion as a temporizing measure until definitive therapy can be provided (Table 12.21). The benefit of vasopressor administration, however, is transient, as intensification of vasospasm may worsen microvascular hypoperfusion and increase the potential for microvascular thrombosis.[35,37,205] Without correcting intravascular volume depletion, the use of vasopressors offers only transient benefit.

Severe complications of vasopressor therapy may result from intense stimulation of systemic and peripheral vascular resistance and include myocardial ischemia and infarction,[33] multiple organ ischemia including the induction of acute renal failure and peripheral tissue ischemia leading to digital and limb ischemia, infarction, and amputation. Once the volume deficit is corrected, vasopressors are to be progressively withdrawn as quickly as possible.

Table 12.21[291] Vasopressors in the treatment of PPH.

Vasopressor	Action	Dose
Dopamine	increased cardiac output, dilates renal and mesenteric vasculature	moderately ill: 2–5 mcg/(kg min); seriously ill: 5 mcg/(kg min) and increase gradually to 20–50 mcg/(kg min)
Isoproterenol	relaxes smooth muscle, increase in heart rate, unchanged stroke volume and increase in ejection velocity	0.02 to 0.06 mg initially, 0.01 to 0.2 mg IV injection according to patient response
Dobutamine	vasodilator effects, increased cardiac output	2.5 to 10 mcg/(kg min); administer according to patient response
Epinephrine	increases strength of ventricular contraction, increases heart rate, relaxes smooth muscle	0.5 to 1 mg administered by IV every 5 minutes
Norepinephrine	vasoconstrictor, increases systolic BP and coronary artery blood flow	8–12 mcg/(kg min) and increase according to patient to establish normal BP (average dose = 0.5 to 1 ml per minute)
Phenylephrine	increases systolic and diastolic BP, vasoconstrictor	mild to moderate hypotension = 2–5 mg
Vasopressin	vasopressor and antidiuretic hormone activity	one 40 mg dose administered by IV

All doses are for IM or SC. Blood volume depletion must be stabilized before administering any of these drugs.

The target for vasopressor therapy is maintenance of the mean arterial pressure of 90 mm Hg, as measured by intraarterial monitoring. The use of these agents should be guided by intraarterial monitoring combined with monitoring of volume resuscitation with central venous and/or pulmonary artery pressure monitoring.[35,37,205,206]

Antibiotics

While the primary etiology of shock in patients with massive PPH is not infection, broad-spectrum antibiotic coverage is recommended.[37,118] At initial presentation, in patients without massive vaginal blood loss, sepsis must be considered in the differential diagnosis. Furthermore, hemorrhagic shock results in gastrointestinal ischemia and predisposes to the translocation of bacteria through the mucosal barrier to enter the systemic circulation.[207] This may then trigger SIRS and complicate hemorrhagic with septic shock.

Monitoring

Resuscitation from PPH requires intensive monitoring of hemodynamic and hematologic parameters. Blood pressure and pulse remain the primary determinants of hemodynamic integrity. Except in abruptio placenta, the primary guide to the degree of intravascular hypovolemia is the blood pressure.[14] The goal of treatment is to achieve the baseline blood pressure and pulse as quickly as possible. When hypovolemia is not accompanied by other features of shock or SIRS, infusion of volume is generally followed by return to baseline blood pressure and pulse quickly. Serial measurement of blood pressure and pulse every 15 minutes is necessary and can be reasonably relied upon to reflect the adequacy of volume replacement. Measurement of urinary output is a sensitive measurement of the adequacy of systemic organ perfusion and close monitoring of output via indwelling urinary catheter is recommended.[14,41] When primary hypovolemia from PPH is not accompanied by shock, volume replacement can be guided by these simple bedside measurements.

As the diagnostic feature of PPH is excessive blood loss, this must be accompanied by serial measurements of the serum Hgb. Although an unreliable measurement of true oxygen carrying capacity,[62] determination of the Hgb must be at least hourly during the early phases of resuscitation, reduced to every 4 hours as it appears that hemorrhage is controlled and gradually reduced in frequency, as clinically indicated. When transfusion is indicated, measurement of hemodynamic parameters such as the mixed venous oxygen content may be more reliable in predicting the need for transfusion, than serial CBCs.[208] Coagulation studies are indicated initially and after every 5–10 units of blood transfused, or as clinically indicated, based upon bedside evaluation for signs of DIC and monitoring for hemodynamic changes which indicate occult hemorrhage. Recommended studies include the Hgb, Hct, platelet count, PT, PTT, fibrinogen, and D-dimer assay.[35]

The patient with massive PPH, and hemorrhagic shock requires immediate transfer to the intensive care unit or other area capable of providing the very highest level of monitoring and intervention available in the hospital. Immediately upon recognition of PPH, emergency consultation should be requested from a critical care specialist, an expert in thrombosis and hemostasis and others, based on the suspected etiology of PPH. As massive crystalloid, blood and blood component administration is required and since hemodynamic changes may occur on a minute-to-minute basis, central venous pressure monitoring is strongly recommended.[37] Insertion of a large central catheter in the internal jugular, subclavian or femoral vein allows the needed access for massive fluid and blood infusion, as well as a port for connection to a central venous pressure monitoring system. Patients with massive PPH, hemorrhagic shock, SIRS, amniotic fluid embolism and DIC have all been documented to have myocardial ischemia and myocardial infarction as consequences.[33] For this reason and because of the limited accuracy of measurements of central venous pressure alone, monitoring with a pulmonary artery catheter capable of measuring cardiac output should be considered.[35,209] It has been noted, however, that randomized controlled trials have not verified superior outcomes with invasive hemodynamic monitoring.[210] The basis for most recommendations remains case series and expert opinions.[37] Clearly, the assessment and management of patients unresponsive to initial fluid resuscitation and those who require therapy with vasoactive medications can be managed with increased accuracy by the use of the pulmonary artery catheter.

Patients who progress to multiple organ dysfunction syndrome (MODS) frequently develop acute respiratory failure and adult respiratory distress syndrome (ARDS).[211] Treatment of ARDS is facilitated by measurement of pulmonary artery and pulmonary capillary wedge pressure and cardiac output.[212] Precise monitoring of intravascular volume is also helpful in avoiding potentially harmful hypervolemia, pulmonary congestion and hypoxemia.[213] Modern pulmonary artery catheter systems provide the additional advantage of multiple ports for venous access and infusion of blood, fluids and medications. In the patient with DIC, the risk of hemorrhage at the insertion site is significant and placement must be performed with every attempt to avoid multiple punctures of the required large vein.

As the early phases of resuscitation frequently require the use of vasopressors to maintain the mean blood pressure above 80 before adequate volume replacement is achieved, intraarterial pressure monitoring is a necessary component of hemodynamic monitoring. Peripheral blood pressure monitoring frequently underestimates the true arterial pressure, due to peripheral vasoconstriction and reduced pulse pressure.[206] Vasopressors are potentially extremely hazardous and must be used with precise monitoring of intraarterial pressure. In addition, the presence of an arterial catheter allows access for the frequent determination of the arterial blood gas and other laboratory studies.[206]

During torrential hemorrhage, a highly efficient laboratory is required for timely measurement of Hgb, Hct, platelet count, fibrinogen, PT, PTT, D-dimer, arterial blood gases, electrolytes and other studies. An important aspect of the initial steps in overall approach to the care of patients with PPH, is to promptly notify the medical diagnostic laboratory of the acuity of the patient's condition and alert the laboratory personnel to the need for close cooperation to facilitate rapid turnaround times with critical laboratory studies. Similarly, the blood bank must be advised of the need for potentially large volumes of blood and blood components over a short period of time, and the need for assistance to maintain a ready supply of the needed units.

Determination of the etiology of post partum hemorrhage

A simple mnemonic of "4 Ts" may be easily remembered as a guide to rapid bedside assessment of the hemorrhaging patient: (1) Tone – uterine atony; (2) Tissue – retained placental tissue; (3) Trauma – genital tract trauma; (4) Thrombin – coagulopathies.[17] The etiology of PPH may be readily apparent from simple inspection of the episiotomy site, lower birth canal or incision after cesarean section. Abdominal examination may reveal findings of uterine atony and suggest uterine origin. A firm uterus with active vaginal hemorrhage suggests a laceration of the birth canal.[41] Examination under anesthesia may be required to identify and allow repair of cervical and vaginal lacerations.[5] Inner myometrial lacerations are a recently described cause of uterine hemorrhage appearing from excessive stress on the uterine cervix resulting from excessively strong uterine contractions at the time of delivery.[214] When bleeding is suspected to originate from the uterus, tamponade techniques may allow both control of hemorrhage and confirmation of the origin. Uterine or hepatic rupture with intraperitoneal bleeding may be suspected by the observation of abdominal swelling without overt vaginal hemorrhage. Delayed postoperative retroperitoneal hemorrhage may present with unexplained hemodynamic collapse. These intraperitoneal and retroperitoneal sources of PPH may be difficult to detect as the peritoneal cavity my hold up to 3,000 ml of blood with minimal change in abdominal girth.[215] Uterine and incisional blood loss may not explain the severity of bleeding if hemorrhagic DIC develops, as bleeding may then be from multiple sites, some of which are clinically occult. Diagnosing DIC and other hemorrhagic diatheses requires laboratory assessment.

Interventional radiology

Although successful transcatheter treatment of vascular hemorrhage was first described over 30 years ago,[216] application for uncontrolled PPH was not reported until 1979.[217] Additional reports have confirmed the importance of transcatheter techniques for the treatment of post partum bleeding.[218–222] A major benefit with transcatheter embolization is the avoidance of a laparotomy in a patient who may have hemodynamic instability and a severe coagulopathy.

In the past 30 years advances in technique have made transcatheter management of vascular hemorrhage highly safe and efficacious. These advances include:

(1) development of preshaped catheters, (2) miniaturization of catheters (microcatheters), used coaxially, (3) new embolic agents, and (4) the use of modern image intensification (fluoroscopy). Advances in embolization materials (polyvinyl chloride particles called Ivalon®) have enabled safe and precise embolization, without clogging of the catheter lumen.

The vascular supply to the uterus (as well as other pelvic viscera) is from the internal iliac arteries, specifically, the uterine artery, a branch of the visceral trunk of the internal iliac artery. All pelvic organs have a dual vascular supply, namely bilateral branches (left and right), supplying each side of the organ. Typically, embolization is of an ipso-lateral arterial branch, and the contra-lateral vascular supply will preclude tissue necrosis. Proximal embolization (similar to the surgical ligation of the vessel) may result in reduced risk of tissue necrosis, due to development of collateral vessels into the distal circulation. However, proximal embolization may be less desired because with collateral vessel development, re-bleeding may occur. In addition, proximal embolization (like surgical ligation) precludes re-catheterization if re-bleeding occurs. Distal embolization increases the likelihood of tissue necrosis, especially if small embolization particles are used. However, distal embolization may be preferable, as collateral vessels are less likely to develop, reducing the risk of re-bleeding. Also, distal embolization will not prevent re-catheterization of the vessel if re-bleeding recurs.

Modern embolization materials include polyvinylchloride particles (Ivalon® particles), which are used for distal embolization techniques. Ivalon® particles are manufactured in various diameters from very small (100-micron diameters), up to relatively large (1,000 micron) diameters. Materials used for proximal embolization include gelfoam and vascular coils. Gelfoam is more often used for elective embolization (pre-surgical embolization) as a technique to temporarily reduce bleeding at the operative site. Gelfoam particles are generally larger than PVC (Ivalon®) particles and are known to be only temporary, with vessel recanalization known to occur in days to weeks. In contradistinction, Ivalon® particles are resistant to arterial recanalization. Vascular coils vary in diameter from very large coils (30 mm), to very small micro-coils designed for interacranial aneurysm embolization. Coils are designed for proximal embolization and often are used as an adjunct to Ivalon® particles (proximal and distal embolization). Transcatheter balloons have also been utilized in massive PPH to temporarily occlude the hypogastric arteries, successfully reducing pulse pressure and allowing correction of hemodynamic instability and coagulopathy.[223]

The technique of transcatheter embolization is straightforward, provided that a qualified practitioner combined with a modern interventional laboratory is available. The common femoral artery is catheterized using a sterile technique, with placement of a standard angiographic, 5 French catheter with an angled tip. The catheter is directed over the distal abdominal aortic bifurcation, distally into the contralateral internal iliac artery (usually the left internal iliac, if the initial vascular puncture was from the right groin approach). The 5 French catheter is directed into the origin of the internal iliac artery and an initial angiogram is performed. If bleeding is brisk, active extravasation will be seen. Angiography may readily identify the source of hemorrhage, including such unanticipated findings as hemorrhage from a false aneurysm of the uterine pedicle,[224] deep vaginal laceration,[225] arteriovenous fistulae, and a uterine artery aneurysm.[226]

Once the 5 French catheter is in place (guiding catheter) in the proximal aspect of the internal iliac artery, a 3 French micro-catheter is advanced through the lumen of the guiding catheter (co-axial technique) into the uterine artery branch. Use of the microcatheter is important because the relatively small diameter of the microcatheter will prevent vasospasm that a larger catheter will often induce. Vasospasm is to be avoided during an embolization procedure, as this will often impede or prevent a successful embolization. Ivalon® particles are then injected through the micro-catheter, thus supra-selectively occluding only the lumen of the uterine artery. Following this, a post-embolization arteriogram is performed to confirm placement. With observation, hemodynamic and clinical stabilization usually follow promptly. If bleeding continues, the ipso-lateral uterine artery is also embolized. This can be accomplished either with recatheterization from the opposite groin or the same groin by looping the initial 5 French catheter (Waltman loop) then pulling the tip of the catheter down into the ipso-lateral internal iliac artery. If rebleeding occurs, embolization can be repeated.[226]

The use of transcatheter embolization for the treatment of post partum hemorrhage has been studied extensively as an alternative to surgery in women with PPH.[225–231] Outcomes are excellent, without reported complications.[226,227] Post partum hemorrhage is controlled in from 91.9%[230] to 94.9%[229] of cases, including 96% of patients with PPH due to uterine artery arteriovenous malformations and 100% of cases with abdominal and cervical pregnancies.[229] As a primary goal of using transcatheter embolization is preservation of uterine function and fertility, long-term outcomes have been studied. Results are excellent, with many reported cases of subsequent successful pregnancy.[232,233] With subsequent pregnancy, recurrence of severe post partum hemorrhage has been reported,[232] as has a single case of intrauterine growth restriction.[234] When modern interventional radiology is available, transcatheter embolization is recommended as the procedure of choice for control of obstetrical hemorrhage.[231] In comparing the choice of bilateral hypogastric artery ligation versus interventional radiologic therapy, transcatheter embolization is preferred in hemodynamically stable patients with birth canal trauma or uterine atony and bilateral hypogastric artery ligation is indicated when PPH occurs after cesarean section, when the patient is hemodynamically unstable.[235]

Surgical management of post partum hemorrhage

Surgical treatment of PPH is indicated when there is evidence of an anatomical cause (uterine rupture, severe cervical or birth canal laceration), when pharmacological medical treatment fails, or when interventional radiology techniques fail or are unavailable. A variety of surgical procedures are available. The choice of procedure depends upon the clinical setting and response to treatment. Options range from uterine packing and uterine artery ligation to hysterectomy (Table 12.22).

Tamponade

Uterine tamponade is a somewhat controversial technique that has been typically achieved by uterine packing with gauze. Newer tamponade techniques include the use of Foley,[236] Sengstaken-Blakemore[237] and Rusch[238] balloon catheters. The "tamponade test" using the Sengstaken-Blakemore tube has emerged as a highly useful technique both for control of hemorrhage and for diagnosis.[239] Vaginal tamponade of severe vaginal hematoma has been achieved with gauze packing and a sterile glove covered blood pressure cuff.[240] Tamponade is indicated with confirmed, active, vaginal or uterine bleeding. Local therapy is emergent and accompanies aggressive resuscitation. Unless other sites of hemorrhage or DIC are present, effective tamponade results in prompt correction of hypotension. Extrinsic compression has also, in effect, been achieved with the use of a pneumatic

Table 12.22 Surgical treatments of PPH.

Uterine tamponade/packing
Gauze packing
Foley catheter
Sengstaken–Blakemore catheter
Rusch catheter
Large-volume balloon
Repair birth canal injuries
Uterine artery ligation
Control uterine hemorrhage
Internal iliac artery ligation
Hemostatic sutures
B-Lynch suture
Modified B-Lynch suture
Multiple square suture
Hysterectomy

anti-shock garment. In a limited study, application of the anti-shock garment combined with volume resuscitation was highly successful at stabilizing vital signs and controlling PPH in women with refractory hemorrhagic shock.[241] Candidates for any tamponade procedure must be chosen carefully as more effective therapy may be potentially delayed.

Vaginal tamponade

Vaginal tamponade with gauze packing has been the treatment of choice to control bleeding after evacuation of a vaginal hematoma associated with active vaginal bleeding.[5] Covering a blood pressure cuff with a sterile glove and inserting this into the vaginal vault has controlled refractory hemorrhage. The cuff is slowly inflated to about 120 mm Hg, 10 mm Hg above systolic pressure. Beginning 8 hours later, the cuff is gradually deflated until removal after 32 hours. Excellent control of hemorrhage, without recurrence or sequelae is reported in 2 cases.[240]

Uterine packing

Uterine packing is a method of controlling uterine hemorrhage, which fell into disfavor in the 1950s primarily due to difficulty monitoring the amount of blood loss and concern regarding infection.[5] A subsequent study demonstrated that with meticulous attention to technique, involving side-to-side packing, avoiding dead space, packing is simple, safe and effective. The indications are confirmed uterine bleeding due to atony, placenta accreta and placenta previa.[242] However, uterine packing is seldom used because it is believed to delay treatment.

Foley catheter

Refractory uterine hemorrhage following spontaneous vaginal delivery has been controlled with the use of a Foley catheter. The technique involves the insertion of a Foley catheter into the uterus, followed by inflation of the balloon with 110 ml of air. The catheter is left in place for 8 hours. While success at controlling bleeding has been achieved, it has also been noted that the volume of the inflated balloon is far less than adequate to fill the large atonic uterus. Continued hemorrhage may occur above the level of the inflated balloon, thereby providing the misleading impression that bleeding has stopped when no additional blood is observed to exit the vagina.[236] It is essential that precise monitoring of vital signs, urine output, fundal height and vaginal blood loss continue. Infusion of oxytocin and prophylactic antibiotics are also indicated.[5]

Sengstaken–Blakemore catheter

The Sengstaken–Blakemore catheter has been used for the control of hemorrhagic esophageal varices. For use as a device to control uterine hemorrhage, the catheter has been modified by cutting off the gastric end of the tube and sterilization.[237] The catheter is carefully inserted with sponge forceps grasping the cervix and the catheter is inserted into the uterus and inflated with 75–300 ml of saline. The distended balloon should then be just visible at the cervical canal and palpable in the uterine fundus. Gentle traction is then applied to verify firm fixation in the uterus. With careful observation it is then noted whether blood continues to drain from the uterine opening or the cervical os.[243] The "tamponade test" is either successful (positive), if blood does not exit the tube or the cervix and unsuccessful (negative) if blood exits either. If the test is negative laparotomy has been advocated.[239,243] Upper vaginal packing may be applied to keep the catheter in place. Patients who stabilize with the Sengstaken–Blakemore tube are carefully monitored in the intensive care unit and oxytocin infusion (40 U/500 ml) is continued for at least 8 hours. Prophylactic antibiotics are administered for at least 24 hours. After approximately 24 hours, and when the patient is hemodynamically stable and disordered coagulation is corrected, half of the inflation volume is removed. If there is no evidence of re-bleeding, the catheter is removed over the subsequent few hours.[243] In a study of the "tamponade test", 87.5% of patients had a positive test associated with the control of hemorrhage and only 12.5% had a negative test, requiring laparotomy.[243]

Rusch catheter

The Rusch catheter, similar to the Foley catheter, is a urologic catheter utilized in the setting of PPH, following spontaneous vaginal delivery. The primary advantage over the Foley catheter is that it can be inflated with as much as 400 to 500 ml of saline.[238] The primary indication is refractory PPH following manual removal of a morbidly adherent placenta or a succentruate lobe.[5] There are reports of success after failure to control hemorrhage with the Sengstaken–Blakemore tube and angiographic uterine artery embolization. This technique is rarely used. Upon controlling the hemorrhage, the catheter is removed after 24 hours. Close monitoring and continued aggressive medical management are required. The technique may be associated with a lower incidence of infection.[238]

Large-volume balloon

A uniquely designed large-volume tamponade balloon, specifically for use in PPH originating from the implantation site of low-lying placenta/placenta previa has proven successful at controlling persistent hemorrhage. The balloon has a therapeutic filling capacity of 500 ml and is used much as other balloon tamponade devices. Drainage ports above the balloon allow careful monitoring for continued bleeding.[244] Application has included use at the time of cesarean section. The large-volume balloon catheter is placed either through the uterus and the distal end pulled through the cervix into the vagina or transvaginally after vaginal delivery.

The primary indication is persistent hemorrhage from the lower uterine segment after repeat cesarean section associated with low lying/placenta previa. Cases did not exhibit features of uterine atony. The primary advantages appear to be ease of application and avoidance of "traumatic friction " at the time of removal.[245]

Laparotomy

Arterial ligation

The objective of ligation of pelvic arteries is to diminish arterial pulse pressure to a degree sufficient to allow control of hemorrhage, without compromising the viability of uterine tissue. Prompt control of hemorrhage with preservation of fertility is the ultimate goal of this and other techniques. The collateral nature of uterine blood flow limits the effectiveness of unilateral procedures.

Uterine artery ligation (O'Leary stitch)

First reported in 1952,[246] ligation of bilateral uterine arteries (O'Leary stitch) is effective at controlling PPH in 40 to 95% of cases.[5,10] It has become the first line procedure for controlling uterine bleeding at laparotomy. It is a more attractive option than internal iliac artery ligation because it is easier, faster and more successful. Figure 12.3 illustrates this procedure. The ascending branches of both uterine arteries are localized and ligated at the level of the vesicouterine reflection.[247] A suture on a large curved needle is passed through the lateral aspect of the uterine segment close to the cervix, then back through the broad ligament just lateral to the uterine vessels. If this step is not successful to control bleeding, the vessels of the utero-ovarian arcade are ligated on both sides by passing a suture through the myometrium just medial to the vessels. The technique requires inclusion of 2–3 cm of myometrium to occlude intramyometrial branches and avoid uterine vessel injury.[49] Limitations of the technique include retained placental fragments, cervical and birth canal lacerations and myometrial pathology such as fibroids.[247]

A variation of the original technique has been developed offering the potential for more precise and effective control of uterine bleeding. In a five-step process, the arterial blood supply of the uterus and ovaries is occluded.[248] One vessel is occluded at a time, observing for bleeding after each. First, the unilateral uterine artery is ligated on the side felt most responsible for hemorrhage. Second, the contralateral uterine artery is ligated. Third, the low uterine arteries are ligated after mobilization of the bladder. Fourth, the unilateral ovarian and fifth, the opposite ovarian artery are ligated.[248] In the initial case series of 103 patients, 100% effectiveness was reported with no patient progressing to hysterectomy.[10] There is no adverse effect in future pregnancies and the risk of uretral injury is small.

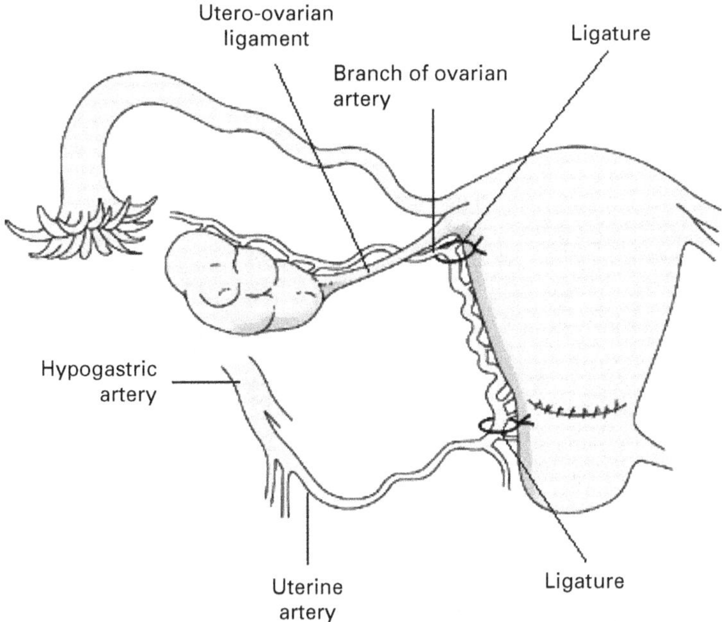

Uterine artery ligation. Sutures are placed to ligate the ascending uterine artery and the anastomotic branch of the ovarian artery. The procedure should be performed on each side.

Figure 12.3 Uterine artery ligation (O'Leary stitch).[292]

Internal iliac (hypogastric) artery ligation

The technique of hypogastric artery ligation significantly reduces pelvic arterial pulse pressure, in effect, converting pelvic circulation to a venous system. Arterial pressure is reduced 14% by contralateral, 77% by homolateral, and 85% by bilateral hypogastric artery ligation.[249] Hypogastric artery ligation is technically more difficult and, if fails, requires hysterectomy. Morbidity and mortality is increased with emergency hysterectomy in this setting and a success rate of only about 42% has been reported.[250] For this reason, the procedure is only indicated in women who are hemodynamically stable and desire future pregnancy.[49] Report of subsequent fertility and pregnancy in 68 patients who underwent bilateral hypogastric artery ligation revealed no evidence of infertility or adverse pregnancy outcomes, except for 3 minor episodes of PPH, treated successfully with medical therapy.[251]

Hemostatic sutures

In order to control uterine hemorrhage with the hope of preserving fertility, a variety of hemostatic suturing techniques have been developed. Consideration of

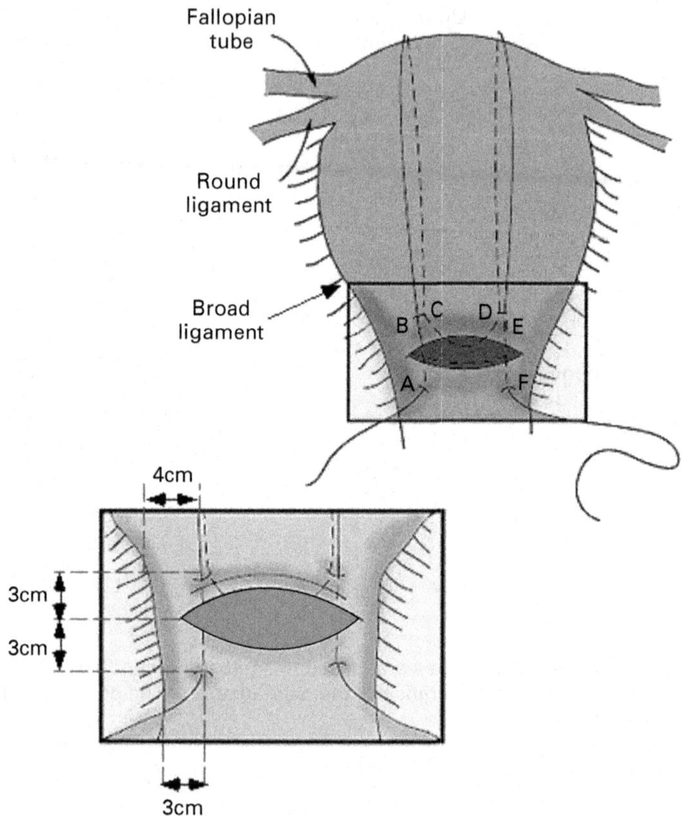

Anterior uterine wall with B–Lynch suture in place and an enlarged drawing (box) of lower uterine segment with B–Lynch suture in place. Adapted from *Obstetrics & Gynecology Case Reports & Reviews*, Vol. 95, Num. 6, June 2000.

Figure 12.4 B-lynch suture.[293]

the use of hemostatic suturing is indicated when the primary source of blood loss is uterine and when pharmacologic therapy, transfusion and factor replacement therapy, tamponade techniques, angiographic arterial embolization (if available) and arterial ligation fail to control bleeding. Success is only likely if bimanual compression of the uterus significantly decreases blood loss.[49,252,253]

B-Lynch suture

The B-Lynch suture is a simplified brace suture designed to control atonic uterine hemorrhage (Figure 12.4). Subsequent to laparotomy the uterus is bimanually compressed and the anterior and posterior wall of the uterus are brought into apposition. If bleeding is controlled by direct compression, the suture is placed.[252] As originally described, a number 2'0 chromic suture on a 75 mm heavy, round-bodied needle is passed through a lower uterine segment hysterotomy from the lower uterine segment over the fundus and returned posteriorly. The suture is continued on the alternate side. Upon completion, the uterus is collapsed into an accordion-like shape.[253] In the initial case series, the technique was 100% effective.[252] Subsequent reports have also indicated good results.[254,255] The primary limitation concerns the need for a hysterotomy and the limited number of reported cases.[49]

Modified B-Lynch suture

Multiple hemostatic simple brace sutures, including an isthmo-cervical stitch are placed in the modified B-Lynch technique. Developed primarily for bleeding at the time of a cesarean section in order to control a morbidly adherent placenta, the modified brace is used to control bleeding from the body of the uterus.[239] A 2'0 Dexon suture on a straight needle is passed through the anterior uterine wall above the bladder reflection, through the uterine cavity and the posterior uterine wall. From another entry 1 cm medial to the initial suture exit point, the needle is passed through the posterior uterine wall, uterine cavity and anterior wall. Both sutures are repeated on the other side. Closed artery forceps are placed between the medial margins of the two sutures to ensure patency of the cervical canal after the apposition sutures are tightened. In addition, a number 2'0 chromic suture on a straight needle is passed through the uterus slightly rostral to the lower horizontal apposition suture from the anterior to the posterior uterine wall and is tied over the fundus, 3–4 cm medial to the cornu. The procedure is repeated on the opposite side. Manual compression is applied and prostaglandin F2 alpha (Hemabate®) 250 mcg is injected intramyometrial.[239] The nature of the procedure and associated operative risk require careful inspection of the bowel, bladder and ureter before closure. A major advantage over the classical B-Lynch is the lack of need for hysterotomy.[5,239]

Multiple square suturing

Another approach to control of PPH at the time of cesarean section is the technique of placing multiple square sutures through the entire uterine wall. The objective is control of bleeding with only the required area of uterine compression. This may be particularly advantageous for patients with a localized site of uterine hemorrhage such as that arising from placenta accreta. Square suturing begins with a suture at the apparent site of bleeding. If bleeding persists, another square suture is placed adjacent to the first. Additional squares are placed until hemorrhage is controlled. Number 1 atraumatic chromic suture on a number 7 or 8 straight surgical needle is used. Sutures are placed by passing the needle from the anterior wall, through the uterine cavity and then the posterior wall. The needle is then passed posterior to anterior from an arbitrary point 2–3 cm lateral. Another suture is placed above or below the first suture point. Once again, lateral, above or below the 2nd suture point, another suture is placed. Sutures are placed such that the points form a small square of about 3 cm on a side. The knot is tied as tightly as possible. The first suture is placed in the area appearing to be the primary site of hemorrhage and additional sutures are placed in other areas, as needed to control bleeding. In cases of uterine atony, 4–5 squares, placed evenly throughout the uterus are required. Success at achieving hemostasis has been 100% and hysterectomy avoided. Women so treated have been confirmed to later have a normal uterine cavity and achieve pregnancy.[256]

Hysterectomy

In developed countries, the incidence of hysterectomy varies from 0.3 to 1.6/1,000 deliveries, and may be higher in tertiary centers[257] and in developing countries.[258] The typical indications are persistent or recurrent bleeding after aggressive medical and transfusion management and conservative surgical intervention.[49,239] In a study of 70 emergency post partum hysterectomies (60 following cesarean section and 10 following vaginal delivery), operated patients included those with uterine atony (43%), placenta accreta (30%), uterine rupture (13%), extension of a low transverse incision (10%), and leiomyomata preventing uterine closure and hemostasis (4%).[259] Subtotal (supracervical) hysterectomy is faster and a safer procedure, associated with a lower risk of intra and postoperative complications and reduced need for transfusion.[260] Active lower uterine segment bleeding is more likely to require total hysterectomy.[5,239] High maternal morbidity is associated with hysterectomy for PPH, regardless of the procedure.[261] Comprehensive monitoring in the intensive care unit with continued attention to manage blood and coagulation factor defects, prophylactic antibiotics and thromboprophylaxis are all required to optimize post-hysterectomy outcome.[239]

Disseminated intravascular coagulation

Disseminated intravascular coagulation (DIC) is a pathological response to a variety of clinical events, which trigger systemic microvascular thrombosis. Any disorder which is associated with the systemic release of thromboplastin or with widespread endothelial injury (as occurs in hemorrhagic shock or any etiology of the systemic inflammatory response syndrome (SIRS)) may trigger DIC.[28,29,173,175,262] During pregnancy and the puerperium a variety of pathological processes may release thromboplastin or by other mechanisms trigger DIC (Table 12.23).[172] Post partum hemorrhage of any etiology, resulting in hemorrhagic shock may trigger DIC.[28,263] Systemic hypoperfusion, acidosis and hypoxia

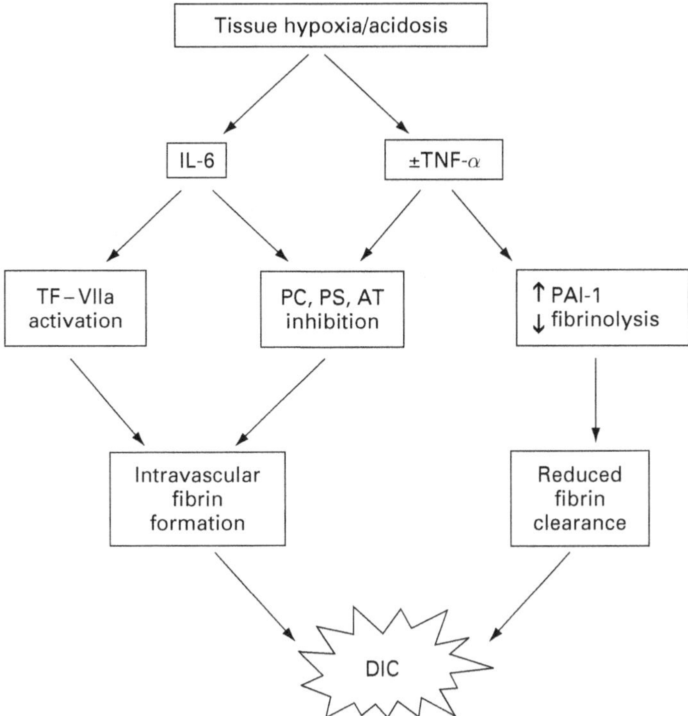

Figure 12.5 Pathogenetic mechanisms of DIC. IL-6 = interleukin-6; TNFα = tumor necrosis factor; TF-VIIa = tissue factor VIIa; PC = protein C, PS = protein S; AT = antithrombin PAI-1 = plasminogen activator inhibitor 1.

provoke the systemic release of cytokines, which activate coagulation and inhibit anticoagulant and fibrinolytic pathways (Figure 12.5). Pro-inflammatory cytokine release initiates SIRS, which further stimulates DIC and results in multiple organ dysfunction syndrome (MODS).[27,28,31,264] The thrombotic stage of DIC is characterized by multiple organ dysfunction due to systemic microvascular fibrin deposition, with clinical evidence of organ failure such as hypoxemia and acute respiratory failure, cardiac dysfunction, acute renal failure and hypoxic encephalopathy or irreversible brain injury (Figure 12.6).[27,28,34,172,173]

Generalized microvascular thrombosis with factor consumption and the production of fibrinogen degradation products may progress to a hemorrhagic phase associated with severe bleeding (Figure 12.6).[27,34,264–266] When PPH is triggered by a cause associated with DIC or when acute hemorrhagic shock leads to DIC, profuse vaginal bleeding is accompanied by hemorrhage from multiple sites, including the abdominal wound in cesarean section, intravenous catheters, urinary tract, gastrointestinal tract, respiratory tract and skin.[34,173,175]

Well-recognized obstetrical complications that trigger DIC include severe preeclampsia and eclampsia,[267,268] amniotic fluid embolism,[116,117,124] placental

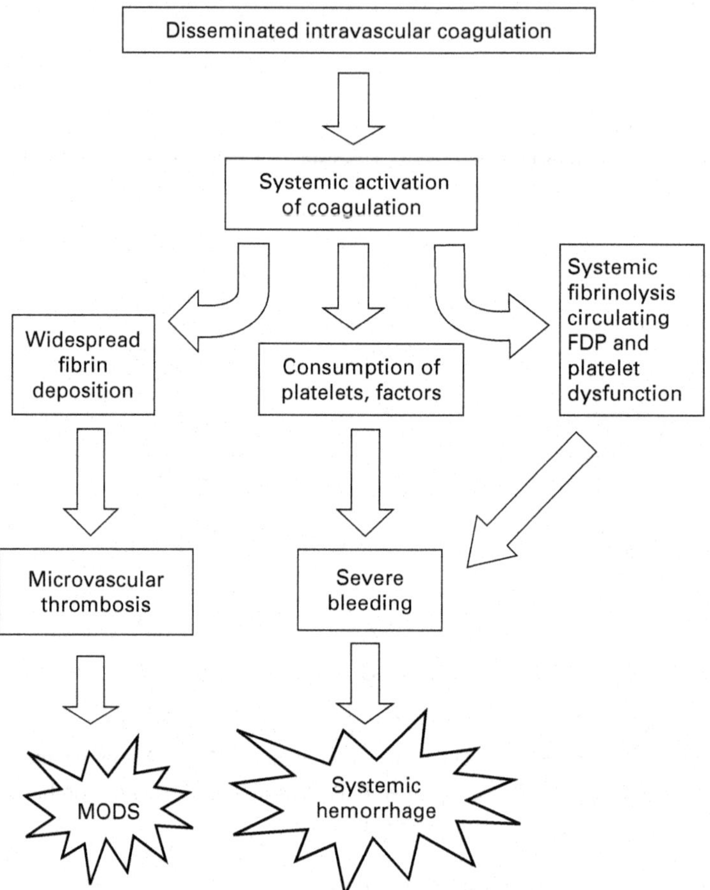

Figure 12.6 Clinical manifestations of DIC.

abruption,[269,270] intrauterine fetal demise, and retained products of conception (Table 12.23).[172,196,271] The syndrome of hemolysis, elevated liver enzymes and low platelets (HELLP syndrome), mimics DIC but is now considered to represent a distinct form of microangiopathy, more closely related to that seen in thrombotic thrombocytopenic purpura and hemolytic uremic syndrome.[27,272] When the primary presentation in an obstetrical patient is that of acute cardiopulmonary decompensation followed quickly by systemic hemorrhage, without another more likely etiology, amniotic fluid embolism is to be strongly considered.[116,117,124,273]

Prevention of DIC

The prevention of DIC rests with the early identification and management of the underlying potential causes and rapid, effective resuscitation from PPH. When acute PPH occurs, avoidance of hemorrhagic shock prevents the additional insult

Table 12.23 Obstetrical disorders associated with DIC.

Amniotic fluid embolism
Placental abruption
Placenta previa
Pre-eclampsia
Eclampsia
Retained fetus syndrome
Retained products of conception
Therapeutic abortion
Hemolysis, elevated liver enzymes and low platelet count syndrome (HELLP) (a thrombotic microangiopathy, mimics DIC)

of DIC. Since a major pathophysiologic trigger for DIC in hemorrhagic shock is acidosis and tissue hypoxia, the maintenance of hemodynamic stability is critical to successful therapy. While amniotic fluid embolism is an unpredictable, event; placental abruption may be identified with proper evaluation of antenatal hemorrhage and DIC averted with evacuation of the uterus.[270] Antenatal identification and aggressive treatment for pre-eclampsia, prompt delivery of a dead fetus and attention to identify and treat retained products of conception are other examples of interventions designed to prevent the development of DIC.

Anticoagulants

Pharmacologic management of DIC may require the use of anticoagulants and coagulation inhibitors to control systemic microvascular thrombosis. In the critically ill patient with PPH who exhibits the hemorrhagic phase of DIC, treatment with anticoagulants and inhibitors must be accompanied by aggressive blood, platelet, fibrinogen, and clotting factor replacement.[172,173,196,274] Patients with DIC and PPH, given the availability of blood and blood product transfusion, are at greatest risk of morbidity and mortality from the consequences of systemic microvascular thrombosis and multiple organ dysfunction syndrome (MODS).[27,28] The potential choices of anticoagulants include intravenous unfractionated heparin, subcutaneous low dose unfractionated heparin, full or prophylactic dose low molecular weight heparin,[172,196,274] and the direct thrombin inhibitors argatroban[275] and hirudin.[196,276,277] The use of any form of heparin requires adequate circulating antithrombin ($\geq$70% of normal human plasma, functional level) to exert pharmacologic effect.[278] The use of the coagulation inhibitors antithrombin[279–285] and recombinant activated protein C (r-aPC)[286–288] to inhibit the microvascular thrombosis associated with DIC has

Table 12.24[123,271] Criteria for diagnosis of DIC.

- Systemic thrombohemorrhagic disorder
- Recognized clinical etiology
- Laboratory evidence of
  - Procoagulant activation
  - Fibrinolytic activation
  - Inhibitor consumption
  - Biochemical evidence of end-organ damage or failure

Table 12.25 The management and treatment of DIC.

- Management of DIC
  - Clinical intervention
  - Manage hemorrhage
  - Manage thrombosis
  - Balance benefit versus risk
  - Monitor response to therapy
- Clinical intervention
  - Complete, accurate diagnosis
  - Treat the "triggering" illness/injury
  - Effectively manage end organ injury
  - Provide effective supportive care designed to avoid new complications
- Management of deranged hemostasis
  - Hemorrhage
    - Local management – surgical
    - Blood replacement
    - Platelet transfusion
    - Factor replacement
      - FFP
      - Cryoprecipitate
  - Thrombosis
    - Maintain hemodynamic stability
    - Inhibit "common pathway"
      - Antithrombin
        - Replace antithrombin deficiency (r-AT)
        - Enhance antithrombin activity (heparin)
      - Activated protein C
        - r-aPC (inhibit factor V "tenase complex")
    - Inhibit thrombin
      - Argatroban
      - Hirudin

been examined in a number of small studies and appears promising. Although published studies indicate efficacy at shortening the course and severity of DIC, conclusive recommendations await additional large-scale trials.[175,196] When utilized, anticoagulation and/or inhibitor therapy should be guided by laboratory evidence of improvement in the levels of platelets, clotting factors, fibrinogen, antithrombin, organ dysfunction, and clinical evidence of improved tissue perfusion.

Comprehensive management of DIC

Proper management of DIC requires early recognition and etiologic diagnosis, followed by prompt and aggressive intervention. Determining the etiology of post partum hemorrhage is essential to effective treatment. Interventional radiology and/or surgical therapy may be required to remove the inciting cause (such as placental abruption, retained products of conception, dead fetus, etc.) and control localized uterine and pelvic hemorrhage. Pharmacologic agents such as ergot derivatives, prostaglandin analogues, inotropic agents, and vasopressors, the administration of blood and blood products, antithrombin and anticoagulants may all be required to prevent or control systemic microvascular thrombosis and control hemorrhage. Consistent clinical and laboratory features are required criteria for diagnosis of DIC (Table 12.24). A plan for the comprehensive management of severe DIC is presented in Table 12.25. The successful treatment of DIC in the course of massive PPH is frequently difficult and requires an experienced team of medical and surgical specialists, a well-equipped intensive care unit, well-trained nursing staff, efficient medical laboratory, and blood bank. Disseminated intravascular coagulation is thoroughly reviewed in Chapter 1 of this text.

Conclusion

All pregnant patients require a thorough history and physical examination and basic laboratory studies as part of standard prenatal care. Investigation of abnormalities and proper planning for delivery are a cornerstone of preventing PPH. Patients with antepartum hemorrhage require careful evaluation, including diagnostic imaging studies in search of placental abnormalities. Active management of the third stage of labor offers perhaps the greatest opportunity to prevent PPH resulting from uterine atony.

The diagnosis of PPH is based on bedside clinical evaluation and the assessment of post partum laboratory studies. Once identified, successful treatment of PPH must include prompt and aggressive resuscitation. Rapid achievement and maintenance of hemodynamic stability are essential to prevent progression to hemorrhagic shock, DIC, and MODS. Concomitant with effective resuscitation and

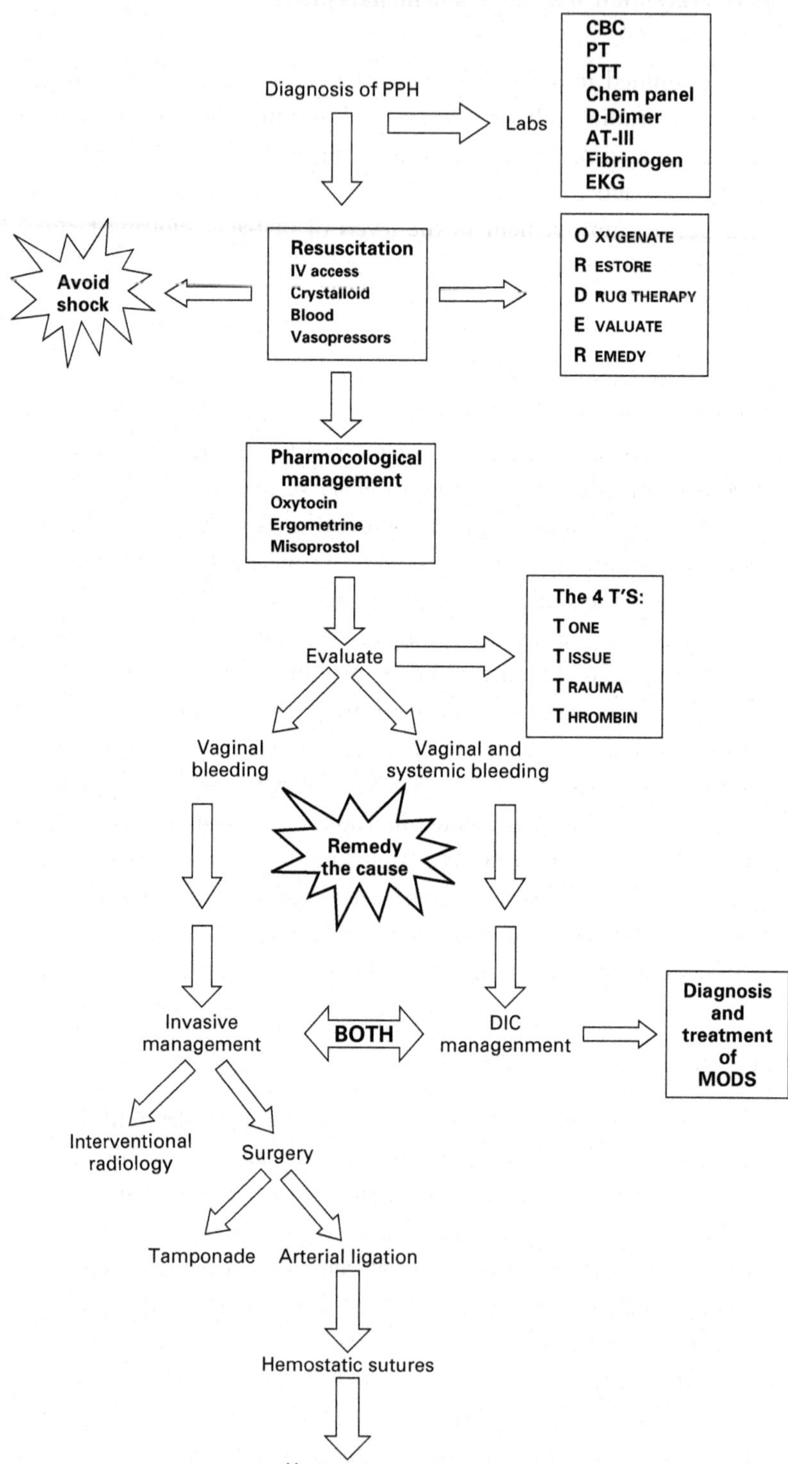

Figure 12.7 Comprehensive diagram of the diagnosis, prevention and management of post partum hemorrhage.

control of deranged hemostasis, identification of the underlying source of hemorrhage and definitive therapy must proceed quickly. Definitive treatment depends on the site of bleeding and may involve uterine tamponade, interventional radiology or surgery.

In patients who develop hemorrhagic shock, DIC, and MODS, survival and the avoidance of permanent organ injury is only possible with a comprehensive approach to correct the underlying cause, maintain hemodynamic stability, correct the deficit in red cells, fibrinogen, clotting factors, and platelets, as well as inhibition of microvascular thrombosis. All of the available medical resources will be required to maintain organ perfusion and sustain life while MODS gradually resolves. Figure 12.7 summarizes the approach to diagnosis and management.

In developing nations, the optimal approaches to prevention and treatment are often unavailable. Efforts to provide education and resources for correction of anemia and the active management of the third stage of labor offer, perhaps the best opportunity for reduction in the incidence and mortality from PPH.[2]

REFERENCES

1 The Department of Health. *Why Mothers Die*. Report on confidential enquiries into maternal deaths in the United Kingdom 1994/96. London: HMSO; 1998.

2 Etuk, S. J., Asuquo, E. E. Effects of community and health facility interventions on postpartum hemorrhage. *Int. J. Gynaecol. Obstet.*, 2000; **70**(3): 381–3.

3 WHO. *Preventing Maternal Deaths*. Geneva: WHO; 1989.

4 Abou Zahr, C. R. E. *Maternal Mortality: A Global Factbook*. Geneva: World Health Organization; 1991.

5 Mousa, H. A., Walkinshaw, S. Major postpartum haemorrhage. *Curr. Opin. Obstet. Gynecol.*, 2001; **13**(6): 595–603.

6 Kraunitz, A., Hughs, J., Grimes, D., *et al.* Causes of maternal mortality in the United States. *Obstet. Gynecol.*, 1985; **65**: 605–12.

7 Chichakli, L. O., Atrash, H. K., MacKay, A. P., *et al.* Pregnancy-related mortality in the United States due to hemorrhage: 1979–1992. *Obstet. Gynecol.*, 1999; **94**(5 Pt 1): 721–5.

8 Combs, C. A., Murphy, E. L., Laros, Jr R. K. Factors associated with postpartum hemorrhage with vaginal birth. *Obstet. Gynecol.*, 1991; **77**: 69–76.

9 Combs, C. A., Murphy, E. L., Laros, Jr R. K. Factors associated with hemorrhage in cesarean deliveries. *Obstet. Gynecol.*, 1991; **77**: 77–82.

10 Pahlavan, P., Nezhat, C. Hemorrhage in obstetrics and gynecology. *Curr. Opin. Obstet. Gynecol.*, 2001; **13**(4): 419–24.

11 Prendiville, W., Elbourne, D., Chalmers, I. The effects of routine oxytocic administration in the management of the third stage of labour: an overview of the evidence from controlled trials. *Br. J. Obstet. Gynaecol.*, 1988; **95**: 3–16.

12 Prendiville, W., Harding, J. E., Elbourne, D., *et al.* The Bristol third stage trial: active versus physiological management of third stage of labour. *BMJ*, 1988; **297**: 1295–300.
13 Etuk, S. J., Itam, I. H., Asuquo, E. E. Morbidity and mortality in booked women who deliver outside orthodox health facilities in Calabar, Nigeria. *Acta Trop.*, 2000; **75**(3): 309–13.
14 Bonnar, J. Massive obstetric haemorrhage. *Baillieres Best Pract. Res. Clin. Obstet. Gynaecol.*, 2000; **14**(1): 1–18.
15 Gerstenfeld, T. S., Wing, D. A. Rectal misoprostol versus intravenous oxytocin for the prevention of postpartum hemorrhage after vaginal delivery. *Am. J. Obstet. Gynecol.*, 2001; **185**(4): 878–82.
16 WHO. *The Prevention and Management of Post Partum Haemorrhage.* Report of a technical working group. Geneva: WHO; 1990.
17 Higgins, S. Obstetric haemorrhage. *Emerg. Med.*, (Fremantle), 2003; **15**(3): 227–31.
18 Pritchard, J. A., Baldwin, R. M., Dickey, J. C., *et al.* Blood volume changes in pregnancy and the puerperium. II. Red blood cell loss and changes in apparent blood volume during and following vaginal delivery, cesarean section, and cesarean section plus total hysterectomy. *Obstet. Gynecol.*, 1962; **84**: 1271–82.
19 El-Refaey, H., Rodeck, C. Post-partum haemorrhage: definitions, medical and surgical management. A time for change. *Br. Med. Bull.*, 2003; **67**: 205–17.
20 McCormick, M. L., Sanghvi, H. C., Kinzie, B., *et al.* Preventing postpartum hemorrhage in low-resource settings. *Int. J. Gynaecol. Obstet.*, 2002; **77**(3): 267–75.
21 Sharma, S., El-Refaey, H. Prostaglandins in the prevention and management of postpartum haemorrhage. *Best Pract. Res. Clin. Obstet. Gynaecol.*, 2003; **17**(5): 811–23.
22 Waterstone, M., Bewley, S., Wolfe, C. Incidence and predictors of severe obstetric morbidity: case-control study. *BMJ*, 2001; **322**(7294): 1089–93; discussion, 93–4.
23 Rangel-Frausto, M. S., Pittet, D., Costignan, M., *et al.* The natural history of the systemic inflammatory response syndrome (SIRS). *JAMA*, 1995; **273**: 117–23.
24 Bone, R. S. Toward a theory of the systemic inflammatory response syndrome: What we do and do not know about cytokine regulation. *Crit. Care Med.*, 1996; **24**: 163–72.
25 Shyu, K. G., Chang, H., Linn, C. C., *et al.* Concentrations of serum interleukin-8 after successful cardiopulmonary resuscitation in patients with cardiopulmonary arrest. *Am. Heart. J.*, 1997; **134**: 551–6.
26 Geppert, A., Zorn, G., Karth, G. D., *et al.* Soluble selectins and the systemic inflammatory response syndrome after successful cardiopulmonary resuscitation. *Crit. Care Med.*, 2000; **28**: 2360–5.
27 Levi, M., de Jonge, E., van der Poll, T., *et al.* Disseminated intravascular coagulation. *Semin. Thromb. Hemost.*, 1999; **82**: 695–705.
28 Gando, S. Disseminated intravascular coagulation in trauma patients. *Semin. Thromb. Hemost.*, 2001; **27**(6): 585–92.
29 Mammen, E. F., Anderson, G. F., Barnard, M. I. Disseminated intravascular coagulation in man. *Thromb. Diath. Haemorrh.*, 1969; **36**(Suppl.): 171–6.
30 Garcia-Fernandez, N., Montes, R., Purroy, A., *et al.* Hemostatic disturbances with systemic inflammatory response syndrome (SIRS) and associated acute renal failure (ARF). *Thromb. Res.*, 2000; **100**: 19–25.

31 Roumen, R. M., Hendricks, T., *et al.* Cytokine patterns in patients after major vascular surgery, hemorrhagic shock, and severe blunt trauma. Relation with subsequent adult respiratory distress syndrome and multiple organ failure. *Ann. Surg.*, 1993; **218**: 769–76.

32 Schrager, S., Sabo, L. Sheehan syndrome: a rare complication of postpartum hemorrhage. *J. Am. Board Fam. Pract.*, 2001; **14**(5): 389–91.

33 Karpati, P. C., Rossignol, M., Pirot, M., *et al.* High incidence of myocardial ischemia during postpartum hemorrhage. *Anesthesiology* 2004; **100**(1): 30–6; discussion, 5 A.

34 Levi, M., ten Cate, H. Disseminated intravascular coagulation. *N. Engl. J. Med.*, 1999; **341**: 586–92.

35 Gynecologists ACoOa. Hemorrhagic shock. *Int. J. Gynaecol. Obstet.*, 1997; **57**: 219–26.

36 Phillips, T. F., Soulier, G., Wilson, R. F. Outcome of massive transfusion exceeding two blood volumes in trauma and emergency surgery. *J. Tramua*, 1987; **27**: 903–10.

37 Smith, H. O., Romero, A. Shock in the gynecologic patient. In Rock, J. A., Jones III, H. W., eds., *Te Linde's Operative Gynecology*. Philadelphia, PA: Lippincott, Williams and Wilkins; 2003: pp. 209–32.

38 Gando, S., Satoshi, N., Osamu, K. Disseminated intravascular coagulation and sustained systemic inflammatory response syndrome predict organ dysfunctions after trauma: Application of clinical decision analysis. *Ann. Surg.*, 1999; **229**: 1–15.

39 Lipitz, S., Admon, D., Menczer, J., *et al.* Midtrimester bleeding: Variables which affect the outcome of pregnancy. *Gynecol. Obstet. Invest.*, 1991; **32**: 24.

40 Ajayi, R. A., Soothill, P. W., Campbell, S., *et al.* Antenatal testing to predict outcome in pregnancies with unexpected antepartum haemorrhage. *Br. J. Obstet. Gynaecol.*, 1992; **99**: 122.

41 Cunningham, F. C., Gant, N. F., Leveno, K. J., eds. *Williams Obstetrics*. 21st edn. New York, NY: McGraw-Hill; 2001.

42 Farine, D., Fox, H. E., Jackobson, S., *et al.* Vaginal ultrasound for diagnosis of placenta previa. *Am. J. Obstet. Gynecol.*, 1988; **159**: 566.

43 Hertzberg, B. S., Bowie, J. D., Carroll, B. A., *et al.* Diagnosis of placenta previa during the third trimester: Role of transperineal sonography. *Am. J. Roentgenol.*, 1992; **159**: 83.

44 Smith, R. S., Lauria, M. R., Comstock, C. H., *et al.* Transvaginal ultrasonography for all placentas that appear to be low-lying or over the internal cervical os. *Ultrasound Obstet. Gynecol.*, 1997; **9**: 22.

45 Wald, D. A. Postpartum hemorrhage resulting from uterine artery pseudoaneurysm. *J. Emerg. Med.*, 2003; **25**(1): 57–60.

46 Davidsen, M. B., Madsen, P. V., Wilken-Jensen, C. True aneurysm of the uterine artery. *Eur. J. Surg.*, 1995; **161**: 775–6.

47 Clark, S. L., Koomings, P. P., Phelan, J. P. Placenta previa/accreta and previous cesarean section. *Obstet. Gynecol.*, 1985; **66**: 89–92.

48 Chesley, L. C. Plasma and red cell volumes during pregnancy. *Am. J. Obstet. Gynecol.*, 1972; **112**: 440–50.

49 Dildy, G. A., 3rd. Postpartum hemorrhage: new management options. *Clin. Obstet. Gynecol.*, 2002; **45**(2): 330–44.

50 Bletka, M., Hlavaty, V., Trnkova, M., *et al.* Volume of whole blood and absolute amount of serum proteins in the early stage of late toxemia of pregnancy. *Am. J. Obstet. Gynecol.*, 1970; **106**: 10–13.

51 Nizzi, F., Mues, G. Hemorrhagic problems in obstetrics, exclusive of disseminated intravascular coagulation. *Hem./Onc. Clinics North Am.*, 2000; **14**: 1171–82.

52 Khan, R., Sharma, S. Use of misoprostol in third stage of labour. *Lancet*, 2002; **359**(9307): 708–9; author reply, 9–10.

53 Kadir, R. A., Economides, D. L., Sabin, C., *et al.* Frequency of inherited bleeding disorders in women with menorrhagia. *Lancet*, 1998; **351**: 485–9.

54 Schuurmans, N., Mac Kinnon, C., Lane, C., *et al.* Prevention and management of postpartum haemorrhage. *J. Soc. Obstet. Gynaecol. Can.*, 2000; **22**: 271–81.

55 Thomas, J. M. The treatment of obstetric haemorrhage in women who refuse blood transfusion. *Ltr. Br. J. Obstet. Gynaecol.*, 1998; **105**: 127–8.

56 Baker, Jr W. F. Iron deficiency in pregnancy, obstetrics and gynecology. *Hem./Onc. Clinics North Am.*, 2000; **14**: 1061–77.

57 Deering, S. H., Landy, H. J., Tchado, N., *et al.* Hypodysfibrinogenemia during pregnancy, labor, and delivery. *Obstet. Gynecol.*, 2003; **101**: 1092–4.

58 Roque, H., Stephenson, M., Lee, M. J., *et al.* Pregnancy-related thrombosis in a woman with congenital afibrinogenemia: a report of two successful pregnancies. *Am. J. Hematol.*, 2004; **76**: 267–70.

59 Nizzi, F., Sapatnekar, S., Bick, R. L. Hereditary coagulation protein defects. In Bick, R. L., ed. *Disorders of Thrombosis and Hemostasis: Clinical and Laboratory Practice.* Third edn. Philadelphia, PA: Lippincott, Williams and Wilkins; 2002: pp. 117–37.

60 Kobayashi, T., Kanayama, N., Tokunaga, N., *et al.* Prenatal and peripartum management of congenital afibrinogenemia. *Br. J. Haematol.*, 2000; **109**: 364–6.

61 Parameswaran, R., Dickinson, J., DeLord, S., *et al.* Spontaneous intracranial bleeding in two patients with congenital afibrinogenaemia and the role of replacement therapy. *Haemophilia*, 2000; **6**: 705–8.

62 Schroeder, M. L. Principles and practice of transfusion medicine. In Lee, G. R., Foerster, J., Lukens, J., *et al.* eds., *Wintrobe's Clinical Hematology.* 10th edn. Baltimore: Lippincott, Williams and Wilkins; 1999: pp. 817–74.

63 Roberts, H. R., White, G. C. Inherited disorders of prothrombin conversion. In Colman, R. W., Hirsh, J., Marder, V. I., *et al.* eds., *Hemostasis and Thrombosis: Basic Principles and Clinical Practice.* Philadelphia, PA: Lippincott, Williams and Wilkins; 2001: pp. 839–53.

64 Rodgers, G. M., Greenberg, G. S. Inherited coagulation disorders. In Lee, G. R., Foerster, J., Lukens, J., *et al.* eds. *Wintrobe's Clinical Hematology.* Baltimore, MD: Lippincott, Williams and Wilkins; 1999: p. 1682.

65 Rogers, G. M., Greenberg, C. S. Inherited coagulation disorders. In Lee, G. R., Foerster, J., Paraskevas, F., *et al.* eds. *Wintrobe's Clinical Hematology.* Baltimore, MD: Lippincott, Williams and Wilkins; 1999: pp. 1682–732.

66 Bick, R. L. Platelet-function defects. In Bick, R. L., ed., *Disorders of Thrombosis and Hemostasis: Clinical and Laboratory Practice.* Philadelphia, PA: Lippincott, Williams and Wilkins; 2002: pp. 59–90.

67 Eskandari, N., Feldman, N., Greenspoon, J. S. Factor VII deficiency in pregnancy treated with recombinant factor VIIa. *Obstet. Gynecol.*, 2002; **99**: 935–7.

68 Fadel, H. E., Krauss, J. S. Factor VII deficiency and pregnancy. *Obstet. Gynecol.*, 1989; **73**: 453–4.

69 Bauer, K. Treatment of factor VIIa deficiency with recombinant factor VII. *Haemostasis*, 1996; **26**(Suppl. 1): 155–8.

70 Jimenez-Yuste, V., Villar, A., Morado, M., *et al.* Continuous infusion of recombinant activated factor VII during cesarean section delivery in a patient with congenital factor VII deficiency. *Haemophilia*, 2000; **6**: 588–90.

71 Arun, B, Kessler, C. M. Clinical manifestations and therapy of the hemophilias. In Colman, R. W., Hirsh, J., Marder, V. I., *et al.* eds., *Hemostasis and Thrombosis: Basic Principles and Clinical Practice.* Philadelphia, PA: Lippincott Williams and Wilkins; 2001: pp. 815–24.

72 Hay, C. R., Negrier, C., Ludlam, C. A. The treatment of bleeding in acquired hemophilia with recombinant factor VIIa: a multicentre study. *Thromb. Haemost.*, 1997; **78**: 1463–7.

73 Green, D., Lechner, K. A survey of 215 nonhemophilic patients with inhibitors to factor VIII. *Thromb. Haemost.*, 1981; **45**: 200.

74 Michiels, J. J. Acquired hemophilia A in women postpartum: clinical manifestations, diagnosis and treatment. *Clin. Appl. Thromb. Hemost.*, 2000; **6**: 82–6.

75 Dhar, P., Abramovitz, S., DiMichele, D. M., *et al.* Management of pregnancy in a patient with severe hemophilia A. *Br. J. Anaesth.*, 2003; **91**: 432–5.

76 DiMichele, D. M., Green, D. Hemophilia-factor VIII deficiency. In Locscalzo, J., Schafer, A. I., eds., *Thrombosis and Hemorrhage.* Baltimore, MD: Williams and Wilkins; 1998: pp. 757–72.

77 Pejsa, V., Grgurevic, I., Kusec, R., *et al.* Rapid decrease in high titer of factor VIII inhibitors upon immunosuppressive treatment in severe postpartum acquired hemophilia. *Croat. Med. J.*, 2004; **45**: 213–16.

78 Bockenstedt, P. L. Laboratory methods in hemostasis. In Loscalzo, J., Schafer, A. I., eds., *Thrombosis and Hemorrhage.* Baltimore: Williams and Wilkins; 1998: pp. 517–80.

79 Grosset, A. B., Rodgers, G. Acquired coagulation disorders. In J.W.P, ed., *Wintrobe's Clinical Hematology.* Baltimore, MD; 1999: pp. 1733–80.

80 Pineda, A. A. Indications for hemapheresis procedures in hematologic disorders. In Bick, R. L., ed., *Hematology: Clinical and Laboratory Practice.* St. Louis,; 1993: 1681–9.

81 Arkel, Y. S., Ku, D. W. Acquired blood coagulation inhibitors. In Bick, R. L., ed., *Disorders of Thrombosis and Hemostasis: Clinical and Laboratory Practice.* 3rd edn. Philadelphia, PA: Lippincott, Williams and Wilkins; 2002: pp. 213–49.

82 Greenberg, C. S., Orthner, C. Blood coagulation and fibrinolysis. In Pine, J. W., ed., *Wintrobe's Clinical Hematology.* Baltimore, MD: LWW; 1999: pp. 684–764.

83 Roberts, N. S., Bingham, M. D. Other coagulation factor deficiencies. In Loscalzo, J., Schafer, A. I., eds., *Thrombosis and Hemorrhage.* Baltimore, MD: Williams and Wilkins; 1998: 773–802.

84 Ozsoylu, S., Ozer, F. L. Acquired factor IX deficiency. *Acta Haematol.*, 1973; **50**: 305–14.

85 Green, D. Factor VIII and other coagulation factor inhibitors. In Loscalzo, J., Schafer, A. I., eds., *Thrombosis and Hemorrhage.* Baltimore, MD: Williams and Wilkins; 1998: pp. 803–15.

86 Romagnolo, C., Burati, S., Ciaffoni, S., *et al.* Severe factor X deficiency in pregnancy: case report and review of the literature. *Haemophilia*, 2004; **10**: 665–8.
87 David, A. L., Paterson-Brown, S., Letsky, E. A. Factor XI deficiency presenting in pregnancy: diagnosis and management. *Br. J. Obstet. Gynaecol.*, 2002; **109**(7): 840–3.
88 Loewy, A. G., McDonagh, J., Mikkola, H., *et al.* Structure and function of factor XIII. In Colman, R. W., Hirsh, J., Marder, V. I., *et al.* eds., *Hemostasis and Thrombosis: Basic Principles and Clinical Practice.* Philadelphia, PA: Lippincott, Williams and Wilkins; 2001: pp. 233–47.
89 Nichols, W. C., Cooney, K. A., Ginsburg, D., *et al.* Von Willebrand disease. In Loscalzo, J., Schafer, A. I., eds., *Thrombosis and Hemorrhage.* Baltimore, MD: Williams and Wilkins; 1998: pp. 729–55.
90 Lak, M., Peyvandi, F., Mannucci, P. M. Clinical manifestations and complications of childbirth and replacement therapy in 385 Iranian patients with type 3 von Willebrand disease. *Br. J. Haematol.*, 2000; **111**(4): 1236–9.
91 Ramsahoye, B. H., Davies, S. V., Dasani, H. Management of pregnancy and delivery in von Willebrand's disease. *Blood*, 1993; **82**(Suppl. 1): 150.
92 Roque, H., Funai, E., Lockwood, C. J. Von Willebrand disease and pregnancy. *J. Matern. Fetal Med.*, 2000; **9**(5): 257–66.
93 Sadler, J. E., Blinder, M. Von Willebrand disease: Diagnosis, classification and treatment. In Colman, R. W., Hirsh, J., Marder, V. I., *et al.* eds., *Hemostasis and Thrombosis: Basic Principles and Clinical Practice.* Philadelphia, PA: Lippincott, Williams and Wilkins; 2001: pp. 826–37.
94 Oshiro, B. T., Branch, W. Maternal hemostasis: coagulation problems in pregnancy. In Loscalzo, J., Schafer, A. I., eds., *Thrombosis and Hemorrhage.* Baltimore, MD: Williams and Wilkins; 1998: pp. 1005–26.
95 Thilaganathan, B., Cutner, A., Latimer, J., *et al.* Management of the third stage of labor in women at low risk of postpartum hemorrhage. *Eur. J. Obstet. Gynecol. Reprod. Biol.*, 1993; **48**: 19.
96 Midwives ICo, Obstetricians IFoGa. Joint Statement: Management of the third stage of labour to prevent post-partum haemorrhage. *J. Midwifery Womens Health* 2004; **49**: 76–7.
97 Prendiville, W. J., Elbourne, D., McDonald, S. Active versus expectant management in the third stage of labour. *Cochrane Database Syst. Rev.*, 2000; **3**: CD000007.
98 Nordstrom, L., Fogelstam, K., Fridman, G., *et al.* Routine oxytocin in the third stage of labour: a placebo controlled randomised trial. *Br. J. Obstet. Gynaecol.*, 1997; **104**: 781–6.
99 Noort, W. A., van Bulck, B., Vereecken, A., *et al.* Changes in plasma levels of PGF2 alpha and PGI2 metabolites at and after delivery at term. *Obstet. Gynecol.*, 1989; **37**: 3–12.
100 Thornton, S., Davison, J. M., Baylis, P. H. Plasma oxytocin during third stage of labour: comparison of natural and active management. *BMJ*, 1988; **297**: 167–9.
101 Jackson, K. W., Jr., Allbert, J. R., Schemmer, G. K., *et al.* A randomized controlled trial comparing oxytocin administration before and after placental delivery in the prevention of postpartum hemorrhage. *Am. J. Obstet. Gynecol.*, 2001; **185**(4): 873–7.
102 Hendricks, C. H., Brenner, W. E. Cardiovascular effects of oxytocic drugs used post partum. *Am. J. Obstet. Gynecol.*, 1970; **108**: 751.

103 Choy, C. M., Lau, W. C., Tam, W. H., *et al.* A randomised controlled trial of intramuscular syntometrine and intravenous oxytocin in the management of the third stage of labour. *Br. J. Obstet. Gynaecol.*, 2002; **109**(2): 173–7.

104 Darney, P. D. Misoprostol: a boon to safe motherhood . . . or not? *Lancet*, 2001; **358**(9283): 682–3.

105 Bugalho, A., Daniel, A., Faundes, A., *et al.* Misoprostol for prevention of postpartum hemorrhage. *Int. J. Gynaecol. Obstet.*, 2001; **73**(1): 1–6.

106 Lokugamage, A. U., Sullivan, K. R., Niculescu, I., *et al.* A randomized study comparing rectally administered misoprostol versus Syntometrine combined with an oxytocin infusion for the cessation of primary post partum hemorrhage. *Acta Obstet. Gynecol. Scand.*, 2001; **80**(9): 835–9.

107 Gulmezoglu, A. M., Villar, J., Ngoc, N. T., *et al.* WHO multicentre randomised trial of misoprostol in the management of the third stage of labour. *Lancet*, 2001; **358**(9283): 689–95.

108 Goldberg, A. B., Greenberg, M. B., Darney, P. D. Misoprostol and pregnancy. *N. Engl. J. Med.*, 2001; **344**(1): 38–47.

109 Dumoulin, J. G. A reappraisal of the use of ergometrine. *J. Obstet. Gynaecol.*, 1981; **1**: 178–81.

110 Carey, M. Adverse cardiovascular sequelae of ergometrine. *Br. J. Obstet. Gynaecol.*, 1981; **100**: 865.

111 Abdel-Aleem, H., El-Nashar, I., Abdel-Aleem, A. Management of severe postpartum hemorrhage with misoprostol. *Int. J. Gynaecol. Obstet.*, 2001; **72**(1): 75–6.

112 Rolfes, D. B., Ishak, K. G. Liver disease in toxemia of pregnancy. *Am. J. Gastroenterol.*, 1986; **81**: 1138.

113 Sheikh, R. A., Yasmeen, S., Pauly, M. P., *et al.* Spontaneous intrahepatic hemorrhage and rupture in the HELLP syndrome: four cases and a review. *J. Clin. Gastroenterol.*, 1999; **28**: 323.

114 Stain, S. C., Woodburn, D. A., Stephens, A. L., *et al.* Spontaneous hepatic hemorrhage associated with pregnancy. Treatment with hepatic arterial ligation. *Ann. Surg.*, 1996; **224**: 72.

115 Smith, L. G., Moise, Jr K. J., Dildy III, G. A., *et al.* Spontaneous rupture of liver during pregnancy: Current therapy. *Obstet. Gynecol.*, 1991; **77**: 171.

116 Davies, S. Amniotic fluid embolism: a review of the literature. *Can. J. Anaesth.*, 2001; **48**: 88–98.

117 Locksmith, G. J. Amniotic flud embolism. *Obstet. Gynecol. Clin. North. Am.*, 1999; **26**: 435–44.

118 Martel, M., MacKinnon, C. J., Arsenault, M., *et al.* Hemorrhagic shock. *J. Obstet. Gynaecol. Can.*, 2002; **24**: 504–11.

119 Smith, H. O. Shock in the gynecologic patient. In Rock, J. A., Thomson, J. D., eds., *Te Linde's Operative Gynecology*, 8th edn. Philadelphia, PA: Lippincott-Raven; 1997: pp. 245–61.

120 Falk, J. L., O'Brien, J. F., Kerr, R. Fluid resuscitation in traumatic hemorrhagic shock. *Crit. Cre. Clin.*, 1992; **8**: 323–40.

121 Assali, N. S. Dynamics of the uteroplacental circulation in health and disease. *Am. J. Perinatol.*, 1989; **6**: 105–9.

122 Marzi, I. Hemorrhagic shock: update in pathophysiology and therapy. *Acta Anaesthesiol. Scand. Suppl.*, 1997; **111**: 42–4.

123 Bick, R. L. Disseminated intravascular coagulation. *Hematol. Oncol. Clin. North Am.*, 1992; **6**(6): 1259–85.

124 Davies, S. Amniotic fluid embolism and isolated disseminated intravascular coagulation. *Can. J. Anaesth.*, 1999; **46**(5 Pt 1): 456–9.

125 Clark, S. L. New concepts of amniotic fluid embolism: a review. *Obstet. Gynecol. Surv.*, 1990; **45**: 360–8.

126 Clark, S. L., Hankins, G. D V, Dudley, D. A., *et al.* Amniotic fluid embolism: analysis of the national registry. *Am. J. Obstet. Gynecol.*, 1995; **172**: 1158–69.

127 Morgan, M. Amniotic fluid embolism. *Anaesthesia*, 1979; **34**: 20–32.

128 Bland, R. D., Shoemaker, W. C., Abraham, E., *et al.* Hemodynamic and oxygen transport patterns in surviving and nonsurviving postoperative patients. *Crit. Care Med.*, 1985; **13**: 85–95.

129 Chiao, J., Minei, J. P., Shires, G. T. In vivo myocyte sodium activity and concentration during hemorrhagic shock. *Am. J. Physiol.*, 1990; **258**: R864.

130 Isbister, J. P. Physiology and pathophysiology of blood volume regulation. *Transus. Sci.*, 1997; **18**: 409–23.

131 Barber, A., Shires III, G. T., Shires, G. T. Shock. In Schwartz, S. I., Shires, G. T., Spencer, F. C., *et al.* eds., *Principles of Surgery*, 7th edn. New York, NY: McGraw-Hill; 1999: p. 101.

132 Bitterman, H., Smith, B. A., Lefer, A. M. Beneficial actions of antagonism of peptide leukotrienes in hemorrhagic shock. *Circ. Shock*, 1988; **24**: 159.

133 Hierholzer, C., Billiar, T. R. Molecular mechanisms in the early phase of hemorrhagic shock. *Langenbeck's Arch. Surg.*, 2001; **386**: 302–8.

134 Afessa, B., Green, B., Delke, I., *et al.* Systemic inflammatory response syndrome, organ failure, and outcome in critically ill obstetric patients treated in an ICU. *Chest*, 2001; **120**: 1271–7.

135 Tamian, F., Richard, V., Bonmarchand, G., *et al.* Induction of hemo-oxygenase-1 prevents the systemic reponses to hemorrhagic shock. *Am. J. Respir. Crit. Care Med.*, 2001; **164**: 1933–8.

136 Muckart, D. J., Bhagwanjee, S. American College of Chest Physicians/Society of Critical Care Medicine Consensus Conference definitions of the systemic inflammatory response syndrome and allied disorders in relation to critically injured patients. *Crit. Care Med.*, 1997; **25**: 1789–95.

137 Shoemaker, W. C., Peitzman, A. B., Bellamy, R., *et al.* Resuscitation from severe hemorrhage. *Crit. Care Med.*, 1996; **24**(2 Suppl.)(S 12–23).

138 Cavanagh, D., Mardsen, D. E. Hemorrhagic shock in the gynecologic patient. *Clin. Obstet. Gynecol.*, 1985; **28**: 383.

139 Shiers, G. T., Barber, A. E., Illner, H. P. Current status of resuscitation: solutions including hypertonic saline. *Adv. Surg.*, 1995; **28**: 133–70.

140 Bickell, W. H., Wall Jr, M. J., Pepe, P. E., *et al.* Immediate versus delayed fluid resuscitation for hypotensive patients with penetrating torso injuries. *N. Engl. J. Med.*, 1994; **331**: 1105–9.

141 Schierhout, G., Roberts, I. Fluid resuscitation with colloid or crystalloid solutions in critically ill patients: a systematic review of randomised trials. *BMJ*, 1998; **316**: 961–4.

142 Bunn, F., Lefebvre, C., Li-Wan-Po, A., *et al.* Human albumin solution for resuscitation and volume expansion in critically ill patients. *Cochrane Database Syst. Rev.*, 2000; **2**: CD001208.

143 Gould, S. A., Sehgal, L. R., Sehgal, H. L., *et al.* Hypovolemic shock. *Crit. Care Clin.*, 1993; **9**: 239–59.

144 Mousa, H. A., Alfirevic, Z. Treatment for primary postpartum haemorrhage. *Cochrane Database Syst. Rev.*, 2003; **1**: CD003249.

145 Lucas, C. E. Update on trauma care in Canada. 4. Resuscitation through the three phases of hemorrhagic shock after trauma. *Can. J. Surg.*, 1990; **33**: 451–6.

146 Macphail, S. F. J. Massive post-partum hemorrhage. *Curr. Opin. Obstet. Gynaecol.*, 2001; **11**: 108–14.

147 Nolan, T. E., Gallup, D. G. Massive transfusion: a current review. *Obstet. Gynecol. Surv.*, 1991; **46**(5): 289–95.

148 Petz, L. D. Red blood cell transfusion. *Clin. Oncol.*, 1983; **2**: 505.

149 Gynecologists ACoOa. Blood component therapy. *Int. J. Gynaecol. Obstet.*, 1995; **48**: 233–8.

150 Wilson, R. F. Trauma. In Shoemaker, W. C., Thompson, W. L., Holbrook, P. R., eds., *Textbook of Critical Care*. Philadelphia, PA: W. B. Saunders Co.; 1984: pp. 877–914.

151 Hewitt, P. E., Machin, S. J. Massive blood transfusion. In *ABC of Transfusion*. London: BMJ Publishing Group; 1998: pp. 49–52.

152 Hiippala, S. Replacement of massive blood loss. *Vox Sang*, 1998; **74** (Suppl. 2): 399–407.

153 Elder, P. T. Accidental hypothermia. In Shoemaker, W. C., Thompson, W. L., Holbrook, P. R., eds., *Textbook of Critical Care*. Philadelphia, PA: W. B. Saunders Co.; 1984: pp. 85–93.

154 Mahajan, W. I., Meyers, T. J., Baldini, M. G. Disseminated intravascular coagulation during rewarming following hypothermia. *JAMA*, 1981; **245**: 2517.

155 Valeri, C. R., Cassidy, G., Khuri, S., *et al.* Hypothermia-induced reversible platelet dysfunction. *Ann. Surg.*, 1987; **205**: 175–81.

156 Luna, G. K., Maier, R. V., Pavlin, E. G., *et al.* Incidence and effect of hypothermia in seriously injured patietns. *J. Trauma*, 1987; **27**: 1014–18.

157 Carmichael, D., Hosty, T., Kastl, D., *et al.* Hypokalemia and massive transfusion. *South Med. J.*, 1984; **77**: 315–17.

158 Durand, F., Duchesne-Gueguen, M., Le Bervet, J. Y., *et al.* Rheologic and cytologic study of autologous blood collected with Cell Saver 4 during cesarean. *Rev. Fr. Transfus. Hemobiol.*, 1989; **32**: 179–91.

159 Zichella, L., Gramolini, R. Autotransfusion during cesarean section. *Am. J. Obstet. Gynecol.*, 1990; **162**: 295.

160 Bernstein, H. H., Rosenblatt, M. A., Gettes, M., *et al.* The ability of haemonetics 4 Cell Saver system to remove tissue factor from blood contaminated with amniotic fluid. *Anesth. Analg.*, 1997; **85**: 831–3.

161 Rebarber, A., Lonser, R., Jackson, S., *et al.* The safety of intraoperative autologous blood collection and autotransfusion during cesarean section. *Am. J. Obstet. Gynecol.*, 1998; **179** (3 Pt 1): 715–20.

162 Hocker, P., Hartmann, T. Management of massive transfusion. *Acta Anaesthesiol. Scand. Suppl.*, 1997; **111**: 205–7.

163 Harigan, C., Lucas, C. E., Ledgerwood, A. M. The effect of hemorrhagic shock on the clotting cascade in injured patients. *J. Trauma*, 1989; **29**(10): 1416–21.

164 Pathologists DTFotCoA. Practice parameter for the use of fresh-frozen plasma, cryoprecipitate, and platelets: fresh frozen plasma, cryoprecipitate and platelets administraton practice guideline. *JAMA*, 1994; **24**: 777–8.

165 Health NIo. Fresh frozen plasma: Indications and risks. In *Consensus Development Conference*; 1985: *JAMA*, 1985; **253**: 551–3.

166 Lundsgard-Hansen, P. Component therapy of surgical hemorrhage: red cell concentrates, colloids and crystalloids. *Bibl. Haematol.*, 1980; **46**: 147.

167 Brugnara, C, Churchill, H. Plasma and component therapy. In Loscalzo, J., Schafer, A. I., eds., *Thrombosis and Hemorrhage.* Baltimore, MD: Williams and Wilkins; 1998: pp. 1135–62.

168 Contreras, M., Ala, F. A., Greaves, M., *et al.* Guidelines for the use of fresh frozen plasma. British Committee for Standards in Haematology, Working Party of the Blood Transfusion Task Force. *Transfus. Med.*, 1992; **2**: 57–63.

169 Miller, R. D., Robbins, T. O., Tong, M. J., *et al.* Coagulation defects associated with massive blood transfusions. *Ann. Surg.*, 1971; **174**: 794–801.

170 Counts, R. B., Haisch, C., Simon, T. L., *et al.* Hemostasis in massively transfused trauma patients. *Ann. Surg.*, 1979; **190**: 91–9.

171 Ciavarella, D., Reed, R. L., Counts, R. B., *et al.* Clotting factor levels and the risk of diffuse microvascular bleeding in the massively transfused patient. *Br. J. Haematol.*, 1987; **67**: 365–8.

172 Bick, R. L. Disseminated intravascular coagulation. In Bick, R. L., ed., *Disorders of Thrombosis and Hemostasis: Clinical and Laboratory Practice*, 3rd edn. Philadelphia, PA: Lippincott, Williams and Wilkins; 2002: pp. 139–64.

173 Baker Jr, W. F. Clinical aspects of disseminated intravascular coagulation: a clinician's point of view. *Semin. Thromb. Hemost.*, 1988; **15**: 1–57.

174 Al-Mondhiry, H. Disseminated intravascular coagulation: experience in a major cancer center. *Thromb. Diath. Haemorrh.*, 1975; **34**: 181.

175 Leung, LLK. Hemorrhagic disorders. In Dale, D. C., Federman, D. D., eds., *ACP Medicine.* New York, NY: WebMD Inc.; 2004: **5**, XIII, pp. 1–22.

176 Kushner, J. P. Normochromic normocytic anemia. In Wyngaarden, J. B., Smith, L. H., eds., *Cecil Textbook of Medicine.* 18th edn. Philadelphia, PA: W. B. Saunders; 1988: pp. 890–2.

177 Baker Jr, W. F. Clinical evaluation of the patient with anemia. In Bick, R. L., ed., *Hematology: Clinical and Laboratory Practice.* St. Louis, MD: Mosby; 1993: pp. 203–29.

178 Bunn, H. F., Federici, A. B., Serchia, G. Anemia. In Wilson, J. D., Braunwald, E., Isselbacher, K. J., *et al.* eds., *Harrison's Principles of Internal Medicine.* 12th edn. New York, NY: McGraw-Hill, Inc.; 1991: pp. 344–8.

179 Manucci, P. M., *et al.* Hemostasis testing during massive blood replacement. *Vox Sang*, 1982; **42**: 113.

180 Noe, D. A., Graham, S. M., Luff, R., *et al.* Platelet counts during rapid massive transfusion. *Transfusion*, 1982; **22**: 392.

181 Kopec, M., Wegrzynowiczy, Z., Budzynski, A., *et al.* Interaction of fibrinogen degradation products with platelets. *Exp. Biol. Med.*, 1968; **3**: 73.

182 Ono, S., Mochizuki, H., Tamakuma, S. A clinical study on the significance of platelet-activating factor in the pathophysiology of septic disseminated intravascular coagulation. *Am. J. Surg.*, 1996; **171**: 409.

183 Harker, L. A., Malpass, T. W., Branson, H. E., *et al.* Mechanism of abnormal bleeding in patients undergoing cardiopulmonary bypass: acquired transient platelet dysfunction associated with selective alpha-granule release. *Blood*, 1980; **56**: 824.

184 Ness, P. M., Perkins, H. A. Cryoprecipitate as a reliable source of fibrinogen replacement. *JAMA*, 1979; **241**: 1690–1.

185 Bouwmeester, F. W., Jonkhoff, A. R., Verheijen, R. H., *et al.* Successful treatment of life-threatening postpartum hemorrhage with recombinant activated factor VII. *Obstet. Gynecol.*, 2003; **101**(6): 1174–6.

186 Boehlen, F., Morales, M. A., Fontana, P., *et al.* Prolonged treatment of massive postpartum haemorrhage with recombinant factor VIIa: case report and review of the literature. *Br. J. Obstet. Gynaecol.*, 2004; **111**(3): 284–7.

187 Segal, S., Shemesh, I. Y., Blumenthal, R., *et al.* Treatment of obstetric hemorrhage with recombinant activated factor VII (rFVIIa). *Arch. Gynecol. Obstet.*, 2003; **268**(4): 266–7.

188 Martinowitz, U., Luboschitz, J., Lubetsky, A., *et al.* New approach for the management of coagulation at the site of injury by recombinant activated factor VII (rVIIa). *Blood*, 2001; **98**: 827–8.

189 Moscardo, F., Perez, F., de la Rubia, J., *et al.* Successful treatment of severe intra-abdominal bleeding associated with disseminated intravascular coagulation using recombinant activated factor VII. *Br. J. Haematol.*, 2001; **114**(1): 174–6.

190 Daro, A. F., Gollin, H. A., Lavieri, V. Management of postpartum hemorrhage by prolonged administration of oxytocics. *Am. J. Obstet. Gynecol.*, 1952; **64**: 1163–4.

191 Abdel-Aleem, H., El Nashar, I., Abdel-Aleem, A. Management of severe postpartum hemorrhage with misoprostol. *Int. J. Gynaecol. Obstet.*, 1998; **92**: 212–14.

192 Kupferminc, M. J., Gull, I., Bar-Am, A., *et al.* Intrauterine irrigation with prostaglandin F2-alpha for management of severe postpartum hemorrhage. *Acta Obstet. Gynecol. Scand.*, 1998; **77**: 548–50.

193 Peyser, M. R., Kupferminc, M. Management of severe post partum hemorrhage by intra-uterine irrigation with prostaglandin E2. *Am. J. Obstet. Gynecol.*, 1990; **162**: 694–6.

194 Mousa, H. A., McKinley, C., Thong, J. Acute post-partum myocardial infarction after ergometrine administration in a woman with familial hypercholesterolemia. *Br. J. Obstet. Gynaecol.*, 2000; **107**: 939–40.

195 Chen, F. G., Koh, K. F., Chong, Y. S. Cardiac arrest associated with sulprostone use during cesarean section. *Anaesth. Intensive Care*, 1998; **26**: 298–301.

196 Feinstein, D. I., Marder, V. I., Colman, R. W. Consumptive thrombohemorrhagic disorders. In Colman, R. W., Hirsh, J., Marder, V. J., eds., *Hemostasis and Thrombosis: Basic Principles and Clinical Practice.* Philadelphia, PA: Lippincott, Williams and Wilkins; 2001: pp. 1197–233.

197 Hedner, U., Hirsh, J., Marder, V. J. Therapy with antifibrinolytic agents. In Colman, R. W., Hirsh, J., Marder, V. I., *et al.* eds., *Hemostasis and Thrombosis: Basic Principles and Clinical Practice.* Philadeplhia, PA: Lippincott, Williams and Wilkins; 2001: pp. 797–813.

198 Scwartz, B. S., Williams, E. C., Conlan, G., *et al.* Epsilon-aminocaproic acid in the treatment of patients with acute promyelocytic leukemia and acquired alpha-2-plasmin inhibtior deficiency. *Ann. Intern. Med.*, 1986; **105**: 873.

199 Gai, M-Y., Wu, L-F., Su, Q-F., *et al.* Clinical observation of blood loss reduced by tranexamic acid during and after cesarean section: a multi-center, randomized trial. *Eur. J. Obstet. Gynecol. Reprod. Biol.*, 2000; **112**: 154–7.

200 Avvisati, G., ten Cate, J. W., Buller, H. R., *et al.* Tranexamic acid for control of hemorrhage in acute promyelocytic leukemia. *Lancet*, 1989; **2**(8655): 122–4.

201 Dunn, C. J., Goa, K. L. Tranexamic acid: a review of its use in surgery and other indications. *Drugs*, 1999; **57**(1005).

202 Peters, D. C., Noble, S. Aprotonin: an update of its pharmacology and therapeutic use in open heart surgery and coronary artery bypass surgery. *Drugs*, 1999; **57**: 23.

203 As, A. K., Hagen, P., Webb, J. B. Tranexamic acid in the management of postpartum haemorrhage. *Br. J. Obstet. Gynaecol.*, 1996; **103**(12): 1250–1.

204 Lurie, S., Appelman, Z., Katz, Z. Subendometrial vasopressin to control intractable placental bleeding. *Lancet*, 1997; **349**: 698.

205 Domsky, M. F., Wilson, R. F. Hemodynamic resuscitation. *Crit. Care Clin.*, 1993; **10**: 715–26.

206 Abboud, F. M. Shock. In Wyngaarden, J. B., Smith, L. H., eds., *Cecil Textbook of Medicine.* Philadelphia, PA: W. B. Saunders Co.; 1988: pp. 236–50.

207 Kale, I. T., Kuzu, M. A., Berkem, H., *et al.* The presence of hemorrhagic shock increases the rate of bacterial translocation in blunt abdominal trauma. *J. Trauma*, 1998; **44**: 171–4.

208 Astiz, M. E., Rackow, E. C. Assessing perfusion failure circulatory shock. *Crit. Care. Clin.*, 1993; **9**: 299–312.

209 Gynecologists ACoOa. *Invasive Hemodynamic Monitoring in Obstetrics and Gynecology.* Washington, D.C.: ACOG; 1992.

210 Conference Pacc. Pulmonary artery consensus conference: consensus statement. *Crit. Care. Med.*, 1997; **25**(6): 910–25.

211 Ware, L. B., Matthay, M. A. The acute respiratory distress syndrome. *N. Engl. J. Med.*, 2000; **341**: 1334.

212 Staton, G. W. Pulmonary edema. In Dale, D. C., Federman, D. D., eds., *ACP Medicine.* New York, NY: WebMD Inc.; 2004: 14:X:1–20.

213 Duane, P. G., Colice, G. L. Impact of noninvasive studies to distinguish volume overload from ARDS in acutely ill patients with pulmonary edema: analysis of the medical literature from 1966–1998. *Chest*, 2000; **118**: 1709.

214 Hayashi, M., Mori, Y., Nogami, K., *et al.* A hypothesis to explain the occurrence of inner myometrial laceration causing massive postpartum hemorrhage. *Acta Obstet. Gynecol. Scand.*, 2000; **79**(2): 99–106.

215 Jones III, H. W., Rock Jr, W. A. Control of pelvic hemorrhage. In Rock, J. A., Jones III, H. W., eds., *Te Linde's Operative Gynecology.* Philadelphia, PA: Lippincott, Williams and Wilkins: pp. 413–46.

216 Rosch, C., Dotter, C. T., Brown, M. J. Selective arterial embolization. *Radiology*, 1972; **102**: 303–6.

217 Brown, B. J., Heaston, D. K., Poulson, A. M., *et al.* Uncontrollable postpartum bldeeding: a new approach to hemostasis through angiographic embolization. *Obstet. Gynecol.*, 1979; **54**: 361–5.

218 Mitty, H., Sterling, K., Alvarez, M., *et al.* Obstetric haemorrhage: prophylactic and emergency arterial catheterization and embolotherapy. *Radiology*, 1996; **188**: 183–7.

219 Merland, J. J., Houdart, E., Herbreteau, D., *et al.* Place of emergency arterial embolization in obstetric hemorrhage about 16 personal cases. *Eur. J. Obstet. Gynecol. Reprod. Biol.*, 1996; **65**: 141–3.

220 Collins, C. D., Jackson, J. E. Pelvic arterial embolization following hysterectomy and bilateral internal iliac artery ligation for intractable post partum hemorrhage. *Clin. Radiol.*, 1995; **50**: 710–3.

221 Reyal, F., Pelage, J. P., Rossignol, M., *et al.* Interventional radiology in managing postpartum hemorrhage. *Presse Med.*, 2002; **31**(20): 939–44.

222 Yamashita, Y., Harada, M., Yamamato, H., *et al.* Transcatheter arterial embolization of obstetric and gynaecological bleeding; efficacy and clinical outcome. *Br. J. Radiol.*, 1994; **67**: 530–4.

223 Oei, S. G., Kho, S. N., ten Broeke, E. D., *et al.* Arterial balloon occlusion of the hypogastric arteries: a life-saving procedure for severe obstetric hemorrhage. *Am. J. Obstet. Gynecol.*, 2001; **185**(5): 1255–6.

224 Descargues, G., Douvrin, F., Gravier, A., *et al.* False aneurysm of the uterine pedicle: an uncommon cause of post-partum haemorrhage after caesarean section treated with selective arterial embolization. *Eur. J. Obstet. Gynecol. Reprod. Biol.*, 2001; **97**(1): 26–9.

225 Murakami, R., Ichikawa, T., Kumazaki, T., *et al.* Transcatheter arterial embolization for postpartum massive hemorrhage: a case report. *Clin. Imaging*, 2000; **24**(6): 368–70.

226 Pelage, J. P., Le Dref, O., Jacob, D., *et al.* Selective arterial embolization of the uterine arteries in the management of intractable post-partum hemorrhage. *Acta Obstet. Gynecol. Scand.*, 1999; **78**(8): 698–703.

227 Pelage, J. P., Soyer, P., Repiquet, D., *et al.* Secondary postpartum hemorrhage: treatment with selective arterial embolization. *Radiology*, 1999; **212**(2): 385–9.

228 Corr, P. Arterial embolization for haemorrhage in the obstetric patient. *Best Pract. Res. Clin. Obstet. Gynaecol.*, 2001; **15**(4): 557–61.

229 Badawy, S. Z., Etman, A., Singh, M., *et al.* Uterine artery embolization: the role in obstetrics and gynecology. *Clin. Imaging*, 2001; **25**(4): 288–95.

230 Tourne, G., Collet, F., Seffert, P., *et al.* Place of embolization of the uterine arteries in the management of post-partum haemorrhage: a study of 12 cases. *Eur. J. Obstet. Gynecol. Reprod. Biol.*, 2003; **110**(1): 29–34.

231 Hong, T. M., Tseng, H. S., Lee, R. C., *et al.* Uterine artery embolization: an effective treatment for intractable obstetric haemorrhage. *Clin. Radiol.*, 2004; **59**(1): 96–101.

232 Salomon, L. J., deTayrac, R., Castaigne-Meary, V., *et al.* Fertility and pregnancy outcome following pelvic arterial embolization for severe post-partum haemorrhage. A cohort study. *Hum. Reprod.*, 2003; **18**(4): 849–52.

233 Ornan, D., White, R., Pollak, J., *et al.* Pelvic embolization for intractable postpartum hemorrhage: long-term follow-up and implications for fertility. *Obstet. Gynecol.*, 2003; **102**(5 Pt 1): 904–10.

234 Cordonnier, C., Ha-Vien, D. E., Depret, S., *et al.* Foetal growth restriction in the next pregnancy after uterine artery embolisation for post-partum haemorrhage. *Eur. J. Obstet. Gynecol. Reprod. Biol.*, 2002; **103**(2): 183–4.

235 Ledee, N., Ville, Y., Musset, D., *et al.* Management in intractable obstetric haemorrhage: an audit study on 61 cases. *Eur. J. Obstet. Gynecol. Reprod. Biol.*, 2001; **94**(2): 189–96.

236 Marcovici, I., Scoccia, B. Postpartum hemorrhage and intrauterine balloon tamponade. A report of three cases. *J. Reprod. Med.*, 1999; **44**(2): 122–6.

237 Katesmark, M., Brown, R., Raju, K. S. Successful use of a Sengstaken–Blakemore tube to control massive postpartum hemorrhage. *Br. J. Obstet. Gynaecol.*, 1994; **101**: 259–60.

238 Johanson, R., Kumar, M., Obhrai, M., *et al.* Management of massive postpartum haemorrhage: use of a hydrostatic balloon catheter to avoid laparotomy. *Br. J. Obstet. Gynaecol.*, 2001; **108**(4): 420–2.

239 Tamizian, O., Arulkumaran, S. The surgical management of postpartum haemorrhage. *Curr. Opin. Obstet. Gynecol.*, 2001; **13**(2): 127–31.

240 Pinborg, A., Bodker, B., Hogdall, C. Postpartum hematoma and vaginal packing with a blood pressure cuff. *Acta Obstet. Gynecol. Scand.*, 2000; **79**(10): 887–9.

241 Hensleigh, P. A. Anti-shock garment provides resuscitation and haemostasis for obstetric haemorrhage. *Br. J. Obstet. Gynaecol.*, 2002; **109**(12): 1377–84.

242 Maier, R. C. Control of postpartum hemorrhage with uterine packing. *Am. J. Obstet. Gynecol.*, 1993; **169**(2 Pt 1): 317–21; discussion, 21–3.

243 Condous, G. S., Arulkumaran, S., Symonds, I., *et al.* The "tamponade test" in the management of massive postpartum hemorrhage. *Obstet. Gynecol.*, 2003; **101**(4): 767–72.

244 Bakri, Y. N. Balloon device for control of obstetrical bleeding. *Eur. J. Obstet. Gynecol. Reprod. Biol.*, 1999; **86**: S84.

245 Bakri, Y. N., Amri, A., Abdul, Jabbar, F. Tamponade-balloon for obstetrical bleeding. *Int. J. Gynaecol. Obstet.*, 2001; **74**(2): 139–42.

246 Waters, E. G. Surgical management of postpartum hemorrhage with particular reference to ligation of uterine arteries. *Am. J. Obstet. Gynecol.*, 1952; **64**: 1143–8.

247 O'Leary, J. A. Uterine artery ligation in the control of postcesarean hemorrhage. *J. Reprod. Med.*, 1995; **40**(3): 189–93.

248 AbdRabbo, S. A. Stepwise uterine devascularization: a novel technique for management of uncontrollable postpartum hemorrhage with preservation of the uterus. *Am. J. Obstet. Gynecol.*, 1994; **171**: 694–700.

249 Burchell, R. C. Internal iliac artery ligation: Hemodynamics. *Obstet. Gynecol.*, 1964; **24**: 737–9.

250 Clark, S. L., Phelan, J. P., Yeh, S. Y., *et al.* Hypogastric artery ligation for obstetric hemorrhage. *Obstet. Gynecol.*, 1985; **66**: 353–6.

251 Nizard, J., Barrinque, L., Frydman, R., *et al.* Fertility and pregnancy outcomes following hypogastric artery ligation for severe post-partum haemorrhage. *Hum. Reprod.*, 2003; **18**(4): 844–8.

252 B-Lynch, C., Coker, A., Lawal, A. H., *et al.* The B-Lynch surgical technique for the control of massive postpartum haemorrhage: an alternative to hysterectomy? Five cases reported. *Br. J. Obstet. Gynaecol.*, 1997; **104**(3): 372–5.

253 Pal, M., Biswas, A. K., Bhattacharya, S. M. B-Lynch Brace Suturing in primary postpartum hemorrhage during cesarean section. *J. Obstet. Gynaecol. Res.*, 2003; **29**(5): 317–20.

254 Dacus, J. V., Busowski, M. T., Busowski, J. D., *et al.* Surgical treatment of uterine atony employing the B-Lynch technique. *J. Matern. Fetal Med.*, 2000; **9**(3): 194–6.

255 Ferguson, J. E., Bourgeois, F. J., Underwood, P. B. B-Lynch suture for postpartum hemorrhage. *Obstet. Gynecol.*, 2000; **95**(6 Pt 2): 1020–2.

256 Cho, J. H., Jun, H. S., Lee, C. N. Hemostatic suturing technique for uterine bleeding during cesarean delivery. *Obstet. Gynecol.*, 2000; **96**(1): 129–31.

257 Zelop, C. M., Harlow, B. L., Frigoletto Jr, F. D., *et al.* Emergency peripartum hysterectomy. *Am. J. Obstet. Gynecol.*, 1993; **168**: 1443–8.

258 Okogbenin, S. A., Gharoro, E. P., Otoide, V. O., *et al.* Obstetric hysterectomy: fifteen years' experience in a Nigerian tertiary centre. *J. Obstet. Gynaecol.*, 2003; **23**(4): 356–9.

259 Clark, S. L., Yeh, S. Y., Phelan, J. P., *et al.* Emergency hysterectomy for obstetric hemorrhage. *Obstet. Gynecol.*, 1984; **64**(3): 376–80.

260 Chanrachakul, B., Chaturachinda, K., Phuapradit, W., *et al.* Cesarean and postpartum hysterectomy. *Intl. J. Gynaecol. Obstet.*, 1996; **54**: 109–13.

261 Wenham, J., Matijevic, R. Post-partum hysterectomies: revisited. *J. Perinat. Med.*, 2001; **29**(3): 260–5.

262 Seckin, N. C., Inegol, I., Turhan, N. O., *et al.* Life-threatening second trimester disseminated intravascular coagulopathy with protein S deficiency. *Clin. Appl. Thromb. Hemost.*, 2004; **10**: 289–91.

263 Cicala, C., Cirino, G. Linkage between inflammation and coagulation: An update on the molecular basis of the crosstalk. *Life Sci.*, 1998; **62**: 1817–24.

264 Muller-Berghaus, G. Pathophysiological and biochemical events in disseminated intravascular coagulation: dysregulation of procoagulant and anticoagulant pathways. *Semin. Thromb. Hemost.*, 1989; **15**: 58–87.

265 Verstraete, M., Vermylen, C., Vermylen, J. Excessive consumption of blood coagulation components as a cause hemorrhagic diathesis. *Am. J. Med.*, 1965; **35**: 899–905.

266 Rodriguez-Erdmann, F. Bleeding due to increased intravascular blood coagulation. Hemorrhagic syndromes caused by consumption of blood-clotting factors (consumption-coagulopathies). *N. Engl. J. Med.*, 1965; **273**: 1370–8.

267 de Boer, K., ten Cate, J. W., Sturk, A., *et al.* Enhanced thrombin generation in normal and hypertensive pregnancy. *Am. J. Obstet. Gynecol.*, 1989; **160**: 95–100.

268 Weiner, C. P. Preeclampsia-eclampsia syndrome and coagulation. *Clin. Perinatol.*, 1991; **18**: 713–26.

269 Weiner, C. P. The obstetric patient and disseminated intravascular coagulation. *Clin. Perinatol.*, 1986; **13**: 705–17.

270 Pritchard, J. A., Brekken, A. L. Clinical and laboratory studies on severe abruptio placentae. *Am. J. Obstet. Gynecol.*, 1967; **97**: 681.

271 Bick, R. L. Disseminated intravascular coagulation and related syndromes: a clinical review. *Semin. Thromb. Hemost.*, 1988; **14**: 299–338.

272 Martin, J. N. J., Stedman, C. M. Imitators of preeclampsia and HELLP syndrome. *Obstet. Gynecol. Clin. North Am.*, 1991; **18**: 181–98.

273 McDougall, R. J., Duke, C. J. Amniotic fluid embolism syndrome. Case report and review. *Anaesthesia Intensive Care*, 1995; **23**: 735–40.

274 Feinstein, D. I. Treatment of disseminated intravascular coagulation. *Semin. Thromb. Hemost.*, 1988; **14**(4): 351–62.

275 Lewis, B. E., Wallis, D. E., Berkowitz, S. D., *et al.* Argatroban anticoagulant therapy in patients with heparin-induced thrombocytopenia. *Circulation*, 2001; **103**: 1838.

276 Munoz, M. C., Montes, R., Hermida, J., *et al.* Effect of the administration of recombinant hirudin and/or tissue-plasminogen activator (t-PA) on endotoxin-induced disseminated intravascular coagulation model in rabbits. *Br. J. Haematol.*, 1999; **105**: 117–22.

277 ten Cate, H., Nurmohamed, M. T., ten Cate, J. W. Developments in antithrombotic therapy: state of the art anno 1996. *Pharmacology World Science* 1996; **18**: 195–203.

278 Bick, R. L. Heparin and low-molecular-weight heparins. In Bick, R. L., ed., *Disorders of Thrombosis and Hemostasis*. Philadelphia, PA: Lippincott, Williams and Wilkins 1992: pp. 359–77.

279 Jochum, M. Influence of high-dose antithrombin concentrate therapy on the release of cellular proteases, cytokines and soluble molecules in acute inflammation. *Semin. Hematol.*, 1995; **32**: 14.

280 Fourier, F., Chopin, C., Huart, J. J., *et al.* Double-blind, placebo-controlled trial of antithrombin III concentrates in septic shock with disseminated intravascular coagulation. *Chest*, 1993; **104**: 882.

281 Laursen, B., Mortensen, J. Z., Frost, L., *et al.* DIC in hepatic failure treated with antithrombin III. *Thromb. Res.*, 1981; **22**: 701.

282 Eisele, B., Lamy, M. Clinical experience with antithrombin III concentrates in critically ill patients with sepsis and multiple organ failure. *Semin. Thromb. Hemost.*, 1998; **24**: 71.

283 Okajima, K., Uchida, M. The anti-inflammatory properties of antithrombin III: new therapeutic implications. *Semin. Thromb. Hemost.*, 1998; **24**: 27.

284 Baluhut, B., Kramar, H., Vinazzer, H., *et al.* Substitution of ATIII in shock and DIC: a randomized study. *Thromb. Res.*, 1985; **39**: 81.

285 von Kries, R., Stannigel, H., Gobel, U. Anticoagulant therapy by continuous heparin-ATIII infusion in newborns with DIC. *Eur. J. Pediatr.*, 1985; **144**: 191.

286 Bernard, G. R., Vincent, J. L., Latere, P. F., *et al.* Efficacy and safety of recombinant human activated protein C for severe sepsis. *N. Engl. J. Med.*, 2001; **344**: 699.

287 Smith, O. P. Protein-C concentrate for meningococcal purpura fulminans. *Lancet*, 1998; **351**: 986.

288 Fijinvandraat, K., Derkx, B., Peters, M., *et al.* Coagulation activation and tissue necrosis in meningococcal septic shock: severely reduced protein C levels predict a high mortality. *Thromb. Haemost.*, 1995; **73**: 15.

289 Shoemaker, W. C. Circulatory pathophysiology of ARDS and its fluid management. In *Textbook of Critical Care*. Philadelphia, PA: W. B. Saunders Company; 1995: p. 312.

290 Urden, L. D., Stacy, K. M., Lough, M. E., Shock. In *Thelan's Critical Care Nursing: Diagnosis and Management*. St. Louis, MO: Mosby; 2002: p. 931.

291 Abrams, J., *et al.* Vassopressors used in shock. In *Drug: Facts and Comparisons*, 1999 edn; Philadelphia, PA: Lippincott, Williams, and Wilkins; 1999: pp. 883–917.

292 *Uterine Artery Ligation*. 2004. (Accessed November 31, 2004, at www.utodol.com/application/image.asp?).

293 *B-Lynch Suture*. 2000. (Accessed November 30, 2004, at www.utdol.com/application/image.asp?).

13

Hemoglobinopathies in pregnancy

Adeboye H. Adewoye, M.D.[1] and Martin H. Steinberg, M.D.[2]

[1]Assistant Professor of Medicine
[2]Professor of Medicine, Pediatrics, Pathology and Laboratory Medicine

From the Department of Medicine, Boston University School of Medicine and the Center of Excellence in Sickle Cell Disease, Boston Medical Center.
Address all correspondence to Dr. Adeboye H. Adewoye, 88 East Newton Street, Boston, MA 02118, USA.
Tel: 617-414-1020; FAX 617-414-1021; adeboye.adewoye@bmc.org

Introduction

All human hemoglobin is composed of two α-globin-like chains and two non-α-globin chains that combine to form a tetramer. Normal adults have three hemoglobin types, HbA ($\alpha 2\beta 2$; ~96%), HbF ($\alpha 2\gamma 2$; ~1%), and HbA_2 ($\alpha_2\delta_2$; ~3%). The amino acid sequence, or primary structure of each globin chain differs; dissimilarities between α- and non-α-globin chains are greater than the variations among the globins of the β-like gene cluster, e.g. γ-, δ-, and β-globin. Despite these differences among globins their similarities are even greater as all have alike secondary and tertiary structure and function similarly. Human hemoglobin is ideally suited for its tasks – primarily oxygen uptake in lungs and delivery in tissues. A sigmoidal shaped curve, so critical for this oxygen transport, is a result of the interactions among the individual globin subunits of the tetramer. As for hemoglobin function, the sigmoidal shape of the oxygen dissociation curve of hemoglobin shows that totally deoxygenated hemoglobin is slow to become oxygenated, but as oxygenation proceeds, the reaction of heme with oxygen accelerates; the reverse is also true. Hemoglobin has other functions in CO_2 exchange and control of vascular tone by nitric oxide (NO) and can modulate oxygen delivery by shifts in its oxygen-hemoglobin dissociation curve caused by temperature, pH, and organic phosphates.

Different classes of mutations can alter the structure, function, and synthesis of hemoglobin. More than 1,000 structurally abnormal hemoglobins have been characterized and the number of thalassemia-causing mutations exceeds 200. Most mutations within the globin genes are innocuous. When mutations involve residues that form important contacts between the α and β chains, so that their

Hematological Complications in Obstetrics, Pregnancy, and Gynecology, ed. R. L. Bick *et al.* Published by Cambridge University Press.

movement relative to one another during oxygenation and deoxygenation is altered, the oxygen affinity of the molecule can be changed. Most often, the hemoglobin is "frozen" in its oxy conformation and therefore has high oxygen affinity and a left-shifted oxygen-hemoglobin dissociation curve described by a low P_{50} (partial pressure at which hemoglobin is half saturated with oxygen). Since oxygen cannot be unloaded satisfactorily in tissues, hypoxia results. One physiologic compensation for hypoxia is the enhanced production of red cells, so that a characteristic of this type of abnormal hemoglobin is polycythemia, or too many red cells. Mutations sometime involve the amino acid residues that surround the heme-binding site. In these cases, heme can be oxidized. The heme group can be lost from globin making the globin unstable, or the oxidized heme fails to bind oxygen and the blood turns blue causing cyanosis. Unstable hemoglobins precipitate, injure the cell membrane, and lead to premature removal of the cell from the circulation. This is the cause of the anemia that is often seen with unstable hemoglobins.

The most common hemoglobin variants are neither unstable nor have abnormal oxygen affinity. These variants, HbS or sickle hemoglobin, HbC, and HbE, have reached very high frequencies in some populations because heterozygotes have a selective advantage in the presence of *Falciparum malaria*. In HbS and HbC the mutations lie at the surface of the molecule, a location not usually associated with abnormal features but, deoxygenated HbS has the almost unique property of polymerizing within the cell, triggering many events that in homozygotes cause severe disease. HbC and HbE, by virtue of their highly positive charge, interact with the cell membrane and cause changes in the ion content of the cytoplasm and in cell shape. Despite this phenomenon, alone, neither variant causes significant disease.

Thalassemias are diseases of insufficient globin synthesis. Normally, nearly equivalent amounts of α and non-α chain are normally produced. If this condition is not met, then redundant globin chains of like type, incapable of forming stable tetramers, precipitate intra-cellularly, injuring the cell. The types of mutations causing thalassemia have been a virtual catalog of what can go wrong in a gene. They include deletions of entire genes or portions of genes; single nucleotide base substitutions in gene promoters that reduce transcription; substitutions of nucleotides that are critical for the faithful excision of introns and re-ligation of exons that impair translation; mutations that fool the normal splicing mechanisms by activating cryptic splice sites; nonsense mutations that interrupt prematurely translation; changes in the 3′ untranslated region of the gene that impair the stability and translatability of the mRNA.

As most hemoglobin variants are rare, problems of pregnancy are nearly always restricted to sickle cell disorders and the thalassemias.

Sickle cell disease

HbS, first of the known hemoglobin gene mutations, is caused by an adenine (A) to thymidine (T) substitution in codon six of the β-globin gene (GAG→GTG), that replaces the normal β^6 glutamic acid residue by a valine. Sickle hemoglobin ($\alpha_2\beta_2{}^S$) polymerizes when it is deoxygenated, a property only of hemoglobin variants that have the $\beta^{6\ glu\rightarrow val}$ substitution. When critical amounts of HbS polymer accumulate within sickle erythrocytes, cellular injury results and a phenotype – notable for its heterogeneity – becomes apparent. Many reviews of the history, pathophysiology, clinical features, and treatment of sickle cell disease have been published.[1–8] DeoxyHbS fibers coalesce to form crystals. When present in sufficiently high concentration, masses of HbS polymer deform and injure the sickle erythrocyte and initiate the pathophysiology of this disease.

Sickle erythrocytes vary in their density and deformability; in some dense cells the mean corpuscular hemoglobin concentration reaches 50 g/dl (normal, 27–38 g/dl) and HbS polymer is always present. Other cells, called irreversibly sickled cells (ISCs), always appear deformed because of irreversible membrane damage even though their HbS may not be polymerized. Hemolysis is greatest in individuals with the highest numbers of ISCs and dense cells. Some intravascular destruction of sickle erythrocytes results from the dissolution of the most damaged cells by mechanical forces, their increased sensitivity to complement-mediated lysis, and microvesiculation that takes place as sickle polymers penetrate the cytoskeleton and is liberated into the circulation as lipid-ensheathed buds. Most red cell destruction occurs by erythrophagocytosis. In blood, erythrophagocytosis takes place mainly in monocytes and to a lesser degree, in neutrophils. Recent studies suggest that liberation of hemoglobin into plasma during hemolysis reduces NO levels and may favor vasoconstriction. Certain disease phenotypes appear to be linked to this intravascular hemolysis.

The vasculopathy of sickle cell disease makes this disorder unique among hemolytic anemias. Vaso-occlusive events are likely to depend on features intrinsic to the sickle erythrocyte – like polymer content and the degree of cellular damage – interacting with factors in the cell's environment – like endothelial injury, vascular tone, and other cells.

The sickle erythrocyte manifests varying abnormalities ranging from puckering of the red cell to abnormal cation homeostasis. These abnormalities result in cellular dehydration, which further increase the concentration of sickle hemoglobin in each cell and the interactions among HbS molecules. Besides these factors there is also accompanying cellular interaction between the red cell membrane and the vascular endothelial wall. The sickle erythrocyte displays receptors allowing it to interact with endothelial cells and circulating blood cells. The exposure of endothelial cell adhesion receptors and endothelial matrix proteins in the subendothelium make the red cell highly adherent to the vessel wall. This further aggravates sludging and creates an impedance to blood flow in the microcirculation. Sludging results in varying degrees of hypoxia in the end-arterioles which result in micro-ischemic events in the end-organs. These micro-ischemic events cause some clinical manifestations of the disease.

The placental circulation and sickle cell disease

The placental circulation, a high pressure circulation, provides a rich capillary bed that specializes in carrying nutrients from the mother to the fetus. The fetus has adapted to this oxygen-depleted environment by having a high level of HbF, which has a high capacity for binding oxygen in the placenta because of its increased Bohr effect (low P_{50}) delivering it to the developing fetal tissues under hypoxic conditions. As HbF predominates in the fetus and since HbS behaves normally in oxygen transport and its polymerization is inhibited by HbF, HbS has little effect on oxygen delivery to the fetus. Erythropoietin rises during pregnancy due to extra-renal production of the hormone by the trophoblast cells of the human placenta, possibly to compensate for the increased demand for oxygen delivery of both the fetus and mother.[9] This change, though physiologically important, has consequences for sickle cell disease patients. An accompanying increase in the production of placental growth factor (PLGF), a member of the VEGF family, activates monocytes and may promote enhanced interactions of blood cells and the endothelium. Expression of PLGF correlates with disease severity in patients with sickle cell disease.[10] In sickle cell disease, endothelial changes can affect the placenta and the umbilical cord.

Placenta and umbilical vein

The placenta of the sickle cell patient weighs less than that of comparable age-matched controls,[11] with histology showing villous sclerosis, intervillous fibrin deposits, and placental infarction. Electron microscopy has shown differences between sickle cell disease umbilical vein endothelial cells compared with normal controls (Figures 13.1a and 13.1b).[12] The morphologic features include irregularly elongated and round, haphazardly elongated cells, both reminiscent of human umbilical vein endothelial cells studied under hypoxic conditions,[13] there also appears to be abnormal proliferation of the smooth muscle cell, absence of an inner elastic lamina in the tunica media and varying thickness of the basement membrane. These changes are possibly related to the production and presence of cytokines in the placenta and umbilical vein secondary to hypoxia.[14]

Pregnancy in sickle cell disease

There are few absolute contraindications to pregnancy in sickle cell disease (poor cardiac reserve, severe pulmonary hypertension). Though patients with sickle cell

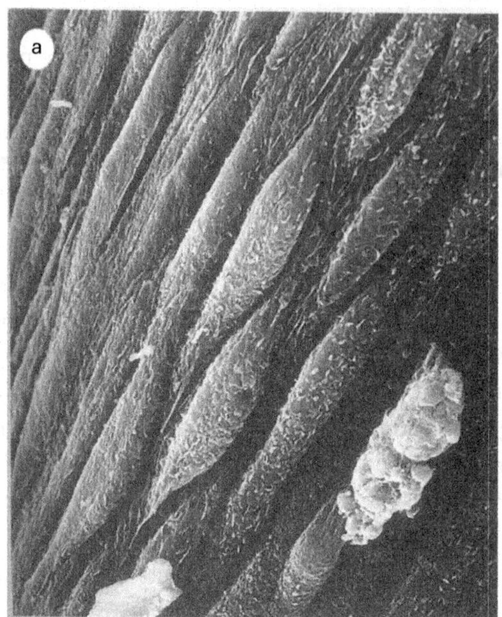

Figure 13.1a Luminal surface of normal umbilical vein. (Scanning electron micrograph, original magnification x2000.)

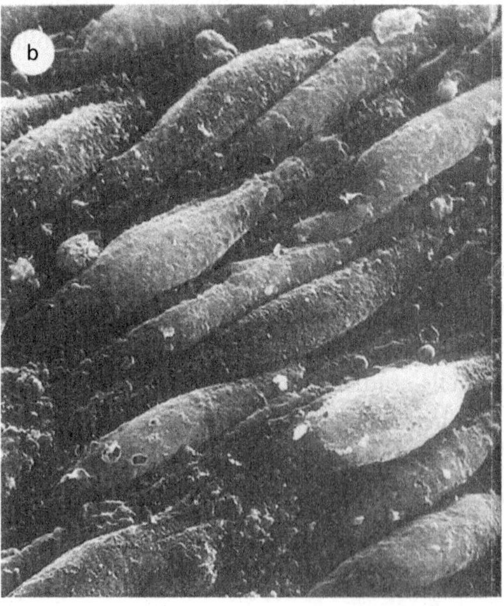

Figure 13.1b Endothelial surface of SCD umbilical vein showing irregularly elongated and rounded cells. (Scanning electron micrograph, original magnification x2000.)

anemia have a delay in sexual maturation,[15] fertility is probably normal if the likelihood that initial sexual encounters occur at a later age in patients compared to controls are accounted for.[16] The low birth rate may be explained in part by the anemia and vasculopathy of sickle cell disease and perhaps poor access to health care. One-hundred twenty-seven deliveries in women with sickle cell anemia and HbSC disease (compound heterozygosity for HbS and HbC) that occurred between 1980 and 1999 were compared with a control group of 129 deliveries by African-American women with normal hemoglobin. Compared with controls, deliveries among women with sickle cell disease were at increased risk for intrauterine growth restriction, antepartum hospital admission, and postpartum infection. They were also more likely to be complicated by low birth weight, prematurity, and preterm labor or preterm premature rupture of membranes. Perinatal deaths were similar and there were no maternal deaths.[15,98]

Pregnancy-related complications in sickle cell disease

Several factors affect the phenotype of sickle cell disease, for example HbF concentration, white blood cell count[95] and pulmonary hypertension[96] and the presence of α thalassemia.[17,18] There is a direct relationship between the severity of sickle cell disease and the likely complication rate the patient will experience while pregnant. Problems in pregnancy are most prevalent in sickle cell anemia and HbS-β^0 thalassemia (compound heterozygosity for HbS and the type of β thalassemia where no normal β-globin is made) and less common in HbSC disease and HbS-β+ thalassemia (compound heterozygosity for HbS and the type of β thalassemia where some normal β-globin is made).

Antenatal care

Antenatal care is best provided by an experienced obstetrician familiar with the care of sickle cell disease patients working with a hematologist. Prenatal visits serve to collect background data, establish the hemoglobin phenotype and catalog the existing complications of the disease. Pertinent is the number of previous pregnancies and their outcomes. Previous complications during pregnancy with emphasis on spontaneous abortions, pre-eclampsia, low-birth weight infants and complications from sickle cell disease like acute chest syndrome, stroke, congestive heart failure, pulmonary hypertension and history of previous blood transfusions including exchange blood transfusion and the presence of alloantibodies. As a group, people with sickle cell anemia have relative hypertension as their blood pressure is higher than expected when compared with a control group with anemia. This is associated with increase risk of stroke. Since even 'normal' blood pressure may be abnormal this should be carefully followed. Similarly, significant renal damage can be present with normal serum creatinine levels because of the very high glomerular filtration rates in young patients with sickle cell anemia.

A medication profile with particular attention to hydroxyurea should be documented. Hydroxyurea is now approved for the treatment of adult sickle cell anemia. A recent longitudinal study reveals a survival advantage in patients maintained on hydroxyurea.[97] An increasing number of patients have become pregnant or fathered children while taking hydroxyurea or having taken hydroxyurea in the past. Hydroxyurea is a teratogen in animals and should not be used if pregnancy is planned. Pregnancy has been reported in at least two-dozen individuals receiving hydroxyurea, usually for myeloproliferative disorders, but sometimes in sickle cell anemia.[22] In this very small experience there have been no adverse outcomes. Developmental defects have not been reported in pregnant patients who took hydroxyurea for other diseases. Contraception should be practiced by both women and men receiving hydroxyurea and the uncertain outcome of unplanned pregnancy discussed frankly. If pregnancy occurs while taking hydroxyurea there is little information besides the above on which to base a decision for continuation or termination. So far, congenital defects have not been described in pregnancies followed to term. This is no cause for complacency. Hydroxyurea is very likely to be teratogenic in humans and should be avoided when pregnancy is planned. Whether or not previous exposure to hydroxyurea affects fertility and the results of pregnancy is unknown.

History, physical examination and laboratory testing provides some indication of the severity of sickle cell disease and focuses attention on elements of the disease that require scrutiny during pregnancy. Though pregnancy in sickle cell patients is *always high risk*, some patients warrant even more intense observation and care. These individuals include patients with frequent hospitalizations for complications from sickle cell disease, like acute chest syndrome, renal failure, hypertension, history of prior spontaneous abortions, frequent blood transfusion, and pulmonary hypertension. Maternal steady-state hematology has little influence on fetal outcome, with the exception that mothers with high HbF levels are less prone to perinatal deaths.

Laboratory testing

A recommended antenatal testing scheme is summarized in Table 13.1. Hemoglobin separation, preferably by HPLC (high-performance liquid chromatography), with quantitation of HbF, is done to establish the hemoglobin phenotype. HPLC is also the preferred method for measuring HbA and HbS concentration in patients being transfused. Besides blood counts and serum chemistries including LDH, other testing should include hepatitis A, B and C testing, HIV status, electrolytes, urinalysis, urine culture, rubella antibody titer and iron status (including serum ferritin). All

Table 13.1 Antenatal testing in sickle cell disease.

Hemoglobin analysis (preferably by HPLC) with HbF quantitation
Parental hemoglobin analysis
CBC with differential cell count
Liver and renal function tests, including LDH.
Hepatitis profile (Hepatitis A, B, C)
HIV testing
Electrolytes, urinalysis (in particular, total protein in urine and urine culture)
Rubella antibody titer
Iron status (including serum ferritin)
RBC screening to identify allo-antibodies (Kell, C, E, S, Fy and Jk)
Echocardiography to detect pulmonary hypertension

patients should have their red cell phenotype recorded (Kell, C, E, S, Fy and Jk) and allo-antibodies identified. This is done so that if the need arises for blood transfusion, phenotypically matched blood can be used. Ultrasound is used to assess fetal growth.

When antenatal diagnosis (see below) is to be done, the parental genotypes must be determined by DNA-based methods because HPLC and other protein-based techniques provide information on hemoglobin phenotype alone and cannot establish a genotypic diagnosis.

Common medications during pregnancy

Folic acid is customarily taken by patients with sickle cell disease even when they are not pregnant. It should be continued during pregnancy at a dose of 1 mg/day. The need for iron supplementation is often questioned. The decision to place a patient with sickle cell disease on iron supplementation during pregnancy depends on the iron status of the patient. For patients already iron overloaded, as judged by an elevated serum ferritin level and history of many transfusions, there is no indication for supplemental iron. When iron stores are judged to be low or marginal, especially in patients transfused infrequently, routine iron supplementation is advisable.[16]

Blood transfusion

Blood transfusion during pregnancy continues to be a debated issue and the practice of transfusion varies according to locale and individual practice customs. A common, but questioned, practice is to place all patients on a transfusion regimen. Available data so far has not shown any benefit resulting from this practice.[23,24,25] The clinical situations where this is warranted are: preoperatively for caesarian section; for acute chest syndrome, acute neurologic events and severe anemia.

Otherwise, lacking a history of complicated pregnancies, prior miscarriage and frequent difficult to manage vaso-occlusive events, like repetitive painful episodes, most pregnancies can be successfully managed without regular transfusions.

Delivery

The mode of delivery of the patient with sickle cell disease depends on the clinical/obstetric indication for delivery, like fetal distress or abruptio placentae and non-obstetric emergencies. If there are definite surgical indications, two important goals must be met:

1. Prophylactic transfusion to reduce the level of HbS to <30% of total hemoglobin. When the hematocrit is <25%, simple transfusion may be used since hyperviscosity is minimal with a hematocrit <30%. Simple transfusion also decreases exposure to blood with its risks of exposure to infectious agents, alloimmunization and iron accumulation. If the baseline hematocrit is higher than 25%, exchange transfusion is preferable.
2. Short induction during anesthesia with adequate oxygenation throughout surgery.

Termination

If pregnancy must be terminated some have advised against using hypertonic saline because of the theoretical possibility of it inducing a vasoocclusive episode. Little information on the choice of method for abortion is available.

Puerperium

During this period, the main concerns are pain control, adequate hydration and the prevention of pulmonary complications, like acute chest syndrome that may be favored by immobility and hypoventilation. Patients should be well hydrated and provided with an incentive spirometer to help lung expansion and prevent atelectasis.

Complications peculiar to sickle cell disease

Acute chest syndrome

This complication is defined as a new chest infiltrate on X-ray, cough, fever, hypoxemia with declining oxygen saturation, and pleuritic chest pain.[26] Its etiology is multifactorial and includes viral and bacterial infection, bone marrow embolization and *in situ* thrombosis. The mortality of acute chest syndrome, if not properly managed, is close to 20%. When hypoxia and respiratory distress exist, the goal of treatment is to reduce the HbS level to less than 30% of total hemoglobin. This is accomplished by either a simple transfusion or an exchange transfusion. If the choice of treatment is a simple transfusion; care must be taken to prevent hyperviscosity syndrome which occurs when the hematocrit approaches 35%. To document if this goal has been reached, a post exchange blood transfusion sample is sent to the laboratory for hemoglobin separation and quantitation of HbS level.

Painful episode

Appropriate analgesics, adequate hydration and treatment of the underlying condition causing the clinical event, if one is detectable, are the mainstays of treatment. Often, patients that present with multi-focal severe pain develop acute chest syndrome because of bone marrow necrosis and fat embolism. For this cohort of patients with severe bone pain crisis, besides adequate appropriate analgesic use and hydration, transfusion may be advisable.[26]

CNS Events

Pregnancy poses a particular high risk period for sickle cell patients because of the increase in metabolic demands, increases in prothrombotic coagulant factors and a decrease in systemic fibrinolysis. Strokes and TIA are the second leading course of morbidity and mortality in patients with sickle cell disease. The overall risk of stroke varies depending on the hemoglobin genotype. Patients homozygous for the HbS gene (sickle cell anemia) or with HbS-β^0 thalassemia have the highest overall risk of 4.01%.[27] Stroke is far less common in HbSC disease or with HbS-β^+ thalassemia. For patients presenting with new onset neurologic events (TIA, full stroke), it is imperative to get appropriate brain imaging by MRI and MRA. Patients with acute chest syndrome and moderate thrombocytopenia have been shown to have a high incidence of stroke.[26] The treatment of acute stroke entails exchange blood transfusion to reduce the level of HbS to <30% followed by initiation of a hypertransfusion regimen throughout pregnancy. Prompt neurological evaluation besides requesting appropriate imaging of the brain is vital. The decision to begin anticoagulant therapy, along with prompt exchange transfusion, should be made in consultation with a neurologist.

Acute anemic episodes

Occasionally, patients with sickle cell disease develop severe acute anemia with a drop in baseline hematocrit by 25–30%. This is a significant health risk for both the mother and the developing fetus and must be managed aggressively with identification of the cause of the anemic episode and the correction of the anemia. Transfusion is indicated when anemia is severe and circulation compromised. Causes of these acute anemic episodes include:

1. Aplastic crisis characterized by reticulocytopenia, and a usually normal baseline LDH. This is usually associated with Parvovirus type B19 infection.

2. Acute splenic or hepatic sequestration. This usually manifests as an acute increase in the size of the spleen or liver with accompanying pain at the site of the enlarging of the organ.
3. Hyperhemolysis characterized by an increase in LDH and total bilirubin level. This is a very rare event and may be associated with severe infection.

Parvovirus B19 infects the erythroid progenitors resulting in transient cessation of erythropoiesis. Its effects are most obvious in patients with reduced red cell survival like sickle cell disease and severe forms of thalassemia. The hallmark of this infection is rapid worsening of anemia with reticulocytopenia. In pregnancy, the B19 parvovirus may also cause fetal loss and hydrops fetalis. In patients with Parvovirus type B19 infection in the general population, the risk of fetal loss approximates 10% before 20 weeks while it falls to 1% afterwards.[28] The incidence and risk in pregnant sickle cell disease patients are unknown. Though some have advocated intra-uterine blood transfusion in these patients,[29] its role in sickle cell patients is not clear; neither is the role of IVIG.[30]

Small for gestational age

Sickle cell fetuses are especially prone to being small for gestational age. Twenty-one percent of infants born to mothers with sickle cell anemia are small for gestational age when compared with the general population;[31] the incidence in mothers with HbSC disease and HbS-β thalassemia is unknown but presumed to be less. Small for gestational age fetuses are likely due to placental insufficiency. Sickle cell patients with preeclampsia and acute anemic events are especially prone to these complications.[31]

Pre-eclampsia

Sickle cell patients have an increased risk of developing pre-eclampsia. This develops when hypertension coexists with edema and proteinuria after 20 weeks of gestation. The pathophysiology of pre-eclampsia lies in utero-placental insufficiency which activates endothelial cells with release of oxygen free radials, endothelial reactive substances and consumption of NO and prostacyclins.[14] Other contributing factors include higher levels of TNF-α,[32] G-CSF, beta subunit HCG and free alpha HCG.[33–35] These cytokines may all contribute to the establishment or progression of the preeclampsia.[36] The treatment of pre-eclampsia includes bed rest, attention to control of blood pressure and careful attention to the growth of the developing fetus. If pre-eclampsia progresses, careful thought should be given to delivery of the fetus depending on the gestational age of the fetus.

Eclampsia

Eclampsia is not an uncommon complication of pregnancy in developing countries. Its hallmark is development of seizures. The treatment of this grave complication includes careful control of blood pressure and immediate delivery of the fetus. Treatment is beyond the scope of this chapter but should definitely include a low threshold for exchange blood transfusion.

Counseling

Sickle cell patients should be adequately counseled about the risk each pregnancy poses but not discouraged from becoming pregnant. The ideal would be for each carrier of the HbS molecule and all sickle cell disease patients to be aware of the risk of having a child with sickle cell disease with each pregnancy. This can only be achieved by the healthcare provider giving adequate genetic counseling before the patient becomes sexually active with constant reinforcement during childbearing years.

Contraception

Any approved form of contraception is acceptable in sickle cell anemia. The dangers and the consequences of unwanted pregnancies outweigh the very small risks of contraceptive devices or drugs and the complications of these methods do not seem to exceed those in the normal population.[37]

Antenatal diagnosis

Antenatal diagnosis is available and is highly accurate. Either chorionic villus sampling or cultured amniotic fluid cells can be used to probe for the presence of heterozygosity or homozygosity for the HbS mutation. Before antenatal diagnosis, the parental mutations must be ascertained and detailed genetic counseling provided as to the risks of bearing an affected fetus, the complications of the procedure and possible causes of error.

Sickle cell trait

Carriers of the HbS gene (sickle cell trait) have few complications of this trait and a normal lifespan. Their blood counts are normal and they have about 40% HbS in their cells, an insufficient amount to cause pathology under most normal circumstances. In Africa, fertility may be increased in women and perhaps men with sickle cell trait.[38] Selected complications of pregnancy may be more frequent in sickle cell trait. The risks for bacteriuria, pyelonephritis, and urinary tract infection may be increased as much as twofold.[39,40] In a prospective study of 162 pregnancies with sickle cell trait and 1,422 controls, the pre-eclampsia rate was doubled in sickle cell trait also.[41] Endometritis occurred more frequently in the sickle cell trait women, and gestational age and birth weights were reduced in their infants. The effect of maternal age on pregnancy outcomes was studied in 157 women with sickle cell trait who were compared with controls by age group. The pregnancy outcomes were similar, but sickle cell trait mothers had offspring whose mean birth weight was almost 200 grams less than that of the controls.[42] Other studies found no differences in mean birth weight, number of low birth-weight infants, five-minute Apgar scores, gestational age, or incidence of delivery complications.[43] Some studies reported increased complications of many types, including prematurity and premature rupture of membranes but they often lacked appropriate controls.[44] While sickle cell trait may be associated with increased risks of certain complications of pregnancy, mainly urinary tract infections, conscientious prenatal care can minimize those risks. Contraception is safe for women with sickle cell trait.

Summary

Obstetricians, working closely with knowledgeable hematologists, should establish strong lines of communication so that care of the pregnant patient with sickle cell disease can be coordinated. A reasonable plan in the primagravida would be to observe the patient carefully and intervene with transfusions only if complications like toxemia, severe anemia, or worsening symptoms of sickle cell disease ensue.[45] Multigravidas have their experience with prior pregnancies to help guide the clinician. Uncomplicated previous pregnancies might be managed like those in primigravidae with transfusions reserved for complications. Individuals who have lost previous pregnancies might benefit from the early use of transfusions aimed at keeping the hemoglobin level above 9 g/dl. Sickle cell complications during pregnancy should be managed as they would be otherwise, with special attention to avoid potentially teratogenic drugs during the first trimester.

Other hemoglobinopathies

Heterozygotes for HbC, HbE and rare structural hemoglobin variants without a clinical phenotype should have no pregnancy-related complications due to the presence of the variant hemoglobin. Homozygous HbC and HbE disease, while associated with characteristic erythrocyte abnormalities and mild anemia, are also unlikely to have complications of pregnancy. In limited studies, fetal wastage did not appear to be in increased. While the mean birthweight of newborns of HbE patients was significantly lower than in HbA patients, the incidence of prematurity was not increased. The incidence of postpartum hemorrhage, preeclampsia, and malaria are not significantly increased in HbE patients but the incidence of abruptio placentae was increased.[46] HbE-β thalassemia should be managed like cases of β thalassemia (see below).

The outcome of pregnancy was recorded for carriers of three high oxygen affinity hemoglobin variants with P_{50} values of 9.5, 9.1, and 12 mm Hg (normal fetal P_{50}, 23 mm Hg). Neither spontaneous abortions nor intrauterine growth retardation was attributable to the presence of high hemoglobin oxygen affinity in the mothers. It was estimated that neither maternal nor fetal polycythemia alone was sufficient to perturb the normal situation and increased uterine and/or fetal blood flow probably provided additional compensation.[47] In other cases of high oxygen affinity hemoglobin, oxygen unloading was reduced, but normal oxygen loading was maintained in the fetus and neither placental abnormalities nor intrauterine growth retardation was present.[48]

While few cases are reported, even when the hemoglobin variant has low oxygen affinity, the outcome of pregnancy may be normal.[47]

Mothers whose hemoglobin is predominantly HbF due to globin gene mutations that allow continued expression of the γ-globin genes probably need no special management during pregnancy despite the high oxygen affinity of HbF.[49]

Little data is available on the management of pregnancy in patients with rare hemoglobinopathies that have a clinical phenotype. If anemia is a feature of these conditions, they might be managed as other cases of anemia in pregnancy.

α thalassemia

Alpha thalassemia results from mutations of the α-globin genes which are present on chromosome 16. Each chromosome 16 carries two α-globin genes that are identical in terms of their amino acid coding regions. Most embryonic, and all fetal and adult hemoglobins contain α-globin chains. Therefore, loss of all α-globin genes usually result in hydrops fetalis due to severe fetal anemia and the inability of that hemoglobin which is present to unload oxygen in the tissues. In general there are two types of mutations that cause α thalassemia; deletional and non-deletional.

Deletional mutations remove one of the two liked α-globin genes are most common and cause either a rightward ($-\alpha^{3.7}$) or leftward ($\alpha^{4.2}$) misalignment of chromosomes and the loss of a single α-globin gene. These mutations are found in 30% of African-Americans and are even more common in Saudi Arabia, Melanesia, Papua New Guinea, Thailand and India.[50,51] Less common deletions remove both α-globin genes from the chromosome and are detailed below. Non-deletional α-globin gene mutations are uncommon and result in mRNA and protein instability and effects on gene transcription, and transcript processing.[52] A major source of diagnostic confusion is the distinction between α thalassemia and iron deficiency anemia. Carriers of α thalassemia with one or two deleted genes ($-\alpha/\alpha\alpha$ and $-/\alpha\alpha$) have mild hypochromic anemia. Pregnancy is unaffected in heterozygotes for these mutations. A helpful distinction is the increase in the soluble transferin receptor which is observed in iron deficiency but not α–thalassemia.

HbH disease

HbH disease (loss of three of four α-globin genes (–/-α) is common in the Middle East, Southeastern Asia, and the Mediterranean. It is very rare in African-Americans. A much smaller number of patients with the phenotype of HbH disease have deletions removing two α-globin genes plus a non-deletional mutation affecting a third α-globin gene (non-deletional HbH disease). This is a more severe disease because the non-deletion mutation is associated with less α-globin protein production. The hallmarks of HbH disease are moderate anemia, hypochromia and marked microcytosis. The excess of β-globin chain in the red cell accumulates as $\beta 4$ tetramers (HbH) which damage the red cell membrane and cause a reduction in red cell survival and ineffective erythropoiesis in the marrow microenvironment. The technique of visualizing subnuclear aggregates using a redox dye (brilliant cresyl blue) has been aided by newer diagnostic techniques based on detection of ζ-globin chains utilizing the polymerase chain reaction or immunocytological assays.[53,54]

Pregnancy

Particular attention should be paid to the pregnant individual with HbH disease with frequent obstetric visits (monthly in the first trimester) and every two weeks thereafter. While there is limited data regarding this disease in pregnancy, the available data show that most patients will have moderate to severe anemia and will require blood transfusions to maintain a healthy placento-uterine circulation. There is a high level of fetal wastage in some published reports indicating that 12% of pregnancies result in miscarriage.[55] Blood transfusion has been recommended for individuals with severe symptomatic anemia or early evidence of fetal compromise by ultrasound.[56]

Hb Bart's ($\gamma 4$) hydrops fetalis

This clinical syndrome develops from complete absence of α-globin chain production. In the developing fetus, it is characterized by generalized edema, hepatosplenomegaly, ascites, pleural and pericardial effusions. Fetal death usually ensues by the 3rd trimester of pregnancy as Hb Portland ($\zeta 2\gamma 2$) levels start to decline. Severe hypoxemia due to anemia and the extremely low P_{50} of Hb Bart's and end-organ failure are present.[57] Chui *et al.* have reviewed the severe α thalassemias.[58,59] The α-globin gene cluster on the short arm of chromosome 16 contains one ζ-globin gene besides two α-globin genes. The ζ-globin gene is the α-like component of Hb Portland. For full expression of the α-globin genes a regulatory region found 40 kb upstream of these genes and called the HS-40 region is required.[60,61]

Common gene deletions causing α thalassemia hydrops fetalis are:

1. South East Asian mutation $(-^{SEA})$ where both α-globin genes are deleted with preservation of the ζ-globin gene.[62] The homozygous state $(-^{SEA}/-^{SEA})$ is the most common cause of Hb Bart's hydrops fetalis. In the United States, the carrier state for this deletion has a frequency of 5.4% in people of Asian descent, 1% are carriers of the Filipino deletion $(-^{FIL})$.[63,64] Other deletions remove both the ζ- and α-globin genes and include:[65,66]
2. Filipino deletion $(-^{FIL})$
3. Thai deletion $(-^{THAI})$
4. $-^{HW}$ deletion recently discovered in a Chinese family.
5. In the Mediterranean region, other deletions have been described and include $(-^{MED})$ and $(\alpha)^{\mathbf{20.5}}$[67,68].

Hydrops fetalis due to α thalassemia has not been reported in Africans or from the Indian subcontinent even though single and double α-globin gene deletions have been described.[50]

Fetal and maternal complications

Fetal death is inevitable in Hb Bart's hydrops due to intra-uterine severe hypoxemia causing multi-organ failure. Anemia is due to ineffective erythropoiesis and shortened red cell life survival.[69] Massive hepatosplenomegaly is caused by extramedullary hematopoiesis and cardiomegaly is caused by high output cardiac failure. As early as the 10th week of pregnancy, anomalies can be detected by ultrasound and include placentomegaly, hydrocephaly, microcephaly, absence of limbs.[70,71,73]

Common maternal complications associated with hydrops fetalis include hypertension, pre-eclampsia, polyhydramnios and antepartum hemorrhage.[72] Other complications include premature labor, disseminated intravascular coagulation, renal failure and congestive heart failure.[74] Because of non-viability of the fetus and these complications, early termination is advisable. Nevertheless, more than one dozen patients with α thalassemia hydrops fetalis survive because of intrauterine transfusions and chronic post-natal transfusion. There is even an example of postnatal "cure" by stem cell allotransplantation. The ethical issues of this practice have yet to be fully explored.

Genetic counseling (for HbH and hydrops fetalis)

Genetic screening is desirable to detect couples at risk for having pregnancies with hydrops fetalis or HbH disease and is imperative in individuals of reproductive age found to have adult HbH disease. Screening for couples at risk includes combinations of blood counts, looking for microcytosis, iron measurements, hemoglobin separation and DNA analysis to detect thalassemia-causing mutations. Properly

Table 13.2 Potential risks of fetuses with inherited α thalassemia syndromes.[59]

α-globin genotypes		Potential risks of fetuses, %	
One parent with Hb H disease	α-globin genotype of the other parent	Hb H disease (–/-α) or (–/$\alpha^{Th}\alpha$)	Homozygous α^0-thalassemia(–/–)
(–/-α) or (–/$\alpha^{Th}\alpha$)	(-α/$\alpha\alpha$) or ($\alpha^{Th}\alpha$/$\alpha\alpha$)	25	Nil
	(-α/-α) or ($\alpha^{Th}\alpha$/-α) or ($\alpha^{Th}\alpha$/$\alpha^{Th}\alpha$)	50	Nil
	(–/$\alpha\alpha$)	25	25
	(–/-α) or (–/$\alpha^{Th}\alpha$)	50	25

done in populations where the risk of α thalassemia is high, this approach should allow early detection of hydropic fetuses and early pregnancy termination. It will also identify fetuses with HbH disease. Table 13.2 stratifies the risk of having an offspring with HbH disease; for example there is a 25% chance of having an affected fetus if the partner is a carrier of a mutation affecting one α-globin gene and a 50% risk with each pregnancy if the partner is homozygous or compound heterozygous for the single α-globin gene.

The following should alert the physician to the risk of a couple having a baby with HbH/hydrops fetalis:

1. A low MCV (<80 fl) on routine screening (iron deficiency and β thalassemia should be excluded).
2. A normal or low Hb A_2 is suggestive of an α thalassemia mutation but by no means definitive. (elevated Hb A_2 suggests β thalassemia).
3. A history of having had a fetus with HbH disease or hydrops fetalis in a family is indicative of an α thalassemia deletion that should prompt thorough DNA analysis in the individual at risk and family members.
4. The presence of HbH inclusion bodies in the red cell.

Prenatal diagnosis

Two options are available for antenatal diagnosis: chorionic villous sampling between 10 and 11 weeks with a 1% risk of a miscarriage; amniocentesis has a 0.5% risk of miscarriage. The material obtained is used to probe for α-globin gene deletions or point mutations, depending on the parental genotype. Recently a novel technique has been described that uses maternal blood that contains fetal nucleated RBCs in early pregnancy.[75,76]

In pregnancies that result in hydropic fetuses the high rate of maternal complications should be actively discussed and early termination advised. There is no reason to terminate pregnancy if the fetus has HbH disease. Patients with HbH disease are usually transfusion-independent and while the spectrum of disease is variable, life is nearly normal for most.

β thalassemia

Beta thalassemia results from a reduction in the production of the β-globin chains, leaving α-globin in excess. The phenotype is very variable and depends partially on the severity of the disease-causing mutation, although as in sickle cell disease, genotype-phenotype correlations are imprecise. Comprising a wide range of disorders with very varying phenotypes, anemia can range from minimal to transfusion-dependent. β thalassemia has recently been reviewed.[77] The management objectives in pregnancy follow the same principles as with patients with sickle cell anemia with certain distinctions. Vasoocclusive crisis is not a feature of thalassemia. A major complication of patients with severe β thalassemia is iron overload resulting from multiple transfusions and increased iron absorption from the gastrointestinal tract. Transfusions are needed to sustain life because of ineffective hematopoiesis and severe anemia. Transfusion-dependency does not appear to hinder the gravid state in patients with β thalassemia as pregnancy can occur, but iron overload affects fertilty.[78,79] In a recent survey of patients with severe thalassemia in North American,[80] in 109 women age 18 years and older, eight had nine term deliveries. None received desferroxamine (Desferal), the major iron chelator, during their pregnancy. During pregnancy, the mean increase in ferritin was 590 ng/ml. In a comparison with non-birthing controls from this same patient group, statistically significant differences in ferritin, diabetes, and hormone replacement treatment were not observed, but the sample size and method of study precluded firm conclusions.

Careful consideration should be given to undertaking pregnancy in patients with severe forms of β thalassemia. It is important to note whether underlying end-organ damage exists prior to conception (or at conception) as this helps with decision to become pregnant and what complications might arise during the course of the pregnancy. Pregnancy in the severe β thalassemias is very high risk because of anemia, iron overload, and iron-induced heart disease.

In the transfusion-dependent individual with β thalassemia, subtle clues to cardiac involvement secondary to iron deposition must be looked for and these may be extraordinarily difficult to detect before the onset of serious arrhythmia and heart failure. Diastolic or systolic dysfunction should be sought by 2-D ECHO cardiography and be part of the initial baseline investigations as the demands of pregnancy have been shown to impair cardiac function.[81] The magnetic relaxation parameter, T2*, measured by magnetic resonance imaging can be a better measure of iron loading in the heart than liver iron content, serum ferritin or transfusion burden. But, its predictive value for heart failure is unknown.[82] During pregnancy, transfusion support should be continued; the decision to continue iron chelation therapy should be weighed against its potential effect on the developing fetus as some animal studies have shown skeletal anomalies. In a study of seven women with β thalassemia major who became pregnant while taking Desferal, all had normal babies.[83,84] If the decision is made to continue chelation during pregnancy, the physician should be alert to the risk of infection with *yersinia* spp. This presents typically with fever, abdominal pain, and diarrhea.[85] Broad spectrum antibiotics should be promptly instituted while iron chelation should be withheld. Stool samples should be sent for *yersinia* spp. culture.

Successful bone marrow transplantation can "cure" β thalassemia but presents another set of problems that affect pregnancy and the ability to conceive. Appropriate sources should be consulted for their management.

Screening and genetic counseling for β thalassemia

Screening and counseling has been shown to decrease the birth of infants with severe β thalassemia when it is carefully applied. The mainstay of this approach relies on the involvement of a willing public, carrier detection, and counseling of individuals who have the disease. Most screening and genetic counseling is based on the Mediterranean model that combines involvement of religious establishments, health-care givers and the state.[86] Screening of populations at risk by combinations of blood counts, HbA_2 measurement and further studies of suspected carriers allows nearly all β thalassemia heterozygotes to be identified. Tables 13.3 and 13.4 are simplified flow charts for β thalassemia carrier detection. Molecular diagnostic techniques have become prevalent in detecting mutations involving the globin genes. Table 13.5 represents commonly employed techniques for the detection of β thalassemia.

β thalassemia heterozygotes

Because of a higher risk of neural tube defects, thalassemia heterozygotes should be given supplemental folic acid. Otherwise, pregnancy in these individuals who are not anemic and do not have clinical phenotype should be uneventful.

Prenatal diagnosis

Couples at risk of bearing affected offspring can be identified by heterozygote screening programs and antenatal diagnosis is available using means similar to

Table 13.3 Flow chart for β thalassemia carrier screening.[86]

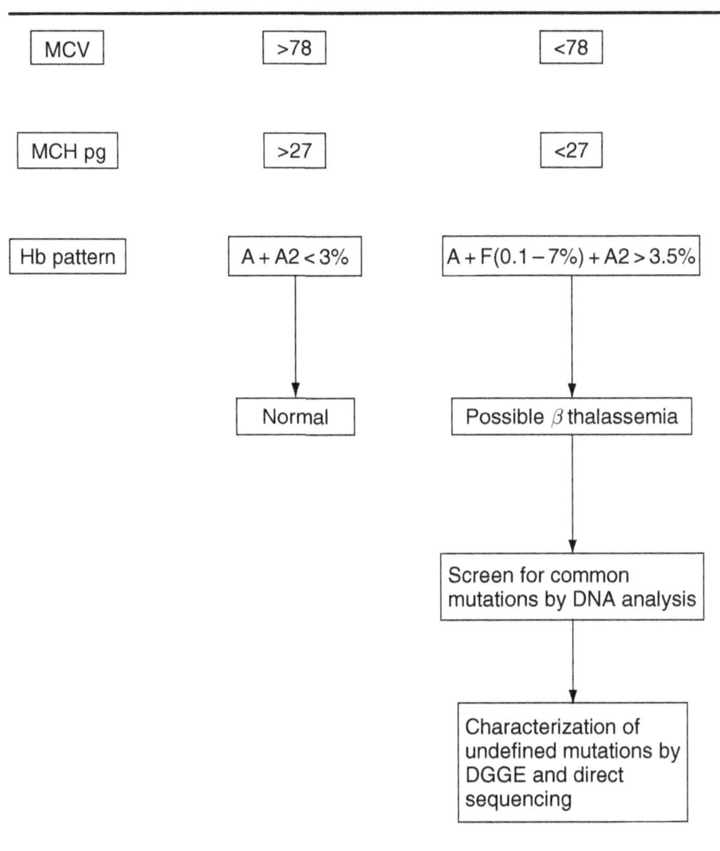

those outlined previously. As β thalassemia is usually due to point mutations in the β-globin gene, antenatal diagnosis centers should know those mutations extant in the population at risk. DNA-based tests then are used to determine the hemoglobin genotype of the fetus.

Conclusions

Hemoglobinopathies and thalassemias are the world's most common genetic disorders. HbS, HbC, HbE and the thalassemias are found in very high frequency in areas of the world where malaria remains and is endemic. Very often, these disorders are found in many combinations so that genetic mixtures of sickle cell disease, α thalassemia, β thalassemia and other inherited erythrocyte disorders occur. Pregnancy in heterozygotes for any of these conditions is usually not

Table 13.4 Flow chart for β thalassemia carrier screening.[86]

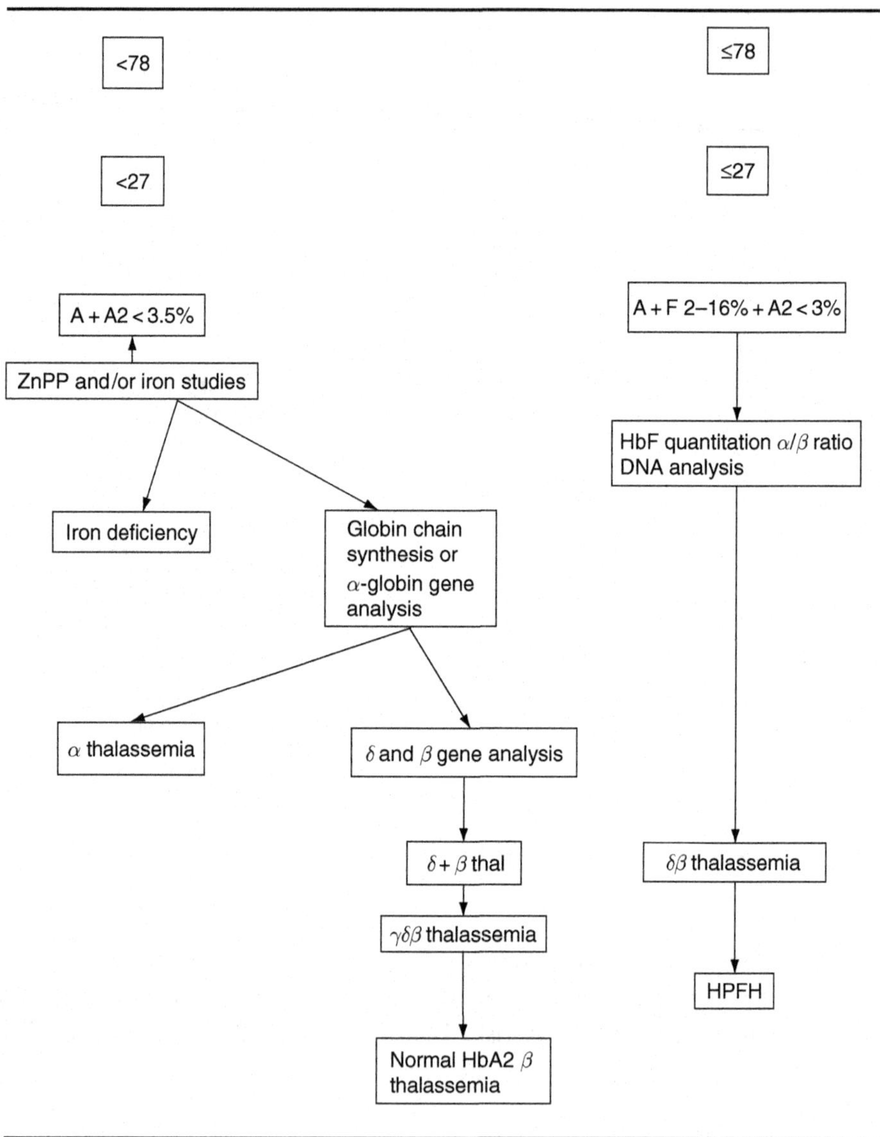

accompanied by complications. When the phenotype of sickle cell disease predominates, its vasoocclusive complications must be attended to and transfusion used judiciously. Well conceived screening programs should alert the physician to the possibilities of fetuses with HbH disease Hb Bart's hydrops fetalis and severe β thalassemia so that antenatal diagnosis can be done.

Table 13.5 PCR-based procedures used for the detection of β thalassemia.[86]

Known mutations
Amplification refractory mutation system (ARMS)[87]
Reverse dot blot analyses
Multiplex primer extension/denaturing high-performance liquid chromatography assay[88]
Oligonucleotide ligation assay[89]
Restriction enzyme digestion[90]
Primer-specific restriction map modification
Unknown mutations
Denaturing gradient gel electrophoresis
Single-strand conformation polymorphism
Protein truncation test[91]
Chemical cleavage method[92]
RNAse cleavage method[93,94]

REFERENCES

1 Steinberg, M. H. Management of sickle cell disease. *N. Engl. J. Med.*, 1999; **340**(13): 1021–30.

2 Embury, S. H. H. R., Mohandas, N., Steinberg, M. H. Sickle Cell Disease: Basic Principles and Clinical Practice, 1st edn. New York, NY: Raven Press; 1994.

3 Brugnara, C. Red cell membrane in sickle cell disease. In Steinberg, M. H. F. D., Nagel, R. L., eds., *Disorders of Hemoglobin: Genetics, Pathophysiology and Clinical Management,* Cambridge: Cambridge University Press; 2001 pp. 550–76.

4 Frempong, K. S. M. Clinical aspects of sickle cell anemia in adults and children. In Steinberg, M. H. F. D., Nagel, R. L., eds., *Disorders of Hemoglobin: Genetics, Pathophysiology and Clinical management*, Cambridge: Cambridge University Press; 2001 pp. 611–710.

5 Fabry, M. E., Nagel, R. L. The effect of deoxygenation on red cell density: significance for the pathophysiology of sickle cell anemia. *Blood*, 1982; **60**(6): 1370–7.

6 Kaul, D. K., Fabry, M. E., Nagel, R. L., The pathophysiology of vascular obstruction in the sickle syndromes. *Blood Rev.*, 1996; **10**(1): 29–44.

7 Nagel, R. The origin of the hemoglobin S gene: Clinical, genetic and anthropological consequences. *Einstein Q Journal Biol. Med.*, 1984; **2**: 53–62.

8 Steinberg, M. H., Pathophysiology of sickle cell disease. *Baillieres Clin. Haematol.*, 1998; **11**(1): 163–84.

9 Conrad, K. P., Benyo, D. F., Westerhausen-Larsen, A., *et al.* Expression of erythropoietin by the human placenta. *Faseb J.*, 1996; **10**(7): 760–8.

10 Perelman, N., Selvaraj, S. K., Batra, S., *et al.* Placenta growth factor activates monocytes and correlates with sickle cell disease severity. *Blood*, 2003; **102**(4): 1506–14.

11 Anyaegbunam, A., Mikhail, M., Axioitis, C., *et al.* Placental histology and placental/fetal weight ratios in pregnant women with sickle cell disease: relationship to pregnancy outcome. *J. Assoc. Acad. Minor Phys.*, 1994; **5**(3): 123–5.

12 Decastel, M., Leborgne-Samuel, Y., Alexandre., L, *et al.* Morphological features of the human umbilical vein in normal, sickle cell trait, and sickle cell disease pregnancies. *Hum. Pathol.*, 1999; **30**(1): 13–20.

13 Kucukcelebi, A., Barmatoski, S. P., Barnhart, M. I. Interactions between vessel wall and perfused sickled erythrocytes: preliminary observations. *Scan. Electron Microsc.*, 1980; **3**: 243–8.

14 Granger, J. P., Alexander, B. T., Llinas, M. T., *et al.* Pathophysiology of preeclampsia: linking placental ischemia/hypoxia with microvascular dysfunction. *Microcirculation*, 2002; **9**(3): 147–60.

15 Alleyne, S. I., Rauseo, R. D., Serjeant, G. R. Sexual development and fertility of Jamaican female patients with homozygous sickle cell disease. *Arch. Intern. Med.*, 1981; **141**(10): 1295–7.

16 Steinberg, M. H. Sickle cell anemia and iron deficiency. *JAMA*, 1982; **248**(17): 2112–3.

17 Steinberg, M. H. The interactions of alpha-thalassemia with hemoglobinopathies. *Hematol. Oncol. Clin. North Am.*, 1991; **5**(3): 453–73.

18 Steinberg, M. H. Modulation of the phenotypic diversity of sickle cell anemia. *Hemoglobin*, 1996; **20**(1): 1–19.

19 Howard, R. J., Tuck, S. M., Pearson, T. C. Pregnancy in sickle cell disease in the UK: results of a multicentre survey of the effect of prophylactic blood transfusion on maternal and fetal outcome. *Br. J. Obstet. Gynaecol.*, 1995; **102**(12): 947–51.

20 Powars, D. R., Sandhu, M., Niland-Weiss, J., *et al.* Pregnancy in sickle cell disease. *Obstet. Gynecol.*, 1986; **67**(2): 217–28.

21 Koshy, M., Burd, L. Management of pregnancy in sickle cell syndromes. *Hematol. Oncol. Clin. North Am.*, 1991; **5**(3): 585–96.

22 Diav-Citrin, O., Hunnisett, L., Sher, G. D., *et al.* Hydroxyurea use during pregnancy: a case report in sickle cell disease and review of the literature. *Am. J. Hematol.*, 1999; **60**(2): 148–50.

23 Mahomed, K. Prophylactic versus selective blood transfusion for sickle cell anaemia during pregnancy. *Cochrane Database Syst. Rev.*, 2000(2): CD000040.

24 El-Shafei, A. M., Kaur Dhaliwal, J., Kaur Sandhu, A., *et al.* Indications for blood transfusion in pregnancy with sickle cell disease. *Aust. N. Z. J. Obstet. Gynaecol.*, 1995; **35**(4): 405–8.

25 Koshy, M., Burd, L., Wallace, D., *et al.* Prophylactic red-cell transfusions in pregnant patients with sickle cell disease. A randomized cooperative study. *N. Engl. J. Med.*, 1988; **319**(22): 1447–52.

26 Vichinsky, E. P., Styles, L. A., Colangelo, L. H., *et al.* Acute chest syndrome in sickle cell disease: clinical presentation and course. Cooperative Study of Sickle Cell Disease. *Blood*, 1997; **89**(5): 1787–92.

27 Ohene-Frempong, K., Weiner, S. J., Sleeper, L. A., *et al.* Cerebrovascular accidents in sickle cell disease: rates and risk factors. *Blood*, 1998; **91**(1): 288–94.

28 Markenson, G. R., Yancey, M. K. Parvovirus B19 infections in pregnancy. *Semin. Perinatol.*, 1998; **22**(4): 309–17.

29 Fairley, C. K., Smoleniec, J. S., Caul, O. E., *et al.* Observational study of effect of intrauterine transfusions on outcome of fetal hydrops after parvovirus B19 infection. *Lancet*, 1995; **346**(8986): 1335–7.

30 Selbing, A., Josefsson, A., Dahle, L. O., *et al.* Parvovirus B19 infection during pregnancy treated with high-dose intravenous gammaglobulin. *Lancet*, 1995; **345**(8950): 660–1.

31 Smith, J. A., Espeland, M., Bellevue, R., *et al.* Pregnancy in sickle cell disease: experience of the Cooperative Study of Sickle Cell Disease. *Obstet. Gynecol.*, 1996; **87**(2): 199–204.

32 Williams, M. A., Farrand, A., Mittendorf, R., *et al.* Maternal second trimester serum tumor necrosis factor-alpha-soluble receptor p55 (sTNFp55) and subsequent risk of preeclampsia. *Am. J. Epidemiol.*, 1999; **149**(4): 323–9.

33 Namiki, A., Hirata, Y., Fukazawa, M., *et al.* Granulocyte-colony stimulating factor stimulates immunoreactive endothelin-1 release from cultured bovine endothelial cells. *Eur. J. Pharmacol.*, 1992; **227**(3): 339–41.

34 Luckas, M., Hawe., J., Meekins, J, *et al.* Second trimester serum free beta human chorionic gonadotrophin levels as a predictor of pre-eclampsia. *Acta Obstet. Gynecol. Scand.*, 1998; **77**(4): 381–4.

35 Huang, S. C., Hsieh, C. Y., Hwang, J. L., *et al.* Free alpha subunit of human chorionic gonadotropin in women with non-trophoblastic tumors. *Taiwan Yi Xue Hui Za Zhi* 1989; **88**(3): 218–25.

36 Polliotti, B. M., Fry, A. G., Saller, D. N., *et al.* Second-trimester maternal serum placental growth factor and vascular endothelial growth factor for predicting severe, early-onset preeclampsia. *Obstet. Gynecol.*, 2003; **101**(6): 1266–74.

37 Serjeant, G. R., Sickle haemoglobin and pregnancy. *BMJ, (Clin. Res. Ed.)*, 1983; **287**(6393): 628–30.

38 Eaton, J. W., Mucha, J. I. Increased fertility in males with the sickle cell trait? *Nature*, 1971; **231**(5303): 456–7.

39 Blattner, P., Dar, H., Nitowsky, H. M. Pregnancy outcome in women with sickle cell trait. *JAMA*, 1977; **238**(13): 1392–4.

40 Sears, D. A. The morbidity of sickle cell trait: a review of the literature. *Am. J. Med.*, 1978; **64**(6): 1021–36.

41 Larrabee, K. D., Monga, M. Women with sickle cell trait are at increased risk for preeclampsia. *Am. J. Obstet. Gynecol.*, 1997; **177**(2): 425–8.

42 Hoff, C., Wertelecki, W., Dutt, J., *et al.* Sickle cell trait, maternal age and pregnancy outcome in primiparous women. *Hum. Biol.*, 1983; **55**(4): 763–70.

43 Kramer, M. S., Rooks, Y., Pearson, H. A. Growth and development in children with sickle-cell trait. A prospective study of matched pairs. *N. Engl. J. Med.*, 1978; **299**(13): 686–9.

44 Rimer, B. A. Sickle-cell trait and pregnancy: A review of a community hospital experience. *Am. J. Obstet. Gynecol.*, 1975; **123**(1): 6–11.

45 Koshy, M., Chisum, D., Burd, L., *et al.* Management of sickle cell anemia and pregnancy. *J. Clin. Apheresis*, 1991; **6**(4): 230–3.

46 Ong, H. C. Maternal and fetal outcome associated with hemoglobin E trait and hemoglobin E disease. *Obstet. Gynecol.*, 1975; **45**(6): 672–4.

47 Charache, S., Catalano, P., Burns, S., *et al.* Pregnancy in carriers of high-affinity hemoglobins. *Blood*, 1985; **65**(3): 713–18.

48 Bard, H., Rosenberg, A., Huisman, T. H. Hemoglobinopathies affecting maternal–fetal oxygen gradient during pregnancy: molecular, biochemical and clinical studies. *Am. J. Perinatol.*, 1998; **15**(6): 389–93.

49 Kaeda, J. S., Prasad, K., Howard, R. J., *et al.* Management of pregnancy when maternal blood has a very high level of fetal haemoglobin. *Br. J. Haematol.*, 1994; **88**(2): 432–4.

50 Dozy, A. M., Kan, Y. W., Embury, S. H., *et al.* Alpha-globin gene organisation in blacks precludes the severe form of alpha-thalassaemia. *Nature*, 1979; **280**(5723): 605–7.

51 Weatherall, D. J., Clegg, J. B. Inherited haemoglobin disorders: an increasing global health problem. *Bull. World Health Organ.*, 2001; **79**(8): 704–12.

52 Russell, J., Liebhaber, S. A. *Advances in Genome Biology*, In Verma, R., ed., Greenwich, CT: JAI Press Inc; 1992.

53 Chan, L. C., So, J. C., Chui, D. H. Comparison of haemoglobin H inclusion bodies with embryonic zeta globin in screening for alpha thalassaemia. *J. Clin. Pathol.*, 1995; **48**(9): 861–4.

54 Chan, A. Y., So, C. K., Chan, L. C. Comparison of the HbH inclusion test and a PCR test in routine screening for alpha thalassaemia in Hong Kong. *J. Clin. Pathol.*, 1996; **49**(5): 411–13.

55 Galanello, R., Aru, B., Dessi, C., *et al.* HbH disease in Sardinia: molecular, hematological and clinical aspects. *Acta Haematol.*, 1992; **88**(1): 1–6.

56 Ong, H. C., White, J. C., Sinnathuray, T. A. Haemoglobin H disease and pregnancy in a Malaysian woman. *Acta Haematol.*, 1977; **58**(4): 229–33.

57 Steinberg, M. H. F. D., Nagel, R. L. Clinical and laboratory features of the alpha thalassemia syndromes. In Steinberg, M. H. F. D., Nagel, R. L., eds., *Disorders of Hemoglobin: Genetics, Pathophysiology, and Clinical Management.* Cambridge: Cambridge University Press; 2001: pp. 431–69.

58 Chui, D. H., Waye, J. S. Hydrops fetalis caused by alpha-thalassemia: an emerging health care problem. *Blood*, 1998; **91**(7): 2213–22.

59 Chui, D. H., Fucharoen, S., Chan, V. Hemoglobin H disease: not necessarily a benign disorder. *Blood*, 2003; **101**(3): 791–800.

60 Higgs, D. R., Wood, W. G., Jarman, A. P., *et al.* A major positive regulatory region located far upstream of the human alpha-globin gene locus. *Genes Dev.*, 1990; **4**(9): 1588–601.

61 Vyas, P., Vickers, M. A., Simmons, D. L., *et al.* Cis-acting sequences regulating expression of the human alpha-globin cluster lie within constitutively open chromatin. *Cell*, 1992; **69**(5): 781–93.

62 Higgs, D. R. Alpha-thalassaemia. *Baillieres Clin. Haematol.*, 1993; **6**(1): 117–50.

63 Monzon, C. M., Fairbanks, V. F., Burgert, E. O., Jr., *et al.* Hematologic genetic disorders among Southeast Asian refugees. *Am. J. Hematol.*, 1985; **19**(1): 27–36.

64 Hofgartner, W. T., West Keefe, S. F., Tait, J. F. Frequency of deletional alpha-thalassemia genotypes in a predominantly Asian-American population. *Am. J. Clin Pathol.*, 1997; **107**(5): 576–81.

65 Fischel-Ghodsian, N., Vickers, M. A., Seip, M., *et al.* Characterization of two deletions that remove the entire human zeta-alpha globin gene complex (- -THAI and - -FIL). *Br. J. Haematol.*, 1988; **70**(2): 233–8.

66 Waye, J. S., Eng, B., Chui, D. H. Identification of an extensive zeta-alpha globin gene deletion in a Chinese individual. *Br. J. Haematol.*, 1992; **80**(3): 378–80.

67 Sophocleous, T., Higgs, D. R., Aldridge, B., *et al.* The molecular basis for the haemoglobin Bart's hydrops fetalis syndrome in Cyprus. *Br. J. Haematol.*, 1981; **47**(1): 153–6.

68 Nicholls, R. D., Higgs, D. R., Clegg, J. B., *et al.* Alpha zero-thalassemia due to recombination between the alpha 1-globin gene and an AluI repeat. *Blood*, 1985; **65**(6): 1434–8.

69 Weatherall, D. J. The thalassemias. In Stamatoyannopoulos, G. M. P., Varmus, H., eds., *The Molecular Basis of Blood Diseases*, Toronto: Saunders; 1994.

70 Chitayat, D., Silver, M. M., O'Brien, K., *et al.* Limb defects in homozygous alpha-thalassemia: report of three cases. *Am. J. Med. Genet.*, 1997; **68**(2): 162–7.

71 Abuelo, D. N., Forman, E. N., Rubin, L. P. Limb defects and congenital anomalies of the genitalia in an infant with homozygous alpha-thalassemia. *Am. J. Med. Genet.*, 1997; **68**(2): 158–61.

72 Liang, S. T., Wong, V. C., So, W. W., *et al.* Homozygous alpha-thalassaemia: clinical presentation, diagnosis and management. A review of 46 cases. *Br. J. Obstet. Gynaecol.*, 1985; **92**(7): 680–4.

73 Ghosh, A., Tang, M. H., Lam, Y. H., *et al.* Ultrasound measurement of placental thickness to detect pregnancies affected by homozygous alpha-thalassaemia-1. *Lancet*, 1994; **344**(8928): 988–9.

74 Mehr, D. S., Rector, J. T., Ngo, K. Y. Pathological case of the month. Hydrops fetalis secondary to homozygous alpha-thalassemia-1 (Bart's hemoglobinopathy). *Arch. Pediatr. Adolesc. Med.*, 1994; **148**(12): 1313–14.

75 Cheung, M. C., Goldberg, J. D., Kan, Y. W. Prenatal diagnosis of sickle cell anaemia and thalassaemia by analysis of fetal cells in maternal blood. *Nat. Genet.*, 1996; **14**(3): 264–8.

76 Williamson, B. Towards non-invasive prenatal diagnosis. *Nat. Genet.*, 1996; **14**(3): 239–40.

77 Rachmilewitz, E. A. S. S. Pathophysiology of beta thalassemia. In Steinberg, M. H. F. D., Nagel, R. L., eds., *Disorders of Hemoglobin: Genetics, Pathophysiology and Clinical Management*, Cambridge: Cambridge University Press; 2001: pp. 233–51.

78 Seracchioli, R., Porcu, E., Colombi, C., *et al.* Transfusion-dependent homozygous beta-thalassaemia major: successful twin pregnancy following in-vitro fertilization and tubal embryo transfer. *Hum. Reprod.*, 1994; **9**(10): 1964–5.

79 Tampakoudis, P., Tsatalas, C., Mamopoulos, M., *et al.* Transfusion-dependent homozygous beta-thalassaemia major: successful pregnancy in five cases. *Eur. J. Obstet. Gynecol. Reprod. Biol.*, 1997; **74**(2): 127–31.

80 Cunningham, M. J. M. E., Muraca, G., Neufeld, E. J. Successful pregnancy in thalassemia major women in the thalassemia clinical research network. In *American Society of Hematology*; 2003: San-Diego, CA.

81 Perniola, R., Magliari, F., Rosatelli, M. C., *et al.* High-risk pregnancy in beta-thalassemia major women. Report of three cases. *Gynecol. Obstet. Invest.*, 2000; **49**(2): 137–9.

82 Wood, J. C. G. N., Carson, S., Tyszka, J., *et al.* Predictors of abnormal myocardial function and T2* in children and young adults with thalassemia major. Session type: Poster session 64-I. In *American Society of Hematology*; 2003; San Diego, CA.

83 Palagiano, A., Pace, L., Pregnancy in women with thalassaemia. *Minerva Ginecol.*, 2001; **53**(3): 203–7.

84 Singer, S. T., Vichinsky, E. P. Deferoxamine treatment during pregnancy: is it harmful? *Am. J. Hematol.*, 1999; **60**(1): 24–6.

85 Adamkiewicz, T. V., Berkovitch, M., Krishnan, C., *et al.* Infection due to Yersinia enterocolitica in a series of patients with beta-thalassemia: incidence and predisposing factors. *Clin. Infect. Dis.*, 1998; **27**(6): 1362–6.

86 Cao, A. R. M., Eckman, J. R. Prenatal diagnosis and screening for thalassemia and sickle cell disease. In Steinberg, M. H. F. D., Nagel, R. L., eds., *Disorders of Hemoglobin: Genetics, Pathophysiology, and Clinical Management*, Cambridge: Cambridge University Press; 2001: pp. 958–78.

87 Agarwal, S., Gupta, A., Gupta, U. R., *et al.* Prenatal diagnosis in beta-thalassemia: an Indian experience. *Fetal Diagn. Ther.*, 2003; **18**(5): 328–32.

88 Wu, G., Hua, L., Zhu, J., *et al.* Rapid, accurate genotyping of beta-thalassaemia mutations using a novel multiplex primer extension/denaturing high-performance liquid chromatography assay. *Br. J. Haematol.*, 2003; **122**(2): 311–16.

89 Chen, X., Livak, K. J., Kwok, P. Y. A homogeneous, ligase-mediated DNA diagnostic test. *Genome Res.*, 1998; **8**(5): 549–56.

90 Chang, J. G., Chen, P. H., Chiou, S. S., *et al.* Rapid diagnosis of beta-thalassemia mutations in Chinese by naturally and amplified created restriction sites. *Blood*, 1992; **80**(8): 2092–6.

91 Powell, S. M. Direct analysis for familial adenomatous polyposis mutations. *Mol. Biotechnol.*, 2002; **20**(2): 197–207.

92 Setianingsih, I. I., Williamson, R., Marzuk, S., *et al.* Molecular basis of beta-thalassemia in Indonesia: Application to prenatal diagnosis. *Mol. Diagn.*, 1998; **3**(1): 11–9.

93 Myers, R. M., Larin, Z., Maniatis, T., Detection of single base substitutions by ribonuclease cleavage at mismatches in RNA:DNA duplexes. *Science*, 1985; **230**(4731): 1242–6.

94 Hiyama, K., Kodaira, M., Satoh, C., Detection of deletions, insertions and single nucleotide substitutions in cloned beta-globin genes and new polymorphic nucleotide substitutions in beta-globin genes in a Japanese population using ribonuclease cleavage at mismatches in RNA:DNA duplexes. *Mutat. Res.*, 1990; **231**(2): 219–31.

95 Platt, O. S., Brambilla, D. J., Rosse, W. F., *et al.* Mortality in sickle cell disease. Life expectancy and risk factors for early death. *N. Engl. J. Med.*, 1994; **330**: 1639–44.

96 Gladwin, M. T., Sachdev, V., Jison, M. L., *et al.* Pulmonary hypertension as a risk factor for death in patients with sickle cell disease. *N. Engl. J. Med.*, 2004; **350**: 886–95.

97 Steinberg, M. H., Barton, F., Castro, O., *et al.* Effect of hydroxyurea on mortality and morbidity in adult sickle cell anemia: risks and benefits up to 9 years of treatment. *JAMA*, 2003; **289**: 1645–51.

98 Sun, P. M., Wilburn, W., Raynor, B. D., *et al.* Sickle cell disease in pregnancy: 20 years at Grady Memorial Hospital, Atlanta, GA. *Am. J. Obstet. Gynecol.*, 2001; **184**(6): 1127–30.

14

Genetic counseling and prenatal diagnosis

Karen Heller, M.S., C.G.C.[1] and Robyn Horsager, M.D.[2]

[1]Faculty Associate, Department of Pathology, University of Texas Southwestern Medical Center at Dallas, Texas, USA
[2]Associate Professor, Division of Maternal Fetal Medicine, Department of Obstetrics and Gynecology, University of Texas Southwestern Medical Center at Dallas, Texas, USA

The purpose of this chapter is to discuss genetic counseling and prenatal diagnosis as it pertains to hematological complications in obstetrics and gynecology. The reader should be aware that, as with any text in a rapidly advancing field, some issues discussed might be outdated or new testing may have become available by the time of publication.

Many of the hematological conditions discussed in this book are hereditary (Table 14.1) and the specific nature of each disorder is discussed in the relevant chapter. It is the responsibility of the practitioner to explain to his or her patient, when applicable, the genetic nature of their condition. The practitioner should point out the increased risk for family members to be similarly affected, and encourage the patient to share this information. In many instances, this can be accomplished in the office of the treating physician. However, when patients have additional questions or concerns or difficulty comprehending or dealing with the genetic information, or there is a question regarding genetic testing, referral to a professional genetic counselor is appropriate.

In this chapter, we will first discuss genetic counseling and prenatal diagnosis in general. This will be followed by a discussion about the specific management of the following conditions:

1. Thrombophilia
2. Hemophilia
3. Hemoglobinopathies
4. Von Willebrand disease
5. Rh isoimmunization

Hematological Complications in Obstetrics, Pregnancy, and Gynecology, ed. R. L. Bick *et al.* Published by Cambridge University Press.

Table 14.1 A sampling of hematologic diseases and their causative genes.

Disease	Gene	Chromosomal location	Inheritance	Clinical DNA testing*
Thrombophilia	Antithrombin III	1q	AD/multi	No
	Factor V	1q	AD/multi	Yes
	Prothrombin	11p	AD/multi	Yes
	Protein C	2q	AD/ multi	No
	Protein S	3p	AD/multi	Yes
	MTHFR	1p	AD/multi	Yes
Hemophilia	Factor VIII	Xq	XLR	Yes
	Factor IX	Xq	XLR	Yes
Hgb S/C	β-globin	11p	AR	Yes
β thalassemia	β-globin	11p	minor-AD	Yes
			major-AR	Yes
α thalassemia	α-globin	16p	AD	Yes
			Hgb Bart's-AR	Yes
Von Willebrand	VW factor	12p	AD/AR/XLR	Yes

Abbreviations: AD = autosomal dominant; AR = autosomal recessive; XLR = X-linked recessive; multi = multifactorial.

*Clinical DNA testing may be available only for certain mutations or limited to linkage analysis. An updated listing of available DNA tests is maintained at genetests.org.

Genetic counselors and genetic counseling

The National Society of Genetic Counselors has about 2,000 members, as of 2003. A directory of genetic counselors is available at the website, www.nsgc.org. Genetic counselors are Masters-level, board certified, health professionals trained in medical genetics and counseling. Some states have licensing requirements for genetic counselors. Construction of the pedigree, using a standardized format,[1] is the cornerstone of the genetic evaluation. Using this information, genetic counselors analyze the inheritance pattern of a particular condition in a family, establish which relatives are at increased risk, discuss the condition and its inheritance with the patient and members of her family, explain the benefits and limitations of genetic testing, coordinate testing with appropriate laboratories and explain the results of such testing. Genetic counselors also provide supportive counseling to families, and make referrals to community support services.

The American Society of Human Genetics has defined genetic counseling as "a communication process which deals with the human problems associated with the occurrence, or the risk of occurrence, of a genetic disorder in the family. This process involves an attempt by one or more appropriately trained persons to help the individual or family to (1) comprehend the medical facts, including the diagnosis, probable course of the disorder, and the available management; (2) appreciate the way heredity contributes to the disorder, and the risk of recurrence in specified relatives; (3) understand the alternatives for dealing with the risk of occurrence; (4) choose the course of action which seems to them appropriate in view of their risk, their family goals, and their ethical and religious standards, to act in accordance with that decision; and (5) to make the best possible adjustment to the disorder in an affected family member and/or the risk of recurrence of that disorder."[2]

We can review each component of the above process in the context of hematological complications in obstetrics and gynecology:

(1) "comprehend the medical facts"

Genetic counselors educate patients about their diagnosis and review treatment plans and prognosis. Education of the patient at her educational level will contribute to patient satisfaction and ensure better compliance with treatment protocols.

(2) "appreciate the way heredity contributes to the disorder, and the risk of recurrence in specified relatives"

The crux of genetic counseling involves determining the inheritance pattern of the particular condition, and based on this predicting the recurrence risk for various relatives. Essential to this process is knowledge of the underlying disorder in the patient. For example, Factor VIII and Factor IX deficiencies are inherited as X-linked traits. However, von Willebrand disease, usually autosomal dominant, can also be autosomal recessive or X-linked. The inheritance pattern for all known genetic disorders is referenced in Victor McKusick's Mendelian Inheritance in Man[3] and the online version is referred to as Online Mendelian Inheritance in Man (OMIM), found at http://www.ncbi.nlm.nih.gov/omim.[4] When different inheritance mechanisms are possible, the pedigree may provide a clue about the likely pattern in that particular family. In some cases, DNA analysis might confirm the type of inheritance, by demonstrating the presence of either one or two mutated genes, on an autosome or on the X-chromosome.

Affected siblings with unaffected parents suggest **autosomal recessive** inheritance (Figure 14.1a). This would be suspected particularly if the parents were consanguineous. Autosomal recessive inheritance can be confirmed by demonstrating that the affected individual inherited a mutation from one unaffected parent and the same or a different mutation in the corresponding gene from the other unaffected parent. Each sibling of the affected individual would have a 25% chance of also inheriting that disorder. However, children of the affected individual could

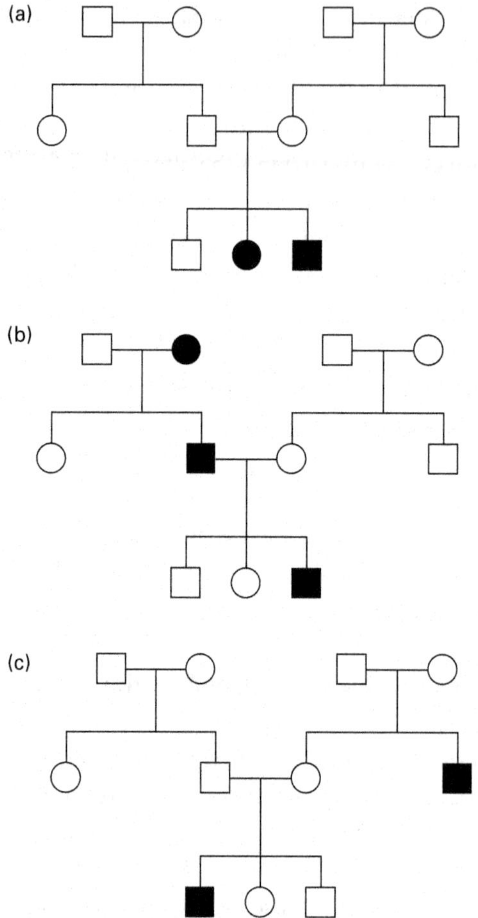

Figure 14.1 Typical pedigrees for (a) autosomal recessive, (b) autosomal dominant, and (c) X-linked recessive conditions.

only be affected if their other parent carried a mutation in the same gene. This would be more likely if the couple is related, if there is a family history of the same condition or if the mutation for the condition is particularly common. If both parents are affected by the same disorder, all offspring would also be affected. The various hemoglobinopathies are examples of autosomal recessive conditions.

A condition occurring in successive generations of a pedigree is likely to be **autosomal dominant** (Figure 14.1b). However, variable expression (that is, a spectrum of disease state from mild to severe) between relatives is typical of autosomal dominant conditions, making pedigree analysis sometimes unreliable. Autosomal dominant inheritance can be confirmed by documenting the presence of a single mutation passed from affected parent to affected child. Each first-degree relative (parent, sibling or child) of a patient would have a 50% chance of being affected with the condition in question. However, as discussed above, the severity may be unpredictable. When an individual is truly the first person in the family affected with an autosomal dominant condition, the condition is the result of a new mutation.

Affected males related through unaffected (or mildly affected) females would suggest **X-linked inheritance** (Figure 14.1c), although a new mutation can result in the presence of a single affected male in the family. Since a father never passes his X chromosome to his sons, observation of male-to-male transmission of a condition would exclude X-linked inheritance. Molecular confirmation of X-linked inheritance involves demonstrating a mutation in a gene on the X chromosome. If the mother of the affected male is determined to be a carrier (based on either the pedigree or testing), then 50% of her sons will be predicted to be affected. Each daughter will have a 50% chance of being a carrier. All daughters of affected males would be "obligate carriers", but the condition could not be passed from father to son. Hemophilia A and B are examples of X-linked conditions.

(3) "understand the alternatives for dealing with the risk of occurrence"

This component of genetic counseling refers to the education of patients regarding options for testing (themselves, their pregnancies, or their children). The benefit of a diagnosis, especially prenatal diagnosis, may be uncertain so patients need to be encouraged to analyze their reasons for pursuing such testing. Invasive prenatal diagnosis is not without risk to the pregnancy so there should be sufficient benefit to outweigh the risk. In some instances, prenatal diagnosis may provide assurance that the fetus is unaffected, and no further evaluation or treatment is needed. In other instances, a prenatal diagnosis may permit prenatal or early neonatal treatment, psychological preparation by the family of an affected fetus, expectant management of a pregnancy or the option for pregnancy termination. When a couple is determined to be at increased risk for having a child with a serious genetic disorder, genetic counseling should include an exploration of various reproductive options. These may encompass pregnancy avoidance, adoption, sperm or oocyte donation, fetal testing, preimplantation genetic diagnosis and pregnancy termination. Ideally, genetic counseling should take place prior to initiation of pregnancy, so that the full range of options can be made available.

(4) "choose the course of action which seems to them appropriate ..."

Patients may be faced with a variety of difficult choices. Decisions about genetic testing, and particularly prenatal testing, are personal and many individuals have strong feelings either for or against testing. In many cases, individuals have not thought through the ramifications of obtaining genetic information.

In assisting a patient to choose the option suitable for them, patient autonomy must be respected and personal factors such as religion and culture should be considered. On the other hand, it may be tempting to make assumptions about the likely choice one would expect from a patient with a particular cultural background. Ideally, genetic counseling should be "non-directive"; the information presented should be balanced, and the counselee should be encouraged to make an autonomous decision without imposition of the counselor's values.[5,6,7]

(5) "to make the best possible adjustment ..."

Supportive counseling and referral to community resources are an integral part of the genetic counseling process. This enables patients to cope with the presence of or risk of genetic conditions.

Prenatal diagnosis

In order to make prenatal diagnosis and other reproductive options available to patients with heritable conditions, they should be referred for genetic counseling prior to pregnancy. Before offering prenatal diagnosis, the impact of a particular condition on a fetus and the availability of prenatal testing must be decided. Making these determinations takes time. In order to offer the widest possible range of options, the process is best undertaken without the time constraints an ongoing pregnancy presents. Most states in this country limit legal termination of pregnancy to the first 24 weeks of gestation. Thus, for patients to have the option of pregnancy termination in the event of diagnosis of a disease with significant morbidity or mortality, final test results must be available prior to this gestational age.

Chromosome analysis of prenatal samples can typically be accomplished in one to two weeks, but DNA testing may depend on a particular technology in which results are not available for several weeks. In addition, DNA testing often requires cells cultured from amniotic fluid or chorionic villi; this will add about 7–14 days to the length of time the test requires.

Prenatal diagnosis is usually considered when the following five tenets can be met (Table 14.2):

1. There is significant risk for the condition in question to occur in the offspring. "Significant" is often defined as greater than 0.5% (the approximate risk of pregnancy loss secondary to a midtrimester amniocentesis). However, the patient must make the decision about whether the risk is significant enough to warrant invasive testing, because the two endpoints (an affected child or a pregnancy loss) may not be equivalent in her mind. Thus, personal factors will influence her decision.

Table 14.2 Prerequisites for prenatal diagnosis.

1. There is significant risk for the condition to occur.
2. The condition has significant morbidity or mortality, particularly during childhood.
3. A suitable assay is available.
4. The test has predictive power.
5. Prenatal knowledge of the diagnosis is beneficial.

2. The condition in question has significant morbidity or mortality. Here too, a judgment is made on the part of the patient. The decision is particularly difficult for conditions of adult onset, since treatment advances cannot be predicted decades in advance. There are ethical imperatives against genetic testing of children unless there is immediate benefit to the child.[8,9]
3. A test is available for the condition in question, and is reproducible on the type of tissue or cells obtained.
4. The test in question has sufficient predictive power; the degree of mortality or morbidity can be predicted by the test result. Some mutations have reduced penetrance, making prenatal predictions impossible. Type 1 Gaucher disease and hemochromatosis are two examples where an individual with two mutated genes may never develop symptoms of the disease.[10,11,12] Performing prenatal diagnosis under these circumstances is of limited benefit.
5. Knowledge of the fetal status is beneficial to the patient or physicians caring for the patient or neonate. The patient may choose to terminate a pregnancy affected with a serious disorder or she may benefit from preparing for the birth of an affected child. There may also be an opportunity for optimal management of the pregnancy, delivery or neonatal care, as in the case of a fetus affected with severe hemophilia at risk for intracranial hemorrhage.

The most commonly utilized procedures of prenatal diagnosis are amniocentesis, followed by chorionic villus sampling and percutaneous umbilical blood sampling. Preimplantation genetic diagnosis (PGD) is also available for a number of conditions.

Amniocentesis is the most widely used technique for prenatal diagnosis. Under real-time ultrasound visualization, a needle is passed through the maternal abdominal wall, uterine wall and amniotic membranes, and amniotic fluid is aspirated. The volume of amniotic fluid removed is dependent on what testing is performed. Various biochemical tests can be performed on the amniotic fluid supernatant. Cells from the fluid, overwhelmingly fetal epithelial cells, can be examined directly or cultured, and used for karyotype analysis as well as DNA testing. Risks of infection or maternal hemorrhage are minimal; the primary risk is for loss of the pregnancy, or early delivery in the case of a later procedure. The risk for procedure-related loss is generally quoted as about 0.3–0.5% when the procedure is performed beyond 15 weeks of pregnancy. The procedure has been performed as early as 11 weeks' gestation, but the rates of pregnancy loss and fetal complications are higher, the sample volume must be smaller, and the cells are less likely to grow in culture.

Chorionic villus sampling (CVS) is performed early in pregnancy (generally around 11–12 weeks), but as there are fewer practitioners skilled in the procedure, it is not as widely available as amniocentesis. Under the guidance of real-time ultrasound, 5–20 mg of chorionic villi are aspirated, depending on the testing required. The procedure can be performed either transabdominally using a needle (similar to amniocentesis) or transcervically with a catheter. The method employed will depend on the position of the placenta and the preference of the clinician. Fetal loss rate following CVS is generally felt to be somewhat higher than that for amniocentesis, in the range of 0.5–1%. Chorionic villus sampling also has a higher rate of maternal cell contamination. Ambiguous cytogenetic findings, such as mosaicism limited to the placenta, may also be problematic.[13] Table 14.3 summarizes the primary differences between CVS and amniocentesis. Most DNA tests can be performed on either amniocytes or chorionic villi, so the choice of procedure will usually depend on its availability and the preference of the patient. Some patients prefer the earlier diagnosis afforded by CVS, despite the higher procedure-related risk, while other patients would prefer to wait for an amniocentesis after 15 weeks of gestation.

Percutaneous umbilical blood sampling (PUBS) or cordocentesis may be employed as a means of prenatal diagnosis when a fetal blood sample is needed for analysis. The technique is similar to amniocentesis, but technically more challenging as the needle must enter an umbilical vessel to obtain a sample of fetal blood. Percutaneous umbilical blood sampling may be used if a rapid karyotype is needed or occasionally to confirm an amniocentesis finding. Percutaneous umbilical blood sampling is also used in the management of fetal hemolytic disease, secondary to maternal isoimmunization. In addition, PUBS may be used if no DNA test is available but fetal blood testing would be diagnostic, for example in some forms of severe von Willebrand disease.[14,15]

Preimplantation genetic diagnosis (PGD) involves in vitro fertilization, testing the embryo for a particular condition, and then attempting pregnancy with only unaffected embryos. The test involved needs to be reproducible as a one-cell assay. Preimplantation genetic diagnosis can be accomplished by sampling the maternal first and second polar bodies (providing indirect evidence of the genetic make-up of the oocyte) or by biopsy of the blastomere. Blastomere biopsy is achieved by removing one or two cells from the 8–10 cell embryo, about 3 days

Table 14.3 Comparison between chorionic villus sampling (CVS) and amniocentesis.

Chorionic villus sampling (CVS)	Amniocentesis
1. Usually performed 10–12 wks after last menstrual period	Usually performed 15–18 weeks after last menstrual period
2. Transcervical and transabdominal methods	Transabdominal method
3. Sample removed from chorionic villi	Sample of amniotic fluid removed
4. Chromosome analysis, DNA and biochemical tests possible	Chromosome analysis, DNA and biochemical tests possible
5. No detection of neural tube defects	90–98% detection of open neural tube defects
6. First trimester ultrasound provides limited anatomical information	Mid-trimester ultrasound provides screen for anatomical anomalies
7. 1 in 100 to 1 in 200 miscarriage risk	1 in 200 to 1 in 300 miscarriage risk
8. Risk for limb defects may be slightly increased, especially if performed before 9 weeks	Risk for limb defects not increased when performed after 15 weeks
9. Repeat CVS or amniocentesis may be needed because of ambiguous chromosome results	Ambiguous results less likely
10. Procedure is technically more difficult and not widely available	More physicians are trained to perform amniocentesis

post-fertilization. The cell can be tested for the disease in question or gender determination can be accomplished using fluorescence *in situ* hybridization (FISH) for the sex chromosomes. Knowledge of the fetal sex may be especially useful in the presence of an X-linked condition. After testing, only unaffected embryos or embryos of a certain gender are selected for implantation. Preimplantation genetic diagnosis will almost double the cost of the IVF procedure and is not widely available. Rates of successful pregnancy appear to be similar to that for IVF without PGD.

Application to specific disorders

1. Thrombophilia

Thrombophilia is a broad term describing a myriad of conditions that predispose an individual to thrombosis. Numerous genetic and environmental factors have been implicated. As discussed in a previous chapter, mutations in various genes have been associated with thrombophilia. These include Factor V, prothrombin, antithrombin III, protein C, protein S and methylenetetrahydrofolate reductase (MTHFR) (Table 14.1). Undoubtedly mutations in other factors will be discovered. Each of these mutations is considered to be a risk factor for venous thromboembolism. The presence of additional mutations or environmental conditions is generally required to provoke disease symptoms. As such, thrombophilia is understood to be a multifactorial condition.

The appropriate work-up of individuals suspected of having inherited thrombophilia is also discussed in a previous chapter. Patients are usually tested for several traits, as the risk for thrombosis is compounded by the presence of multiple factors. Special attention should be paid to the pedigree.[16] A positive family history of thrombosis, bleeding or pregnancy loss suggests a possible genetic basis for a thrombotic event in a patient. The pedigree also identifies relatives who may be at risk for similar mutations. Although thrombophilia has a multifactorial basis, the deficiency of each protein is inherited in an autosomal dominant fashion. Therefore, each of the patient's first-degree relatives (parents, siblings or children) would be at 50% risk for carrying the same trait. The patient should be advised to notify her relatives, who may consider genetic testing for the relevant mutation if this information would benefit their medical care. A patient undergoing testing should understand that a positive test result in itself may not affect her health, but it may alter therapeutic approaches, (for example, the use of antithrombotic prophylaxis in high risk situations) as well as lead to further testing for other potential risk factors.[17] The appropriateness of testing (that is, whether the results will impact the medical management of the individual) should be considered.[16] Particularly in the case of an asymptomatic individual considering testing, the possibility of insurance and/or job discrimination should be discussed. However concerns about discrimination appear to be largely theoretical at this time[18] and legal protections are being created.[19,20]

The benefit of testing children for these mutations is not clear at present. The American College of Medical Genetics and the National Society of Genetic Counselors have recommended against genetic testing of minors, unless there is medical benefit to the child during childhood.[8,9] However, the above mutations have been associated with pediatric thrombosis,[21] so a family history of thromboembolic events in children may warrant testing of related children. Because thrombophilias have a multifactorial etiology, predictions of disease severity from prenatal diagnosis would be problematic. Thus, prenatal diagnosis is usually not indicated for these mutations.[22]

2. Hemophilia

Factors VIII and IX are produced by two different genes, both on the X chromosome. Hemophilia A (deficiency of Factor VIII) and hemophilia B (deficiency of

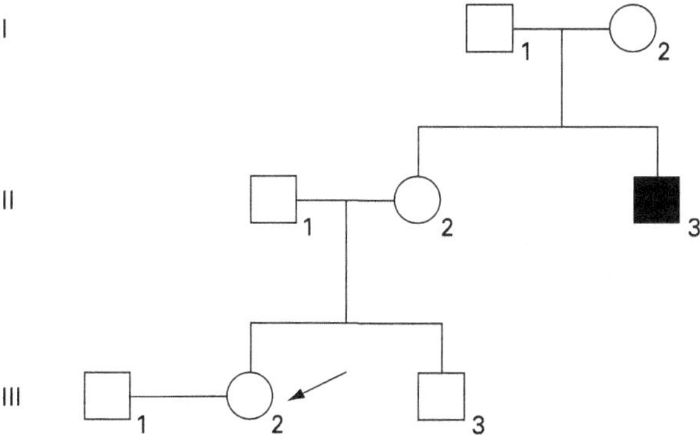

Figure 14.2 Pedigree of consultand (III-2) with a family history of an isolated case of hemophilia (II-3). See text and Appendix for details.

Factor IX) are therefore inherited in an X-linked fashion (Table 14.1). While it is rare for them to be affected, women frequently present with a family history of hemophilia. A woman whose father is affected will be an "obligate" carrier. A woman with a maternal family history of hemophilia is at risk of being a carrier; this risk can be calculated based on the pedigree and the patient's relationship to the affected individual(s). When the pedigree includes only one case of hemophilia, the affected individual may represent a new mutation or there may be members of the family who are undiagnosed carriers. Bayesian analysis[23] is frequently employed in calculating carrier risks, since this method takes into consideration prior risk and conditional risks. Figure 14.2 provides a typical example of a woman at risk to be a carrier of hemophilia (III-2) because she has an affected maternal uncle (II-3). The woman's chance of being a carrier is about 10%. The calculation of this number is detailed in the Appendix at the end of this chapter and takes into consideration the chance that the affected uncle represents a new mutation, as well as the fact that the woman has an unaffected brother. Thus, without performing any testing, we can say that each of this woman's sons will have a $1/10 \times 1/2 = 1/20$ or 5% chance of having hemophilia. Even if no testing is pursued, prenatal ultrasound can be performed in the second trimester of pregnancy to determine the gender of the baby. If it is male, the patient and delivery staff can be prepared for the possibility of an affected child.

DNA testing can provide more definitive information. Factor levels may be unreliable, particularly during pregnancy, so carrier testing should depend on DNA analysis. This is performed either by direct analysis of the gene in question, or if a mutation in the gene cannot be identified in the family, by linkage analysis. Online resources are available to determine whether clinical testing is available for particular gene mutations.[24] At this time, the vast majority of clinical laboratories offering DNA testing for factor VIII test for a specific inversion within the gene.

This inversion accounts for about half of all mutations in severe cases of hemophilia A (Factor VIII activity less than 1%). Sequencing of the factor VIII gene, available on only a limited basis and with great cost, would be required to detect the other half of the mutations. Once a specific mutation has been identified in an affected male within the family, it is relatively simple to test female relatives and their fetuses (by means of CVS or amniocentesis). In families without a detectable mutation, a linkage study is performed by obtaining blood for DNA samples from various relatives and tracking the mutation indirectly. This is performed by testing DNA markers, which are easily identifiable sequences in and around the gene in question. Using information about which relatives inherited which markers, one can deduce who is likely to have inherited the mutation. As an indirect method, linkage analysis can never be 100% accurate, but depending on the available markers, the structure of the family and the willingness of family members to cooperate, accuracy can approach 95–99%. An informative linkage study will determine whether a woman has a very high or a very low risk of being a carrier. In the case of a high risk, CVS or amniocentesis can be offered and the same linkage study performed on a male fetus to determine if he is likely to be affected. If the fetus is determined to be female, either by ultrasound or by chromosome analysis, a decision to pursue carrier testing can be considered.

Direct mutation analysis of the Factor IX gene currently depends on sequencing, an expensive procedure performed by few labs. Therefore DNA testing for hemophilia B usually consists of linkage analysis.

Because it is time-consuming to obtain blood from family members and perform linkage, patients desiring evaluation for a family history of hemophilia should be referred for genetic counseling prior to initiation of pregnancy.

3. Hemoglobinopathies

Normal adult hemoglobin (Hgb A) is formed from the combination of 2 α- and 2 β-globin peptide chains. Mutations in the genes that control synthesis of α- and β-globin cause abnormal globin formation or decreased production of specific globin chains. The diagnosis and management of the woman with a hemoglobinopathy is discussed in a separate chapter. Because of the heritable nature of these conditions and the significant risk to offspring, once a hemoglobinopathy has been diagnosed a woman should receive genetic counseling. The exact risk to her offspring will depend on the genotype of her partner; the initial step in the evaluation of a woman with a known or suspected hemoglobinopathy is evaluation of the partner's complete red blood count with red cell indices and hemoglobin fractionation. Optimally this would occur prior to pregnancy and in conjunction with genetic counseling. This approach allows a discussion of complete reproductive options; preimplantation genetic diagnosis has been performed successfully for sickle cell disease and other hemoglobinopathies.[25,26] Figure 14.3 demonstrates the evaluation of a couple when the woman has a variant hemoglobin, β thalassemia or α thalassemia.

Sickle cell disease is caused by a mutation in the gene encoding β-globin production on the short arm of chromosome 11. The mutation causes valine to replace glutamic acid in the 6th amino acid position of β-globin. The resulting abnormal hemoglobin chains (Hgb S) cause "sickle" shaped red blood cells. About 8% of African-Americans carry this mutation. A woman who carries one copy of the mutation will produce both Hgb A and Hgb S and remain relatively asymptomatic (sickle cell "trait" or carrier). On average, half of her children will inherit the mutation. A woman with sickle cell disease carries this mutation in both her β-globin genes, so all her children will inherit at least one copy of the abnormal gene. If the fetus also inherits a mutation in its paternal copy of the β-globin gene, there is a possibility for a hemoglobinopathy in the fetus. A complete blood count and hemoglobin fractionation of the partner can demonstrate the presence of Hgb S, Hgb C, another hemoglobin variant or thalassemia. If the woman is a sickle cell carrier, and the partner is a carrier of one of the hemoglobin variants or β thalassemia, there is a 25% chance for the fetus to have Hgb SS, Hgb SC, sickle-β thalassemia disease or another combination. If the woman has sickle cell disease and the partner is a carrier, the risk to the fetus is 50%. The effect of various combinations of hemoglobin genotypes can be found in other resources.[27,28] When the risk to the fetus is for disease with significant morbidity, prenatal diagnosis is usually possible. Chorionic villi or amniocytes can be used for DNA analysis, or direct evaluation of fetal hemoglobin can be performed on fetal blood obtained through PUBS.

Other mutations in the β-globin gene may result in **beta thalassemia**, in which there is a reduction in the number of β-globin chains produced. A carrier of a mutation in one copy of the β-globin gene has beta thalassemia minor. As in the case of sickle cell disease, the status of the partner should be evaluated with a complete blood count and hemoglobin fractionation (Figure 14.3(b)). DNA analysis for β thalassemia is available from specialized molecular laboratories[24] and can confirm the presence of a mutation. If both parents carry a β thalassemia mutation, prenatal diagnosis of β thalassemia major (Cooley's anemia) is possible by amniocentesis, CVS or PUBS.

Alpha-globin production is regulated by two pairs of genes located on the short arm of chromosome 16. A normal individual therefore has a total of four α-globin genes. The spectrum of **alpha thalassemias** corresponds directly with the number of deletions an individual carries (Figure 14.4). Persons from South and Southeast Asia as well as the Mediterranean area are at high risk for being a carrier of one or more gene deletions.

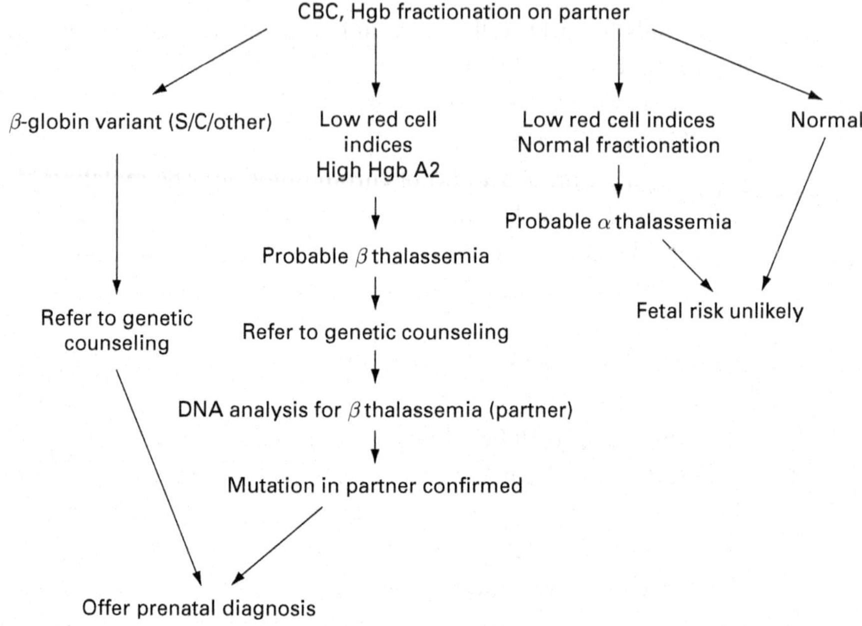

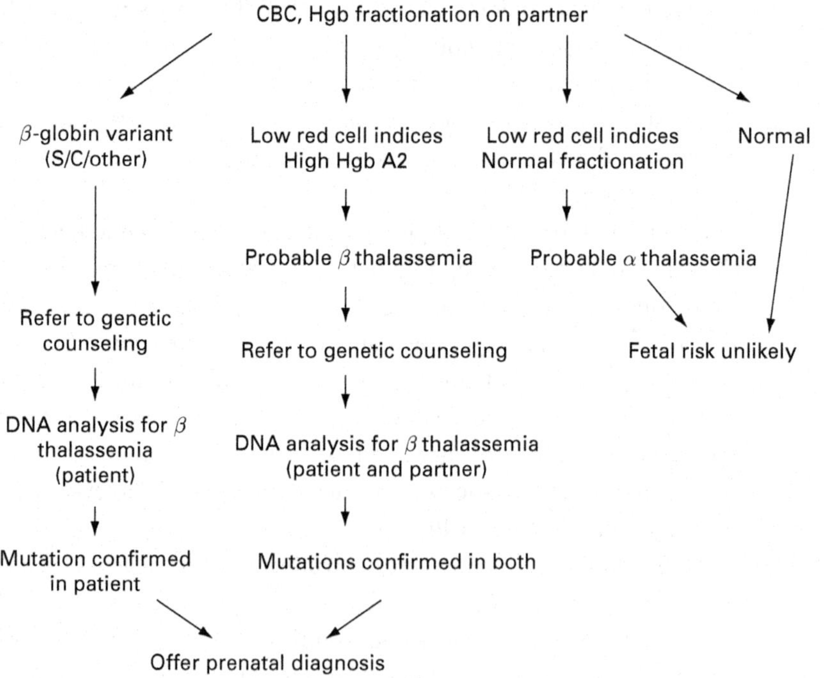

Figure 14.3 Flowchart for evaluation of a couple when the woman has a hemoglobinopathy.

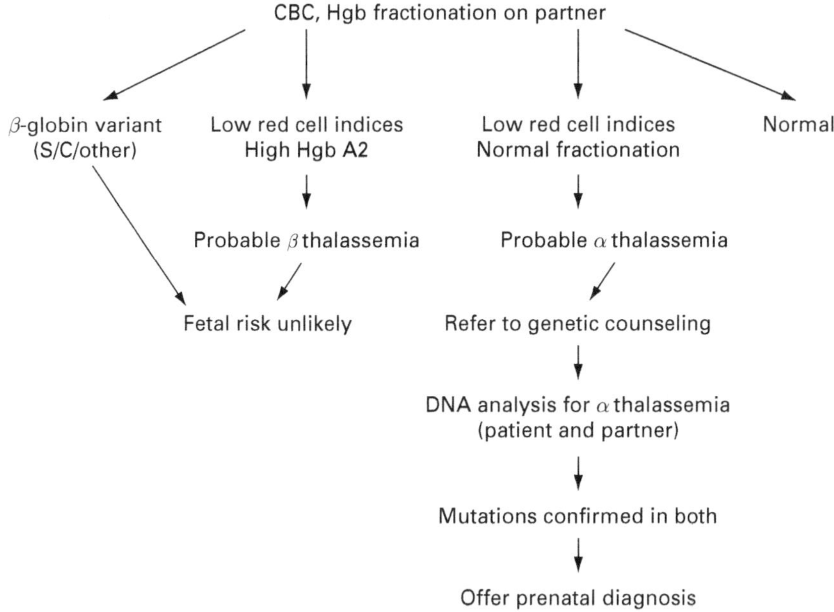

Figure 14.3 (cont.)

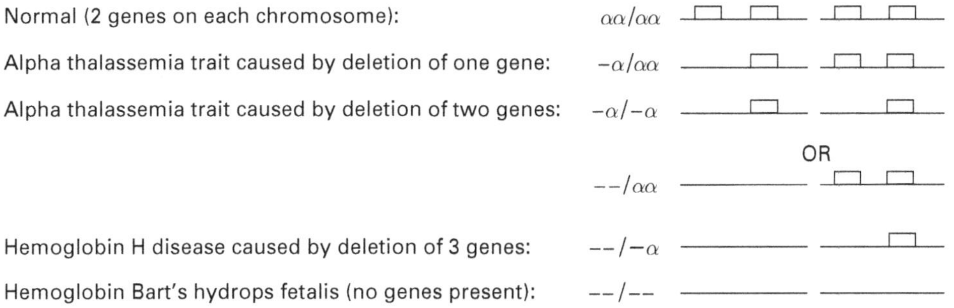

Figure 14.4 Deletional mutations in the α-globin gene complex. The number of α-globin genes present on each chromosome is depicted in a normal individual, as well as in individuals with α thalassemia trait, Hgb H disease, and Hgb Bart's hydrops fetalis.

The absence of one α-globin gene, $-\alpha/\alpha\alpha$, is not associated with clinical signs of α thalassemia. When two gene deletions are present they may be arranged on the same chromosome, $--/\alpha\alpha$ ("*cis*"), or on opposite chromosomes, $-\alpha/-\alpha$ ("*trans*"). Hemoglobin H disease results when only one α-globin gene is functional. The paramount concern for pregnancy occurs when both parents carry at least

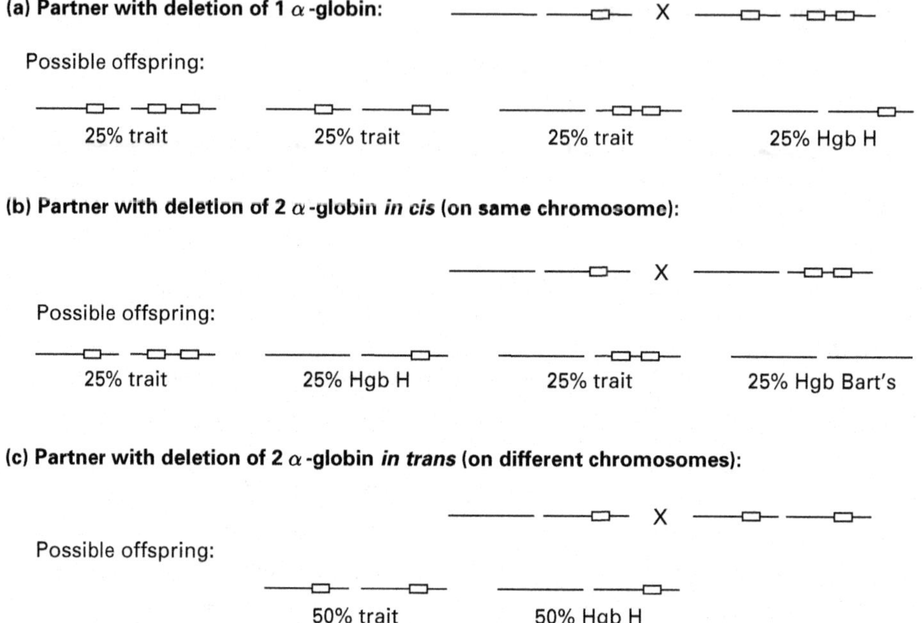

Figure 14.5 Possible outcomes for offspring of a woman with Hgb H disease and a partner with α thalassemia trait.

two α-globin gene deletions; in this situation there is a possibility that the fetus will not inherit any functional α-globin genes, – –/– –. Hemoglobin Bart's is then formed as a tetramer of γ-globin genes and has a high affinity for oxygen. Hgb Bart's disease presents with fetal hydrops, and in utero or neonatal death. DNA testing for α-globin deletions is available through specialized molecular laboratories.[24] Once the deletions have been identified in the patient and her partner, the couple can be offered definitive prenatal diagnosis. Figure 14.5 describes three possible scenarios for offspring between a woman with Hgb H disease and a partner with varying numbers of deletions.

4. Von Willebrand disease

The diagnosis and management of von Willebrand disease are discussed in a separate chapter. The von Willebrand factor gene is near the tip of the short arm of chromosome 12. The von Willebrand factor has a complex multimeric structure and various mutations in the gene cause absent to decreased levels of the factor or aberrant structure of the factor. The disease is divided into 3 broad types: Type 1, the most common, is autosomal dominant and involves reduced levels of the factor. Type 2, also autosomal dominant, occurs due to qualitative changes in the structure of the factor and is further classified into several subtypes. Type 3, more severe, is autosomal recessive and results from absent factor. A rare, X-linked form has also been reported.[4] DNA testing for von Willebrand disease is complex, due to the variety of different mutations and the various types and subtypes. In general, one can determine the inheritance pattern from the pedigree and counsel the family about recurrence risk. Autosomal dominant forms result in affected individuals in consecutive generations, although, as with other autosomal dominant conditions, the severity may vary. Autosomal recessive forms tend to be more severe and affect siblings; parents are usually asymptomatic.

DNA testing may be useful to confirm a diagnosis in a relative. At this time, clinical DNA testing is usually available by linkage; direct mutation analysis is limited to a few of the Type II subtypes.[24] Ideally, the family mutation should be documented, but linkage analysis can be employed for families where the mutation has not been identified. In families with severe disease, prenatal diagnosis may be desired. This can often be accomplished by DNA linkage analysis on amniocytes or chorionic villi, or by testing factor levels in fetal blood obtained by PUBS.[14,15]

5. Rh isoimmunization

The Rhesus blood group system consists of 5 main antigens that are found on the cell membrane of erythrocytes. While the Rh-D antigen receives the most attention and is the most investigated, C, c, E, and e antigens are also clinically significant in pregnancy. There is no d antigen; the absence of D antigen is equivalent to Rh-D negative status. Two genes encode the Rh blood group system and are found on the short arm of chromosome one. The first is responsible for the production of the Cc and Ee polypeptides while the second encodes D antigen production.

Exposure of an Rh-D negative woman to Rh-D positive blood cells may occur with a transfusion of unmatched blood or during pregnancy. Rh-D positive fetal erythrocytes may gain entrance to the maternal circulation during pregnancy termination, trauma, delivery or invasive prenatal testing. Asymptomatic transplacental passage may also occur in the absence of these events. After the initial exposure to Rh-D positive cells, the woman's immune system produces IgM antibodies that are large and do not cross the maternal–fetal interface; subsequent exposures prompt IgG antibody formation. These antibodies are smaller and readily cross the placenta and gain access to the fetal circulation. Once present in the fetus, the IgG antibodies bind to the fetal erythrocytes and cause hemolysis.

All pregnant women should have a blood type and indirect Coombs' test performed at the first prenatal visit. If a woman has a "positive" antibody screen reported, further investigation into the nature of the antibody and the titer of the antibody is mandatory. Anti-D antibodies rarely cause fetal compromise at titers less than 1:16. If the first titer is 1:8 or less, it is reasonable to measure titers on a monthly basis. However, if the titer is greater than or equal to 1:16, further evaluation is warranted. The first step is determination of the paternal Rh-D status. In most Caucasians, the incidence of Rh-D negativity is about 15%; it is lower for other groups. If the partner is Rh-D negative, the fetal erythrocytes will not have D antigen present on the cell membrane and therefore not be adversely affected by the presence of the antibodies. An Rh-D positive partner will be heterozygous for the D antigen about 55% of the time and homozygous about 45% of the time.[29] If he is homozygous, then all of his offspring will be Rh-D positive. If he is a heterozygote, then 50% of his offspring (with a partner who is Rh-D negative) will be Rh-D positive and 50% will be Rh-D negative. With currently available molecular technology, it is not possible to distinguish between homozygous and heterozygous Rh-D positive individuals, although the production of an Rh-D negative child would confirm a partner in the above scenario to be heterozygous. Because certain combinations of antigens are more prevalent than others, determination of the partner's C/c and E/e type would suggest whether he is likely to be hetero- or homozygous for D.[29]

If the possibility exists that the fetus is Rh-D positive, determination of the fetal Rh-D status should be made by means of amniocentesis or chorionic villus sampling. DNA analysis, utilizing polymerase chain reaction testing, can be performed on chorionic villi or amniocytes and is available at many commercial molecular laboratories in the United States.[24] At the same time, a fetal karyotype is usually obtained to rule out common chromosomal anomalies. As stated earlier, a fetus that is Rh-D negative is not vulnerable to attack by maternal anti-D IgG antibodies, so no further treatment is necessary with this result. However, the Rh-D positive fetus is at significant risk for hemolysis, anemia and hydrops fetalis. The management of affected pregnancies in this situation is discussed in a previous chapter.

In the 1960s, it was reported that injecting anti-D immune globin blocked the formation of anti-D antibodies in persons exposed to Rh-D positive cells. Rh immune globulin is now administered to all Rh-D negative women at 28 weeks of gestation and after delivery of an Rh-D positive infant, in an attempt to prevent sensitization due to asymptomatic exposure to fetal Rh-D positive red blood cells. If a woman experiences vaginal bleeding, undergoes invasive testing, or terminates a pregnancy, Rh immune globulin is also prescribed. This has led to a marked reduction in anti-D isoimmunization and a relative rise in the importance of atypical red blood cell antigens in isoimmunization and hemolytic disease of the newborn.

The most important atypical antigen is the Kell antigen. The Kell gene, located on chromosome 7, has been demonstrated to have 24 different polymorphisms, producing 24 serologically distinct Kell antigens.[4] Fortunately, approximately 90% of the general population is Kell antigen negative and therefore partners of Kell isoimmunized women are very likely to be Kell negative, placing their offspring at no risk. The maternal Kell antibody titer does not correlate well with the risk of hemolysis and fetal anemia. Therefore if the father of the baby is Kell antigen positive and the maternal titer is greater than 1:4, determination of the fetal Kell status is recommended. As with Rh isoimmunization, this can be accomplished by chorionic villus sampling or amniocentesis, and DNA testing.

Antigens such as Rh-C, Rh-c, Rh-E, Rh-e, Duffy, Kidd and MNS are some of the other more frequently seen atypical antigens that can cause hemolytic disease in the fetus. A complete listing of atypical antigens and their risk for hemolytic disease in the fetus is useful in the evaluation of abnormal antibody screens in pregnancy.[30]

Conclusion

In summary, the approach to genetic counseling and testing depends on the specific disease and its inheritance pattern, and relies on the determination of whether molecular testing is clinically available and useful for the patient. The availability of testing for a particular disease in a particular family must be established, preferably prior to initiation of pregnancy. For diseases that are treatable, patients will benefit from diagnostic work-up. For the majority of genetic conditions where there is potential for significant morbidity or mortality in affected offspring, prenatal diagnosis may be desired. For diseases that have adult onset, particularly if they are treatable, prenatal diagnosis is generally not considered. In cases where invasive prenatal testing may lead to altered management of the mother or fetus, as in the case of a fetus with Hgb Bart's disease or severe isoimmunization, counseling may be more directive.

REFERENCES

1 Bennett, R. L., Steinhaus, K. A., Uhrich, S. B., *et al.* Recommendations for Standardized Human Pedigree Nomenclature. *Am. J. Hum. Genet.*, 1995; **56**: 745.

2 Ad Hoc Committee on Genetic Counseling. Genetic Counseling. *Am. J. Hum. Genet.*, 1975; **27**: 240.

3 McKusick, V. *Mendelian Inheritance in Man*, 12th edn. Baltimore, MD: Johns Hopkins University Press; 1998.

4 Online *Mendelian Inheritance in Man.* Accessed August 25, 2003, at http://www.ncbi.nlm.nih.gov/omim.

5 Kessler, S. Psychological aspects of genetic counseling. IX. Teaching and counseling. *J. Genet. Counseling*, 1997; **6**: 287.

6 Michie, S., Bron, F., Bobrow, M., *et al.* Nondirectiveness in genetic counseling: An empirical study. *Am. J. Hum. Genet.*, 1997; **60**: 40.
7 Weil, J. Psychosocial genetic counseling in the post-nondirective era: A point of view. *J. Genet. Counseling*, 2003; **12**: 199.
8 American Society of Human Genetics/American College of Medical Genetics Report. Points to consider: Ethical, legal, and psychosocial implications of genetic testing in children and adolescents. *Am. J. Hum. Genet.*, 1995; **57**: 1233.
9 National Society of Genetic Counselors. *Prenatal and Childhood Testing for Adult-Onset Disorders*. Adopted 1995. Accessed August 25, 2003, at http://www.nsgc.org/newsroom/position.asp.
10 Beutler, E., Nguyen, N. J., Henneberger, M. W., *et al.* Gaucher disease: Gene frequencies in the Ashkenazi Jewish population. *Am. J. Hum. Genet.*, 1993; **52**: 85.
11 Grabowski, G. A. Gaucher disease: Gene frequencies and genotype/phenotype correlations. *Genet. Testing*, 1997; **1**: 5.
12 Burke, W., Imperatore, G., McDonnell, S. M., *et al.* Contribution of different HFE genotypes to iron overload disease: a pooled analysis. *Genetics in Medicine*, 2000; **2**: 271.
13 Ledbetter, D. H., Zachary, J. M., Simpson, J. L., *et al.* Cytogenetic results from the US Collaborative Study on CVS. *Prenatal Diag.*, 1992; **12**: 317.
14 DeVore, G. R., Mahoney, M. J., Hobbins, J. C. Antenatal diagnosis of haemoglobinopathies, haemophilia, von Willebrand's disease, Duchenne's muscular dystrophy, and chronic granulomatous disease by fetal blood analysis. *Clin. Obstet. Gynaecol.*, 1980; **7**: 41.
15 Rothschild, C., Foresteir, F., Daffos, F., *et al.* Prenatal diagnosis in type IIA von Willebrand disease. *Nouv. Rev. Fr. Hematol.*, 1990; **32**: 125.
16 Reich, L. M., Bower, M., Key, N. S. Role of the geneticist in testing and counseling for inherited thrombophilia. *Genetics in Medicine*, 2003; **5**: 133.
17 Olson, J. D. College of American Pathologists Consensus Conference XXXVI: Diagnostic issues in thrombophilia. *Arch. Pathol. Lab. Med.*, 2002; **126**: 1277.
18 Wertz, D. C. Genetic discrimination: an overblown fear. *Nat. Rev. Gen.*, 2002; **3**: 496.
19 Genetic Information Nondiscrimination Act of 2003. Senate Bill 1053, May 13, 2003. Accessed November 11, 2003 at http://www.theorator.com/bills108/s1053.html.
20 Health Insurance Portability and Accountability Act of 1996, Public Law 104–191, US Statutes at Large 110 (1996).
21 Manco-Johnson, M. J., Grabowski, E. F., Hellgreen, M., *et al.* Laboratory testing for thrombophilia in pediatric patients. On behalf of the Subcommittee for Perinatal and Pediatric Thrombosis of the Scientific and Standardization Committee of the International Society of Thrombosis and Haemostasis (ISTH). *Thromb. Haemost.*, 2002; **88**: 155.
22 Grody, W. W., Griffin, J. H., Taylor, A. K., *et al.* American College of Medical Genetics consensus statement on factor V Leiden mutation testing. *Genet. Med.*, 2001; **3**: 139.
23 Hodge, S. E. A simple, unified approach to Bayesian risk calculations. *J. Genet. Counseling*, 1998; **7**: 235.
24 GeneTests. Accessed September 10, 2003, at http://www.genetests.org/.
25 Xu, K., Shi, Z. M., Veeck, L. L., *et al.* First unaffected pregnancy using preimplantation genetic diagnosis for sickle cell anemia. *JAMA*, 1999; **281**: 1701.

26 Kanavakis, E., Vrettou, C., Palmer, G., *et al.* Preimplantation genetic diagnosis in 10 couples at risk for transmitting beta-thalassaemia major: clinical experience including the initiation of six singleton pregnancies. *Prenat. Diagn.*, 1999; **19**: 1217.
27 Steinberg, M. H. Compound heterozygous and other sickle hemoglobinopathies. In Steinberg, M. H., Forget, B. G., Higgs, D. R., *et al.*, eds., *Disorders of Hemoglobin. Genetics, Pathophysiology, and Clinical Management.* Cambridge: Cambridge University Press; 2001. pp. 786–810.
28 Old, J. M. Prenatal diagnosis of the hemoglobinopathies. In Milunsky, A., ed., *Genetic Disorders and the Fetus: Diagnosis, Prevention, and Treatment*, 4th edn. Baltimore, MD: Johns Hopkins University Press; 1998. p. 583.
29 Bowman, J. M. Hemolytic disease (erythroblastosis fetalis). In Creasy, R. K., and Resnik, R., eds., *Maternal Fetal Medicine*, 4th edn. Philadelphia, PA: WB Saunders Co.; 1999, p. 737.
30 Bowman, J. M. Hemolytic disease (erythroblastosis fetalis). In Creasy, R. K., and Resnik, R., eds., *Maternal Fetal Medicine*, 4th edn. Philadelphia, PA: WB Saunders Co.; 1999, pp. 764–5.

APPENDIX: CALCULATION OF HEMOPHILIA CARRIER RISKS IN FIGURE 14.2 USING BAYESIAN ANALYSIS

Figure 14.2 provides an example of a woman at risk to be a carrier of hemophilia (III-2) because she has an affected maternal uncle (II-3). The affected relative is the only known case in the family; it is assumed that there is approximately a 1/3 chance that he represents a new mutation and a 2/3 chance that his mother (I-2) is a carrier. (This is the assumption made for an X-linked, genetically lethal condition.) The a priori risk therefore that the consultand's mother, II-2, is a carrier is $1/2 \times 2/3$, or one-half the risk that her mother is a carrier. Since II-2 has an unaffected son, (III-3), Bayes' Theorem must be applied to properly reduce her carrier risk. Only then can her daughter's risk be calculated. The Bayesian analysis is as follows:

Probability that II-2:	Inherited the mutation	Did not inherit the mutation
Prior probability:	$1/2 \times 2/3 = 1/3$	$1-1/3 = 2/3$
Conditional probability: (the chance of having an unaffected son)	1/2	1
Joint probability:	$1/3 \times 1/2 = 1/6$	$2/3 \times 1 = 2/3$
Posterior probability:	$\frac{1/6}{1/6 + 2/3} = 1/5$	$\frac{2/3}{1/6 + 2/3} = 4/5$

Thus, the fact that II-2 has an unaffected son reduces her chance of being a carrier from 1/3 to 1/5. Using this, we can calculate the consultand's chance of being a carrier, which would be half that of her mother, that is, $1/2 \times 1/5$ or 1/10. In other words, the consultand has a 1/10 or 10% chance of being a carrier, and she can be advised that each of her sons would have a $1/10 \times 1/2 = 1/20$ or 5% chance of having hemophilia.

15

Thrombocytopenia in pregnancy

Ravindra Sarode, M.D.[1] and Eugene P. Frenkel, M.D.[2]

[1]Professor of Pathology, University of Texas Southwestern Medical Center, Director: Transfusion Medicine and Hemostasis, Dallas, Texas, USA
[2]Professor of Medicine and Radiology, Harold C. Simmons Comprehensive Cancer Center, University of Texas Southwestern Medical School, Dallas, Texas, USA

Thrombocytopenia is a common hematological disorder that has classically been evaluated in an orderly clinical and laboratory approach. When thrombocytopenia is identified in the patient who is pregnant, important clinical differences and therapeutic implications exist when compared to the non-pregnant patient. These relate to the safety of the mother during pregnancy, viability of the fetus, the proper approach to parturition, and post-delivery care of the mother and the baby.

The recognition of thrombocytopenia is quite common in pregnancy, occurring in nearly 10% of patients.[1–3] An unusual aspect of most of these events is that the majority are physiological. Thus the term "gestational thrombocytopenia" has been applied to this group of patients. This physiologic event must be differentiated from the less common, but clinically significant occurrence of a pathological mechanism for the thrombocytopenia. Such pathologic events are commonly associated with an evident clinical presentation and are potentially serious issues in the maintenance of the pregnancy and the health of the mother. In some circumstances, the thrombocytopenia is actually part of a more complex clinical disorder. The causes of thrombocytopenia in pregnancy are delineated in Table 15.1.

Gestational or physiological thrombocytopenia

Clearly, the most common cause of thrombocytopenia in pregnancy is a physiological event, since it is seen in 5 to 7% of all pregnancies, and actually accounts for more than 75% of all cases of thrombocytopenia during pregnancy.[4–6] The decrease in platelet count occurs predominantly in the third trimester of pregnancy;[4,5] and, the degree of platelet reduction is mild and is not associated with a hemorrhagic diathesis. In general, platelet counts are only slightly reduced to a range of

Hematological Complications in Obstetrics, Pregnancy, and Gynecology, ed. R. L. Bick *et al.* Published by Cambridge University Press.

Table 15.1 Causes of thrombocytopenia during pregnancy.

A. Physiological: gestational
B. Decreased production:
  1. Aplastic anemia
  2. Myelodysplasia
  3. Severe megaloblastic anemia
C. Destruction:
  1. ITP
  2. Drug-induced thrombocytopenia
    a. Heparin-induced thrombocytopenia
D. Consumption:
  1. Pregnancy related
    a. HELLP syndrome
    b. Preeclampsia
    c. Acute fatty liver
  2. Non-pregnancy related
    a. TTP-microangiopathic hemolysis
    b. HUS-microangiopathic hemolysis
    c. DIC

100–150,000/μl with a normal mean platelet volume. Clinically, platelet counts above 70,000/μl, with no other explanation in an otherwise healthy pregnant woman can be considered physiological.[3] However, if the platelet count is below 70,000/μl, a pathological cause of thrombocytopenia should be sought. The exact mechanism of gestational thrombocytopenia is not known, but it has been postulated to be related to expansion of blood volume and thus related to a dilutional effect.[2,7] Additional theories are an increased clearance of platelets (both immune and non-immune).[2] Neither proposed mechanism appears to cogently explain the finding, its incidence or clinical pattern. Gestational thrombocytopenia does not have pathophysiologic sequalae, and there is no increased risk of bleeding. The platelet count should be compared with pre-pregnancy level(s) and followed carefully during pregnancy, especially if counts fall below 100,000/μl. Fetal outcome is not affected and neonatal thrombocytopenia generally does not occur.

Pathological thrombocytopenia

Of the mechanisms of thrombocytopenia that are disease-related, some are particularly related to pregnancy, and these will be reviewed herein.

Immune thrombocytopenia

Of the various pathophysiologic mechanisms and diseases producing thrombocytopenia during pregnancy, immune/idiopathic thrombocytopenic purpura (ITP) is the most common, although the projected incidence is less than 0.1% of all pregnancies. Its usual occurrence is during the first trimester,[2,8,9] thereby producing a clinical issue of significance throughout the pregnancy, with implications relative to the management of parturition and the potential of neonatal thrombocytopenia in the infant.

The clinical presentation can be explosive with evidence of mucous membrane, vaginal, or gastrointestinal bleeding, ecchymosis and/or hematuria. More commonly, it is recognized because of unexplained mucosal bleeding that is mild but persistent. Virtually all of the symptoms are the result of bleeding. No constitutional symptoms or evidence of underlying systemic disease is present. There may be a past history of ITP, which then provides aid in the diagnosis and the management of the current pregnancy.

Laboratory findings include the presence of a low platelet count often under 20,000/μl and an increased mean platelet volume (MPV). The latter finding provides evidence of increased platelet production and turnover, which is consistent with immune destruction of platelets. The remainder of the laboratory findings are normal. If anemia is present, it relates only to the identified amount of blood loss. Since ITP can be associated with systemic lupus erythematosus, confirmatory relevant laboratory studies should be done.

Idiopathic thrombocytopenic purpura results from the formation of IgG autoantibodies against platelet glycoprotein (GP) receptors GPIIb/IIIa and GPIb/V/IX.[10–13] These antibodies coat platelets, which results in their removal by the reticuloendothelial system (RES), especially the spleen.

Idiopathic thrombocytopenic purpura is still a diagnosis of exclusion even though the etiology is known. Applicable tests to identify platelet GP autoantibodies are not yet accurate or reliable and continue to be available only in selected research laboratories.[11,12] Similarly, testing for increased platelet-bound IgG is non-specific because platelet associated IgG is known to be increased in a variety of clinical conditions associated with thrombocytopenia.[14] Since platelet counts are usually noted to be reduced in ITP in the first half of the pregnancy and are commonly less than 50,000/μl with an elevated MPV, it can be differentiated from gestational thrombocytopenia which is usually noted in the second half of the pregnancy with only slight reductions in platelet numbers (i.e. generally above 70,000/μl). In addition, the platelet counts in ITP generally decline as the pregnancy progresses, whereas they are stable in gestational thrombocytopenia.[15,16]

Idiopathic thrombocytopenic purpura affects not only the mother but also the fetus as well, due to the transplacental passage of IgG anti-platelet antibodies; therefore, the management of ITP becomes very critical during the third trimester.[2] Most of the neonates born to ITP mothers have mild to moderate thrombocytopenia,[17] however, significant neonatal thrombocytopenia <50,000/μl is seen in 10–25% newborns, and severe thrombocytopenia <20,000/μl is seen in approximately 5% neonates.[18,19] The greatest concern in neonates at the time of delivery is bleeding, which is seen in 25–50% neonates with severe thrombocytopenia.[18,19] Therefore, there is a serious concern about head trauma resulting in intracranial bleeding during vaginal delivery in neonates with severe thrombocytopenia. Unfortunately, the severity of maternal thrombocytopenia or platelet associated IgG does not clearly correlate with the presence or degree of the neonatal thrombocytopenia.[2,9] This is well documented in the case of dizygotic twins where the platelet counts were widely different in each of the two newborns.[20] However, one reliable indicator of neonatal thrombocytopenia would be a history of thrombocytopenia in previous pregnancy and women who had splenectomy prior to pregnancy.[19,21,22]

Since the fetal platelet count does not correlate with either the clinical or laboratory features in the mother,[2,9] a percutaneous umbilical cord sampling (PUBS) may be performed before labor to define the severity of fetal thrombocytopenia; since recognition of a platelet count <50,000/μl heralds the decision for a cesarean section as the desirable mode of delivery.[23,24] In part, this is based on the complication rate of PUBS, which is similar to (or slightly higher than) the incidence of intracranial hemorrhage encountered in neonates born to a mother with severe thrombocytopenia.[24] Therefore, clearly the role of PUBS is controversial and many neonatologists oppose its use.[25] An older approach, that of fetal scalp blood sampling early in the delivery (i.e., at early presentation), is no longer used because of the difficulty in achieving an accurate and reliable platelet count.

The cord blood platelet count should be immediately performed on all neonates born to mothers with ITP. Since platelet counts may continue to fall after birth due to persistent maternal (passive) antibody, daily platelet counts must be performed until stable normal values occur, generally by day 4.[26,27,28] When severe thrombocytopenia with active bleeding is identified, platelets should be transfused (10–15 cm^3/kg). Other treatments include IVIg and steroid.

The management of ITP in pregnancy is based on the severity of thrombocytopenia and the previous or present history of bleeding.[29] In general, if the platelet count is above 30,000/μl and active bleeding is not present; there is no need to institute therapy.[3] The treatment of ITP during pregnancy is not different from the approach in non-pregnant patients. The goal of therapy is to eliminate bleeding and maintain platelet counts greater than 30,000/μl.[9,27,30] Although a variety of newer therapeutic approaches exist for ITP, corticosteroid treatment is effective, less expensive, and more predictable. Thus corticosteroids continue as the first line of therapy in most cases.[2,27,30] However, they may induce or worsen gestational diabetes and hypertension and/or induce osteoporosis and weight gain.[3] These risks must be considered when selecting treatment. Glucocorticoids are given at 1–2 mg/kg/day for 2–3 weeks.[15,27] A response is usually seen in 3–7 days, and a maximum effect is reached in 2–3 weeks. If the platelet counts reach >50,000/μl, the steroids can be tapered by 10–20% per week to an approximately 10 mg/day maintenance dose.[30] If this treatment fails, then high dose intravenous gamma globulin (IVIg) therapy is the next choice (1–2 g/kg).[9,15] The response rate is 60–70% and the effect is commonly seen within a few days. Its major drawbacks are expense and transient efficacy usually necessitating multiple courses. The side effects of IVIg are usually mild but are common and include headache, chills, nausea, back-pain, liver dysfunction and flushing. Two rare complications include (1) alloimmune hemolytic anemias due to passive transfer of high titer red cell antibody from a donor; and, (2) anaphylaxis in patients with IgA deficiency.[31]

An important alternative to IVIg therapy is now available and has largely replaced it. It is intravenous anti-D IgG (WinRho). It is highly effective, and at a dosage of 50–75/(μg kg), the platelet count usually increases within 24–48 hours.[32–34] The response rate is approximately 75%.[33] A durable response status may require a second dose after 4–6 weeks. It merits important emphasis that anti-D therapy is to be given *only* to patients whose red cells are Rh positive. The anti-D antibodies bind to the D antigen on red cells and appear to result in alteration (engage/blockade) of the reticuloendothelial system.[32] The result is that the platelets coated with anti-platelet antibodies are not cleared.

Currently anti-D is not used in patients with significant anemia (hemoglobin <10 g/dl), because occasionally severe hemolysis occurs and the hemoglobin may decrease by 4–6 g/dl. In the uncommon event of occurrence of acute hemolysis, ABO compatible Rh-positive (*not Rh negative*) red cells should be transfused. Either IVIg or anti-D treatment is particularly useful when a rapid rise in platelet count is required. This is particularly relevant before delivery and surgery. Presently, anti-D therapy is clearly the preferred approach because of ease of administration, rapid response, and relatively low cost. In refractory patients a combination of corticosteroids and anti-D or IVIg may be required. Patients refractory to these treatments may be offered splenectomy, which has approximately 70–80% success rate,[35] though the long-term durability of response is uncertain. Splenectomy is safest during the second trimester[36] because, when performed during the first trimester, there is an increased risk of spontaneous abortion. When performed during the third trimester, the surgical field is obstructed by the large, gravid uterus. In addition, splenectomy during the third trimester is confounded by an increased risk of spontaneous labor.[2] Laparoscopic splenectomies have been performed successfully during pregnancy.[37,38] Although a variety of other treatment approaches have been used in non-pregnant patients (vincristine, danazol and azathioprine), these should be avoided in pregnancy due to their toxicity and potential untoward effects on fetuses.[27] Platelet transfusion may be required if the platelet count is $<30{,}000/\mu l$. Platelets should be transfused just before surgery is scheduled because anti-platelet antibodies destroy transfused platelets very rapidly. The complex picture of a pregnant woman with ITP requires that team approach to her management between the obstetrician, hematologist and transfusion medicine specialist.

Finally, the recent association of ITP with *Helicobacter pylori* infection has been identified.[39] Although the present data are insufficient to prove this hypothesis correct,[40] eradication of *H. pylori* infection has been reported to be associated with cure of ITP. Since this is a simple and expedient approach, *H. pylori* should be ruled out when the initial diagnosis of ITP is made.

Preeclampsia and eclampsia

Preeclampsia is encountered in 4–6% of all pregnancies, usually during the third trimester.[2] It is seen most often in nulliparous women or multiparous women with a change in partners.[2,12] The diagnostic criteria include new onset of hypertension and proteinuria (>300 mg/24 hours) after the 20th week of gestation. The exact etiology is unknown, but a genetic predisposition and association with the presence of thrombophilia (tendency to clot) has been proposed.[41,42] Central to the pathogenesis is generalized endothelial cell activation likely due to enhanced lipid peroxidation,[43] vascular endothelial growth factor release,[44] expression of adhesion molecules,[45] or activation of metalloproteases.[46] This endothelial cell "alteration" then leads to activation of platelets and coagulation cascade.

About 50% of patients with preeclampsia have thrombocytopenia and other markers that define disseminated intravascular coagulation (DIC) such as elevated d-dimers, thrombin-anti-thrombin complex levels, and often altered tests of coagulation (prothrombin time, partial Thromboplastin time and thrombin time).[2,12,47] All of these abnormalities and the related clinical symptoms revert to normal immediately after the delivery of the fetus. Therefore, patients with mild to moderate preeclampsia are managed conservatively.[47] However, patients with severe eclampsia who have moderate to severe thrombocytopenia and evidence of DIC commonly require aggressive management, especially before cesarean section. This requires correction of the coagulopathy by transfusing platelets to maintain platelet counts $>50{,}000/\mu l$, fresh frozen plasma (FFP, 10 cm^3/kg) to provide clotting factors and cryoprecipitate (10–15 units) to maintain fibrinogen >100 mg/dl. Commonly, cryoprecipitate infusion is forgotten or not used until continued or excessive bleeding is seen. Since hypofibrinogenemia will not be corrected by FFP alone, cryoprecipitate is paramount in the prevention of bleeding in these patients.

HELLP syndrome (hemolysis, elevated liver function tests, low platelets)

This syndrome occurs in approximately 10% of patients with severe preeclampsia.[12] It is usually seen in the third trimester in multiparous white women. It merits emphasis that HELLP can occur in patients who do not have hypertension and proteinuria thereby resulting in the failure to recognize the correct diagnosis.[48] HELLP can worsen in the immediate postpartum period or even present for the first time within 48 hours after delivery. The presenting symptoms include nausea, malaise, and epigastric or right upper quadrant abdominal pain and edema. It is important to have historical data, since it recurs in approximately 3% of subsequent pregnancies.[49] The diagnostic criteria include (a) microangiopathic hemolytic anemia (MAHA), which is characterized by the presence of fragmented RBCs and elevated lactate dehydrogenase; (b) elevated transaminases (AST, SGOT > 70 U/l); and (c) thrombocytopenia (<100,000/μl). The central nervous system and renal involvement are generally not seen in HELLP, and this is in sharp contrast to thrombotic thrombocytopenic purpura (TTP) or hemolytic uremic syndrome (HUS) (described later). Disseminated intravascular coagulation is encountered in approximately 20% of HELLP patients and abruption in 16%.[50] The neonatal mortality with HELLP is 10–20%,[12] and is usually due to placental ischemia, abruption, prematurity, and asphyxia. The maternal mortality is less than 1%.

The pathophysiology of HELLP is well understood. There is evidence for generalized damage/alteration of endothelium that results in microthromboses. However, since the exact etiology of this syndrome is unknown, the management presently is empirical. In general, patients with severe disease and evidence of DIC require (a) platelet transfusion to maintain counts >50,000/μl, (b) FFP to correct clotting factor deficiencies, and (c) cryoprecipitate transfusion to correct the hypofibrinogenemia. The coagulopathy worsens as the degree of liver damage increases. Steroids given, both in ante- and post-partum period, have been shown to be helpful.[51,52] Since the syndrome reverts to normal after delivery, prompt delivery is the treatment of choice. Following delivery most patients have a complete recovery within 24–48 hours. For those rare patients who have a persistent or worsening of the syndrome beyond 48–72 hours plasma exchange therapy should be instituted.[53,54] This is accomplished by an exchange of 1 to 1.5 volume of plasma replaced with FFP daily for 2–4 days.

Acute fatty liver of pregnancy (AFLP)

This is a rare condition affecting one in 10,000 pregnancies. It is almost always seen during the third trimester of pregnancy. Acute fatty liver of pregnancy is characterized by malaise, nausea, epigastric and right upper quadrant pain, dyspnea, and sometimes changes in mental status. Laboratory studies show moderate to severe abnormal liver function tests, hypoglycemia that can be severe, and electrolyte imbalance. Coagulopathy ensues due to depressed clotting factor synthesis. The associated liver damage leads to release of tissue factor that initiates acute DIC. During acute DIC, there is a major consumption of clotting factors, especially fibrinogen and antithrombin. Although thrombocytopenia is present, there is virtually no associated microangiopathic hemolytic anemia (MAHA). The exact etiology is unknown; however, fetal deficiency of long-chain 3-hydroxy-acyl CoA dehydrogenase or mitochondrial enzymes involved in fatty acid oxidation have been associated with AFLP.[55,56]

Although the diagnosis of AFLP can be made clinically, confirmation can be achieved by a liver biopsy stained with oil red O showing fat in hepatocytes.[57,58] Management of AFLP involves correcting hypoglycemia and electrolyte imbalance. Disseminated intravascular coagulation is corrected after the delivery of the fetus. Rarely, it may persist in the postpartum period. The appropriate treatment of DIC includes (a) FFP infusion (10 cm^3/kg) to correct clotting factor deficiencies; (b) cryoprecipitate (10–15 units) to replace fibrinogen (not present in sufficient quantity in FFP); and (c) platelets. Fresh frozen plasma should be given in a timely manner to prevent bleeding or fetal demise. The fetal mortality in AFLP is approximately 15%, and the maternal mortality is less than 5%.[59]

Thrombotic thrombocytopenic purpura (TTP)

TTP is a rare disease that is characterized by a triad of MAHA (fragmented RBCs on blood smear and elevated LDH), thrombocytopenia, and neurological symptoms that can vary from headaches to serious paresis and even coma.[60,61] Sometimes renal dysfunction or fever may also be present; this constellation was previously termed the pentad of TTP. Presently, a "triad" is diagnostic, because the disease is generally very far advanced if one waits for all five findings.[61]

The etiology of TTP has been identified recently to be due to a severe deficiency of von Willebrand factor cleaving protease (VWF-CP), now known as ADAMTS13.[62–67] Two clinical forms have been described. The most common is due to an acquired deficiency of this enzyme, resulting from an autoantibody or drug-induced antibody.[67,68] Less common is congenital deficiency, which is due to a rare genetic defect.[69–71] Deficiency of ADAMTS13, regardless of the mechanism,

Table 15.2 Consumptive thrombocytopenia syndromes.

Characteristics	Preeclampsia	HELLP syndrome	Acute fatty liver	Thrombotic thrombocytopenic purpura	Hemolytic uremic syndrome
Onset	3rd TM	3rd TM	3rd TM	Anytime/postpartum	Usually postpartum
Hypertension	++++	+−	+−	−	−
MAHA	+−	++	+	++++	++
Thrombocytopenia	+	+++	+++	++++	++
Coagulopathy (DIC)	+−	++	++++	−	+−
Liver involvement	−	+++	++++	−	−
CNS involvement	+	−	−	++++	+−
Renal involvement	++	+	−	+−	+++
Etiology	Unknown	Unknown	Unknown	Deficiency of ADAMTS13	Unknown
Management	Delivery of the fetus	Delivery of the fetus	Delivery of the fetus	Plasma exchange	Supportive
Transfusion therapy	−	FFP, CRYO, platelets	FFP, CRYO, platelets	Platelet transfusion absolute contraindication	−
Fetal mortality	Good	Good	Approximately 15%		

leads to persistence of ultra large sized multimers of VWF, which undergo unfolding under high shear rate that occurs in the microcirculation (arteriole and capillaries). These unfolded ultra large VWF multimers are capable of interacting with the platelet receptors GPIb and GPIIb/IIIa resulting in platelet–VWF rich microthrombi in many organs, especially the brain, kidney and heart. These microthrombi cause MAHA and thrombocytopenia.[72,73] The incidence of TTP was thought to be higher in pregnancy than in the general population. However, recent study and personal experience does not support this hypothesis.[74–76] The basis for this increased incidence is uncertain but a decrease in VWF-CP during late pregnancy has been reported.[77] This has been thought to be due to increased FWF during an acute phase reaction that then consumes VWF-CP. The apparent higher incidence of TTP in pregnancy appears to be due an overlap of a TTP-like syndrome with the hemolytic uremic syndrome (HUS), HELLP and severe preeclampsia that share some clinical and laboratory features. In HUS, there is predominant renal involvement and VWF-CP is normal.[78] Actually, the differential diagnosis of TTP with HUS, HELLP and severe preeclampsia can be very difficult at times (Table 15.2).

Although diagnostic specificity may be difficult, good clinical judgment supports urgent plasma exchange (PE) therapy. Daily PE is performed by replacing 1–1.5 plasma volume by fresh frozen plasma until the platelet count becomes normal for at least two days and LDH returns to near normal.[61,79,80] During PE, there is removal of ADAMTS13 antibody from the patient's plasma and replacement of the deficient enzyme by the FFP. On an average 9–11 treatments are necessary to achieve a clinical remission, however, some patients may require up to 85 treatments. About 25–30% patients have recurrences of the disease requiring further PE.[79] Because of the autoimmune nature of the disease steroids and other immunosuppression therapy has been used in conjunction with PE. By contrast, IVIg is not effective. Recently rituximab has been used successfully in the management of TTP.[81,82] Rituximab is a humanized monoclonal mouse antibody against the CD20 molecule on B-cells. By destroying B-cells, the antibody producing cells are eliminated. It is given as a 375 mg/(m week dose).

Recurrent TTP can be precipitated in patients with previous disease when they become pregnant. This is especially true in congenital TTP.[76] Congenital TTP is treated by the infusion of FFP rather than PE,[83] because patients with congenital TTP do not have an antibody inhibitor to the ADAMTS13. Plasma infusions are given every 3–4 weeks because the enzyme has a long half life.[84,85]

Platelet transfusions are absolutely contraindicated in TTP. Platelet transfusions are well known to be associated with either the appearance or worsening of CNS symptoms in patients with TTP.[86,87] This is likened to "adding fuel to the fire", since the microthrombi in TTP are composed of platelets. Even though TPE requires a central line insertion, it can be placed safely in the femoral vein with platelet counts as low as 5,000/μl. Similarly, because a unit of packed RBCs contains an abundance of platelets and platelet microparticles, red cell transfusions are also "relatively" contraindicated. Red cells should be transfused only to treat clinically symptomatic anemia.

Hemolytic uremic syndrome (HUS)

Hemolytic uremic syndrome is characterized by MAHA, thrombocytopenia and renal involvement. Childhood HUS is generally associated with *E. coli* (H7:O157) infection where shiga-like toxin is responsible for renal damage.[88] The microthrombi in HUS are composed of fibrin-platelet clots and little or no von Willebrand factor-like DIC lesions.[78,89] Childhood HUS resolves with conservative management.[79] Adult onset and pregnancy associated HUS has poorer outcome. The response to plasma exchange is poor, probably because the deficiency of ADAMTS13 seen in TTP does not occur in HUS.[78] However, a trial of PE should be considered, because some success has been reported.[90] The reports of HUS responsive to PE are thought to be due to the "removal of an unknown toxin." During a 1.0–1.5 volume plasma exchange, the replacement fluid used is FFP.

It is interesting that HUS has been known to recur in subsequent pregnancies.[91] The long-term prognosis of HUS is not good and many patients develop hypertension and chronic renal failure.[74]

The prognosis for the fetus in TTP, HUS and preeclampsia is poor due to extensive placental ischemia that results from the thrombotic microangiopathy.[92] In addition, premature parturition commonly further adds to fetal morbidity and mortality.[92]

REFERENCES

1 Burrows, R. F., Kelton, J. G. Incidentally detected thrombocytopenia in healthy mothers and their infants. *N. Engl. J. Med.*, 1988; **319**: 142–5.

2 McCrae, K. R., Samuels, P., Schreiber, A. D. Pregnancy-associated thrombocytopenia: pathogenesis and management. *Blood*, 1992; **80**: 2697–714.

3 McCrae, K. R., Bussel, J. B., Mannucci, P. M., *et al.* Platelets: an update on diagnosis and management of thrombocytopenic disorders. *Hematology (Am. Soc. Hematol. Educ. Program)*, 2001: 282–305.

4 Boehlen, F., Hohlfeld, P., Extermann, P., *et al.* Platelet count at term pregnancy: a reappraisal of the threshold. *Obstet. Gynecol.*, 2000; **95**: 29–33.

5 Saino, S., Kekomaki, R., Riikonen, S., *et al.* Maternal thrombocytopenia at term: a population-based study. *Acta Obstet. Gynecol. Scand.*, 2000; **79**: 744–9.

6 Shehata, N., Burrows, R., Kelton, J. G. Gestational thrombocytopenia. *Clin. Obstet. Gynecol.*, 1999; **42**: 327–34.

7 Verdy, E., Bessous, V., Dreyfus, M., *et al.* Longitudinal analysis of platelet count and volume in normal pregnancy. *Thromb. Haemost.*, 1997; **77**: 806–7.

8 Crowther, M. A., Burrows, R. F., Ginsberg, J., *et al.* Thrombocytopenia in pregnancy: diagnosis, pathogenesis and management. *Blood Rev.*, 1996; **10**: 8–16.

9 Gill, K. K., Kelton, J. G. Management of idiopathic thrombocytopenic purpura in pregnancy. *Semin. Hematol.*, 2000; **37**: 275–89.

10 Berchtold, P., Wenger, M. Autoantibodies against platelet glycoproteins in autoimmune thrombocytopenic purpura: their clinical significance and response to treatment. *Blood*, 1993; **81**: 1246–50.

11 Warner, M. N., Moore, J. C., Warkentin, T. E., *et al.* A prospective study of protein-specific assays used to investigate idiopathic thrombocytopenic purpura. *Br. J. Haematol.*, 1999; **104**: 442–7.

12 Guidelines for the investigation and management of idiopathic thrombocytopenic purpura in adults, children and in pregnancy. *Br. J. Haematol.*, 2003; **120**: 574–96.

13 Chan, H., Moore, J. C., Finch, C. N., *et al.* The IgG subclasses of platelet-associated autoantibodies directed against platelet glycoproteins IIb/IIIa in patients with idiopathic thrombocytopenic purpura. *Br. J. Haematol.*, 2003; **122**: 818–24.

14 Kelton, J. G., Murphy, W. G., Lucarelli, A., *et al.* A prospective comparison of four techniques for measuring platelet-associated IgG. *Br. J. Haematol.*, 1989; **71**: 97–105.

15 Burrows, R. F., Kelton, J. G. Thrombocytopenia during pregnancy. In Greer, I., Turpie, A. G. G., Forbes, C. D., eds. *Haemostasis and Thrombosis in Obstetrics and Gynaecology.* London: Chapman & Hall, 1992, pp. 407–29.

16 Burrows, R. F. Platelet disorders in pregnancy. *Curr. Opin. Obstet. Gynecol.*, 2001; **13**: 115–19.

17 Song, T. B., Lee, J. Y., Kim, Y. H., *et al.* Low neonatal risk of thrombocytopenia in pregnancy associated with immune thrombocytopenic purpura. *Fetal Diagn. Ther.*, 1999; **14**: 216–19.

18 Burrows, R. F., Kelton, J. G. Pregnancy in patients with idiopathic thrombocytopenic purpura: assessing the risks for the infant at delivery. *Obstet. Gynecol. Surv.*, 1993; **48**: 781–8.

19 Webert, K. E., Mittal, R., Sigouin, C., *et al.* A retrospective 11-year analysis of obstetric patients with idiopathic thrombocytopenic purpura. *Blood*, 2003; **102**: 4306–11.

20 Moise, K. J., Jr., Cotton, D. B. Discordant fetal platelet counts in a twin gestation complicated by idiopathic thrombocytopenic purpura. *Am. J. Obstet. Gynecol.*, 1987; **156**: 1141–2.

21 Christiaens, G. C., Nieuwenhuis, H. K., Bussel, J. B. Comparison of platelet counts in first and second newborns of mothers with immune thrombocytopenic purpura. *Obstet. Gynecol.*, 1997; **90**: 546–52.

22 Yamada, H., Kato, E. H., Kobashi, G., *et al.* Passive immune thrombocytopenia in neonates of mothers with idiopathic thrombocytopenic purpura: incidence and risk factors. *Semin. Thromb. Hemost.*, 1999; **25**: 491–6.

23 Berry, S. M., Leonardi, M. R., Wolfe, H. M., *et al.* Maternal thrombocytopenia. Predicting neonatal thrombocytopenia with cordocentesis. *J. Reprod. Med.*, 1997; **42**: 276–80.

24 Stamilio, D. M., Macones, G. A. Selection of delivery method in pregnancies complicated by autoimmune thrombocytopenia: a decision analysis. *Obstet. Gynecol.*, 1999; **94**: 41–7.

25 Peleg, D., Hunter, S. K. Perinatal management of women with immune thrombocytopenic purpura: survey of United States perinatologists. *Am. J. Obstet. Gynecol.*, 1999; **180**: 645–9.

26 Yamada, H., Kato, E. H., Kishida, T., *et al.* Risk factors for neonatal thrombocytopenia in pregnancy complicated by idiopathic thrombocytopenic purpura. *Ann. Hematol.*, 1998; **76**: 211–14.

27 Letsky, E. A., Greaves, M. Guidelines on the investigation and management of thrombocytopenia in pregnancy and neonatal alloimmune thrombocytopenia. Maternal and Neonatal Haemostasis Working Party of the Haemostasis and Thrombosis Task Force of the British Society for Haematology. *Br. J. Haematol.*, 1996; **95**: 21–6.

28 Iyori, H., Fujisawa, K., Akatsuka, J. Thrombocytopenia in neonates born to women with autoimmune thrombocytopenic purpura. *Pediatr. Hematol. Oncol.*, 1997; **14**: 367–73.

29 Silver, R. M. Management of idiopathic thrombocytopenic purpura in pregnancy. *Clin. Obstet. Gynecol.*, 1998; **41**: 436–48.

30 George, J. N., Woolf, S. H., Raskob, G. E., *et al.* Idiopathic thrombocytopenic purpura: a practice guideline developed by explicit methods for the American Society of Hematology. *Blood*, 1996; **88**: 3–40.

31 Schiavotto, C., Ruggeri, M., Rodeghiero, F. Adverse reactions after high-dose intravenous immunoglobulin: incidence in 83 patients treated for idiopathic thrombocytopenic purpura (ITP) and review of the literature. *Haematologica*, 1993; **78**: 35–40.

32 Bussel, J. B., Graziano, J. N., Kimberly, R. P., *et al.* Intravenous anti-D treatment of immune thrombocytopenic purpura: analysis of efficacy, toxicity, and mechanism of effect. *Blood*, 1991; **77**: 1884–93.

33 Michel, M., Novoa, M. V., Bussel, J. B. Intravenous anti-D as a treatment for immune thrombocytopenic purpura (ITP) during pregnancy. *Br. J. Haematol.*, 2003; **123**: 142–6.

34 Blanchette, V., Carcao, M. Intravenous immunoglobulin G and anti-D as therapeutic interventions in immune thrombocytopenic purpura. *Transfus. Sci.*, 1998; **19**: 279–88.

35 Bussel, J. B. Splenectomy-sparing strategies for the treatment and long-term maintenance of chronic idiopathic (immune) thrombocytopenic purpura. *Semin. Hematol.*, 2000; **37**: 1–4.

36 Gottlieb, P., Axelsson, O., Bakos, O., *et al.* Splenectomy during pregnancy: an option in the treatment of autoimmune thrombocytopenic purpura. *Br. J. Obstet. Gynaecol.*, 1999; **106**: 373–5.

37 Anglin, B. V., Rutherford, C., Ramus, R., *et al.* Immune thrombocytopenic purpura during pregnancy: laparoscopic treatment. *JSLS*, 2001; **5**: 63–7.

38 Iwase, K., Higaki, J., Yoon, H. E., *et al.* Hand-assisted laparoscopic splenectomy for idiopathic thrombocytopenic purpura during pregnancy. *Surg. Laparosc. Endosc. Percutan. Tech.*, 2001; **11**: 53–6.

39 Gasbarrini, A., Franceschi, F., Tartaglione, R., *et al.* Regression of autoimmune thrombocytopenia after eradication of Helicobacter pylori. *Lancet*, 1998; **352**: 878.

40 Jarque, I., Andreu, R., Llopis, I., *et al.* Absence of platelet response after eradication of Helicobacter pylori infection in patients with chronic idiopathic thrombocytopenic purpura. *Br. J. Haematol.*, 2001; **115**: 1002–3.

41 Broughton, Pipkin, F., Roberts, J. M. Hypertension in pregnancy. *J. Hum. Hypertens.*, 2000; **14**: 705–24.

42 Kupferminc, M. J., Eldor, A., Steinman, N., *et al.* Increased frequency of genetic thrombophilia in women with complications of pregnancy. *N. Engl. J. Med.*, 1999; **340**: 9–13.

43 Hubel, C. A. Oxidative stress in the pathogenesis of preeclampsia. *Proc. Soc. Exp. Biol. Med.*, 1999; **222**: 222–35.

44 Hayman, R., Brockelsby, J., Kenny, L., *et al.* Preeclampsia: the endothelium, circulating factor(s) and vascular endothelial growth factor. *J. Soc. Gynecol. Investig.*, 1999; **6**: 3–10.

45 Zhou, Y., Damsky, C. H., Chiu, K., *et al.* Preeclampsia is associated with abnormal expression of adhesion molecules by invasive cytotrophoblasts. *J. Clin. Invest.*, 1993; **91**: 950–60.

46 Graham, C. H., McCrae, K. R. Altered expression of gelatinase and surface-associated plasminogen activator activity by trophoblast cells isolated from placentas of preeclamptic patients. *Am. J. Obstet. Gynecol.*, 1996; **175**: 555–62.

47 McCrae, K. R., Cines, D. B. Thrombotic microangiopathy during pregnancy. *Semin. Hematol.*, 1997; **34**: 148–58.

48 Martin, J. N., Jr., Files, J. C., Blake, P. G., *et al.* Plasma exchange for preeclampsia. I. Postpartum use for persistently severe preeclampsia–eclampsia with HELLP syndrome. *Am. J. Obstet. Gynecol.*, 1990; **162**: 126–37.

49 Sibai, B. M., Ramadan, M. K., Chari, R. S., *et al.* Pregnancies complicated by HELLP syndrome (hemolysis, elevated liver enzymes, and low platelets): subsequent pregnancy outcome and long-term prognosis. *Am. J. Obstet. Gynecol.*, 1995; **172**: 125–9.

50 Sibai, B. M., Ramadan, M. K., Usta, I., *et al.* Maternal morbidity and mortality in 442 pregnancies with hemolysis, elevated liver enzymes, and low platelets (HELLP syndrome). *Am. J. Obstet. Gynecol.*, 1993; **169**: 1000–6.

51 Magann, E. F., Bass, D., Chauhan, S. P., *et al.* Antepartum corticosteroids: disease stabilization in patients with the syndrome of hemolysis, elevated liver enzymes, and low platelets (HELLP). *Am. J. Obstet. Gynecol.*, 1994; **171**: 1148–53.

52 Magann, E. F., Perry, K. G., Jr., Meydrech, E. F., *et al.* Postpartum corticosteroids: accelerated recovery from the syndrome of hemolysis, elevated liver enzymes, and low platelets (HELLP). *Am. J. Obstet. Gynecol.*, 1994; **171**: 1154–8.

53 Martin, J. N., Jr., Files, J. C., Blake, P. G., *et al.* Postpartum plasma exchange for atypical preeclampsia–eclampsia as HELLP (hemolysis, elevated liver enzymes, and low platelets) syndrome. *Am. J. Obstet. Gynecol.*, 1995; **172**: 1107–25; discussion, 1125–7.

54 Roberts, G., Gordon, M. M., Porter, D., *et al.* Acute renal failure complicating HELLP syndrome, SLE and anti-phospholipid syndrome: successful outcome using plasma exchange therapy. *Lupus*, 2003; **12**: 251–7.

55 Ibdah, J. A., Bennett, M. J., Rinaldo, P., *et al.* A fetal fatty-acid oxidation disorder as a cause of liver disease in pregnant women. *N. Engl. J. Med.*, 1999; **340**: 1723–31.

56 Ibdah, J. A., Yang, Z., Bennett, M. J. Liver disease in pregnancy and fetal fatty acid oxidation defects. *Mol. Genet. Metab.*, 2000; **71**: 182–9.

57 Schapiro, L., Thorp, J. M., Jr. Diagnosis of early acute fatty liver of pregnancy. *J. Matern. Fetal Med.*, 1996; **5**: 314–16.

58 Minakami, H., Takahashi, T., Tamada, T. Should routine liver biopsy be done for the definite diagnosis of acute fatty liver of pregnancy? *Am. J. Obstet. Gynecol.*, 1991; **164**: 1690–1.

59 Bacq, Y. Acute fatty liver of pregnancy. *Semin. Perinatol.*, 1998; **22**: 134–40.

60 Amorosi, E. L., Ultmann, J. E. Thrombotic thrombocytopenic purpura: report of 16 cases and review of the literature. *Medicine*, 1966; **45**: 139–59.

61 Sarode, R., Gottschall, J. L., Aster, R. H., *et al.* Thrombotic thrombocytopenic purpura: early and late responders. *Am. J. Hematol.*, 1997; **54**: 102–7.

62 Furlan, M., Robles, R., Galbusera, M., *et al.* Von Willebrand factor-cleaving protease in thrombotic thrombocytopenic purpura and the hemolytic–uremic syndrome. *N. Engl. J. Med.*, 1998; **339**: 1578–84.

63 Tsai, H. M., Lian, E. C. Antibodies to von Willebrand factor-cleaving protease in acute thrombotic thrombocytopenic purpura. *N. Engl. J. Med.*, 1998; **339**: 1585–94.

64 Veyradier, A., Obert, B., Houllier, A., *et al.* Specific von Willebrand factor-cleaving protease in thrombotic microangiopathies: a study of 111 cases. *Blood*, 2001; **98**: 1765–72.

65 Furlan, M., Lammle, B. Aetiology and pathogenesis of thrombotic thrombocytopenic purpura and haemolytic uraemic syndrome: the role of von Willebrand factor-cleaving protease. *Best Pract. Res. Clin. Haematol.*, 2001; **14**: 437–54.

66 Fujikawa, K., Suzuki, H., McMullen, B., *et al.* Purification of human von Willebrand factor-cleaving protease and its identification as a new member of the metalloproteinase family. *Blood*, 2001; **98**: 1662–6.

67 Tsai, H. M. Is severe deficiency of ADAMTS-13 specific for thrombotic thrombocytopenic purpura? Yes. *J. Thromb. Haemost.*, 2003; **1**: 625–31.

68 Tsai, H. M., Rice, L., Sarode, R., *et al.* Antibody inhibitors to von Willebrand factor metalloproteinase and increased binding of von Willebrand factor to platelets in ticlopidine-associated thrombotic thrombocytopenic purpura. *Ann. Intern. Med.*, 2000; **132**: 794–9.

69 Furlan, M., Robles, R., Solenthaler, M., *et al.* Deficient activity of von Willebrand factor-cleaving protease in chronic relapsing thrombotic thrombocytopenic purpura. *Blood*, 1997; **89**: 3097–103.

70 Allford, S. L., Harrison, P., Lawrie, A. S., *et al.* Von Willebrand factor-cleaving protease activity in congenital thrombotic thrombocytopenic purpura. *Br. J. Haematol.*, 2000; **111**: 1215–22.

71 Levy, G. G., Nichols, W. C., Lian, E. C., *et al.* Mutations in a member of the ADAMTS gene family cause thrombotic thrombocytopenic purpura. *Nature*, 2001; **413**: 488–94.

72 Moschcowitz, E. An acute febrile pleiochromic anemia with hyaline thrombosis of the terminal arterioles and capillaries. *Arch. Intern. Med.*, 1925; **36**: 89–93.

73 Tsai, H. M. Advances in the pathogenesis, diagnosis, and treatment of thrombotic thrombocytopenic purpura. *J. Am. Soc. Nephrol.*, 2003; **14**: 1072–81.

74 Dashe, J. S., Ramin, S. M., Cunningham, F. G. The long-term consequences of thrombotic microangiopathy (thrombotic thrombocytopenic purpura and hemolytic uremic syndrome) in pregnancy. *Obstet. Gynecol.*, 1998; **91**: 662–8.

75 McMinn, J. R., George, J. N. Evaluation of women with clinically suspected thrombotic thrombocytopenic purpura-hemolytic uremic syndrome during pregnancy. *J. Clin. Apheresis*, 2001; **16**: 202–9.

76 George, J. N. The association of pregnancy with thrombotic thrombocytopenic purpura-hemolytic uremic syndrome. *Curr. Opin. Hematol.*, 2003; **10**: 339–44.

77 Mannucci, P. M., Canciani, M. T., Forza, I., *et al.* Changes in health and disease of the metalloprotease that cleaves von Willebrand factor. *Blood*, 2001; **98**: 2730–5.

78 Tsai, H. M., Chandler, W. L., Sarode, R., *et al.* Von Willebrand factor and von Willebrand factor-cleaving metalloprotease activity in *Escherichia coli* O157:H7-associated hemolytic uremic syndrome. *Pediatr. Res.*, 2001; **49**: 653–9.

79 George, J. N., Sadler, J. E., Lammle, B. Platelets: thrombotic thrombocytopenic purpura. *Hematology (Am. Soc. Hematol. Educ. Program)*, 2002: 315–34.

80 George, J. N. How I treat patients with thrombotic thrombocytopenic purpura-hemolytic uremic syndrome. *Blood*, 2000; **96**: 1223–9.

81 Tsai, H. M., Shulman, K. Rituximab induces remission of cerebral ischemia caused by thrombotic thrombocytopenic purpura. *Eur. J. Haematol.*, 2003; **70**: 183–5.

82 Zheng, X., Pallera, A. M., Goodnough, L. T., *et al.* Remission of chronic thrombotic thrombocytopenic purpura after treatment with cyclophosphamide and rituximab. *Ann. Intern. Med.*, 2003; **138**: 105–8.

83 Moake, J. L., Byrnes, J. J., Troll, J. H., *et al.* Effects of fresh-frozen plasma and its cryosupernatant fraction on von Willebrand factor multimeric forms in chronic relapsing thrombotic thrombocytopenic purpura. *Blood*, 1985; **65**: 1232–6.

84 Chintagumpala, M. M., Hurwitz, R. L., Moake, J. L., *et al.* Chronic relapsing thrombotic thrombocytopenic purpura in infants with large von Willebrand factor multimers during remission. *J. Pediatr.*, 1992; **120**: 49–53.

85 Furlan, M., Robles, R., Morselli, B., *et al.* Recovery and half-life of von Willebrand factor-cleaving protease after plasma therapy in patients with thrombotic thrombocytopenic purpura. *Thromb. Haemost.*, 1999; **81**: 8–13.

86 Gordon, L. I., Kwaan, H. C., Rossi, E. C. Deleterious effects of platelet transfusions and recovery thrombocytosis in patients with thrombotic microangiopathy. *Semin. Hematol.*, 1987; **24**: 194–201.

87 Harkness, D. R., Byrnes, J. J., Lian, E. C., *et al.* Hazard of platelet transfusion in thrombotic thrombocytopenic purpura. *JAMA*, 1981; **246**: 1931–3.

88 Milford, D. V., Taylor, C. M., Guttridge, B., *et al.* Haemolytic uraemic syndromes in the British Isles 1985–8: association with verocytotoxin producing *Escherichia coli*. Part 1: Clinical and epidemiological aspects. *Arch. Dis. Child.*, 1990; **65**: 716–21.

89 Hosler, G. A., Cusumano, A. M., Hutchins, G. M. Thrombotic thrombocytopenic purpura and hemolytic uremic syndrome are distinct pathologic entities. A review of 56 autopsy cases. *Arch. Pathol. Lab. Med.*, 2003; **127**: 834–9.

90 Downes, K. A., Allen, K., Sarode, R., *et al.* Consanguinous hemolytic uremic syndrome secondary to *Escherichia coli* O157:H7 infection treated with aggressive therapeutic plasma exchange. *J. Clin. Apheresis*, 2001; **16**: 155–6.

91 Hebisch, G., Bernasconi, M. T., Gmuer, J., *et al.* Pregnancy-associated recurrent hemolytic uremic syndrome with fetal thrombotic vasculopathy in the placenta. *Am. J. Obstet. Gynecol.*, 2001; **185**: 1265–6.

92 Esplin, M. S., Branch, D. W. Diagnosis and management of thrombotic microangiopathies during pregnancy. *Clin. Obstet. Gynecol.*, 1999; **42**: 360–7.

16

Neonatal immune thrombocytopenias

Katharine A. Downes, M.D.[1] and Ravindra Sarode, M.D.[2]

[1]Assistant Professor, Department of Pathology, University Hospitals of Cleveland, Cleveland, Ohio, USA
[2]Professor of Pathology, University of Texas Southwestern Medical Center; Director: Transfusion Medicine and Hemostasis, Dallas, Texas, USA

Introduction

Platelets first appear in the fetal circulation at approximately 5–6 weeks of gestational age. By the end of the first trimester, the mean fetal platelet count is greater than 150×10^9/l[1] and this is maintained for the remainder of the gestation.[2,3] Thus, at birth full term infants have normal platelet counts.

Thrombocytopenia in the full term, healthy neonate is defined as a platelet count of less than 150×10^9/l.[4] The frequency of neonatal thrombocytopenia has been estimated at 1–4%.[5,6] Approximately 1–2% of term infants born to mothers with normal platelet counts are thrombocytopenic at birth.[7,8] There are numerous causes of neonatal thrombocytopenia, and a severe form of the disorder may result from increased consumption or destruction, deficient production, or abnormal splenic sequestration of platelets.[9,10]

The major causes of neonatal thrombocytopenia are non-immune and related to infection, sepsis *etc.* Immune mediated platelet destruction resulting from transplacental passage of maternal antibodies remains an important cause of thrombocytopenia at birth. Up to 15% of neonatal thrombocytopenias that occur at birth result from maternal auto- or alloantibodies directed against fetal platelet antigens.[11] Neonatal thrombocytopenia can be a devastating clinical condition and requires systematic evaluation of the cause and its management. It is also important to address the possibility of recurrence of thrombocytopenia in subsequent pregnancies. This chapter focuses on immune mediated thrombocytopenia in the fetus and neonate.

Hematological Complications in Obstetrics, Pregnancy, and Gynecology, ed. R. L. Bick *et al.* Published by Cambridge University Press.

Neonatal alloimmune thrombocytopenia (NAITP)

Overview

NAITP is defined as thrombocytopenia (platelet count $< 150 \times 10^9$/l) due to transplacentally acquired maternal platelet alloantibodies. First described in 1957,[12] NAITP results from the development of maternal IgG antibodies directed against fetal platelet antigens inherited from the father but that are absent on platelets in the mother. Fetal platelets and platelet microparticles that cross the placental barrier are recognized as foreign by the maternal immune system and then stimulate formation of maternal IgG anti-platelet antibodies directed against the fetal platelet antigens. Transplacental passage of the IgG antibody results in fetal platelet destruction.[13–15]

NAITP caused by human platelet antigens

Incidence

The incidence of NAITP varies between different ethnic/racial populations.[16–20] Neonatal alloimmune thrombocytopenia[21,22] occurs in approximately 1 per 1,000 live births in a Caucasian population with greater than 75% of cases due to fetomaternal incompatibility for the human platelet antigen (HPA), HPA-1a (P1A1, Zwa). Incompatibility for the HPA-5[23] antigen is the next most frequent cause. In the Asian population HPA-1a incompatibility rarely causes NAITP and other alloantigens such as HPA-4 and HPA-3a are implicated.[24–27] Platelet alloantibody specificities in frequently transfused patients (predominantly anti-HPA-5b and -1b, with antigen frequencies <30% among Caucasians) differ significantly from those observed in patients with NAITP or post transfusion purpura, where anti-HPA-1a (antigen frequency >95%) is the most prevalent specificity.[28]

HPA polymorphisms

Development of maternal antibodies to fetal antigens is directly related to the frequency of different platelet antigens in a given population and to the presence of certain polymorphisms in the HPA DNA. Polymorphisms are stable DNA sequence variations in which two or more alleles for a given locus each occur in greater than 1% of the population. Platelet antigen names were initially derived from the names of patients in whom the antigen was first described. To standardize the nomenclature, in 1990 the HPA system was developed[29,30] in which each platelet antigen is determined by anti-sera designed to identify the target antigen. To date, 24 platelet-specific antigens have been characterized; 12 are grouped into six bi-allelic systems (HPA-1, -2, -3, -4, -5, -15) and the molecular basis of 22 has been determined.[31] The HPA polymorphisms[32] relevant to NAITP are discussed below and organized by the HPA system in which the polymorphism occurs.

HPA-1 system: HPA-1a (Pl^{A1}) and HPA-1b (Pl^{A2}) polymorphism

The polymorphism affecting the HPA-1a (Pl^{A1}) antigen[33] is the most frequent cause of NAITP in the Caucasian population.[34] The prevalence of HPA-1a and HPA-1b varies by ethnic background and geography[35] with a gene frequency of HPA-1a of 0.84–0.89 and HPA-1b of 0.11–0.15 in the Caucasian population.[36–39] Maternal alloimmunization to HPA-1a has been reported in <1%[40]–11.4%[41–44] of HPA-1a-negative women. HPA-1 antigen polymorphisms result in the most severe form of the reported cases of alloimmune thrombocytopenia.[25]

HPA-3 system: HPA-3a (Bak^a, Lek^a) and HPA-3b (Bak^b) polymorphism

Antibodies directed against HPA-3a[45] and HPA-3b have been described in NAITP. Anti-HPA-3a generally causes mild to moderate thrombocytopenia in affected neonates but may rarely induce NAITP[46,47] with severe thrombocytopenia at birth (platelet count $< 20 \times 10^9$/l)[48] similar in severity to disease caused by anti-HPA-1a.

HPA-5 system: HPA-5a (Br^a) and HPA-5b (Br^b) polymorphism

HPA-5a (Br^a) and HPA-5b (Br^b) reside on the platelet GP Ia/IIa complex. Incompatibility for HPA-5 is the second most frequent cause of NAITP in the Caucasian population; HPA-5 frequencies have been studied in other populations.[49] HPA-5 polymorphisms correlate with the number of GPIa molecules on the platelet surface.[50,51] Anti-HPA-5b is common among pregnant women, but it does not usually cause severe fetal-neonatal alloimmune thrombocytopenia in the majority of affected infants. In one study anti-HPA-5b was titrated in specimens obtained at the third trimester and antibody-positive women and their neonates were HPA-5 genotyped.[51] It suggested that a high titer (>/= 64) of anti-HPA-5b was associated with an increased risk of neonatal thrombocytopenia, though severe thrombocytopenia rarely occurred.

Clinical presentation/natural history[41]

While often considered the platelet equivalent of hemolytic disease of the newborn (HDN), NAITP differs from the erythrocyte induced Rh(D) HDN in that about 50% of NAITP cases occur in the first pregnancy with a recurrence rate in subsequent pregnancies of 75 to 85%, with a tendency toward increasing disease severity.[52] Hemolytic disease of the newborn does not occur in the first pregnancy unless patient made red cell alloantibodies following blood transfusion. Rarely, HDN and NAITP have been reported in the same patient.[53] *Not all pregnancies in which a mother has formed HPA alloantibodies will result in the delivery of a thrombocytopenic infant.* Serial antibody titers may vary considerably during the evolution of the antibody response during the course of the pregnancy.[25] In some patients, antibodies present early in the pregnancy and then later become undetectable only to appear again in the postnatal period. Neither antibody titer nor its subclass composition is predictive of the occurrence of thrombocytopenia in a newborn whose mother is alloimmunized against HPA,[54–56] though some assert that the level of maternal anti-HPA-1a antibodies is predictive for fetal thrombocytopenia and may be used in decisions related to time and mode of delivery.[57] The maternal platelet count is normal but the fetus may suffer from severe thrombocytopenia.

Maternal history

Prior pregnancy complicated by fetal hydrocephalus, unexplained fetal thrombocytopenia, or recurrent miscarriages may suggest NAITP; multiparous women with a history of giving birth to at least one alloimmune thrombocytopenic infant should be carefully monitored in subsequent pregnancies.[44,58] Maternal history should be reviewed to rule out the effect of drugs taken during pregnancy, maternal autoimmune thrombocytopenia (ITP), and for familial causes of thrombocytopenia.

Diagnosis

The diagnosis is typically suspected either at the time of delivery of the neonate with petechiae, purpura, and large cephalhematoma or *in utero* if intracranial hemorrhage (ICH) occurs. The neonate has thrombocytopenia and the mother has a normal platelet count. Diagnostic testing is implemented after a woman has had an affected pregnancy or in a woman known to have anti-HPA antibodies and a previously affected fetus or neonate (see below).[59] The diagnosis is made by 1) detection and identification of platelet-specific maternal IgG antibody and by 2) identification of the implicated platelet antigen by performing platelet genotyping of the mother and/or father and fetus/neonate.[60]

Maternal antibody detection

Serologic tests to detect platelet specific IgG maternal antibodies include the enzyme-linked immunosorbent assay (ELISA), the platelet suspension immunofluorescence test (PSIFT), the mixed red cell adherence assay (solid-phase red cell assay (SPRCA)), and the monoclonal antibody specific immobilization of platelet antigens assay (MAIPA).[61] Detection is usually performed using an antigen capture *ELISA* methodology, where maternal serum is incubated with sensitized platelets or platelet-specific antigen bound to specific antibody (double capture or sandwich), followed by addition of an enzyme linked antiglobulin reagent, which is used to detect bound IgG.[62] In *PSIFT* platelets are treated with paraformaldehyde, incubated with the maternal serum, washed and then incubated with antiglobulin serum labeled with a fluorescent dye, washed again and then viewed under a fluorescent microscope;[29] this methodology has been modified for flow cytometry analysis. In *SPRCA* donor platelets are fixed to microtiter plate wells that have been coated with monoclonal anti-platelet antibody and maternal serum is added to the well, incubated and washed, then followed by addition of anti-IgG coated erythrocytes. If a platelet antibody is present in the maternal serum, the indicator red cells will cover the plate as an even monolayer; if no antibody is present, the erythrocytes will collect in a small circle in the center of the plate. In *MAIPA* donor platelets are incubated with maternal serum, washed, incubated with platelet specific murine monoclonal antibodies and then placed in microtiter plates coated with polyclonal anti-murine IgG capture antibody, which fixes the donor platelet with the bound maternal antibody to the well. Alkaline phosphatase labeled anti-human IgG is added to detect bound maternal antibody to the donor platelet. The second-generation platelet serological assays, PSIFT and SPRCA may demonstrate only the presence of HLA class-I antibodies of limited specificities and not detect platelet-specific antibodies, while the use of a third generation assay (MAIPA) has detected the additional presence of anti-HPA-5b.[63] In one study, antibodies were detected in the majority of the cases by the platelet suspension immunofluorescence test (PSIFT) and the monoclonal antibody immobilization of platelet antigens (MAIPA) assay; in approximately 20% cases, antibodies were detectable by MAIPA only; in approximately 11% of cases, no antibodies were detectable.[64] *Thus, the negative result of a maternal antibody test does not necessarily exclude NAITP*. In such cases genotyping of maternal, paternal, and fetal/neonatal platelet antigens may allow for identification of NAITP. Antibodies detected in early gestation may require confirmation with a later specimen, because early antibodies may be transient and/or of no clinical significance.

Platelet antigen genotyping[65]

Identification of the locations of HPA antigens on the platelet membrane, cloning of the platelet glycoproteins gene, and the discovery that most of the human platelet-specific alloantigen systems are based on a single nucleotide polymorphism in the DNA sequence led to development of polymerase chain reaction- (PCR) based techniques for platelet antigen genotyping.[66] PCR with sequence-specific primers (PCR-SSP) is used to genotype single nucleotide polymorphisms (SNPs) in both routine diagnosis and medical research. HPAs represent SNPs in platelet-specific glycoproteins. Conventional PCR techniques for HPA antigen genotyping rely on SSPs and detection by gel electrophoresis; new PCR technology measures the match of a hybridization probe with its target thereby allowing simultaneous detection of both alleles for genotyping of the HPA systems.[67] These techniques may be used to genotype platelets from an affected fetus, the mother, or the father.[68] Genotyping studies may be more accurate for platelet alloantigen determination than conventional serologic methods.[69] Genotyping methods also include restriction fragment length polymorphism (RFLP) and Dot-Blot hybridization.[70] Prenatal fetal HPA genotyping is often limited by the restricted amounts of fetal DNA that are obtainable. Modified PCR-SSP technique enables the identification of fetal HPA genotypes using only 0.5 ml amniotic fluid (from week 16 of gestation) and from a maternal plasma sample (from week 38 of gestation).[71]

Management of pregnancy in alloimmunized mother

Management of prenatally diagnosed NAITP is both controversial and challenging and continues to be debated.[72] The optimal treatment of NAITP remains to be elucidated. Treatment approaches have included intrauterine platelet transfusions, some in combination with intravenous gamma globulin (IVIG) to the mother and others in combination with IVIG and prednisone.[73] For the moment, the treatment of choice is a combination of maternal IVIG and/or glucocorticosteroids with intrauterine platelet transfusions in severely affected cases. The results obtained by American and European investigators vary, and at this time no randomized large clinical trials have been conducted. Consequently, there are no definitive recommendations in the literature.

Prenatal screening

While routine screening procedures do not exist at this time to detect NAITP, the value of such programs to detect 'at risk' alloimmunized women during pregnancy continues to be debated.[74] Limited understanding of the relationship between the presence of alloantibodies and clinical disease, lack of reliable platelet typing and antibody detection assays, lack of predictors as to which cases will have a severe outcome, and controversy as to the optimal antenatal therapy have limited the implementation of screening programs.[75] Also, the incidence is not well predicted on the basis of antigen screening tests. Once a woman has had an affected fetus her risk of having a subsequent affected pregnancy will range from 50–100% depending on the heterozygosity or homozygosity of the father for the allele. Hence, prenatal diagnosis and management are now available only for subsequent siblings following diagnosis of a previously affected infant. Because severe fetal alloimmune thrombocytopenia does not always occur in subsequent fetuses either fetal antigen status or platelet counts or both are necessary to determine whether treatment is needed.[76]

Paternal platelet genotyping is recommended to assist in risk counseling following an affected pregnancy.[52] Affected families should be counseled and considered for antenatal therapy. It is suggested that in cases of paternal heterozygosity for the HPA-1a allele, amniocentesis be performed to allow platelet-antigen genotyping of the fetus. If the fetus lacks the incompatible antigen then NAITP will not occur. However, if the incompatible antigen is present on the fetal platelets then percutaneous umbilical vein sampling (PUBS) (see below) at 20 to 24 weeks may be considered with transfusion of antigen negative platelets during the procedure to minimize the risk of fetal hemorrhage.

Prenatal therapeutic strategies are aimed at elevating the fetal platelet count in affected pregnancies in order to prevent hemorrhagic sequelae. A major challenge is the prenatal management of pregnant women alloimmunized to HPA-1a who have a history of a previously affected infant with severe thrombocytopenia and/or ICH. The risk of *in utero* ICH in such women is high enough to merit intervention; however, the optimal treatment is yet to be determined.

Intravenous gamma globulin (IVIG)

There have been encouraging results reported on the use of maternal IVIG.[77] IVIG has been used to treat thrombocytopenia in the fetus via administration to the mother[78,79] as well as in the newborn to treat NAITP.[77,80] Treatment with IVIG has significantly decreased the risk of fetal and neonatal neurological events. Similarly, treatment with only antenatal complementary platelet transfusions increased the likelihood of a neurologically normal outcome.[81] However, some authors assert that maternal IVIG treatment does not always prevent ICH and that the treatment of choice for severely affected cases is serial fetal blood sampling combined with transfusion of compatible platelets.[82] Although IVIG appears to reduce the risk of ICH, the dosage and timing of IVIG treatment is varied.[83] In North America either weekly infusion of high-dose IVIG (1 g/kg) with or without corticosteroids is given to the mother. For some patients who have not responded to IVIG alone, dexamethasone has been used (4 mg/day). In some European hospitals the preferred treatment approach is a repeated *in utero* fetal platelet transfusion.[84]

Fetus and neonate

Clinical presentation

The clinical presentation of the fetus and neonate may reflect the presence and degree of thrombocytopenia. The full term neonate may range from being asymptomatic with thrombocytopenia discovered as an incidental finding to exhibiting widespread purpura to having ICH in severe cases. Generalized petechiae may appear minutes to hours after delivery. Typically, though, other than such sequelae the NAITP full term infant is healthy; gastrointestinal bleeding or hematuria is less commonly observed.[10] Thrombopoietin plasma concentrations in fetuses with alloimmune thrombocytopenia are normal or slightly elevated.[85] Thrombocytopenia may increase in the first 2 days of life and may last for several weeks after birth.

Intracranial hemorrhage (ICH)

The most serious complication of NAITP is ICH,[86–88] which occurs in 10%–20% of severely affected neonates with 25%–50% of ICH occurring *in utero*.[25,52,89] Intracranial hemorrhage may lead to severe hydrocephalus,[90] hydrops fetalis,[91] and fetal death. These infants have elevated risk of neurological complications, including cerebral palsy, hypotonia, developmental delay, seizures,[92] and psychomotor retardation.[93] ICH may occur at birth or for as long as the newborn remains thrombocytopenic. Antenatal or early postnatal neuroradiologic imaging showing hemispheric porencephaly and lateral ventriculomegaly has been suggested as a recognizable pattern of cerebral injury suggestive of the diagnosis of NAITP.[94] The majority of hemorrhages are either intraventricular or intraparenchymal; a rare case of fourth ventricle hemorrhage with extension into the spinal column down the spinal cord has been reported.[95] Infants with ICH should be monitored in the first years of life for persistent neurological damage.

Management of fetus with NAITP in utero

Prenatal management of alloimmune thrombocytopenia of the fetus is by no means standardized and some argue that there is currently less consensus of opinion concerning its management than 10 years ago.[96] If a fetus is at risk of NAITP (i.e. maternal history of NAITP in previous pregnancy) the obstetrician may elect to measure and/or follow the fetal platelet count and/or administer IVIG with or without corticosteroids to the mother. Of these treatment modalities the one that carries the greatest risk is measuring the fetal platelet count.

Determination of fetal platelet count

Confirmation of the severity of NAITP in the fetus requires fetal blood sampling during pregnancy or cord blood samples after birth.[42] Performing a fetal blood sampling carries with it certain risks such as fetal distress, bradycardia, hemorrhage, and death. Diagnostic fetal blood sampling has resulted in fetal mortality due to severe fetal thrombocytopenia where platelets were not transfused during the procedure. If the procedure is performed by an experienced, trained practitioner, the risks may be minimized. If the fetal blood sampling was performed within 5 days of delivery, there was a correlation at birth of fetal platelet count with neonatal platelet count.[97,98]

Fetal scalp sampling removes blood using a heparinized capillary tube from a small scalp laceration. Platelet counts obtained with this method may be inaccurate due to platelet clumping, and/or contamination with maternal blood or amniotic fluid. This procedure also has the risk of scalp hematoma.

Percutaneous umbilical blood sampling (PUBS) cordocentesis provides a more accurate platelet count and requires an experienced, technically skilled physician to minimize the risk of bleeding which may necessitate emergency C-section and may cause fetal death in 1%.[99] If the fetal platelet count is less than 100,000/μl then maternal treatment with IVIG at a dose of 1 g/kg/week may be initiated and continued throughout the pregnancy.[83] Repeat PUBS may be performed 3–6 weeks after starting IVIG to document improvement in platelet count. If the platelet count remains low, high-dose prednisone (60 mg/day) or dexamethasone (4 mg/day) along with weekly IVIG may increase the platelet count. Percutaneous umbilical blood sampling should then be repeated to determine the fetal platelet count. During PUBS, antigen negative platelets should be kept on hand for transfusion if counts are less than 75,000/μl. It is important to communicate with the blood bank prior to performing PUBS regarding the need for platelets in order to allow for the time required to obtain and prepare platelets.[100]

Intrauterine platelet transfusion (IUPT)

The number of transfusions should be limited because of the high cumulative risk associated with repeated procedures. IUPT may be associated with prolonged fetal bradycardia after the transfusion. Transfusion may need to be repeated each week because of the short half-life of the transfused platelets. The dose of platelets in intrauterine transfusion in NAITP is not standardized but rather is based on the gestational age, estimated fetal weight, total blood volume, and the platelet numbers in each platelet concentrate; a dose of 5–10 cm^3/kg may be used. Other equations used to calculate the volume of platelets for IUPT include:

(1) volume = [desired platelet increment/platelet count of concentrate] × estimated fetal blood volume

(2) volume = [VSF (C3-C1)]/C2

Where VSF = estimated fetal blood volume according to fetal weight estimation; C1 = fetal platelet concentration before transfusion; C2 = platelet concentration in component preparation; and C3 = fetal platelet concentration to be obtained.[101]

Platelets should be gamma irradiated to avoid graft-versus-host-disease (GVHD) in the fetus. Platelets should be selected from CMV-negative donors or should be leukocyte reduced to decrease the risk of CMV transmission to the fetus.

Platelets must be negative for the implicated antigen. For intrauterine transfusion, platelets are generally concentrated to provide more platelets in a smaller volume. This also reduces the amount of anti-A and/or anti-B antibodies in plasma, though ABO matching is generally not an issue as A and B blood group antigens are not well developed on fetal red cells. However, a recent case report suggests that transfused platelets should be ABO compatible though it may be very difficult to get ABO and HPA matched platelets.[101]

A recent study of 56 fetuses that all had a sibling affected by NAITP due to anti-HPA-1a found that cases with a sibling history of antenatal ICH or severe thrombocytopenia (platelet counts $< 20 \times 10^9/l$) had significantly lower pretreatment platelet counts than cases whose siblings had less severe thrombocytopenia or postnatal ICH.[99] None of the fetuses managed by serial platelet IUPT suffered ICH following treatment but serious complications arose with fetal blood sampling. The results of this study suggest that a sibling history of NAITP may be used to stratify treatment in future pregnancy.

Management of the neonate

Transfusion therapy

To prevent or to treat hemorrhagic complications from NAITP, the treatment of choice is platelet transfusion. Transfusion therapy in the neonate affected by NAITP consists of selecting platelets that lack the platelet antigen against which the mother has an antibody.[102,103] Hence, postpartum management of severely affected infants focuses on obtaining antigen-negative platelets for transfusion for the neonate. Platelets may be collected from a phenotyped allogeneic donor or from the affected infant's mother for transfusion. Transfusion management in these patients requires close collaboration between the obstetrician, hematologist, and transfusion medicine specialist and the blood center/supplier.

Because of the high frequency of the HPA-1a antigen in the Caucasian population, platelets that lack HPA-1a may be difficult to find. One study found approximately 2.5% of 557 units to be HPA-1a negative.[104] A screening program of over 60,000 blood donations, found only 45 HPA-1a-negative donors with no antibodies to HPA, HLA, RBC antigens, granulocytes or lymphocytes, and with low titer anti-A and/or -B.[105] To facilitate management of NAITP, some blood collection agencies create a panel of platelet donors, to provide timely transfusion support for fetal and neonatal therapy, who are fully genotyped for HPA-1, -2, -3 and -5.

Sometimes, a mother may also have HLA alloantibodies that cross placenta and cause a poor response to platelet transfusion in the fetus due to immune destruction of transfused platelets. In such a scenario an improved transfusion response is seen when HLA compatible HPA-1a negative platelets are transfused.[106] Cross-matching platelets with patient serum may be needed to circumvent platelet-specific antibodies of unknown specificity.[107]

While the optimal approach to postnatal management is to transfuse compatible platelets promptly, lack of awareness of the potential seriousness of the condition among clinical staff, and non-availability of HPA-1a negative platelets may complicate effective management of these patients.[108,109] Since antigen-negative platelets are not always available for transfusion, one should transfuse whatever platelets are available in the blood bank, i.e. HPA-1a positive platelets.[110]

Use of maternal platelets for transfusion

By definition maternal platelets lack the antigen and would be appropriate to transfuse to the neonate provided certain conditions are met. The mother should be healthy, afebrile, and fulfill all allogeneic blood donor criteria other than being pregnant/post-partum. Coordination between the obstetrical service, blood collection facility and transfusion service is critical in orchestrating the collection, processing and administration of maternal platelets. Administration of high-dose IVIG may interfere with the immunoassays used for infectious disease testing and may result in false positive immunoassays for the routine infectious disease tests performed on the mother. Thus, it is preferable to perform the infectious disease tests on the mother prior to administration of IVIG. Maternal platelets are collected by apheresis technology and before transfusion to the neonate should be washed to remove plasma that contains platelet alloantibodies. Maternal platelets must be irradiated to eliminate the risk of GVHD and should be leukocyte reduced.

Other treatment modalities

In an emergency, whole blood exchange has been tried to remove passive antibodies; however its efficacy is somewhat limited as it removes primarily IgM antibodies and not IgG antibodies that cause NAITP.[111] The neonate can be given IVIG therapy but its effect is delayed for up to 18 hours after the administration.[112]

NAITP caused by human leukocyte antigens (HLA) antibody

Overview

HLA antigens are cell-surface glycoproteins encoded by a series of linked genes on chromosome 6. Platelets express MHC (major histocompatibility) Class I but not Class II antigens. The highly polymorphic Class I antigens are further classified into A, B, or C antigens. On platelets there is at least ten times greater expression of the HLA-A or HLA-B antigen as compared to the HLA-C antigen.

Diagnosis

The presence of HLA antibodies in NAITP can be determined by reactions of the maternal sera with lymphocytes and beads from an HLA antibody screening test as well as adsorption and elution tests with paternal cells.[113]

Anti-HLA antibodies

The role of HLA antibodies in NAITP has not yet been clearly delineated.[114] The role of maternal anti-human leukocyte antigen (HLA) antibodies in NAITP is not yet firmly established though neonatal thrombocytopenia induced by maternal IgG anti-HLA antibody has been documented.[115] Neither titers nor IgG subclass could explain the occurrence of NAITP. The factors that contribute to NAITP induced by maternal anti-HLA antibodies remain to be identified. Anti-HLA antibodies reportedly exist in 31% of pregnant women; however cases of NAITP caused by anti-HLA are relatively rare.[116]

Neonatal thrombocytopenia due to HLA alloantibodies is generally mild to moderate and does not pose clinical problems in the neonate. Anti-HLA antibodies have often been seen in conjunction with anti-HPA-3a (Bak^a) antibodies in NAITP cases. While the majority of reported anti-HPA-3a antibodies have co-existing anti-HLA antibodies, anti-HPA-3a is most likely the cause of thrombocytopenia.

Immune thrombocytopenic purpura (ITP)

Clinical presentation

Immune thrombocytopenic purpura is a common autoimmune disorder that often affects women in the child-bearing years but is an uncommon cause of thrombocytopenia during pregnancy.[117] It typically presents as a chronic condition characterized by easy bruisability and with a low platelet count.

Pathophysiology

Maternal antibodies directed against platelets are IgG and cross the placenta, but the binding of antibodies to fetal platelets varies, resulting in a wide range of platelet counts in the affected fetus. Severity of maternal thrombocytopenia does not correlate with that of the fetus. Interventions to raise maternal platelet count may not necessarily increase the fetal platelet count.

Differential diagnosis

Thrombocytopenia is the most common hemostatic abnormality identified in pregnancy[118] and it presents difficult diagnostic and management problems. ITP is a diagnosis of exclusion and must be distinguished from other causes of thrombocytopenia in pregnancy such as infection (HIV), thrombotic thrombocytopenic purpura,[119,120] hemolytic uremic syndrome, preeclampsia, hemolysis elevated liver enzymes low platelets (HELLP) syndrome,[121] and especially the much more common gestational thrombocytopenia (see Chapter 15).[122]

History

A clinical history of thrombocytopenia or bleeding with petechiae and epistaxis prior to conception suggests the diagnosis of ITP. To differentiate between ITP and gestational thrombocytopenia, it is important to review the patient's record for evidence of thrombocytopenia before pregnancy. If previous maternal platelet counts are not available, then the distinction rests upon the timing and severity of thrombocytopenia with more severe thrombocytopenia that occurs earlier in pregnancy more likely to be ITP.

Laboratory values

In the absence of a hypertensive disorder, a moderate asymptomatic thrombocytopenia with platelet count from 50,000/μl–75,000/μl in the first trimester is most likely to be ITP.[123] A patient with thrombocytopenia due to ITP would likely have normal blood pressure, liver enzymes, white and red blood cell indices, no splenomegaly, no drug exposures, and negative HIV testing. Platelet counts less than 50,000/μl are more commonly found secondary to ITP. Patients may be identified before pregnancy or early on using routine complete blood counts. Antiplatelet antibody testing is not recommended because assays have high false positive and false negative rates.

Management

ITP in pregnancy requires the management of two patients, the mother and her fetus. Thus, collaboration between hematologist, obstetrician, anesthesiologist, and neonatologist is critical.[124] *American Society of Hematology* practice guidelines on the management of ITP include recommendations for the care of the pregnant patient and her newborn infant.[125] Intravenous anti-D (WinRho SDF; Nabi, Boca Raton, FL) has been used to treat ITP in the pediatric[126] and non-pregnant Rh (D) positive adult patient;[127–130] its role in the pregnant patient has yet to be delineated.[131] Management strategies during pregnancy may include IVIG and/or glucocorticoids.[98,132–137] For a detailed discussion see Chapter 15.

Neonate

Incidence and degree of thrombocytopenia

While maternal autoantibodies may occur in 2 of every 1000 pregnant women, neonatal thrombocytopenia occurs in only about 10% of neonates born to such mothers and serious hemorrhage occurs in only up to 1%. Large prospective studies show that among infants born to women with ITP, 8.9–14.7% have platelet counts less than 50,000/μl[6] with ICH occurring in 0–1.5% of infants.[138] Only 4% have counts less than 20,000/μl and are therefore at risk for hemorrhage at birth. Infants born to mothers with ITP may have further decrements in platelet count in the first week postpartum. At this time the strongest predictor of severe neonatal thrombocytopenia in a pregnant woman with ITP is a previous pregnancy with a severely thrombocytopenic neonate.

Management

A neonate born to a mother with ITP should have a cord blood platelet count performed at birth and repeated at 24 hours. If thrombocytopenia is severe, IVIG is recommended with platelet transfusion support in cases of active bleeding. The ITP antibody has broad-spectrum reactivity against platelets with shortened survival of all sources of platelets. Thus, in a bleeding or at risk neonate any source of ABO compatible platelets can be transfused. In severe cases exchange transfusion may be considered to remove the circulating anti-platelet antibodies.

REFERENCES

1 Pahal, G. S., Jauniaux, E., Kinnon, C., *et al.* Normal development of human fetal hematopoiesis between eight and seventeen weeks' gestation. *Am. J. Obstet. Gynecol.*, 2000; **183**(4): 1029–34.

2 Forestier, F., Daffos, F., Galacteros, F., *et al.* Hematological values of 163 normal fetuses between 18 and 30 weeks of gestation. *Pediatr. Res.*, 1986; **20**(4): 342–6.

3 Forestier, F., Daffos, F., Catherine, N., *et al.* Developmental hematopoiesis in normal human fetal blood. *Blood*, 1991; **77**(11): 2360–3.

4 Roberts, I. A., Murray, N. A. Thrombocytopenia in the newborn. *Curr. Opin. Pediatr.*, 2003; **15**(1): 17–23.

5 Kaplan, C. Immune thrombocytopenia in the foetus and the newborn: diagnosis and therapy. *Transfus. Clin. Biol.*, 2001; **8**(3): 311–14.

6 Dreyfus, M., Kaplan, C., Verdy, E., *et al.* Frequency of immune thrombocytopenia in newborns: a prospective study. Immune Thrombocytopenia Working Group. *Blood*, 1997; **89**(12): 4402–6.

7 Burrows, R. F., Kelton, J. G. Incidentally detected thrombocytopenia in healthy mothers and their infants. *N. Engl. J. Med.*, 1988; **319**(3): 142–5.

8 Burrows, R. F., Kelton, J. G. Thrombocytopenia at delivery: a prospective survey of 6715 deliveries. *Am. J. Obstet. Gynecol.*, 1990; **162**(3): 731–4.
9 Blanchette, V. S., Rand, M. L. Platelet disorders in newborn infants: diagnosis and management. *Semin. Perinatol.*, 1997; **21**(1): 53–62.
10 Sola, M. C., Del Vecchio, A., Rimsza, L. M. Evaluation and treatment of thrombocytopenia in the neonatal intensive care unit. *Clin. Perinatol.*, 2000; **27**(3): 655–79.
11 Sainio, S., Jarvenpaa, A. L., Renlund, M., *et al.* Thrombocytopenia in term infants: a population-based study. *Obstet. Gynecol.*, 2000; **95**(3): 441–6.
12 Moulinier, J. Iso-immunisation maternelle antiplaquettaire et purpura neo-natal. Le systeme de groupe plaquettaire "Duzo". In *Proc. 6th Cong. Europe Soc. Haematol.*, Copenhagen, p. 817.
13 Simister, N. E. Placental transport of immunoglobulin G. *Vaccine*, 2003; **21**(24): 3365–9.
14 Simister, N. E., Story, C. M. Human placental Fc receptors and the transmission of antibodies from mother to fetus. *J. Reprod. Immunol.*, 1997; **37**(1): 1–23.
15 Saji, F., Samejima, Y., Kamiura, S., *et al.* Dynamics of immunoglobulins at the feto-maternal interface. *Rev. Reprod.*, 1999; **4**(2): 81–9.
16 Chiba, A. K., Bordin, J. O., Kuwano, S. T., *et al.* Platelet alloantigen frequencies in Amazon Indians and Brazilian blood donors. *Transfus. Med.*, 2000; **10**(3): 207–12.
17 Davoren, A., McParland, P., Barnes, C. A., *et al.* Neonatal alloimmune thrombocytopenia in the Irish population: a discrepancy between observed and expected cases. *J. Clin. Pathol.*, 2002; **55**(4): 289–92.
18 Romphruk, A. V., Akahat, J., Srivanichrak, P., *et al.* Genotyping of human platelet antigens in ethnic Northeastern Thais by the polymerase chain reaction-sequence specific primer technique. *J. Med. Assoc. Thai.*, 2000; **83**(11): 1333–9.
19 Mojaat, N., Halle, L., Proulle, V., *et al.* Gene frequencies of human platelet antigens in the Tunisian population. *Tissue Antigens* 1999; **54**(2): 201–4.
20 Santoso, S., Kiefel, V., Masri, R., *et al.* Frequency of platelet-specific antigens among Indonesians. *Transfusion*, 1993; **33**(9): 739–41.
21 Bussel, J. B., Zabusky, M. R., Berkowitz, R. L., *et al.* Fetal alloimmune thrombocytopenia. *N. Engl. J. Med.*, 1997; **337**(1): 22–6.
22 Hohlfeld, P., Forestier, F., Kaplan, C., *et al.* Fetal thrombocytopenia: a retrospective survey of 5,194 fetal blood samplings. *Blood*, 1994; **84**(6): 1851–6.
23 Kaplan, C., Morel-Kopp, M. C., Kroll, H., *et al.* HPA-5b (Br(a)) neonatal alloimmune thrombocytopenia: clinical and immunological analysis of 39 cases. *Br. J. Haematol.*, 1991; **78**(3): 425–9.
24 Shih, M. C., Liu, T. C., Lin, I. L., *et al.* Gene frequencies of the HPA-1 to HPA-13, Oe and Gov platelet antigen alleles in Taiwanese, Indonesian, Filipino and Thai populations. *Int. J. Mol. Med.*, 2003; **12**(4): 609–14.
25 Ohto, H. Neonatal alloimmune thrombocytopenia. *Nippon Rinsho*, 1997; **55**(9): 2310–14.
26 Kunicki, T. J. Platelet antigen polymorphism in platelets: New understanding of platelet glycoproteins and their role in disease. *American Society of Hematology*, 2000: 225.
27 Mueller-Eckhardt, C., Kiefel, V., Grubert, A., *et al.* 348 cases of suspected neonatal alloimmune thrombocytopenia. *Lancet*, 1989; **1**(8634): 363–6.
28 Kiefel, V., Konig, C., Kroll, H., *et al.* Platelet alloantibodies in transfused patients. *Transfusion*, 2001; **41**(6): 766–70.

29 Von dem Borne, A. E., van Leeuwen, E. F., von Riesz, L. E., *et al.* Neonatal alloimmune thrombocytopenia: detection and characterization of the responsible antibodies by the platelet immunofluorescence test. *Blood*, 1981; **57**(4): 649–56.

30 Von dem Borne, A. E., Decary, F. ICSH/ISBT Working Party on platelet serology. Nomenclature of platelet-specific antigens. *Vox Sang*, 1990; **58**(2): 176.

31 Metcalfe, P., Watkins, N. A., Ouwehand, W. H., *et al.* Nomenclature of human platelet antigens. *Vox Sang*, 2003; **85**(3): 240–5.

32 Rozman, P. Platelet antigens. The role of human platelet alloantigens (HPA) in blood transfusion and transplantation. *Transpl. Immunol.*, 2002; **10**(2–3): 165–81.

33 Kunicki, T. J., Aster, R. H. Isolation and immunologic characterization of the human platelet alloantigen, P1A1. *Mol. Immunol.*, 1979; **16**(6): 353–60.

34 Davoren, A., McParland, P., Crowley, J., *et al.* Antenatal screening for human platelet antigen-1a: results of a prospective study at a large maternity hospital in Ireland. *BJOG* 2003; **110**(5): 492–6.

35 Seo, D. H., Park, S. S., Kim, D. W., *et al.* Gene frequencies of eight human platelet-specific antigens in Koreans. *Transfus. Med.*, 1998; **8**(2): 129–32.

36 Simsek, S., Faber, N. M., Bleeker, P. M., *et al.* Determination of human platelet antigen frequencies in the Dutch population by immunophenotyping and DNA (allele-specific restriction enzyme) analysis. *Blood*, 1993; **81**(3): 835–40.

37 Kim, H. O., Jin, Y., Kickler, T. S., *et al.* Gene frequencies of the five major human platelet antigens in African-American, white, and Korean populations. *Transfusion*, 1995; **35**(10): 863–7.

38 Kekomaki, S., Partanen, J., Kekomaki, R. Platelet alloantigens HPA-1, -2, -3, -5 and -6b in Finns. *Transfus. Med.*, 1995; **5**(3): 193–8.

39 Merieux, Y., Debost, M., Bernaud, J., *et al.* Human platelet antigen frequencies of platelet donors in the French population determined by polymerase chain reaction with sequence-specific primers. *Pathol. Biol. (Paris)*, 1997; **45**(9): 697–700.

40 Panzer, S., Auerbach, L., Cechova, E., *et al.* Maternal alloimmunization against fetal platelet antigens: a prospective study. *Br. J. Haematol.*, 1995; **90**(3): 655–60.

41 Williamson, L. M., Hackett, G., Rennie, J., *et al.* The natural history of fetomaternal alloimmunization to the platelet-specific antigen HPA-1a (PlA1, Zwa) as determined by antenatal screening. *Blood*, 1998; **92**(7): 2280–7.

42 Doughty, H. A., Murphy, M. F., Metcalfe, P., *et al.* Antenatal screening for fetal alloimmune thrombocytopenia: the results of a pilot study. *Br. J. Haematol.*, 1995; **90**(2): 321–5.

43 Blanchette, V. S., Chen, L., de Friedberg, Z. S., *et al.* Alloimmunization to the PlA1 platelet antigen: results of a prospective study. *Br. J. Haematol.*, 1990; **74**(2): 209–15.

44 Durand-Zaleski, I., Schlegel, N., Blum-Boisgard, C., *et al.* Screening primiparous women and newborns for fetal/neonatal alloimmune thrombocytopenia: a prospective comparison of effectiveness and costs. Immune Thrombocytopenia Working Group. *Am. J. Perinatol.*, 1996; **13**(7): 423–31.

45 Takada, H., Nakamura, S., Nishiguchi, T., *et al.* Neonatal alloimmune thrombocytopenia associated with anti-human platelet antigen-3a antibody. *Acta Paediatr. Jpn.*, 1997; **39**(3): 371–4.

46 Harrison, C. R., Curtis, B. R., McFarland, J. G., *et al.* Severe neonatal alloimmune thrombocytopenia caused by antibodies to human platelet antigen 3a (Baka) detectable only in whole platelet assays. *Transfusion*, 2003; **43**(10): 1398–402.

47 Boehlen, F., Kaplan, C., de Moerloose, P. Severe neonatal alloimmune thrombocytopenia due to anti-HPA-3a. *Vox Sang*, 1998; **74**(3): 201–4.

48 Glade-Bender, J., McFarland, J. G., Kaplan, C., *et al.* Anti-HPA-3A induces severe neonatal alloimmune thrombocytopenia. *J. Pediatr.*, 2001; **138**(6): 862–7.

49 Covas, D. T., Biscaro, T. A., Nasciutti, D. C., *et al.* Gene frequencies of the HPA-3 and HPA-5 platelet antigen alleles among the Amerindians. *Eur. J. Haematol.*, 2000; **65**(2): 128–31.

50 Corral, J., Rivera, J., Gonzalez-Conejero, R., *et al.* The number of platelet glycoprotein Ia molecules is associated with the genetically linked 807 C/T and HPA-5 polymorphisms. *Transfusion*, 1999; **39**(4): 372–8.

51 Ohto, H., Yamaguchi, T., Takeuchi, C., *et al.* Anti-HPA-5b-induced neonatal alloimmune thrombocytopenia: antibody titre as a predictor. Collaborative Study Group. *Br. J. Haematol.*, 2000; **110**(1): 223–7.

52 Dickinson, J. E., Marshall, L. R., Phillips, J. M., *et al.* Antenatal diagnosis and management of fetomaternal alloimmune thrombocytopenia. *Am. J. Perinatol.*, 1995; **12**(5): 333–5.

53 Schild, R. L., Hoch, J., Plath, H., *et al.* Perinatal management of fetal hemolytic disease due to Rh incompatibility combined with fetal alloimmune thrombocytopenia due to HPA-5b incompatibility. *Ultrasound Obstet. Gynecol.*, 1999; **14**(1): 64–7.

54 McFarland, J. G., Frenzke, M., Aster, R. H. Testing of maternal sera in pregnancies at risk for neonatal alloimmune thrombocytopenia. *Transfusion*, 1989; **29**(2): 128–33.

55 Proulx, C., Filion, M., Goldman, M., *et al.* Analysis of immunoglobulin class, IgG subclass and titre of HPA-1a antibodies in alloimmunized mothers giving birth to babies with or without neonatal alloimmune thrombocytopenia. *Br. J. Haematol.*, 1994; **87**(4): 813–17.

56 Kurz, M., Stockelle, E., Eichelberger, B., *et al.* IgG titer, subclass, and light-chain phenotype of pregnancy-induced HPA-5b antibodies that cause or do not cause neonatal alloimmune thrombocytopenia. *Transfusion*, 1999; **39**(4): 379–82.

57 Jaegtvik, S., Husebekk, A., Aune, B., *et al.* Neonatal alloimmune thrombocytopenia due to anti-HPA 1a antibodies; the level of maternal antibodies predicts the severity of thrombocytopenia in the newborn. *BJOG*, 2000; **107**(5): 691–4.

58 Kaplan, C. Alloimmune thrombocytopenia of the fetus and the newborn. *Blood Rev.*, 2002; **16**(1): 69–72.

59 Hurd, C., Lucas, G. Human platelet antigen genotyping by PCR-SSP in neonatal/fetal alloimmune thrombocytopenia. *Methods Mol. Med.*, 2004; **91**: 71–8.

60 Panzer, S. Report on the Tenth International Platelet Genotyping and Serology Workshop on behalf of the International Society of Blood Transfusion. *Vox Sang*, 2001; **80**(1): 72–8.

61 Berry, J. E., Murphy, C. M., Smith, G. A., *et al.* Detection of Gov system antibodies by MAIPA reveals an immunogenicity similar to the HPA-5 alloantigens. *Br. J. Haematol.*, 2000; **110**(3): 735–42.

62 Kiefel, V., Santoso, S., Weisheit, M., *et al.* Monoclonal antibody specific immobilization of platelet antigens (MAIPA): a new tool for the identification of platelet-reactive antibodies. *Blood*, 1987; **70**(6): 1722–6.

63 Allen, D. L., Floyd, A. P., Billson, A. L., *et al.* Neonatal alloimmune thrombocytopenia due to anti-HPA-5b (Br(a), Zav(a), Hca): the importance of third-generation platelet antibody detection techniques, a case report. *Transfus. Med.*, 1992; **2**(4): 277–81.
64 Uhrynowska, M., Maslanka, K., Zupanska, B. Neonatal thrombocytopenia: incidence, serological and clinical observations. *Am. J. Perinatol.*, 1997; **14**(7): 415–18.
65 Kroll, H., Kiefel, V., Santoso, S. Clinical aspects and typing of platelet alloantigens. *Vox Sang*, 1998; **74** (Suppl. 2): 345–54.
66 Kretzschmar, E., Von Ahsen, N., Trobisch, H. Rapid genotyping of human platelet antigen 5 with fluorophore-labelled hybridization probes on the LightCycler. *Br. J. Haematol.*, 2001; **114**(2): 397–9.
67 Randen, I., Sorensen, K., Killie, M. K., *et al.* Rapid and reliable genotyping of human platelet antigen (HPA)-1, -2, -3, -4, and -5 a/b and Gov a/b by melting curve analysis. *Transfusion*, 2003; **43**(4): 445–50.
68 Hurd, C. M., Cavanagh, G., Schuh, A., *et al.* Genotyping for platelet-specific antigens: techniques for the detection of single nucleotide polymorphisms. *Vox Sang*, 2002; **83**(1): 1–12.
69 Schuh, A. C., Watkins, N. A., Nguyen, Q., *et al.* A tyrosine703serine polymorphism of CD109 defines the Gov platelet alloantigens. *Blood*, 2002; **99**(5): 1692–8.
70 McFarland, J. G. Platelet and neutrophil alloantigen genotyping in clinical practice. *Transfus. Clin. Biol.*, 1998; **5**(1): 13–21.
71 Bugert, P., Lese, A., Meckies, J., *et al.* Optimized sensitivity of allele-specific PCR for prenatal typing of human platelet alloantigen single nucleotide polymorphisms. *Biotechniques*, 2003; **35**(1): 170–4.
72 Kaplan, C., Murphy, M. F., Kroll, H., *et al.* Feto-maternal alloimmune thrombocytopenia: antenatal therapy with IvIgG and steroids – more questions than answers. European Working Group on FMAIT. *Br. J. Haematol.*, 1998; **100**(1): 62–5.
73 Sainio, S., Teramo, K., Kekomaki, R. Prenatal treatment of severe fetomaternal alloimmune thrombocytopenia. *Transfus. Med.*, 1999; **9**(4): 321–30.
74 Gopel, W., Fehlau, K., Kohl, M., *et al.* HPA-1 carrier status and thrombocytopenia in preterm infants with a birth weight below 1500 grams. *J. Perinat. Med.*, 2002; **30**(2): 176–8.
75 Williamson, L. M. Screening programmes for fetomaternal alloimmune thrombocytopenia. *Vox Sang*, 1998; **74** (Suppl. 2): 385–9.
76 Silver, R. M., Porter, T. F., Branch, D. W., *et al.* Neonatal alloimmune thrombocytopenia: antenatal management. *Am. J. Obstet. Gynecol.*, 2000; **182**(5): 1233–8.
77 Herrero, R. J., Chitrit, Y., Caubel, P., *et al.* Feto-maternal alloimmune thrombocytopenia due to HPA-5b incompatibility: a case report. *Eur. J. Obstet. Gynecol. Reprod. Biol.*, 2003; **110**(2): 240–1.
78 Lucas, G. F., Hamon, M., Carroll, S., *et al.* Effect of IVIgG treatment on fetal platelet count, HPA-1a titre and clinical outcome in a case of feto-maternal alloimmune thrombocytopenia. *BJOG*, 2002; **109**(10): 1195–8.
79 Nathan, F. E., Herman, J. H., Keashen-Schnell, M., *et al.* Anti-Bak(a) neonatal alloimmune thrombocytopenia: possible prevention by intravenous immunoglobulin. *Pediatr. Hematol. Oncol.*, 1994; **11**(3): 325–9.

80 Winters, J. L., Jennings, C. D., Desai, N. S., *et al.* Neonatal alloimmune thrombocytopenia due to anti-HPA-1b (PLA2)(Zwb). A case report and review. *Vox Sang*, 1998; **74**(4): 256–9.

81 Spencer, J. A., Burrows, R. F. Feto-maternal alloimmune thrombocytopenia: a literature review and statistical analysis. *Aust. NZ J. Obstet. Gynaecol.*, 2001; **41**(1): 45–55.

82 Kroll, H., Kiefel, V., Giers, G., *et al.* Maternal intravenous immunoglobulin treatment does not prevent intracranial haemorrhage in fetal alloimmune thrombocytopenia. *Transfus. Med.*, 1994; **4**(4): 293–6.

83 Zuppa, A. A., Cota, F., De Luca, D., *et al.* Incidental diagnosis and tempestive therapy in a case of neonatal alloimmune thrombocytopenia due to anti-HPA-5b. *Pediatr. Hematol. Oncol.*, 2002; **19**(8): 587–91.

84 Blanchette, V. S., Johnson, J., Rand, M. The management of alloimmune neonatal thrombocytopenia. *Baillieres Best Pract. Res. Clin. Haematol.*, 2000; **13**(3): 365–90.

85 Cremer, M., Dame, C., Schaeffer, H. J., *et al.* Longitudinal thrombopoietin plasma concentrations in fetuses with alloimmune thrombocytopenia treated with intrauterine PLT transfusions. *Transfusion*, 2003; **43**(9): 1216–22.

86 Meyer-Heim, A. D., Boltshauser, E. Spontaneous intracranial haemorrhage in children: aetiology, presentation and outcome. *Brain Dev.*, 2003; **25**(6): 416–21.

87 Sia, C. G., Amigo, N. C., Harper, R. G., *et al.* Failure of cesarean section to prevent intracranial hemorrhage in siblings with isoimmune neonatal thrombocytopenia. *Am. J. Obstet. Gynecol.*, 1985; **153**(1): 79–81.

88 Naidu, S., Messmore, H., Caserta, V., *et al.* CNS lesions in neonatal isoimmune thrombocytopenia. *Arch. Neurol.*, 1983; **40**(9): 552–4.

89 Dean, L. M., McLeary, M., Taylor, G. A. Cerebral hemorrhage in alloimmune thrombocytopenia. *Pediatr. Radiol.*, 1995; **25**(6): 444–5.

90 Murphy, M. F., Hambley, H., Nicolaides, K., *et al.* Severe fetomaternal alloimmune thrombocytopenia presenting with fetal hydrocephalus. *Prenat. Diagn.*, 1996; **16**(12): 1152–5.

91 Stanworth, S. J., Hackett, G. A., Williamson, L. M. Fetomaternal alloimmune thrombocytopenia presenting antenatally as hydrops fetalis. *Prenat. Diagn.*, 2001; **21**(5): 423–4.

92 Sadowitz, P. D., Balcom, R. Intrauterine intracranial hemorrhage in an infant with isoimmune thrombocytopenia. *Clin. Pediatr.* (Phila), 1985; **24**(11): 655–7.

93 Sharif, U., Kuban, K. Prenatal intracranial hemorrhage and neurologic complications in alloimmune thrombocytopenia. *J. Child. Neurol.*, 2001; **16**(11): 838–42.

94 Dale, S. T., Coleman, L. T. Neonatal alloimmune thrombocytopenia: antenatal and postnatal imaging findings in the pediatric brain. *AJNR Am. J. Neuroradiol.*, 2002; **23**(9): 1457–65.

95 Abel, M., Bona, M., Zawodniak, L., *et al.* Cervical spinal cord hemorrhage secondary to neonatal alloimmune thrombocytopenia. *J. Pediatr. Hematol. Oncol.*, 2003; **25**(4): 340–2.

96 Engelfriet, C. P., Reesink, H. W., Kroll, H., *et al.* Prenatal management of alloimmune thrombocytopenia of the fetus. *Vox Sang*, 2003; **84**(2): 142–9.

97 Moise, K. J., Jr., Carpenter, R. J., Jr., Cotton, D. B., *et al.* Percutaneous umbilical cord blood sampling in the evaluation of fetal platelet counts in pregnant patients with autoimmune thrombocytopenia purpura. *Obstet. Gynecol.* 1988; **72**(3 Pt 1): 346–50.

98 Kaplan, C., Daffos, F., Forestier, F., *et al.* Fetal platelet counts in thrombocytopenic pregnancy. *Lancet*, 1990; **336**(8721): 979–82.

99 Birchall, J. E., Murphy, M. F., Kaplan, C., *et al.* European collaborative study of the antenatal management of feto-maternal alloimmune thrombocytopenia. *Br. J. Haematol.*, 2003; **122**(2): 275–88.

100 Morales, W. J., Stroup, M. Intracranial hemorrhage in utero due to isoimmune neonatal thrombocytopenia. *Obstet. Gynecol.*, 1985; **65**(3 Suppl): 20–21S.

101 Yeast, J. D., Plapp, F. Fetal anemia as a response to prophylactic platelet transfusion in the management of alloimmune thrombocytopenia. *Am. J. Obstet. Gynecol.*, 2003; **189**(3): 874–6.

102 Kekomaki, S., Volin, L., Koistinen, P., *et al.* Successful treatment of platelet transfusion refractoriness: the use of platelet transfusions matched for both human leucocyte antigens (HLA) and human platelet alloantigens (HPA) in alloimmunized patients with leukaemia. *Eur. J. Haematol.*, 1998; **60**(2): 112–18.

103 Pappalardo, P. A., Secord, A. R., Quitevis, P., *et al.* Platelet transfusion refractoriness associated with HPA-1a (Pl(A1)) alloantibody without coexistent HLA antibodies successfully treated with antigen-negative platelet transfusions. *Transfusion*, 2001; **41**(8): 984–7.

104 Denomme, G., Horsewood, P., Xu, W., *et al.* A simple and rapid competitive enzyme-linked immunosorbent assay to identify HPA-1a (PlA1)-negative donor platelet units. *Transfusion*, 1996; **36**(9): 805–8.

105 Ranasinghe, E., Walton, J. D., Hurd, C. M., *et al.* Provision of platelet support for fetuses and neonates affected by severe fetomaternal alloimmune thrombocytopenia. *Br. J. Haematol.*, 2001; **113**(1): 40–2.

106 Murphy, M. F., Metcalfe, P., Waters, A. H., *et al.* Antenatal management of severe feto-maternal alloimmune thrombocytopenia: HLA incompatibility may affect responses to fetal platelet transfusions. *Blood*, 1993; **81**(8): 2174–9.

107 Kekomaki, R. Use of HLA- and HPA – matched platelets in alloimmunized patients. *Vox Sang*, 1998; **74**(Suppl. 2): 359–63.

108 Murphy, M. F., Knechtli, C., Downie, C., *et al.* Serendipity and the use of random donor platelets in fetomaternal alloimmune thrombocytopenia (FMAIT). *Br. J. Haematol.*, 2001; **113**(4): 1077–8.

109 Murphy, M. F., Verjee, S., Greaves, M. Inadequacies in the postnatal management of fetomaternal alloimmune thrombocytopenia (FMAIT). *Br. J. Haematol.*, 1999; **105**(1): 123–6.

110 Win, N. Provision of random-donor platelets (HPA-1a positive) in neonatal alloimmune thrombocytopenia due to anti HPA-1a alloantibodies. *Vox Sang*, 1996; **71**(2): 130–1.

111 Bussel, J., Kaplan, C., McFarland, J. Recommendations for the evaluation and treatment of neonatal autoimmune and alloimmune thrombocytopenia. The Working Party on Neonatal Immune Thrombocytopenia of the Neonatal Hemostasis Subcommittee of the Scientific and Standardization Committee of the ISTH. *Thromb. Haemost.*, 1991; **65**(5): 631–4.

112 Massey, G. V., McWilliams, N. B., Mueller, D. G., *et al.* Intravenous immunoglobulin in treatment of neonatal isoimmune thrombocytopenia. *J. Pediatr.*, 1987; **111**(1): 133–5.

113 Saito, S., Ota, M., Komatsu, Y., *et al.* Serologic analysis of three cases of neonatal alloimmune thrombocytopenia associated with HLA antibodies. *Transfusion*, 2003; **43**(7): 908–17.

114 Taaning, E. HLA antibodies and fetomaternal alloimmune thrombocytopenia: myth or meaningful? *Transfus. Med. Rev.*, 2000; **14**(3): 275–80.

115 Del Rosario, M. L., Fox, E. R., Kickler, T. S., *et al.* Neonatal alloimmune thrombocytopenia associated with maternal anti-HLA antibody: a case report. *J. Pediatr. Hematol. Oncol.*, 1998; **20**(3): 252–6.

116 Sasaki, M., Yagihashi, A., Kobayashi, D., *et al.* Neonatal alloimmune thrombocytopenia due to anti-human leukocyte antigen antibody: a case report. *Pediatr. Hematol. Oncol.*, 2001; **18**(8): 519–24.

117 Burrows, R. F., Kelton, J. G. Fetal thrombocytopenia and its relation to maternal thrombocytopenia. *N. Engl. J. Med.*, 1993; **329**(20): 1463–6.

118 Burrows, R. Hemorrhagic complications in the obstetric patient. In Hirsch, J., ed., *Hemostasis and Thrombosis*, 4th edn. Philadelphia, PA: Lippincott, Williams and Wilkins; 2001. pp. 1045–51.

119 Lattuada, A., Rossi, E., Calzarossa, C., *et al.* Mild to moderate reduction of a von Willebrand factor cleaving protease (ADAMTS-13) in pregnant women with HELLP microangiopathic syndrome. *Haematologica*, 2003; **88**(9): 1029–34.

120 Nabhan, C., Kwaan, H. C. Current concepts in the diagnosis and management of thrombotic thrombocytopenic purpura. *Hematol. Oncol. Clin. North Am.*, 2003; **17**(1): 177–99.

121 Martin, J. N., Jr., Thigpen, B. D., Rose, C. H., *et al.* Maternal benefit of high-dose intravenous corticosteroid therapy for HELLP syndrome. *Am. J. Obstet. Gynecol.*, 2003; **189**(3): 830–4.

122 Al-Kouatly, H. B., Chasen, S. T., Kalish, R. B., *et al.* Causes of thrombocytopenia in triplet gestations. *Am. J. Obstet. Gynecol.*, 2003; **189**(1): 177–80.

123 Shehata, N., Burrows, R., Kelton, J. G. Gestational thrombocytopenia. *Clin. Obstet. Gynecol.*, 1999; **42**(2): 327–34.

124 Ali, R., Ozkalemkas, F., Ozcelik, T., *et al.* Idiopathic thrombocytopenic purpura in pregnancy: a single institutional experience with maternal and neonatal outcomes. *Ann. Hematol.*, 2003; **82**(6): 348–52.

125 George, J. N., Woolf, S. H., Raskob, G. E., *et al.* Idiopathic thrombocytopenic purpura: a practice guideline developed by explicit methods for the American Society of Hematology. *Blood*, 1996; **88**(1): 3–40.

126 Freiberg, A., Mauger, D. Efficacy, safety, and dose response of intravenous anti-D immune globulin (WinRho SDF) for the treatment of idiopathic thrombocytopenic purpura in children. *Semin. Hematol.*, 1998; **35**(1 Suppl. 1): 23–7.

127 Cooper, N., Woloski, B. M., Fodero, E. M., *et al.* Does treatment with intermittent infusions of intravenous anti-D allow a proportion of adults with recently diagnosed immune thrombocytopenic purpura to avoid splenectomy? *Blood*, 2002; **99**(6): 1922–7.

128 Sagripanti, A., Ferretti, A., Giannessi, D., *et al.* Anti-D treatment for chronic immune thrombocytopenic purpura: clinical and laboratory aspects. *Biomed. Pharmacother.*, 1998; **52**(7–8): 293–7.

129 Newman, G. C., Novoa, M. V., Fodero, E. M., *et al.* A dose of 75 microg/kg/d of i.v. anti-D increases the platelet count more rapidly and for a longer period of time than 50 microg/kg/d in adults with immune thrombocytopenic purpura. *Br. J. Haematol.*, 2001; **112**(4): 1076–8.

130 Scaradavou, A., Bussel, J. B. Clinical experience with anti-D in the treatment of idiopathic thrombocytopenic purpura. *Semin. Hematol.*, 1998; **35**(1 Suppl. 1): 52–7.

131 Michel, M., Novoa, M. V., Bussel, J. B. Intravenous anti-D as a treatment for immune thrombocytopenic purpura (ITP) during pregnancy. *Br. J. Haematol.*, 2003; **123**(1): 142–6.

132 David, M., Chevalier, I. Alternatives to intravenous immunoglobulins in the treatment of immune thrombocytopenic purpura. *Vox Sang*, 2002; **83** (Suppl. 1): 443–5.

133 Payne, S. D., Resnik, R., Moore, T. R., *et al.* Maternal characteristics and risk of severe neonatal thrombocytopenia and intracranial hemorrhage in pregnancies complicated by autoimmune thrombocytopenia. *Am. J. Obstet. Gynecol.*, 1997; **177**(1): 149–55.

134 Gill, K. K., Kelton, J. G. Management of idiopathic thrombocytopenic purpura in pregnancy. *Semin. Hematol.*, 2000; **37**(3): 275–89.

135 Boehlen, F., Hohlfeld, P., Extermann, P., *et al.* Maternal antiplatelet antibodies in predicting risk of neonatal thrombocytopenia. *Obstet. Gynecol.*, 1999; **93**(2): 169–73.

136 Valat, A. S., Caulier, M. T., Devos, P., *et al.* Relationships between severe neonatal thrombocytopenia and maternal characteristics in pregnancies associated with autoimmune thrombocytopenia. *Br. J. Haematol.*, 1998; **103**(2): 397–401.

137 Gandemer, V., Kaplan, C., Quelvennec, E., *et al.* Pregnancy-associated autoimmune neonatal thrombocytopenia: role of maternal HLA genotype. *Br. J. Haematol.*, 1999; **104**(4): 878–85.

138 Guidelines for the investigation and management of idiopathic thrombocytopenic purpura in adults, children and in pregnancy. *Br. J. Haematol.*, 2003; **120**(4): 574–96.

17

The rational use of blood and its components in obstetrical and gynecological bleeding complications

Katharine A. Downes, M.D.[1] and Ravindra Sarode, M.D.[2]

[1]Assistant Professor, Department of Pathology, University Hospitals of Cleveland, Cleveland, Ohio, USA
[2]Professor of Pathology, University of Texas Southwestern Medical Center; Director: Transfusion Medicine and Hemostasis, Dallas, Texas, USA

Introduction

Hemorrhagic complications in obstetrical practice are frequently encountered that require specific blood component therapy. This chapter presents an overview of the rational use of blood components in pregnancy, for obstetrical bleeding complications, and in general gynecology practice. Section I discusses blood collection, transfusion risk, and pretransfusion compatibility testing. Section II describes the preparation, contents, storage, and indications for blood and its components. Section III focuses on the use of new pharmacological therapeutic agents in lieu of blood and component therapy in specific patient populations. Section IV reviews transfusion of blood components in clinical situations involving the obstetrical patient.

I Blood collection, transfusion risk, and pretransfusion testing

Blood collection

Each year in the United States over 12 million units of whole blood are collected.[1] Blood donors are qualified for donation based on an initial history and physical examination using eligibility criteria established by the Food and Drug Administration (FDA). Blood donation is performed using two different methods: (1) *whole blood donation* where a single unit of whole blood (WB) is collected into a plastic bag and then separated *at a later time* into components, or (2) *apheresis donation* via an automated technology where the donor is connected to an instrument which selectively collects either red blood cells (RBCs), platelets or plasma. The blood components are RBCs, plasma, cryoprecipitate, and platelets. The donor is tested for

Hematological Complications in Obstetrics, Pregnancy, and Gynecology, ed. R. L. Bick *et al.* Published by Cambridge University Press.

Table 17.1 Current infectious disease testing of allogeneic blood donors.

	Agent	Tests performed on donor blood	Estimated risk
Viral	HIV	anti-HIV-1 and HIV-2	~1:2,000,000
	HBV	anti-HBc, HBSAg	~1:200,000
	HVC	anti-HCV; NAT for HCV RNA	~1:1,900,000
	HTLV-I/II	anti HTLV-I; anti-HTLV-II	~1:2,990,000
Bacterial	Syphilis	Serologic test	Extremely rare

Key: HIV = Human immunodeficiency virus; NAT = nucleic acid testing; HBV = hepatitis B virus; anti-HBc = anti-hepatitis B core; HBSAg = hepatitis B surface antigen; HCV = hepatitis C virus; HTLV-I/II = Human T-cell lymphocytotrophic virus-I/II.

infectious diseases (see Table 17.1), ABO blood group, Rh(D) type, and red cell alloantibodies. Whole blood and its components are stored in a variety of different anticoagulant-preservative solutions that may include *dextrose* for ATP generation by the glycolytic pathway, *adenine* to serve as substrate for ATP synthesis, *citrate* as anticoagulant, and *sodium diphosphate* to maintain pH.

Risks of transfusion therapy

The blood supply has never been safer in its history than it is today.[2–10] Transfusion risks may be infectious (see Table 17.1) or non-infectious (see Table 17.2).

Infectious risks

Blood collecting agencies, the Food and Drug Administration (FDA), physicians, and scientists have tiers of protective layers to interdict transfusion-transmitted diseases (TTD).[11–13] Before any blood component unit is released, pre-donation screening of the donor and post-donation infectious disease testing has occurred. Nevertheless, each transfusion carries with it a slight risk of transmitting a known infectious agent for which testing is performed if the infection is in an undetectable phase known as the window period. Also, there is an additional risk of an unknown or an emerging infection for which testing is not performed.[14] The recent discovery that West Nile virus is transmissible by transfusion is the latest reminder that the blood supply continues to be vulnerable to emerging pathogens.[15–20] Another example involves transmissible spongiform encephalopathy [Creutzfeldt-Jakob Disease (CJD) and new variant CJD (nCJD) or mad cow disease], which have theoretical but unproven transmission of their infectious prion particles.[21,22] At present, there is no test to detect the infectious prion particle in blood donors, nor do current viral inactivation methods definitively eliminate the abnormal prion

Table 17.2 Noninfectious risks of transfusion.

Transfusion reactions
Hemolytic
Immediate or delayed
Allergic
Moderate to severe – anaphylactic, bronchospasm, etc.
Mild – urticarial, itching
Febrile nonhemolytic
Volume overload
Transfusion-related acute lung injury
Citrate reactions
Alloimmunization
Transfusion-associated graft vs. host disease
Post-transfusion purpura

protein. Those involved in Transfusion Medicine are constantly monitoring new pathogens and developing strategies to keep the blood supply as safe as possible.

Non-infectious risks

The current, single greatest transfusion threat of immediate mortality from a non-infectious cause is the administration of ABO incompatible blood to a patient.[23–25] Patient identification and/or clerical errors may be made at the time of initial sample collection, during laboratory testing, or at the bedside at the time of transfusion.[26] Other noninfectious risks of blood and component therapy[27] include mild urticarial to severe allergic[28] reactions such as anaphylaxis to plasma proteins, febrile nonhemolytic transfusion reactions due to cytokines, acute and delayed hemolytic transfusion reactions due to red cell alloantibodies, volume overload, transfusion related acute lung injury[29,30] and alloimmunization against erythrocyte, leukocyte or platelet antigens.[31] Large volumes of plasma infusions,[32] as seen in massive transfusion, may have complications of citrate reaction (from tingling numbness to parasthesias), hypothermia and metabolic acidosis. Transfusion associated graft-versus-host disease (GVHD) is a rare complication seen in immunocompromised patients, and in immunocompetent patients who are getting transfusions from first-degree relatives.[33–35]

Pretransfusion compatibility testing

When a blood product or component is requested, a series of immunohematology tests are performed on a patient's blood in order to provide compatible blood. This pretransfusion testing is performed to prevent immune mediated hemolytic transfusion reactions.[36] Hemolytic transfusion reactions may have serious sequelae including hemoglobinemia, disseminated intravascular coagulation (DIC), renal failure, and death.

Before transfusion, ABO blood group and Rh(D) type are determined on the patient's blood. If within the preceding 3 months the patient has been transfused with blood, has been pregnant, or if the history is unknown, it is necessary to obtain a sample from the patient within 3 days of the scheduled transfusion with the day of the draw considered Day 0 (zero).[37] Additionally, an antibody screen is performed on the patient's plasma or serum to determine if any antibody is present. If the antibody screen is positive, antibody identification is performed in order to determine the specificity of the antibody, after which RBC donor units are selected that lack the antigen(s) to which the antibody is directed. ABO/Rh(D) type is also determined for each individual unit of RBCs destined for transfusion. Both ABO Group and Rh(D) type must be compatible between the recipient and donor. This is accomplished by (1) a clerical check of all the records as well as (2) a cross-match where the donor RBCs and patient serum or plasma are mixed together and upon examination if RBC agglutination or hemolysis is absent, compatibility of donor RBC with patient serum or plasma is indicated.

II Blood and its components: Preparation, contents, storage, volume, indications, and administration

The following section reviews the preparation, contents, storage, and indications of Whole Blood (WB) and its components; thereafter, some practical aspects of blood administration are presented. Whole blood and its components are listed in parallel to how they are produced in actuality (see Table 17.3).

Whole blood

Preparation and storage

Whole blood (450 ml ± 10%) is collected into a closed system consisting of a phlebotomy needle, tubing, and attached polyvinyl resin bags. Each of the bags contains approximately 63 ml–70 ml of a citrate-based anticoagulant. Whole blood is stored at 1–6 °C and the expiration date depends upon the composition of the anticoagulant used. Additive solutions cannot be added to whole blood to increase the storage time. After 24 hours of storage, WB essentially becomes red cells suspended (38% hematocrit) in a protein solution equivalent to liquid plasma. This is due to significant loss of labile coagulation factors (FV and VIII), and platelets that become dysfunctional.[38]

Table 17.3 Blood and its components: Preparation, contents, storage, volume, indications, and administration.

Blood/blood component	Approximate volume/unit	Storage conditions	Composition/ constituents in each unit	Expiration of unit and storage media	Major indications (see chapter for detailed description)	Other considerations	Rate of infusion of blood/component
Whole blood	500 ml	1 °C–6 °C	Red blood cells, plasma, (hematocrit ~40%). Functional platelets are virtually absent	ACD/CPD/CP2D 21 days CPDA-1 35 days	Massive hemorrhage	Must be ABO identical	For massive hemorrhage as rapidly as tolerated. Must be within 4 hours
Packed red blood cells (PRBCs)	250–330 ml	1 °C–6 °C	RBCs suspended mostly in anticoagulant and very small amount of plasma	CPD/CP2D 21 days CPDA-1 35 days (250 ml with Hct ~80%) Additive solution 42 days (~330 ml with Hct 52–60%)	Symptomatic anemia	Must be ABO compatible	Must be within 4 hours
Platelets, random donor	50 ml	20 °C–24 °C with continuous agitation/rotation	Greater than 5.5×10^{10} platelets	5 days after collection	Hemorrhage secondary to thrombocytopenia or platelet dysfunction	For adults 4–6 units pooled for a single dose	Must be within 4 hours
Platelets, apheresis/ single donor platelets (SDP)	200–300 ml	20 °C–24 °C with continuous agitation/rotation	Greater than 3×10^{11} platelets/unit	5 days after collection	See platelets, RDP	For children it can be divided into smaller doses	Less than 4 hours

Fresh frozen plasma (FFP)	~200 ml	<−18 °C	Plasma proteins All of the coagulation factors	≤18 °C 12 months ≤65 °C 7 years	Deficiency of plasma coagulation factors	Must be frozen within 8 hours if collected in CPD, CP2D, CPDA-1. Must be frozen within 6 hours if collected in ACD. Must be ABO-compatible	Must be within 4 hours
FFP thawed	See FFP	1 °C–6 °C	See FFP	24 hours	See FFP		Less than 4 hours
Thawed plasma	See FFP	1 °C–6 °C	Reduced levels of Factor VIII and Factor V	5 days	See FFP		Less than 4 hours
Cryoprecipitate (CRYO)	15 ml	<−18 °C	Fibrinogen, Factor VIII, von Willebrand factor, FXIII, fibronectin	12 months	Replacement of fibrinogen, Factor XIII	Thaw at 30 °C–37 °C and 5–20 units pooled	Within 4 hours

Key: Anticoagulant storage solution abbreviations: ACD = adenine citrate dextrose; CPD = citrate phosphate dextrose; CP2D = citrate phosphate 2 dextrose; CDPA-1 citrate phosphate dextrose adenine-1.

Indications

While WB was the first product transfused in the United States, the development of centrifugation technology and storage bags allowed for its breakdown into multiple specific components. Today whole blood is rarely used in clinical practice in the United States. Whole blood has limited efficacy and use in clinical practice. Its limitations include (1) circulatory/volume overload in patients who require only the oxygen-carrying capacity of RBCs, (2) loss of platelet function, (3) loss of labile coagulation factors, and (4) ***the requirement that whole blood must be ABO identical to the patient's ABO type***. Some physicians elect to transfuse whole blood in cardiovascular surgery. Whole blood is indicated for patients with massive hemorrhage (active bleeding and loss of >25% of their total blood volume – see Section IV) and for patients undergoing an exchange transfusion.[39] One unit of whole blood will increase hemoglobin by 1 g/dl or the hematocrit by 3%. In one study of patients undergoing liver transplantation, the use of WB provided effective therapy for blood loss comparable to the use of components, while allowing fewer donor exposures.[40] In cases of massive hemorrhage, WB transfusion may be more expeditious as compared to packed red cells and fresh frozen plasma, which require time to be thawed.

Packed red blood cells (PRBC)

Preparation and storage

PRBCs are units of whole blood with most of the plasma removed. WB is collected and centrifuged at a slow spin; RBCs settle at the bottom of the bag and platelet rich plasma (PRP) is expressed off into a satellite bag. Additive solution (AS-1, AS-3, AS-5) may be added to the PRBCs to extend the shelf life by providing additional nutrients. PRBCs collected via apheresis are similar in efficacy to PRBCs prepared from a WB donation.[41] A PRBC unit contains a small volume of plasma (~15 cc) and mostly anticoagulant solution. Each PRBC unit raises the adult patient's hemoglobin concentration by 1 g/dl or the hematocrit by 3%. PRBCs are stored at 1–6 °C with the storage time based on the anticoagulant and additive solution used. The volume of one PRBC unit is between 220–350 ml with a hematocrit of ~80%. In those units which contain an additive solution, the hematocrit decreases to ~55% in a volume of about 300–400 ml.

Indications

PRBC transfusion is indicated when tissue oxygenation is compromised by either acute or chronic blood loss or anemia. RBC transfusion is commonly used to increase oxygen-carrying capacity for patients who are anemic or undergoing chemotherapy or radiation therapy, trauma victims, surgical patients, end-stage renal disease patients, premature infants, or patients with sickle cell disease.[42] Adequate oxygenation can be maintained with a hemoglobin content of 7 g/dl in the normovolemic patient without cardiac disease; however, co-morbid factors often necessitate transfusion at a higher threshold. Blood and its components must only be transfused when clinically indicated. *The physician should document on each patient's chart the clinical necessity for transfusion.* The decision to transfuse a patient should not be based solely on a numerical value but rather on (1) patient's age as related to her health, (2) severity of anemia, (3) etiology of anemia, (4) duration of anemia, (5) estimated blood loss, and (6) vital signs. RBCs should not be transfused to treat anemia(s) that might be corrected with medications such as iron, vitamin B_{12}, or folic acid, nor should they be used as volume expanders or to increase oncotic pressure.

Platelets

Random donor platelets (RDPs)

Preparation

RDPs are obtained from PRP (collected during PRBC preparation) as described above. PRP is centrifuged at high speed at room temperature, which creates a platelet pellet; platelet poor plasma (PPP) is then siphoned off to another bag. The platelet pellet is re-suspended and constitutes one random donor platelet unit. For transfusion in adults, 4–6 RDP units are pooled together in a single large bag. It is important to note that once pooled, the unit must be transfused within 4 hours. After 4 hours, the unit is considered expired (due to increased risk of bacterial growth because pooling is done in an open system) and it must be discarded. One unit of RDP contains at least 5.5×10^{10} platelets in $\sim$50 cm^3 of plasma. Depending on the collection technique, platelet units may contain numerous leukocytes. Some RBCs are present in each unit, which may result in a pink tinge/coloration if the concentration of RBC exceeds 1 cm^3 in the pool of six RDPs.

Single donor platelets (SDPs)

Preparation

SDPs, also known as apheresis platelets, are collected by apheresis machine during an approximately two-hour donor session. SDP contain at least 3×10^{11} platelets in 200–300 cm^3 a unit, which includes a small amount of anticoagulant solution. This number of platelets is equivalent to a pool of 4–6 RDP units. The apheresis techniques used generally produce leukocyte reduced SDPs whereas RDPs can be leukoreduced by leukoreduction filters either at the collection facility or in the hospital blood bank.

Storage

RDP and SDP are stored at 20–24 °C with gentle agitation and expire 5 days from the day of the collection.

Indications and dose

The objective of platelet transfusion is to provide an adequate number of functioning platelets to prevent and/or stop hemorrhage.[43] Therefore, platelet transfusion is indicated for the management of patients with quantitative and qualitative platelet disorders. Thrombocytopenia may be due to increased consumption or decreased production.[44] With normal platelet function, a platelet count of 10,000/μl is hemostatic in an otherwise stable patient. One adult dose of platelet (1 SDP or 4–6 pooled RDP) increases the platelet count by 25–50,000/μl. For large adults (>80 kg) the dose is usually 1 RDP per 10 kg of body weight. Because of the platelet's short life span, frequent (2–3 days) platelet transfusion may be required to maintain an adequate platelet count. Inadequate increment at 60 minutes post transfusion may suggest refractoriness to platelet transfusion due to HLA alloantibodies. Other causes of platelet refractoriness include alloantibodies against platelet specific antigens, DIC, idiopathic thrombocytopenic purpura (ITP), drugs, hypersplenism, fever and sepsis.

Other considerations

The A and B blood group antigens are weakly expressed on platelets. Therefore, ABO compatibility of platelets generally is not an issue unless the patient seems to be refractory to platelet transfusion in which case ABO identical transfusion should be tried. When platelets need to be transfused to infants or for large volume transfusion in an adult, donor plasma in the platelets should be ABO compatible with the recipient's red cells. Care should be taken in transfusing O platelets (which can have extremely high titer anti-A antibodies) to a Group A patient.

While the Rh(D) antigen is not expressed on platelets, contaminating Rh(D) positive RBCs (6-pooled RDP may have up to 0.5–1 cc and SDP up to 0.5 cc) may stimulate an immune response in a patient who is Rh(D) negative. Thus, there is a potential for development of anti-D in an Rh(D)-negative woman of childbearing age or in a young female who receives platelets from an Rh(D) positive donor.[45] Therefore, when Rh(D) positive platelets are given to an Rh(D) negative female the use of intravenous Rh(D) immune globulin (300 μg single dose; WinRho SDF® Nabi Biopharmaceuticals Boca Raton, FL) is recommended, since the intramuscular route (i.e. RhoGAM®, Ortho-Clinical Diagnostics Inc, Raritan, New Jersey) is contraindicated in thrombocytopenic patients. Administration of RhIg is a conservative therapy with little risk to the patient. Efficacy lasts for 4–6 weeks, thus allowing for platelet transfusion with Rh(D)-positive platelets.[46]

Fresh frozen plasma

Preparation and storage

Supernatant plasma, separated during RDP preparation and frozen within 8 hours of whole blood collection at –18 °C, is known as fresh frozen plasma (FFP).[47] The volume of one unit of FFP varies depending on the method used to collect and prepare the unit and may range from 200–250 ml if WB derived and 400–600 ml if collected by apheresis technique. FFP is stored at or below 18 °C for one year. Since plasma must be ABO compatible with the patient's RBCs, the ABO blood group must be known. FFP must be thawed in a water bath at 30 °C–37 °C and transfused within 4 hours if kept at room temperature or within 24 hours if stored at 4 °C. If it is not used within 24 hours it is relabeled as thawed plasma and must be refrigerated at 4 °C and it may be used for up to 5 days. Thawing 2–4 units of plasma may take 15–30 minutes. FFP contains all of the coagulation proteins including the heat labile coagulation factors V and VIII, which degrade over time if stored unfrozen. With the exception of Factor VIII, levels of clotting factor activity are stable for up to 5 days in thawed plasma.[48] One international unit (IU) of each coagulation factor is present in each ml of undiluted plasma.

Indications and dose

Liver Disease: In liver disease decreased production of clotting factors and anti-plasmin, increased levels of tissue plasminogen activator (TPA) and abnormal or decreased fibrinogen production may lead to bleeding.[49,50] If a liver disease patient with coagulopathy (prothrombin time >5 seconds above normal) requires surgery or is bleeding, 10–15 cm^3/kg FFP should be given. Factor VII has a half-life of about 6 hours; consequently, a patient may require FFP every 6–8 hours to correct coagulopathy or stop bleeding.

Reversal of warfarin effect

Fresh frozen plasma is used for the reversal of warfarin effect before surgery or to treat warfarin overdose when the patient is bleeding or is at a greater risk of bleeding. Warfarin decreases the vitamin K-dependent clotting factors (FII, VII, IX, and X) that are present in FFP. It is given as a 10–15 cm^3/kg dose that may need to be repeated after 6–8 hours.

Replacement of isolated coagulation factor deficiencies:[51–53] FFP is indicated for the replacement of isolated deficiencies of Factors II, V, X and XI for which purified concentrates are not available. These factors have long half-lives of 24–72 hours and hence need to be treated at 24–48 hour intervals after a loading dose of 10–15 cm^3/kg. Factor VII deficiency can be treated with either FFP or recombinant FVIIa, which is generally used for the treatment of patients with acquired hemophilia or congenital hemophilia, who have developed inhibitors. Acquired deficiencies of these factors, having a wide range in the severity of bleeding, are seen in a variety of conditions ranging from autoimmune disorders to malignancy. Diagnosis depends on demonstration of decreased factor activity.[54]

Massive transfusion

FFP is used in the setting of massive blood transfusion[55–57] or major blood loss to replace depleted clotting factors that are not present in PRBCs. Generally in the setting of massive transfusion, one unit of FFP is given for each 5 PRBC units transfused, but the dose may vary with the clinical situation.

Disseminated intravascular coagulation (DIC)

The management of DIC includes treating the primary cause; however, FFP should be given to patients with acute DIC who are bleeding in order to replace consumed clotting factors along with cryoprecipitate and platelets. If the patient is not bleeding, then FFP should not be transfused simply to correct laboratory values; in such a case adding FFP would be like *adding fuel to the fire* and can worsen microvascular thromboses. FFP *should not* be used when a coagulopathy might be corrected more effectively with a specific therapy (i.e. vitamin K, cryoprecipitate) nor should it be used solely as a volume expander.

Other indications of FFP include plasma exchange therapy for thrombotic thrombocytopenic purpura and HELLP syndrome.

Cryoprecipitate (CRYO)

Preparation and storage

CRYO is prepared by thawing FFP at 1 °C–6 °C, a procedure which produces an insoluble precipitate. After centrifugation at 4 °C this precipitate is separated from cryosupernatant and then re-frozen within 1 hour. The volume of CRYO is 15–20 cm^3 in each unit. For transfusion, the CRYO units are thawed at 30 °C–37 °C, and 5–15 units are pooled, based upon the patient's weight and the substance that is being replaced. After pooling, CRYO must be transfused within 4 hours. In adults CRYO units are not necessarily ABO compatible due to very small volume of plasma; however, the ABO group is honored in a neonate.

CRYO contains fibrinogen, von Willebrand factor (VWF), FVIII, FXIII, and fibronectin. Each unit of CRYO should contain at least ≥80 IU Factor VIII: C units and at least ≥150 mg of fibrinogen. CRYO is stored at or <−18 °C for up to 12 months from the date of collection. CRYO must be transfused within 6 hours of thawing and pooling.

Indications and dose

Fibrinogen replacement: The hemostatic level of fibrinogen is ≥100 mg/dl. A single unit of CRYO will increase the fibrinogen level by ~5–10 mg/dl in an adult who is not bleeding. In a patient who is bleeding, the target fibrinogen level is >150 mg/dl. CRYO is indicated for congenital afibrinogenemia,[58,59] congenital or acquired hypofibrinogenemia,[60] and dysfibrinogenemia. FXIII and fibrinogen play an essential role in placental implantation and maintenance of pregnancy. Maternal fibrinogen maintains hemostatic balance during pregnancy and may play a role in stabilizing uteroplacental attachment at the fetal–maternal junction.[61] Congenital low fibrinogen levels may be associated with placental abruption.[62] Deficiencies of FXIII and/or of fibrinogen are the only coagulation deficiencies associated with pregnancy loss.[63] Acquired hypofibrinogenemia is encountered in acute DIC, liver disease or massive transfusion. Generally, CRYO is given as a pool of 10–15 bags for hypofibrinogenemia. In the steady state, the half-life of fibrinogen is 3–5 days. Dosing schedules of CRYO infusions of every 3 days for patients with congenital a/hypofibroginemia is appropriate during hemostatic challenge. The patients receiving cryoprecipitate as fibrinogen replacement in conditions with rapid fibrinogen turnover should be monitored with fibrinogen assays.

Von Willebrand disease (VWD): CRYO contains von Willebrand factor (VWF) (>80 units/bag) and is used to treat VWD; however, it is a second line therapy for VWD because of availability of a safer, purified product, Humate-P® (Aventis-Behring, Marburg, Germany). The loading dose of CRYO is 20–30 units (depending on the weight of the patient) followed by half of that every 12 hours (t/2 is 12 hours).

Factor XIII replacement: FXIII catalyzes cross-linking between fibrin monomers, which increases the strength of the fibrin clot.[64–66] Since FXIII may play a critical role in uterine hemostasis and maintenance of the placenta during gestation,[67] a deficiency of FXIII would result in a weakened fibrin clot with hemostatic abnormalities. FXIII level required to maintain hemostasis is very small (>1–2%) and it has a very long half-life (~96 hours), therefore CRYO is given for treatment of FXIII deficiency at a dose of 10–15 units every 2–3 weeks.[68,69]

Uremia

CRYO is given at a dose of 10–15 units every 12–24 hours to treat the coagulopathy associated with uremia.[70,71] The precise mechanism leading to the benefit is unknown; however, abnormality of VWF is postulated. Its use should be restricted to patients who do not respond to non-transfusion therapy (DDAVP, desmopressin) or have shown tachyphylaxis to DDAVP.

Modifications to whole blood and its components

Leukocyte reduction, irradiation and/or washing of blood components are performed to prevent adverse effects of transfusion. *Leukocyte reduction* removes leukocytes that may carry CMV or induce febrile non-hemolytic transfusion reactions or alloimmunization to HLA antigens.[72,73] RBC, SDP and RDP units may be leukocyte-reduced at the time of or immediately after collection at the collection centers or in the blood bank before sending the unit to the floor for transfusion. Pre-storage leukocyte reduction at blood centers is preferred because this results in less cytokine release from the lymphocytes in platelets that are stored at room temperature.[74] *Irradiation* is indicated for the prevention of transfusion-associated graft-versus-host disease in immunocompromised patients such as neonates, intrauterine transfusion, congenital immunodeficiency syndromes, and blood transfusions from first-degree blood relatives (directed donation) in immunocompetent patients.

Plasma proteins, which may cause severe allergic reactions, can be removed from cellular blood components by *washing*; this is especially indicated to prevent anaphylaxis in a patient with absolute IgA deficiency or occasional intractable severe allergic reactions not responding to antihistamines and steroids.

Blood administration

The unit of blood or blood component *may only be administered* to the patient after both recipient and blood/component have been properly identified. All blood components must be transfused through a filter designed to remove small clots and microaggregates (170–260 micron filter). With the exception of a 0.9% sodium chloride injection (USP), no medications or solutions may be added to or infused through the same tubing with blood or components unless such a solution has specific approval from the FDA for this use. Avoid infusing solutions containing calcium (i.e., Lactated Ringer's, Injection ISP) through the same tubing used for the transfused blood; the addition of calcium may reverse the anti-coagulant effect of citrate and cause clotting in the tubing. Except in cases of massive hemorrhage, the infusion rate should be slow, e.g. 2 cc/minute (one unit in ∼2 hours). The patient must be monitored carefully and vital signs must be recorded. In the event of a transfusion reaction as described in Table 17.2 **the transfusion should be stopped.** Transfusion should not be restarted until the transfusion service has evaluated the patient. The only exception is mild allergic reactions like rash and/or urticaria, where a transfusion can be stopped, and re-started once antihistamine/steroids have controlled the reaction.

III Use of new pharmacological agents in lieu of blood and component therapy

Red blood cell substitutes

The development of a blood substitute would be invaluable for patients requiring emergent transfusion or patients unwilling to receive transfusions. There is a persistent search for a red blood cell substitute with the oxygen carrying capacity of hemoglobin. The two classes of red blood cell substitutes are hemoglobin-containing fluids and Perfluoro compound emulsions. Inherent difficulties with these hemoglobin-based products include high oxygen affinity, a short plasma half-life, and auto-oxidation.[75] The Perfluoro compounds are water insoluble. More studies are needed to determine the efficacy of these compounds and the side-effect profile for pregnancy.[76–78]

Erythropoietin (EPO)

Erythropoietin regulates red cell production and is secreted by renal peritubular cells in adult and fetal hepatocytes. EPO increases erythrocyte survival and causes maturation and proliferation of erythroid progenitor cells. In normal pregnancy maternal EPO levels may increase 2–4× of normal[79–83] EPOGEN® (rHuEPO; Epoetin Alfa) is a recombinant EPO that stimulates RBC production. It was initially used in the treatment of anemia associated with chronic renal failure (50–100 units/kg) for patients on dialysis. Its uses have expanded to treat anemias due to other causes, as well as perioperative surgical patients (300 units/kg/day for 10 days preoperatively), and autologous blood donors.[84] EPO has been used to treat iron deficiency anemia during pregnancy[85] as well as anemic women in the puerperium (20,000 units in one time single dose).[86] EPO has been used with some success in pregnant women with renal failure[87] and renal transplantation (50–150 units/kg/week).[88,89] For a detailed discussion of the role of EPO in the management of anemia in pregnancy, see Chapter 9.

A novel erythropoiesis-stimulating factor (NESP, Darbepoetin Alfa (Aranesp) Amgen Inc, Thousand Oak, CA)[90–92] has been synthesized. When compared with rHuEPO, NESP has a higher carbohydrate content (52% vs. 40%), a longer plasma half-life[93,94] and has been reported to maintain hemoglobin levels just as effectively in patients with chronic renal failure as rHuEPO but at less frequent dosing.[95] It has not yet been studied in pregnant women and its effects on the fetus are unknown.

Although EPO has been used in some patients, many Jehovah's Witness patients refuse EPO because it contains albumin, which some consider to be a prohibited blood product.

Recombinant Factor VIIa (Novoseven)

Recombinant activated FVII (NovoSeven, Novo Nordisk, Princeton NJ; rFVIIa) is a hemostatic agent that complexes *in vivo* with tissue factor to activate Factor X, thereby initiating the clotting cascade by bypassing requirements for Factors VIII and IX. It has been used as a universal hemostatic agent because of its potent thrombin generating power in patients with trauma.

rVIIa is used to treat patients with hemophilia A or hemophilia B who have inhibitors to Factor VIII or Factor IX.[96,97] There are no well-controlled studies of rVIIa in pregnant women; rVIIa should be used in pregnancy only when the potential benefits justify the potential risk to the fetus. It has been successfully used in pregnant patients with congenital FVII deficiency (an off-label use).[98] Because of its universal hemostatic effect and recombinant preparation, it may be used in obstetric patients with trauma or severe hemorrhage who are Jehovah's Witnesses. Glanzmann's Thrombasthenia is a rare, autosomal recessive bleeding disorder resulting from a deficiency of the platelet glycoprotein IIb-IIIa complex.[99] rFVIIa has been used in the management of two pregnant women with Glanzmann's Thrombasthenia.[100] rFVIIa has also been used to treat severe obstetric hemorrhage due to placental accreta, uterine rupture, and preeclampsia with HELLP.[101]

Individuals who are Jehovah's Witnesses pose a unique challenge for the obstetrician in the management of labor and delivery and their potential complications.[102,103] A pregnant Jehovah's Witness patient requires a thoughtful multidisciplinary approach that unites obstetricians, transfusion medicine specialists, anesthesiologists, and interventional radiologists in proactive and preventive management. Women who are Jehovah's Witnesses may refuse transfusions, even when the transfusion is life saving for them. Maternal deaths have occurred in cases related to refusal of blood transfusion.[104] One retrospective cohort study found that in 391 deliveries by 332 Jehovah's Witness women, there was a 6% obstetric hemorrhage rate resulting in two maternal deaths.[105] This translates into a rate of 512 maternal deaths per 100,000 live births versus 12 maternal deaths per 100,000 live births in the non-Jehovah's Witness population, leading to a conclusion that women who are Jehovah's Witnesses may be at a 44-fold increased risk of maternal death from obstetric hemorrhage. Each institution should have clearly defined consent procedures and documentation regarding the transfusion wishes of such a patient. Many adult Jehovah's Witnesses carry a wallet-sized advance directive card stating that they refuse blood;[106] however, the patient's decision with regards to receipt of blood and its components should be reviewed with her at the time of admission. Limiting the amount and frequency of phlebotomy during a hospital stay may help to minimize blood loss in these patients.[107] Intra-operative blood salvage with cell savers and auto-transfusion may be used in these patients; collection devices can be modified to ensure a continuous closed connection with the patient's own circulation. Jehovah's Witnesses may accept synthetic blood substitutes but may refuse hemoglobin-based substitutes composed of animal or human protein. For anemic patients EPO is an option to increase hemoglobin values before delivery, and, if there is massive hemorrhage, then rFVIIa can be used at 70 μg/kg dose (4800 μg/vial dose).

IV Special clinical conditions encountered in obstetrics and use of blood components

Overview

Hemorrhagic disorders during pregnancy and the puerperium create a challenge for the obstetrician in management of both mother and fetus. Hemorrhagic disorders may be inherited,[108] acquired, or related to the physiology of pregnancy.

Anemia

Anemia is the most common hematologic complication of pregnancy and is associated with increased rates of premature birth, low birth weight and perinatal mortality. Detection of anemia beyond the physiologic anemia of pregnancy is important because anemia at the time of delivery may increase the need for a blood transfusion. Hemoglobin should be maintained >7–8 g/dl.

Etiologies

Iron deficiency is the most common cause of anemia, and iron supplementation will both prevent and treat iron deficiency anemia. Most pregnant women benefit from daily elemental iron supplementation of 30 to 60 mg.[109]

Obstetric hemorrhage

Common hemorrhagic complications of pregnancy remain among the leading causes of maternal mortality, e.g., abruptio placenta, DIC, placenta previa, uterine rupture, and postpartum hemorrhage.[110–112] While maternal hemorrhage is a primary cause of maternal mortality world-wide,[113–118] the mortality rate from major hemorrhage is lower in developed countries and has been reported from 1.4 to 2.0 pregnancy-related-deaths due to hemorrhage per 100,000 live births in the

United States.[119,120] The risk of death from obstetric hemorrhage has been minimized by the availability of blood products for transfusion. A recent study found an overall maternal mortality rate of 9.5 per 100,000 live births in Japan, with hemorrhage the most common cause of death.[121]

Transfusion management

Guidelines

Each obstetric unit should have protocols and guidelines to manage intra or postpartum hemorrhage.[122,123] Such guidelines should encompass the management of patients who agree to transfusion as well as those patients who object to blood transfusions.[124]

Transfusion therapy

The degree of hypotension is the first guide to the degree of blood loss, except in abruptio placentae. Delays in correcting hypovolemia, diagnosing and treating coagulopathy, and surgical correction of bleeding are potentially avoidable. Rapid, immediate correction of hypovolemia with crystalloids and red cells is then followed by blood component therapy guided by hematocrit, PT, APTT, fibrinogen, platelet count and clinical features. The management of massive hemorrhage is described below.

Massive transfusion

Definition and pathophysiology

Massive transfusion is defined as the replacement of one or more blood volumes within 24 hours due to hemorrhage. The blood volume of a 70 kg adult is approximately 5,000 ml, which is the equivalent of 10 units of whole blood. Rapid hemorrhage initiates complex interrelated physiologic responses or hemorrhagic shock, which complicates the management of acute hemorrhage. Hypotension, tachycardia, oliguria, pallor, cyanosis, decreased hematocrit and central venous pressure are characteristic signs and symptoms of shock. Severe hemorrhage affects electrolyte balance and oxygen transport.

Laboratory investigation

In a patient with massive hemorrhage laboratory studies should be drawn as STAT and include coagulation studies (PT, APTT, fibrinogen and platelet count), blood type and Screen, blood gases or pulse-oximetry, as well as a biochemical profile.

Samples should be collected at the earliest opportunity, as results may be affected by colloid infusion.

Treatment

Successful treatment requires immediate action and excellent communication between the obstetrical service, the transfusion medicine service and the blood bank. The objectives of treatment of massive hemorrhage are to restore blood volume and to maintain tissue perfusion and oxygenation, as well as to achieve hemostasis by correcting coagulopathy by the rational use of blood component therapy. The most important goal in treating acute hemorrhage is to prevent or correct hypovolemic shock. Adequate fluid volume should be infused to maintain adequate blood flow and blood pressure for tissue oxygenation. Immediate volume restoration with crystalloid or colloid solutions is recommended through wide-bore peripheral cannulae (14 gauge or larger). The use of albumin versus crystalloids for volume replacement has been debated; further trials are needed before definitive recommendations may be made.[125,126] The clinician should aim to maintain a normal blood pressure and a urine output of greater than 30 ml/hour. The patient's hematocrit, vital signs, and clinical situation determine the requirement and urgency for transfusion of red blood cells.

Transfusion considerations

Emergency release, uncrossmatched RBCs

Acute hemorrhage often does not permit the time needed to perform a Type and Screen and therefore necessitates the transfusion of uncrossmatched, "emergency release": Group O Rh(D) negative red blood cells. Similarly, if the patient's ABO blood type is not current, then Group O Rh(D) negative RBCs and or Group AB plasma must be transfused. In an emergency platelets of any blood type can be transfused.

Whole blood

In a situation of massive hemorrhage, a physician may select WB, if available, for transfusion to restore simultaneously both red cell mass and blood volume. *To transfuse Whole Blood, the patient's ABO type must be known.* Typically, however, PRBCs are administered with a crystalloid solution to restore oxygen carrying capacity and blood volume. If the patient has a known alloantibody to RBC antigen(s) and if time permits, PRBC or WB units should be antigen negative for the specificity of the antibody. In cases where time does not permit identification of the antigen negative donor unit, potentially incompatible blood might be transfused after weighing the risk of hemolysis versus patient exsanguinating. As WB does not require thawing, it is prepared more quickly than FFP.

Platelets

The clinician should allow time for platelet preparation (i.e., pooling) and delivery from the blood bank (15–30 minutes). After a 2-volume blood replacement, dilutional thrombocytopenia should be anticipated and hence after every 10 units of PRBC, a dose of platelets should be given. Target platelet counts are $>100 \times 10^9$/l for CNS trauma, and $>50 \times 10^9$/l for other situations.

FFP

An ABO Type is needed to transfuse. During massive transfusion 1–2 units FFP is given for each 5 units of PRBCs. Allow least 15–30 minutes for thawing of FFP.

CRYO

During massive transfusion therapy, generally CRYO is ignored till bleeding is uncontrolled due to hypofibrinogenemia! FFP does not contain enough fibrinogen to correct hypofibrinogenemia due to dilution or consumption during massive hemorrhage and has to be supplemented by CRYO. After every 10–15 PRBCs, 10 units of CRYO should be given to achieve good hemostasis. Again, allow ~30 minutes to thaw and pool the component.

Complications

Transfusion of a large volume of stored blood over a short time interval may result in adverse metabolic effects including citrate toxicity, hypothermia, and coagulation abnormalities resulting in microvascular bleeding. Citrate toxicity results from a decrease in ionized calcium from the effect of anticoagulant in blood products. Often rapid infusion of blood and its components may cause hypothermia in the recipient; using high-flow blood warmers may prevent this complication.

Disseminated intravascular coagulation (DIC)

Etiology

Obstetric conditions that may induce DIC include abruptio placentae[127,128] placenta previa, retained dead fetus syndrome, amniotic fluid embolism,[129] uterine atony, therapeutic abortion, and toxemia of pregnancy. Tissue factor (TF) and tissue factor pathway inhibitor (TFPI) are present in amniotic fluid. The level of TF has been found to be almost 45 times higher than in blood plasma. Amniotic fluid present in the circulation may influence the plasmatic TFPI-TF equilibrium resulting in intravascular blood coagulation.[130]

Management and transfusion therapy

To treat DIC the underlying cause of the DIC must be treated. A patient may present in labor with massive bleeding and clinical and laboratory findings consistent with DIC. The appropriate treatment is to evacuate the uterus. The diagnosis of DIC is clinopathological based on signs and symptoms and abnormalities of coagulation laboratory tests. If the patient is bleeding, then transfusion therapy should be considered. If however she is not bleeding, then it may be prudent to observe and hold off on transfusion of platelets, FFP and CRYO to prevent adding "*fuel to the fire*" effect where these products may aggravate intravascular micro or macrovascular thromboses.

Intra-uterine transfusion

For a discussion of this topic, see **Chapter 4**.

Pregnancy in a patient with sickle cell disease

Transfusion therapy is used to prevent and treat the complications of sickle cell disease (SCD). PRBCs are the preferred blood component. Transfusion risks unique to the SCD patient are iron overload and the hyperhemolytic transfusion syndrome. Additionally, SCD patients are sensitive to increased blood viscosity and blood pressure; thus, a transfusion might potentially trigger a sickle cell complication such as stroke and pulmonary complication.[131] Delayed hemolytic transfusion reactions, which are often seen in SCD patients and have been reported in a pregnant woman with SCD,[132,133] occur via an anamnestic immune response in patients previously alloimmunized by certain RBC antigens. Pretransfusion compatibility testing does not detect certain antibodies that cause these reactions because the antibody may be present in low concentrations, or its corresponding indicator rare antigen may be absent from the tested RBCs.

Red blood cell exchange (RBCx) is used to reduce the percentage of cells containing sickle hemoglobin while decreasing volume overload and minimizing hyperviscosity that may occur with RBC transfusion.[134] RBCx is indicated on an emergent basis for acute complications of SCD, e.g., stroke or acute chest syndrome. Approximately 2–4 hours are required to arrange for this procedure since it requires 5–8 units of fresh RBCs (<7 days old) that are partial phenotype-matched (see below).

Some authors assert that prophylactic red cell transfusions reduce maternal morbidity and perinatal mortality appreciably, although perinatal morbidity is not eliminated; transfusion therapy is justifiably started early in pregnancy for women with hemoglobin SS disease but may be withheld until the end of the second trimester for women with hemoglobin SC or sickle cell-beta-thalassemia disease.[135]

Antigen-matched RBCs: Alloimmunization to red cell antigens is a significant risk in chronically transfused SCD patients. Providing RBC units that are matched for erythrocyte antigens may prevent the development of RBC alloantibodies. To provide an erythrocyte antigen-matched RBC unit, the laboratory first must determine the SCD patient's erythrocyte antigen phenotype. Secondly, in order to prevent alloimmunization, RBC donor units are selected that are negative for the antigens that the patient lacks. In one study, none (0%) of the 40 sickle cell disease patients who received antigen-matched transfusions showed any evidence of alloimmunization, while 16 (34.8%) of the 46 patients who received both antigen-matched and non-antigen-matched transfusions developed clinically significant alloantibodies.[136] Therefore, chronically transfused sickle cell anemia patients should get antigen-matched units to prevent alloimmunization. Limited matching for at least Rh and Kell group antigens is sufficient to prevent alloimmunization for those antigens.

Atypical, life-threatening hyperhemolysis in patients with SCD has been well described in the literature. Continuing transfusion may be fatal, as it can further exacerbate hemolysis in these patients where both autologous and transfused cells may be hemolyzed.[137] Holding transfusion and giving steroids (1–2 mg/kg/day) is helpful.

REFERENCES

1 Goodnough, L. T., Brecher, M. E., Kanter, M. H., *et al.* Transfusion medicine. First of two parts – blood transfusion. *N. Engl. J. Med.*, 1999; **340**(6): 438–47.

2 Bausch, M. Blood safety in the new millennium. In Stramer, S., ed., *American Association of Blood Banks*. Bethesda, MD: 2001; Closing the windows on viral transmission by blood transfusion. pp. 33–54.

3 Busch, M. P., Kleinman, S. H., Jackson, B., *et al.* Committee report. Nucleic acid amplification testing of blood donors for transfusion-transmitted infectious diseases: Report of the Interorganizational Task Force on Nucleic Acid Amplification Testing of Blood Donors. *Transfusion*, 2000; **40**(2): 143–59.

4 Roth, W. K., Weber, M., Seifried, E. Feasibility and efficacy of routine PCR screening of blood donations for hepatitis C virus, hepatitis B virus, and HIV-1 in a blood-bank setting. *Lancet*, 1999; **353**(9150): 359–63.

5 Kuhns, M., McNamara, A., Peterson, B., *et al.* Detection of hepatitis B seroconversion by highly sensitive assays for surface antigen and HBV DNA (abstract). *Transfusion*, 1998; **3**(Suppl.): 91S.

6 Peddada, L., Heldebrant, C., Smith, R., *et al.* HBV viremia preceding HbsAg positivity: Implications for minipool (MP) and individual donation (ID) HBV nucleic acid testing (NAT) (abstract). *Transfusion*, 2000; **40**(Suppl.): 14–15S.

7 Stramer, S. L. Nucleic acid testing for transfusion-transmissible agents. *Curr. Opin. Hematol.*, 2000; **7**(6): 387–91.

8 Kleinman, S. H., Busch, M. P. The risks of transfusion-transmitted infection: direct estimation and mathematical modelling. *Baillieres Best Pract. Res. Clin. Haematol.*, 2000; **13**(4): 631–49.

9 Saldanha, J. Validation and standardisation of nucleic acid amplification technology (NAT) assays for the detection of viral contamination of blood and blood products. *J. Clin. Virol.*, 2001; **20**(1–2): 7–13.

10 Holmes, H., Davis, C., Heath, A., *et al.* An international collaborative study to establish the 1st international standard for HIV-1 RNA for use in nucleic acid-based techniques. *J. Virol. Methods*, 2001; **92**(2): 141–50.

11 Downes, K. A., Yomtovian, R. Advances in pretransfusion infectious disease testing: ensuring the safety of transfusion therapy. *Clin. Lab. Med.*, 2002; **22**(2): 475–90.

12 Dodd, R. Y. Emerging infections, transfusion safety, and epidemiology. *N. Engl. J. Med.*, 2003; **349**(13): 1205–6.

13 Goodman, C., Chan, S., Collins, P., *et al.* Ensuring blood safety and availability in the US: technological advances, costs, and challenges to payment – final report. *Transfusion*, 2003; **43**(8 Suppl.): 3S–46S.

14 Dodd, R. Y., Leiby, D. A. Emerging infectious threats to the blood supply. *Annu. Rev. Med.*, 2004; **55**: 191–207.

15 Pealer, L. N., Marfin, A. A., Petersen, L. R., *et al.* Transmission of West Nile virus through blood transfusion in the United States in 2002. *N. Engl. J. Med.*, 2003; **349**(13): 1236–45.

16 Mather, T., Takeda, T., Tassello, J., *et al.* West Nile virus in blood: stability, distribution, and susceptibility to PEN110 inactivation. *Transfusion*, 2003; **43**(8): 1029–37.

17 Harrington, T., Kuehnert, M. J., Kamel, H., *et al.* West Nile virus infection transmitted by blood transfusion. *Transfusion*, 2003; **43**(8): 1018–22.

18 Biggerstaff, B. J., Petersen, L. R. Estimated risk of transmission of the West Nile virus through blood transfusion in the US, 2002. *Transfusion*, 2003; **43**(8): 1007–17.

19 Biggerstaff, B. J., Petersen, L. R. Estimated risk of West Nile virus transmission through blood transfusion during an epidemic in Queens, New York City. *Transfusion*, 2002; **42**(8): 1019–26.

20 Centers for Disease Control and Prevention CfDCaP. Detection of West Nile virus in blood donations – United States. *MMRR*, 2003; **52**(32): 769–72.

21 Yap, P. L., Leaver, H. A., Gillon, J. Prions: properties, occurrence, modes of transmission and relevance for blood transfusion and blood derivatives. *Vox Sang*, 1998; **74** (Suppl. 2): 131–4.

22 Brown, P., Rohwer, R. G., Dunstan, B. C., *et al.* The distribution of infectivity in blood components and plasma derivatives in experimental models of transmissible spongiform encephalopathy. *Transfusion*, 1998; **38**(9): 810–16.

23 Linden, J. V. Errors in transfusion medicine. Scope of the problem. *Arch. Pathol. Lab. Med.*, 1999; **123**(7): 563–5.

24 Myhre, B. A. Fatalities from blood transfusion. *JAMA*, 1980; **244**(12): 1333–5.

25 Dzik, W. H., Corwin, H., Goodnough, L. T., *et al.* Patient safety and blood transfusion: new solutions. *Transfus. Med. Rev.*, 2003; **17**(3): 169–80.

26 Voak, D., Chapman, J. F., Phillips, P. Quality of transfusion practice beyond the blood transfusion laboratory is essential to prevent ABO-incompatible death. *Transfus. Med.*, 2000; **10**(2): 95–6.

27 Janatpour, K., Holland, P. V. Noninfectious serious hazards of transfusion. *Curr. Hematol. Rep.*, 2002; **1**(2): 149–55.

28 Domen, R. E., Hoeltge, G. A. Allergic transfusion reactions: an evaluation of 273 consecutive reactions. *Arch. Pathol. Lab. Med.*, 2003; **127**(3): 316–20.

29 Silliman, C. C. Transfusion-related acute lung injury. *Transfus. Med. Rev.*, 1999; **13**(3): 177–86.

30 Kopko, P. M., Marshall, C. S., MacKenzie, M. R., *et al.* Transfusion-related acute lung injury: report of a clinical look-back investigation. *JAMA*, 2002; **287**(15): 1968–71.

31 Perrotta, P. L., Snyder, E. L. Non-infectious complications of transfusion therapy. *Blood. Rev.*, 2001; **15**(2): 69–83.

32 Popovsky, M. A. Breathlessness and blood: a combustible combination. *Vox Sang*, 2002; **83** (Suppl. 1): 147–50.

33 Moroff, G., Luban, N. L. The irradiation of blood and blood components to prevent graft-versus-host disease: technical issues and guidelines. *Transfus. Med. Rev.*, 1997; **11**(1): 15–26.

34 Schroeder, M. L. Transfusion-associated graft-versus-host disease. *Br. J. Haematol.*, 2002; **117**(2): 275–87.

35 Wagner, F. F., Flegel, W. A. Transfusion-associated graft-versus-host disease: risk due to homozygous HLA haplotypes. *Transfusion*, 1995; **35**(4): 284–91.

36 Shulman, I. A., Downes, K. A., Sazama, K., *et al.* Pretransfusion compatibility testing for red blood cell administration. *Curr. Opin. Hematol.*, 2001; **8**(6): 397–404.

37 Gorlin, J, ed. XXII edn. *Standards for Blood Banks and Transfusion Services*. Bethesda, MD: American Association of Blood Banks; 2003.

38 Blood component preparation, storage, shipping, and transportation. In *American Association of Blood Banks Technical Manual*. Bethesda, MD: AABB Press; 1999. p. 169.

39 Practice guidelines for blood component therapy: A report by the American Society of Anesthesiologists Task Force on Blood Component Therapy. *Anesthesiology*, 1996; **84**(3): 732–47.

40 Laine, E., Steadman, R., Calhoun, L., *et al.* Comparison of RBCs and FFP with whole blood during liver transplant surgery. *Transfusion*, 2003; **43**(3): 322–7.

41 Holme, S., Elfath, M. D., Whitley, P. Evaluation of in vivo and in vitro quality of apheresis-collected RBC stored for 42 days. *Vox Sang*, 1998; **75**(3): 212–17.

42 Consensus conference. Perioperative red blood cell transfusion. *JAMA*, 1988; **260**(18): 2700–3.

43 Consensus conference. Platelet transfusion therapy. *JAMA*, 1987; **257**(13): 1777–80.

44 Schiffer, C. A., Anderson, K. C., Bennett, C. L., *et al.* Platelet transfusion for patients with cancer: clinical practice guidelines of the American Society of Clinical Oncology. *J. Clin. Oncol.*, 2001; **19**(5): 1519–38.

45 Lozano, M., Cid, J. The clinical implications of platelet transfusions associated with ABO or Rh(D) incompatibility. *Transfus. Med. Rev.*, 2003; **17**(1): 57–68.

46 Menitove, J. E. Immunoprophylaxis for D− patients receiving platelet transfusions from D+ [correction of D−] donors? *Transfusion*, 2002; **42**(2): 136–8.

47 Practice parameter for the use of fresh-frozen plasma, cryoprecipitate, and platelets. Fresh-Frozen Plasma, Cryoprecipitate, and Platelets Administration Practice Guidelines Development Task Force of the College of American Pathologists. *JAMA*, 1994; **271**(10): 777–81.

48 Downes, K. A., Wilson, E., Yomtovian, R., *et al.* Serial measurement of clotting factors in thawed plasma stored for 5 days. *Transfusion*, 2001; **41**(4): 570.

49 Kaul, V. V., Munoz, S. J. Coagulopathy of liver disease. *Curr. Treat. Options. Gastroenterol.*, 2000; **3**(6): 433–8.

50 Amitrano, L., Guardascione, M. A., Brancaccio, V., *et al.* Coagulation disorders in liver disease. *Semin. Liver Dis.*, 2002; **22**(1): 83–96.

51 Dhar, P., Abramovitz, S., DiMichele, D., *et al.* Management of pregnancy in a patient with severe haemophilia A. *Br. J. Anaesth.*, 2003; **91**(3): 432–5.

52 Lao, T. T., Lewinsky, R. M., Ohlsson, A., *et al.* Factor XII deficiency and pregnancy. *Obstet. Gynecol.*, 1991; **78**(3 Pt 2): 491–3.

53 Schved, J. F., Gris, J. C., Neveu, S., *et al.* Variations of factor XII level during pregnancy in a woman with Hageman factor deficiency. *Thromb. Haemost.*, 1988; **60**(3): 526–7.

54 DiPaola, J., Nugent, D., Young, G. Current therapy for rare factor deficiencies. *Haemophilia*, 2001; **7** (Suppl. 1): 16–22.

55 Bianco, C. Choice of human plasma preparations for transfusion. *Transfus. Med. Rev.*, 1999; **13**(2): 84–8.

56 Consensus conference. Fresh-frozen plasma. Indications and risks. *JAMA*, 1985; **253**(4): 551–3.

57 Downes, K., Sarode, R. Massive blood transfusion. *Indian J. Pediatr.*, 2001; **68**(2): 145–9.

58 Kobayashi, T., Asahina, T., Maehara, K., *et al.* Congenital afibrinogenemia with successful delivery. *Gynecol. Obstet. Invest.*, 1996; **42**(1): 66–9.

59 Thompson, H. W., Touris, S., Giambartolomei, S., *et al.* Treatment of congenital afibrinogenemia with cryoprecipitate collected through a plasmapheresis program using dedicated donors. *J. Clin. Apheresis*, 1998; **13**(4): 143–5.

60 Deering, S. H., Landy, H. J., Tchabo, N., *et al.* Hypodysfibrinogenemia during pregnancy, labor, and delivery. *Obstet. Gynecol.*, 2003; **101**(5 Pt 2): 1092–4.

61 Iwaki, T., Sandoval-Cooper, M. J., Paiva, M., *et al.* Fibrinogen stabilizes placental–maternal attachment during embryonic development in the mouse. *Am. J. Pathol.*, 2002; **160**(3): 1021–34.

62 Ness, P. M., Budzynski, A. Z., Olexa, S. A., *et al.* Congenital hypofibrinogenemia and recurrent placental abruption. *Obstet. Gynecol.*, 1983; **61**(4): 519–23.

63 Inbal, A., Muszbek, L. Coagulation factor deficiencies and pregnancy loss. *Semin. Thromb. Hemost.*, 2003; **29**(2): 171–4.

64 Ichinose, A., Izumi, T., Hashiguchi, T. The normal and abnormal genes of the a and b subunits in coagulation factor XIII. *Semin. Thromb. Hemost.*, 1996; **22**(5): 385–91.

65 Duckert, F. Documentation of the plasma factor XIII deficiency in man. *Ann. NY Acad. Sci.*, 1972; **202**: 190–9.

66 Lak, M., Peyvandi, F., Ali Sharifian, A., *et al.* Pattern of symptoms in 93 Iranian patients with severe factor XIII deficiency. *J. Thromb. Haemost.*, 2003; **1**(8): 1852–3.

67 Koseki-Kuno, S., Yamakawa, M., Dickneite, G., *et al.* Factor XIII A subunit-deficient mice developed severe uterine bleeding events and subsequent spontaneous miscarriages. *Blood*, 2003; **102**(13): 4410–12.

68 Burrows, R. F., Ray, J. G., Burrows, E. A. Bleeding risk and reproductive capacity among patients with factor XIII deficiency: a case presentation and review of the literature. *Obstet. Gynecol. Surv.*, 2000; **55**(2): 103–8.

69 Boda, Z., Pfliegler, G., Muszbek, L., *et al.* Congenital factor XIII deficiency with multiple benign breast tumours and successful pregnancy with substitutive therapy. A case report. *Haemostasis*, 1989; **19**(6): 348–52.

70 Janson, P. A., Jubelirer, S. J., Weinstein, M. J., *et al.* Treatment of the bleeding tendency in uremia with cryoprecipitate. *N. Engl. J. Med.*, 1980; **303**(23): 1318–22.

71 Remuzzi, G. Bleeding in renal failure. *Lancet*, 1988; **1**(8596): 1205–8.

72 The Trial to Reduce Alloimmunization to Platelets (TRAP) Study Group. Leukocyte reduction and ultraviolet irradiation of platelets to prevent alloimmunization and refractoriness to platelet transfusions. *N. Eng. J. Med.*, 1997; **337**: 1861–9.

73 Seftel, M. D., Growe, G. H., Petraszko, T., *et al.* Universal prestorage leukoreduction in Canada decreases platelet alloimmunization and refractoriness. *Blood*, 2004; **103**(1): 333–9.

74 Aye, M. T., Palmer, D. S., Giulivi, A., *et al.* Effect of filtration of platelet concentrates on the accumulation of cytokines and platelet release factors during storage. *Transfusion*, 1995; **35**(2): 117–24.

75 Jahr, J. S., Nesargi, S. B., Lewis, K., *et al.* Blood substitutes and oxygen therapeutics: an overview and current status. *Am. J. Ther.*, 2002; **9**(5): 437–43.

76 Levy, J. H. Hemoglobin-based oxygen-carrying solutions: close but still so far. *Anesthesiology*, 2000; **92**(3): 639–41.

77 Vlahakes, G. J. Hemoglobin solutions come of age. *Anesthesiology*, 2000; **92**(3): 637–8.

78 Winslow, R. M. New transfusion strategies: red cell substitutes. *Annu. Rev. Med.*, 1999; **50**: 337–53.

79 Widness, J. A., Clemons, G. K., Garcia, J. F., *et al.* Plasma immunoreactive erythropoietin in normal women studied sequentially during and after pregnancy. *Am. J. Obstet. Gynecol.*, 1984; **149**(6): 646–50.

80 Harstad, T. W., Mason, R. A., Cox, S. M. Serum erythropoietin quantitation in pregnancy using an enzyme-linked immunoassay. *Am. J. Perinatol.*, 1992; **9**(4): 233–5.

81 Widness, J. A., Sawyer, S. T., Schmidt, R. L., *et al.* Lack of maternal to fetal transfer of 125I-labelled erythropoietin in sheep. *J. Dev. Physiol.*, 1991; **15**(3): 139–43.

82 Koury, M. J., Bondurant, M. C., Graber, S. E., *et al.* Erythropoietin messenger RNA levels in developing mice and transfer of 125I-erythropoietin by the placenta. *J. Clin. Invest.*, 1988; **82**(1): 154–9.

83 Braga, J., Marques, R., Branco, A., *et al.* Maternal and perinatal implications of the use of human recombinant erythropoietin. *Acta Obstet. Gynecol. Scand.*, 1996; **75**(5): 449–53.

84 Goodnough, L. T. Erythropoietin therapy versus red cell transfusion. *Curr. Opin. Hematol.*, 2001; **8**(6): 405–10.

85 Harris, S. A., Payne, G., Jr., Putman, J. M. Erythropoietin treatment of erythropoietin-deficient anemia without renal disease during pregnancy. *Obstet. Gynecol.*, 1996; **87**(5 Pt 2): 812–14.

86 Hatzis, T., Cardamakis, E., Tsapanos, V., *et al.* The effects of recombinant human erythropoietin given immediately after delivery to women with anaemia. *Curr. Med. Res. Opin.*, 2003; **19**(4): 346–9.

87 Hou, S., Orlowski, J., Pahl, M., *et al.* Pregnancy in women with end-stage renal disease: treatment of anemia and premature labor. *Am. J. Kidney Dis.*, 1993; **21**(1): 16–22.

88 Szurkowski, M., Wiecek, A., Kokot, F., *et al.* Safety and efficiency of recombinant human erythropoietin treatment in anemic pregnant women with a kidney transplant. *Nephron*, 1994; **67**(2): 242–3.

89 Yankowitz, J., Piraino, B., Laifer, S. A., *et al.* Erythropoietin in pregnancies complicated by severe anemia of renal failure. *Obstet. Gynecol.*, 1992; **80**(3 Pt 2): 485–8.

90 Smith, R. Applications of darbepoietin-alpha, a novel erythropoiesis-stimulating protein, in oncology. *Curr. Opin. Hematol.*, 2002; **9**(3): 228–33.

91 Smith, R. E., Jr., Jaiyesimi, I. A., Meza, L. A., *et al.* Novel erythropoiesis stimulating protein (NESP) for the treatment of anaemia of chronic disease associated with cancer. *Br. J. Cancer*, 2001; **84** (Suppl. 1): 24–30.

92 Glaspy, J., Jadeja, J. S., Justice, G., *et al.* A dose-finding and safety study of novel erythropoiesis stimulating protein (NESP) for the treatment of anaemia in patients receiving multicycle chemotherapy. *Br. J. Cancer*, 2001; **84** (Suppl. 1): 17–23.

93 Overbay, D. K., Manley, H. J. Darbepoetin-alpha: a review of the literature. *Pharmacotherapy*, 2002; **22**(7): 889–97.

94 Joy, M. S. Darbepoetin alfa: a novel erythropoiesis-stimulating protein. *Ann. Pharmacother.*, 2002; **36**(7–8): 1183–92.

95 Fisher, J. W. Erythropoietin: physiology and pharmacology update. *Exp. Biol. Med. (Maywood)*, 2003; **228**(1): 1–14.

96 Dutton, R. P., Hess, J. R., Scalea, T. M. Recombinant factor VIIa for control of hemorrhage: early experience in critically ill trauma patients. *J. Clin. Anesth.*, 2003; **15**(3): 184–8.

97 Hedner, U., Ingerslev, J. Clinical use of recombinant FVIIa (rFVIIa). *Transfus. Sci.*, 1998; **19**(2): 163–76.

98 Eskandari, N., Feldman, N., Greenspoon, J. S. Factor VII deficiency in pregnancy treated with recombinant factor VIIa. *Obstet. Gynecol.*, 2002; **99**(5 Pt 2): 935–7.

99 Sherer, D. M., Lerner, R. Glanzmann's thrombasthenia in pregnancy: a case and review of the literature. *Am. J. Perinatol.*, 1999; **16**(6): 297–301.

100 Bell, J. A., Savidge, G. F. Glanzmann's thrombasthenia proposed optimal management during surgery and delivery. *Clin. Appl. Thromb. Hemost.*, 2003; **9**(2): 167–70.

101 Segal, S., Shemesh, I. Y., Blumenthal, R., *et al.* Treatment of obstetric hemorrhage with recombinant activated factor VII (rFVIIa). *Arch. Gynecol. Obstet.*, 2003; **268**(4): 266–7.

102 Sacks, D. A., Koppes, R. H. Caring for the female Jehovah's Witness: balancing medicine, ethics, and the First Amendment. *Am. J. Obstet. Gynecol.*, 1994; **170**(2): 452–5.

103 Gyamfi, C., Gyamfi, M. M., Berkowitz, R. L. Ethical and medicolegal considerations in the obstetric care of a Jehovah's Witness. *Obstet. Gynecol.*, 2003; **102**(1): 173–80.

104 Drew, N. C. The pregnant Jehovah's Witness. *J. Med. Ethics*, 1981; **7**(3): 137–9.

105 Singla, A. K., Lapinski, R. H., Berkowitz, R. L., *et al.* Are women who are Jehovah's Witnesses at risk of maternal death? *Am. J. Obstet. Gynecol.*, 2001; **185**(4): 893–5.

106 Migden, D. R., Braen, G. R. The Jehovah's Witness blood refusal card: ethical and medicolegal considerations for emergency physicians. *Acad. Emerg. Med.*, 1998; **5**(8): 815–24.

107 Smoller, B. R., Kruskall, M. S. Phlebotomy for diagnostic laboratory tests in adults. Pattern of use and effect on transfusion requirements. *N. Engl. J. Med.*, 1986; **314**(19): 1233–5.

108 Lusher, J. M. Systemic causes of excessive uterine bleeding. *Semin. Hematol.*, 1999; **36**(3 Suppl. 4): 10–20.

109 Lops, V. R., Hunter, L. P., Dixon, L. R. Anemia in pregnancy. *Am. Fam. Physician*, 1995; **51**(5): 1189–97.

110 Pahlavan, P., Nezhat, C. Hemorrhage in obstetrics and gynecology. *Curr. Opin. Obstet. Gynecol.*, 2001; **13**(4): 419–24.

111 Crane, S., Chun, B., Acker, D. Treatment of obstetrical hemorrhagic emergencies. *Curr. Opin. Obstet. Gynecol.*, 1993; **5**(5): 675–82.

112 Bonnar, J. Massive obstetric haemorrhage. *Baillieres Best Pract. Res. Clin. Obstet. Gynaecol.*, 2000; **14**(1): 1–18.

113 Van den Broek, N. R., White, S. A., Ntonya, C., *et al.* Reproductive health in rural Malawi: a population-based survey. *BJOG*, 2003; **110**(10): 902–8.

114 Pattinson, R. C., Buchmann, E., Mantel, G., *et al.* Can enquiries into severe acute maternal morbidity act as a surrogate for maternal death enquiries? *BJOG*, 2003; **110**(10): 889–93.

115 Ronsmans, C., Etard, J. F., Walraven, G., *et al.* Maternal mortality and access to obstetric services in West Africa. *Trop. Med. Int. Health*, 2003; **8**(10): 940–8.

116 Fenton, P. M., Whitty, C. J., Reynolds, F. Caesarean section in Malawi: prospective study of early maternal and perinatal mortality. *BMJ*, 2003; **327**(7415): 587.

117 Adamu, Y. M., Salihu, H. M., Sathiakumar, N., *et al.* Maternal mortality in Northern Nigeria: a population-based study. *Eur. J. Obstet. Gynecol. Reprod. Biol.*, 2003; **109**(2): 153–9.

118 Okogbenin, S. A., Gharoro, E. P., Otoide, V. O., *et al.* Obstetric hysterectomy: fifteen years' experience in a Nigerian tertiary centre. *J. Obstet. Gynaecol.*, 2003; **23**(4): 356–9.

119 Chichakli, L. O., Atrash, H. K., MacKay, A. P., *et al.* Pregnancy-related mortality in the United States due to hemorrhage: 1979–1992. *Obstet. Gynecol.*, 1999; **94**(5 Pt 1): 721–5.

120 Chang, J., Elam-Evans, L. D., Berg, C. J., *et al.* Pregnancy-related mortality surveillance – United States, 1991–1999. *MMWR Surveill. Summ.*, 2003; **52**(2): 1–8.

121 Nagaya, K., Fetters, M. D., Ishikawa, M., *et al.* Causes of maternal mortality in Japan. *JAMA*, 2000; **283**(20): 2661–7.

122 Chamberlain, G., Steer, P. ABC of labour care: obstetric emergencies. *BMJ*, 1999; **318**(7194): 1342–5.

123 Stainsby, D., MacLennan, S., Hamilton, P. J. Management of massive blood loss: a template guideline. *Br. J. Anaesth.*, 2000; **85**(3): 487–91.

124 Shevell, T., Malone, F. D. Management of obstetric hemorrhage. *Semin. Perinatol.*, 2003; **27**(1): 86–104.

125 Schierhout, G., Roberts, I. Fluid resuscitation with colloid or crystalloid solutions in critically ill patients: a systematic review of randomised trials. *BMJ*, 1998; **316**(7136): 961–4.

126 Reviewers CIGA. Human albumin administration in critically ill patients: systematic review of randomized trials. *Br. J. Med.*, 1998; **317**: 235–40.

127 Chen, C. Y., Chen, C. P., Wang, K. G., *et al.* Factors implicated in the outcome of pregnancies complicated by acute respiratory failure. *J. Reprod. Med.*, 2003; **48**(8): 641–8.

128 Mechem, C. C., Knopp, R. K., Feldman, D. Painless abruptio placentae associated with disseminated intravascular coagulation and syncope. *Ann. Emerg. Med.*, 1992; **21**(7): 883–5.

129 Clark, S. L., Hankins, G. D., Dudley, D. A., *et al.* Amniotic fluid embolism: analysis of the national registry. *Am. J. Obstet. Gynecol.*, 1995; **17**(4 Pt 1): 1158–67; discussion, 1167–9.

130 Uszynski, M., Zekanowska, E., Uszynski, W., *et al.* Tissue factor (TF) and tissue factor pathway inhibitor (TFPI) in amniotic fluid and blood plasma: implications for the mechanism of amniotic fluid embolism. *Eur. J. Obstet. Gynecol. Reprod. Biol.*, 2001; **95**(2): 163–6.

131 Vichinsky, E. P. Current issues with blood transfusions in sickle cell disease. *Semin. Hematol.*, 2001; **38**(1, Suppl. 1): 14–22.

132 Anderson, R. R., Sosler, S. D., Kovach, J., *et al.* Delayed hemolytic transfusion reaction due to anti-Js(a) in an alloimmunized patient with a sickle cell syndrome. *Am. J. Clin. Pathol.*, 1997; **108**(6): 658–61.

133 Plante, L. A. Transfusion issues in a gravida with sickle cell disease. *Obstet. Gynecol.*, 1998; **92**(4 Pt 2): 712.

134 Eckman, J. R. Techniques for blood administration in sickle cell patients. *Semin. Hematol.*, 2001; **38**(1, Suppl. 1): 23–9.

135 Cunningham, F. G., Pritchard, J. A., Mason, R. Pregnancy and sickle cell hemoglobinopathies: results with and without prophylactic transfusions. *Obstet. Gynecol.*, 1983; **62**(4): 419–24.

136 Tahhan, H. R., Holbrook, C. T., Braddy, L. R., *et al.* Antigen-matched donor blood in the transfusion management of patients with sickle cell disease. *Transfusion*, 1994; **34**(7): 562–9.

137 Win, N., Doughty, H., Telfer, P., *et al.* Hyperhemolytic transfusion reaction in sickle cell disease. *Transfusion*, 2001; **41**(3): 323–8.

18

Heparin-induced thrombocytopenia in pregnancy

Barbara B. Haley, M.D.,[1] Rodger L. Bick, M.D., Ph.D.[2] and Eugene P. Frenkel, M.D.[3]

[1]Professor of Medicine, Sherry Wigley Crow Cancer Research Endowed Chair in Honour of Robert Lewis Kirby, M.D., University of Southwestern Medical School, Dallas, Texas, USA
[2]Clinical Professor of Medicine and Pathology, University of Taxas Southwestern Medical Center; Director: Dallas Thrombosis Hemostasis and Vascular Medicine Clinical Center, Dallas, Texas, USA
[3]Professor of Medicine and Radiology, Harold C. Simmons Comprehensive Cancer Center, University of Texas Southwestern Medical School, Dallas, TX, USA

Heparin is the most commonly used pharmacologic intervention to prevent or treat thrombosis in pregnancy. Both unfractionated heparin and low molecular weight heparins have been used successfully for therapeutic and prophylactic anticoagulation during gestation. Conversely, the use of coumadin in pregnancy is not advised as the drug crosses transplacentally and has been associated with a risk of fetal embryopathy and hemorrhage.[1] The use of heparin, however, can have adverse clinical side effects for the pregnant female that include heparin-associated osteoporosis, eosinophilia, allergic reactions, ski rashes, and alopecia.[2,3] However, the most significant and potentially devastating consequence is the development of heparin-induced thrombocytopenia.[2,3] This is particularly true when the thrombocytopenia is paradoxically associated with either a venous or arterial thrombosis. Although heparin and low-molecular-weight (LMW) heparins are generally considered safe during pregnancy, a recent adverse reaction MedWatch report has been issued regarding the use of enoxaparin in pregnancy. This MedWatch report, issued January 9 2002 states the following: PRECAUTIONS:

Pregnancy

Teratogenic effects

There have been reports of congenital anomalies in infants born to women who received enoxaparin during pregnancy including cerebral anomalies, limb anomalies, hypospadias, peripheral vascular malformation, fibrotic dysplasia, and cardiac defect. A cause and effect relationship has not been established nor has the incidence been shown to be higher than in the general population.

Hematological Complications in Obstetrics, Pregnancy, and Gynecology, ed. R. L. Bick *et al.* Published by Cambridge University Press.

Non-teratogenic effects

There have been post-marketing reports of fetal death when pregnant women received Lovenox Injection. Causality for these cases has not been determined. Pregnant women receiving anti-coagulants, including enoxaparin, are at increased risk for bleeding. Hemorrhage can occur at any site and may lead to death of mother and/or fetus. Pregnant women receiving enoxaparin should be carefully monitored. Pregnant women and women of child-bearing potential should be apprised of the potential hazard to the fetus and the mother if enoxaparin is administered during pregnancy.

In a clinical study of pregnant women with prosthetic heart valves given enoxaparin (1 mg/kg bid) to reduce the risk of thromboembolism, 2 of 7 women developed clots resulting in blockage of the valve and leading to maternal and fetal death. There are postmarketing reports of prosthetic valve thrombosis in pregnant women with prosthetic heart valves while receiving enoxaparin for thromboprophylaxis. These events resulted in maternal death or surgical interventions. The use of Lovenox Injection is not recommended for thromboprophylaxis in pregnant women with prosthetic heart valves.

Adverse reactions

Ongoing Safety Surveillance: Since 1993, there have been over 80 reports of epidural or spinal hematoma formation with concurrent use of Lovenox Injection and spinal/epidural anesthesia or spinal puncture.[4]

The syndrome of heparin-induced thrombocytopenia

Two clinical syndromes of heparin-induced thrombocytopenia (HIT) are seen, each with different pathophysiologic mechanisms and distinct clinical events and potential sequelae. One termed Type I HIT (with features highlighted in Table 18.1) is a non-immunologic event occurring early within hours to a few days after heparin exposure.[3]

The degree of thrombocytopenia is mild, usually a 10 to 30% decrease of platelets from baseline counts. There are no accompanying clinical manifestations. Though uncertain, the mechanism is thought secondary to a heparin-platelet

Table 18.1 Heparin-induced thrombocytopenia Type I.

- Non immune
- Thrombocytopenia occurs early after heparin exposure
- Thrombocytopenia mild: 10–30% decrease in platelet numbers
- No clinical manifestation
- Mechanism – heparin-induced platelet aggregation
- Therapy – none; episode transient and counts normalize even if heparin continued

Table 18.2 Clinical features of heparin-induced thrombocytopenia Type II.

- Usual onset day 3–14 (median day 6) – onset within hours if previous heparin exposure
- Nadir platelet count – usually 30,000–60,000 but can be <10,000
- Risk – heparin exposure of any type (subcutaneous, IV, heparin coated catheter)
  Risk > with continuous infusion vs. subcutaneous dosing
  Risk > with Unfractionated vs. LMW heparin
  Risk: bovine > porcine > LMW
- Mechanism – immune mediated platelet destruction
- Clinical manifestation – spectrum including thrombosis (arterial and venous), DVT, PE, CVA, MI, visceral infarction including mesenteric

interaction leading to platelet activation, aggregation, sequestration and consumption. The episode is transient and the platelet count returns to normal even with continued heparin exposure. Unfractionated (high molecular weight) heparin is more likely to cause a Type I HIT as opposed to a low molecular weight heparin. No specific therapy is required for this lesion, which usually goes clinically unrecognized and is commonly diagnosed retrospectively.

By contrast, clinically significant HIT, commonly termed Type II HIT represents a disease spectrum that is due to an immune mediated destruction of platelets in response to heparin. To emphasize its clinical potential it has often been further subdivided into HIT (heparin-induced thrombocytopenia) and HITT (heparin-induced thrombocytopenia and thrombosis syndrome). Type II HIT/T can have significant clinical sequelae with severe morbidity and mortality.[5] Deep vein thrombosis, pulmonary embolism, arterial thrombosis, mesenteric ischemia and cerebral and myocardial infarction are some of the potentially devastating consequences of this lesion. Therefore it is important to recognize the characteristics of a Type II HIT/T that distinguishes it from Type I HIT. Table 18.2 lists the common clinical features of Type II HIT/T.[6]

These characteristics include a later onset, usually day 3 to 14 (median day 6), after exposure to either an unfractionated or low molecular weight heparin. However, the onset may be earlier (within hours) after a heparin infusion in the patient who has had recent heparin exposure of any type. Since this lesion is immunologically mediated, some have felt that the temporal relationship to the exposure can be quantified, since antibody disappearance commonly occurs by 3 to 4 months following heparin exposure. Although this is commonly seen (i.e. decreased risk after 100 days), episodes of rapid onset have been seen and this 100 day rule appears relative.[7] Type II nadir-platelet counts are in a much lower-range than Type I HIT, usually 30,000 to 60,000 but can be <10,000.

No individual platelet value mandates the diagnosis of Type II HIT/T. Although no absolute number exists, a 50% decrease in the platelet count from initial baseline should be considered diagnostic. Less than 50% drop in baseline counts should arouse suspicion of HIT/T and prompt further investigation. A drop of 30% from baseline in any 24-hour period, unless otherwise explained, should be considered strongly suspicious for HITT.[5]

HIT/T frequency

The overall frequency of Type II HIT/T has been estimated at 3 to 5% in a general population exposed to unfractionated heparin.[5] These are clearly estimates. Nevertheless the incidence with low molecular weight heparin is clearly less than that with unfractionated heparin. In pregnancy, heparin-induced thrombocytopenia is much rarer and occurs less frequently than in the non-pregnant heparin exposed woman. The basis for this reduced frequency is not certain. However, the explanation for the decreased incidence of HIT/T in pregnancy may center on the altered immune response of the pregnant female to the antigenic heparin platelet factor 4 (PF4) complex, presumably the most frequent basis for HIT.[8]

HIT/T pathophysiology

The most commonly defined mechanism to explain heparin-induced thrombocytopenia and thrombosis is based on the development of antibody to the heparin platelet factor 4 complex (PF4). Platelet factor 4 (PF4) is a protein released from platelet alpha granules. PF4 binds to heparin forming a complex antigen that induces antibody formation. The Fab region of the antibody binds to the heparin-PF4 complex; and, the Fc portion of the antibody binds to the FcγRIIA receptor on the platelets. Complexes of heparin-PF4-antibody accumulate on the platelet surface, activate the platelet which then releases more PF4 thereby perpetuating further platelet activation and aggregation in a positive feedback cycle.[9]

The antibody is not heparin specific and reacts with other highly sulfated materials such as dextran sulfate, pentosan sulfate and endothelial heparin. Heparin itself can also bind to peptides, proteins and glycoproteins on platelet and endothelial cell surfaces. PF4 can bind to heparan sulfate on the endothelial cell surface, and this complex can be bound by the antibody causing endothelial cell damage and localized platelet activation and tissue factor release. The damaged endothelial cell serves as a nidus for the thrombotic cascade with tissue factor release, monocyte recruitment, platelet microparticle release, further platelet aggregation, thrombin generation and resultant thrombosis.

It is now recognized that heparin antibodies are heterogeneous in function. The antibody generated against the heparin platelet factor 4 complex is most often an

IgG2 isotype, but IgA and IgM antibodies have also been described. A complex issue relative to HIT/T antibodies is that they may be functional or nonfunctional in terms of platelet activation. Thus, the laboratory recognition of an antibody does not absolutely define the existence of HIT, which presently is a clinical diagnosis. In addition, they may be dependent or independent of heparin to produce the actual platelet activation. For these reasons, the actual antibody titer has a poor correlate with the clinical manifestations.[10,11] Furthermore, the antibodies are heterogeneous in specificity and affinity for the target epitope thereby explaining the variability of clinical consequences noted in patients. Finally heparin itself varies in amino acid and protein content and degree of sulfation from different laboratories and manufacturers further contributing to the heterogeneity of the spectrum of HIT/T antibody induction.

Although antibodies generated against the heparin platelet factor 4 complex account for the great majority of cases of HITT, there are two rarer forms which are equally catastrophic. One is due to heparin induced antibodies against the platelet membrane interleukin 8 (IL 8) site and the other is due to a heparin induced antibody directed against the platelet membrane bound neutrophil activating peptide 2 (NAP – 2).[12,13] These rarer forms of HIT/T may not follow the usual timeline pattern of 3–14 days and may lead to HITT either before or after the usually expected occurrence of HIT/T; however, fortunately, these forms of HIT/T are very rare.

Risk factors for the development of HIT/T

Heparin-induced thrombocytopenia can develop after exposure to any amount or type of heparin administered by any route, although it is most common during the continuous infusion of unfractionated heparin. However, HIT has been reported even after a subcutaneous heparin dose, following heparin flushes of catheters, and with heparin-coated catheters.[14,15] A hierarchy of risk has been noted relative to the frequency of HIT. Thus, bovine unfractionated heparins have a higher incidence then those made from porcine; and regarding the source low molecular heparin has a significantly lower risk than unfractionated heparin.[16] Although the low molecular weight heparins differ from one another, a clear hierarchy of incidence for them is not yet known. For reasons that are uncertain an interesting observation is that patients with the platelet FcγRIIA receptor genotype appear to have a slightly higher degree of risk of developing HIT.[17]

HIT-associated thrombosis

In the presence of a clinically defined episode of HIT there is an estimated probability of 35% of developing a significant thrombosis. Thrombi can occur in either the venous or arterial vessels.[18] When these occur in the extremities the seriousness is emphasized by an estimated 20% risk of limb amputation. Thromboembolism occurs in 10% of patients and other clinical consequences include recurrent pulmonary embolism, stroke, myocardial infarction, and mesenteric ischemia. The mortality of HIT/T with a thromboembolic event in some series has been 30%.[19,20]

Clinical management

Since the diagnosis of HIT predicts a high risk of developing thrombosis with serious morbidity and mortality, patients on heparin require careful monitoring of the platelet count. The most recent guidelines of the North American Consensus Conference Committee (American College of Chest Physicians/ ACCP) recommend a daily or every other day platelet count while on heparin therapy.[21] However, although this recommendation is mandatory for short-term intravenous or subcutaneous thrombotherapeutic heparin dosing use, this is impractical for use of thromboprophylactic doses during gestation. One of the authors (RLB) chooses to monitor weekly platelet counts for the first trimester and monthly platelet counts during the second and third trimesters.[22] If a presumptive diagnosis of HIT/T is made, all heparin exposure must be stopped immediately including subcutaneous and flush doses and heparin-coated catheters should be removed. The patient should be assessed physically for limb swelling, discoloration or pain. Dyspnea, chest pain, subtle neurologic symptoms, and abdomen discomfort, unexplained acidosis (due to ischemia) or elevated white count must all be evaluated.

Differential diagnosis

Development of thrombocytopenia in a pregnant patient being treated with heparin demands a prompt an immediate evaluation as to cause. Aspects of the differential diagnosis relative to the thrombocytopenia are delineated in Table 18.3 and further reviewed by Sarode *et al.* in Chapter 15.

Table 18.3 Thrombocytopenia in pregnancy – differential diagnosis.

DIC	Drugs
AIDS	Autoimmune (lupus, RA, etc.)
HIT	Malignancy
ITP	Hemorrhage
Gestational thrombocytopenia	Preeclampsia
Septicemia	

The diagnosis of HIT is a clinical one which utilizes commonly accepted diagnostic criteria that include:

- Thrombocytopenia – platelet count <100,000 or a 50% decrease from baseline (initial) pre-heparin count. HIT/T should be strongly suspected if the platelet count drops >30% in any 24 hour period.
- Exclusion of other causes of thrombocytopenia.
- Confirmation by a heparin-associated antibody assay.
- Restoration of a normal platelet count with cessation of heparin.[3]

It cannot be emphasized too strongly that the diagnosis of HIT is a clinical one and that the physician should not await extensive laboratory testing before proceeding with appropriate management. Indeed, no single laboratory assay for the relevant antibodies identifies all cases, which have the classical clinical characteristics. The present availability of excellent agents to manage a thrombotic or prothrombotic state allows the clinician to make an immediate discontinuation of the heparin and an abrupt change to one of these newer agents.

Clinical testing

Specific antibody assays are not routinely available in most laboratories. Delays of therapy waiting confirmatory testing can be catastrophic to the patient. Both functional and quantitative antibody tests have been developed, but no single highly sensitive and specific assay exists. In clinical practice functional platelet aggregation assays or quantitative antibody testing are available for diagnostic confirmation.

Functional tests These include the platelet aggregation assay and the serotonin release assay (SRA). The platelet aggregation assay uses a mixture of reactive normal donor platelets, patient serum, and heparin to evaluate platelet aggregation. A lumi aggregometer can be used to measure platelet activation with aggregation. The platelet aggregation assay has a high false negative rate and a sensitivity of about 40%.[23,24]

The serotonin release assay (SRA) measures platelet activation. Normal donor platelets pre-incubated with radio labeled serotonin are mixed with patient serum and heparin. Platelet activation is a function of the released radiolabeled serotonin. The SRA has a higher sensitivity (60% to 80%) but requires greater technical expertise in the lab for handling of the radioisotope. It has long been considered the "gold standard" of diagnosis.[25]

Quantitative tests These tests measure antibodies to the heparin PF4 complex. Several Elisa assays have been developed.[26] Unfortunately, heparin can induce measurable antibody that does not induce thrombocytopenia; and, conversely patients with a clear clinical picture of HIT do not always have measurable antibody. Thus, the antibody titer may not correlate with clinical manifestations. The most important issue is that a patient with the classical clinical picture of HIT may have a negative test in all of the assays. Therefore the clinical diagnosis must take precedence over any laboratory test in the decision to treat.

Clinical treatment of HIT/T

The treatment of HIT/T in pregnancy can be complex and some controversy as to approach exists. Once the diagnosis is suspected, the prompt discontinuation of heparin is mandatory. However, simply stopping heparin does not reduce the thrombotic event rate. Indeed, the risk may persist as long as 3 weeks following the discontinuation of heparin. For patients who have experienced an actual thrombus, no question exists relative to the need for further anticoagulation. For patients with HIT and no clinically recognized thrombus, prophylactic anticoagulation is appropriate until the platelet count increases to normal and the antibody titer declines because these patients are at high risk for developing thrombotic complications for at least 3 weeks.[18,27]

There are various alternative anticoagulant drugs available. Many of these are of limited value. The current state of the art treatment for the therapy of HIT/T is the use of a direct thrombin inhibitor as these drugs are rapid acting and do not cross react with the HIT antibody.

Alternative anticoagulants

Low molecular weight heparins These drugs have high rates of cross reactivity with heparin dependent antibodies (80–100%) and have absolutely *no* significant role in treating HIT/T![28]

Anacrod (Arvin; Knoll) – This is a defibrinating enzyme derived from snake venom. It has an indirect action against fibrin and high risks of bleeding. Prolonged use is associated with tachyphylaxis and thrombosis. The safety profile for use in pregnancy is unknown and is therefore considered *contra-indicated* for use in pregnancy.

Coumadin This drug, even if started immediately after the diagnoses of HIT/T requires 48–120 hours to achieve full anticoagulant effect. This requirement means that the patient is without protection for a prolonged period. In addition, large loading doses are contra-indicated as they inhibit Protein C and may result in a prothrombotic state and tissue necrosis. Finally, Coumadin also crosses the placenta and carries a risk of malformation or fetal hemorrhage. Indeed, it is this observation that lead to the standard utilization of heparin in the management of thrombotic or prothrombotic states in pregnancy.

Danaparoid (Organon) This drug is a heparinoid, a mixture of heparin sulfate, dermatan sulfate, chondroitin sulfate and LMW heparin. It differs in sulfation and molecular weight from unfractionated and LMW heparins. It has at least a 20% cross-reactivity with heparin dependent antibodies. Although there are reports of its successful use to treat HIT/T in pregnancy it has largely been replaced by other agents.[29,30] Because of this cross-reactivity, the absence of an antagonist to reverse its action, and a long half-life there is a significant risk of bleeding with it. Danaparoid (Organon®) is not available in the USA, but is available in Canada and Europe.

Direct thrombin inhibitors These are the most effective drugs presently available for the prophylactic and therapeutic treatment of HIT/T. These agents are direct inhibitors of thrombin. They are rapid acting, have a short half-life, and have no immunologic similarity to heparin and do not cross react with heparin antibodies.[30] Their level of anticoagulation can be conveniently monitored with the activated partial thromboplastin time (aPTT). The FDA has approved hirudin (Lepirudin, Refludan®) and argatroban (Argatroban®) for treating HIT-associated thrombosis. Argatroban has also been FDA approved for prophylactic treatment of HIT-associated thrombosis.

Hirudin (Lepirudin, Refludan®) This drug is a protein naturally derived from leech saliva but now produced by recombinant technology. Hirudin irreversibly binds to thrombin and has a long terminal half-life (80 min.). Its protein structure induces antibodies that can either enhance or diminish its anticoagulant activity. The dosing recommendation is 0.4 mg/kg bolus followed by a continuous IV of 0.15 mg/kg/hr. The dose must be adjusted for renal failure:

- Decrease by 50% for Creatinine 1.6–2.0
- By 70% for Creatinine 2.1–3.0
- By 85% for Creatinine 3.0–6.0

Monitoring is by the aPTT adjusted to keep the aPTT 1.5 to 2.5 of control. Unfortunately no antidote is available for episodes of bleeding.[31,32] Hirudin has also been used clinically at doses of 10 to 20 mg s.c. every 12 hours in patients requiring prophylactic therapy with heparin but who have a prior or current history of HIT/HITT.[33] Hirudin is designated Pregnancy Category B. By definition this indicates that: no evidence of risk in humans: adequate, well controlled studies in pregnant women have not shown increased risk of fetal abnormalities despite adverse findings in animals, or, in the absence of adequate human studies, animal studies show no fetal risk. The chance of fetal harm is remote, but remains a possibility. It is not known if hirudin crosses the placenta or is excreted into breast milk. Clinical studies[34] have included one prospective and three historically controlled trials in combination including 1,700 HITT patients. These studies have demonstrated that Refludan was associated with a relative risk reduction (RR) of 62.9%, p = 0.005[35,36] and the combined clinical endpoint of death, limb amputation, and recurrent thrombosis was associated with a 55.4% risk reduction p = 0.004.[37]

Argatroban This drug is a synthetically derived, reversible, direct thrombin inhibitor, with a rapid onset of action (30 minutes). Steady state plasma concentration is achieved in 1 to 3 hours after initiating a continuous infusion. The terminal half-life is 39–51 minutes. The argatroban dose is 2 micrograms/kg/min (not to exceed 10 μ/kg/min or aPTT of 100 seconds). It does not induce antibody formation and is metabolized by the liver. Therefore, dose reduction is required for hepatic dysfunction, but not for renal impairment. Monitoring is by the aPTT with a therapeutic goal of 1.5 to 2.5 of control.[29,38,39] Like Refludan, unfortunately no antidote is available for episodes of bleeding with Argatroban. Argatroban is also designated Pregnancy Category B with no clinical studies evaluating use in pregnancy. It is unknown if it is excreted in human breast milk. One prospective historically controlled study has evaluated the efficacy of Argatroban in 304 HITT patients.[40] For the composite endpoint of death, amputation, and new thrombosis, argatroban significantly reduced the composite endpoints by a 34% relative reduction (25.6% versus 38.8%, p = 0.014). However, when individual components of the endpoints were assessed separately, the incidence of new thrombosis was significantly reduced in the argatroban group versus controls (6.9% versus 15.0%, p = 0.027, RR = 54.0%), however the limb amputation rate was not significantly different for argatroban (1.9%) versus controls (2.0%) nor was there a significant difference in all-cause death (16.9% versus 21.8%).[34,40]

A comparison of the two drugs is shown in Table 18.4.

Bivalirudin A synthetic peptide with reversible thrombin inhibition, metabolized by the liver. It is not FDA-approved for the treatment of HIT. There is no safety data on use in pregnancy. It is currently used only in interventional cardiology procedures.

Antiplatelet agents Since HIT/T involves both thrombin generation and platelet activation, the use of anti-platelet agents are currently being evaluated. Traditional anti-platelet agents like dextran or aspirin are not effective as single agents in the acute treatment of HIT/T. Newer anti-platelet agents like the glycoprotein 11b/111a inhibitor (Abciximab, ReoPro®), or Tirofiban (Aggrastat®) and the ADP platelet receptor inhibitor Clopidrogel (Plavix®) can inhibit platelet activation, aggregation, and microparticle formation in vitro using HIT serum and heparin. However very limited clinical studies in HIT/T using combinations of

Table 18.4 Comparison of drug characteristics of Hirudin and Argatroban.

Drug characteristics	Hirudin	Argatroban
Thrombin binding	Irreversible	Reversible
Half-life	90 min	40 min
Antibody induction	Yes	No
Dosing		
• Bolus	0.4 mg/kg IV	No
• Continuous infusion	0.15 mg/(kg hr)	2 micrograms/(kg min) (do not exceed 10 μ/(kg min) or PTT >100 s)
Dose-adjusted renal impairment	Yes	No
Hepatic impairment	No	Yes
Monitoring	aPTT (1.5–2.5 × control)	aPTT (1.5–2.5 × control)
FDA approved therapeutic use HIT/T	Yes	Yes
Prophylactic use HIT/T	No	Yes
FDA pregnancy designation	Category B	Category B
Placental crossage	Unknown	Unknown
Breast milk excretion		

thrombin inhibitors and newer anti-platelet agents are reported.[41] Hence no dosing regimen, clinical trial or safety data are available as a guideline for use in pregnancy.

A clinically relevant approach to the patient with suspected HIT or HIT/T can be summarized as described:

Quick guideline for direct thrombin inhibitor use in HIT/T with pregnancy

1. Stop heparin immediately.
2. Start rapid onset antithrombotic therapy while assessing for evidence of occult thrombosis.
   a. Hirudin (Refludan/Lepirudin) @ 0.4 mg/kg bolus followed by 0.15 mg/kg/hr constant infusion IV or subcutaneous dose.
   b. Argatroban @ 2 micrograms/kg/min (not to exceed 10 micrograms/kg/min).
3. For prophylaxis, continue Argatroban or Refludan until thrombocytopenia resolves. Some would then add low-dose aspirin.
4. For therapeutic treatment of HIT/T, continue Argatroban or Refludan until the platelet count rises. Begin Coumadin once the platelet count rises. Start Coumadin at expected daily maintenance dose without use of a loading dose. Taper off Argatroban or Refludan once stable INR is reached.

REFERENCES

1 Bates, S. M., Ginsberg, J. S. Anticoagulants in pregnancy: fetal effects. *Baillieres Clin. Obstet. Gynaecol.*, 1997; **11**: 479–88.

2 Nelson-Piercy, C. Hazards of heparin: allergy, heparin-induced thrombocytopenia and osteoporosis. *Baillieres Clin. Obstet. Gynaecol.*, 1997; **11**: 489–509.

3 Bick, R. L., Frenkel, E. P. Clinical aspects of heparin-induced thrombocytopenia and thrombosis and other side effects of heparin therapy. *Clin. Appl. Thromb. Hemost.*, 1999; **5** (Suppl. 1): S7–15.

4 LOVENOX (enoxaparin sodium) Injection [January 9, 2002: Aventis]: *WARNINGS* FDA MedWatch 1/9/2002 http://www.fda.gov/medwatch/SAFETY/2002/jan02.htm#lovenox.

5 Walenga, J. M., Bick, R. L. Heparin-induced thrombocytopenia, paradoxical thromboembolism, and other side effects of heparin therapy. *Med. Clin. North Am.*, 1998; **82**: 635–58.

6 Walenga, J. M., Frenkel, E. P., Bick, R. L. Heparin-induced thrombocytopenia, paradoxical thromboembolism, and other adverse effects of heparin-type therapy. *Hematol. Oncol. Clin. North Am.*, 2003; **17**: 259–82, viii–ix.

7 Warkentin, T. E., Kelton, J. G. Temporal aspects of heparin-induced thrombocytopenia. *N. Engl. J. Med.*, 2001; **344**: 1286–92.

8 Fausett, M. B., Vogtlander, M., Lee, R. M., *et al.* Heparin-induced thrombocytopenia is rare in pregnancy. *Am. J. Obstet. Gynecol.*, 2001; **185**: 148–52.

9 Amiral, J., Vissac, A. M. Generation and pathogenicity of anti-platelet factor 4 antibodies: diagnostic implications. *Clin. Appl. Thromb. Hemost.*, 1999; **5** (Suppl. 1): S28–31.

10 Ahmad, S., Walenga, J. M., Jeske, W. P., *et al.* Functional heterogeneity of antiheparin-platelet factor 4 antibodies: implications in the pathogenesis of the HIT syndrome. *Clin. Appl. Thromb. Hemost.*, 1999; **5** (Suppl. 1): S32–7.

11 Amiral, J., Pouplard, C., Vissac, A. M., *et al.* Affinity purification of heparin-dependent antibodies to platelet factor 4 developed in heparin-induced thrombocytopenia: biological characteristics and effects on platelet activation. *Br. J. Haematol.*, 2000; **109**: 336–41.

12 Regnault, V., de Maistre, E., Carteaux, J. P., *et al.* Platelet activation induced by human antibodies to interleukin-8. *Blood*, 2003; **101**: 1419–21.

13 Amiral, J. Antigens involved in heparin-induced thrombocytopenia. *Seminars Hematology*, 1999; **36**: 7–11.

14 Hirsh, J., Raschke, R., Warkentin, T. E., *et al.* Heparin: mechanism of action, pharmacokinetics, dosing considerations, monitoring, efficacy, and safety. *Chest*, 1995; **108**: 58–75S.

15 Moberg, P. Q., Geary, V. M., Sheikh, F. M. Heparin-induced thrombocytopenia: a possible complication of heparin-coated pulmonary artery catheters. *J. Cardiothorac. Anesth.*, 1990; **4**: 226–8.

16 Warkentin, T. E., Levine, M. N., Hirsh, J., *et al.* Heparin-induced thrombocytopenia in patients treated with low-molecular-weight heparin or unfractionated heparin. *N. Engl. J. Med.*, 1995; **332**: 1330–5.

17 Carlsson, L. E., Santoso, S., Baurichter, G., *et al.* Heparin-induced thrombocytopenia: new insights into the impact of the FcgammaRIIa-R-H131 polymorphism. *Blood*, 1998; **92**: 1526–31.

18 Wallis, D. E., Workman, D. L., Lewis, B. E., *et al.* Failure of early heparin cessation as treatment for heparin-induced thrombocytopenia. *Am. J. Med.*, 1999; **106**: 629–35.

19 Warkentin, T. E., Kelton, J. G. A 14-year study of heparin-induced thrombocytopenia. *Am. J. Med.*, 1996; **101**: 502–7.

20 Weismann, R. E., Tobin, R. W. Arterial embolism occurring during systemic heparin therapy. *AMA Arch. Surg.*, 1958; **76**: 219–25; discussion, 217–25.

21 Hirsh, J., Warkentin, T. E., Shaugnassey, S. G., *et al.* Heparin and low molecular weight heparin: mechanisms of action, pharmacokinetics, dosing, monitoring, efficacy and safety. *Chest*, 2001; **119**: 64–94.

22 Bick, R. L. Recurrent miscarriage syndrome and infertility caused by blood coagulation protein or platelet defects. *Hematol. Oncol. Clin. North Am.*, 2000; **14**: 1117–32.

23 Look, K. A., Sahud, M., Flaherty, S., *et al.* Heparin-induced platelet aggregation vs. platelet factor 4 enzyme-linked immunosorbent assay in the diagnosis of heparin-induced thrombocytopenia-thrombosis. *Am. J. Clin. Pathol.*, 1997; **108**: 78–82.

24 Walenga, J. M., Jeske, W. P., Fasanella, A. R., *et al.* Laboratory diagnosis of heparin-induced thrombocytopenia. *Clin. Appl. Thromb. Hemost.*, 1999; **5** (Suppl. 1): S21–27.

25 Sheridan, D., Carter, C., Kelton, J. G. A diagnostic test for heparin-induced thrombocytopenia. *Blood*, 1986; **67**: 27–30.

26 Collins, J., Aster, R., Moghaddam, M., *et al.* Diagnostic testing for heparin-induced thrombocytopenia (HIT): an enhanced platelet factor 4 complex enzyme linked immunosorbent assay (PF4 ELISA). *Blood*, 1997; **90**: 761a.

27 Wallis, D. E., Lewis, B. E., Messmore, H. L., *et al.* Inadequacy of current prevention strategies for heparin-induced thrombocytopenia. *Clin. Appl. Thromb. Hemost.*, 1999; **5** (Suppl. 1): S16–20.

28 Hirsh, J., Warkentin, T. E., Shaughnessy, S. G., *et al.* Heparin and low-molecular-weight heparin: mechanisms of action, pharmacokinetics, dosing, monitoring, efficacy, and safety. *Chest*, 2001; **119**: 64–94S.

29 Alving, B. M. How I treat heparin-induced thrombocytopenia and thrombosis. *Blood*, 2003; **101**: 31–7.

30 Fareed, J., Lewis, B. E., Callas, D. D., *et al.* Antithrombin agents: the new class of anticoagulant and antithrombotic drugs. *Clin. Appl. Thromb. Hemost.*, 1999; **5** (Suppl. 1): S45–55.

31 Vanholder, R., Camez, A., Veys, N., *et al.* Pharmacokinetics of recombinant hirudin in hemodialyzed end-stage renal failure patients. *Thromb. Haemost.*, 1997; **77**: 650–5.

32 Eichler, P., Friesen, H. J., Lubenow, N., *et al.* Antihirudin antibodies in patients with heparin-induced thrombocytopenia treated with lepirudin: incidence, effects on aPTT, and clinical relevance. *Blood*, 2000; **96**: 2373–8.

33 Eriksson, B. I., Ekman, S., Kalebo, P., *et al.* Prevention of deep-vein thrombosis after total hip replacement: direct thrombin inhibition with recombinant hirudin, CGP 39393 *Lancet*, 1996; **347**: 635–9.

34 Larned, Z. L., O'Shea, S. I., Ortel, T. L. Heparin-induced thrombocytopenia: clinical presentations and therapeutic management. *Clinical Advances Hematology/Oncology*, 2003; **1**: 356–64.

35 Gerinacher, A., Volpel, H., Janssens, U. for the HIT Investigators Group. Recombinant hirudin (lepirudin) provides sage and effective anticoagulation in patients with heparin-induced thrombocytopenia: a prospective study. *Circulation*, 1999; **99**: 73–80.

36 Gerinacher, A., Janssens, U., Berg, G. for the Heparin-Induced Thrombocytopenia Study HAT Investigators. Lepirudin (recombinant hirudin) for parenteral anticoagulation in patients with heparin-induced thrombocytopenia. *Circulation*, 1999; **100**: 587–93.
37 Gerinacher, A., Eichler, R., Lubenow, N., *et al.* Heparin-induced thrombocytopenia with thromboembolic complications: meta-analysis of 2 prospective trials to assess the value of parenteral treatment with lepirudin and its therapeutic range. *Blood*, 2000; **96**: 846–51.
38 Jeske, W., Walenga, J., Lewis, B., *et al.* Pharmacology of argatroban. *Exp. Opin. Invest. Drugs*, 1999; **8**: 625–54S.
39 Lewis, B. E., Wallis, D. E., Leya, F., *et al.* Argatroban anticoagulation in patients with heparin-induced thrombocytopenia. *Arch. Intern. Med.*, 2003; **163**: 1849–56.
40 Lewis, B. E., Wallis, D. E., Berkowitz, S. D. Argatroban anticoagulant therapy in patients with heparin-induced thrombocytopenia. *Circulation*, 2001; **103**: 1838–43.
41 Walenga, J., Lewis, B., Jeske, W., *et al.* Combined thrombin and platelet inhibition treatment for HIT patients. *Hamostaseologie*, 1999; **19**: 128–33.

19

Coagulation defects as a cause for menstrual disorders

Albert J. Phillips, M.D., F.A.C.O.G.

Clinical Professor of Obstetrics and Gynecology, University of Southern California, School of Medicine, 1301 20th Street, Suite 270, Santa Monica, California 90404, USA. Tel: 3108288585; Fax 310 453-4844; ajphillips@pol.net

Menorrhagia

Introduction

Normal menstruation occurs every 21–35 days lasting on average 7 days. Normal blood loss is between 25 and 69 ml per cycle.[1] Menstrual abnormalities can be characterized by their flow and regularity. Menorrhagia is defined as bleeding of over 80 ml with menstruation. Menometrorrhagia is irregular heavy menstruations. Menstrual abnormalities can be caused by multiple etiologies. These include gynecological abnormalities of the uterus, hormonal disorders, and systemic disorders. Prior reports have identified causes for excessive bleeding in only 50% of patients.[2] The estimated prevalence of menorrhagia in healthy women is between 9% and 14%.[3] Menorrhagia has been found to be a reliable predictor for coagulation and platelet disorders.[4] In the absence of a readily identifiable cause, all adolescents with menorrhagia, especially those with anemia, should be examined for an undiagnosed coagulation defect.

Quality of life evaluations were shown to be poorer in all areas in women who had inherited bleeding disorders. As compared to controls, women with menorrhagia found that they accomplished less than they would like during menses, and their heavy flow limited their activities and the kind of work they could do.[5] Forty-six percent of type 1 von Willebrand disease (VWD) patients reported losing on average 4 days from work or school due to menorrhagia.[6]

The gynecologist has a unique role in being the primary care giver, who generally is the first practitioner to whom the patient presents with menstrual bleeding problems. Unfortunately, many patients do not get evaluated for coagulation defects when other obvious causes of menorrhagia are not found. Often a patient's coagulopathy is first diagnosed when they are evaluated for excessive menstrual bleeding. With proper assessment and diagnosis, appropriate treatment can begin.

Hematological Complications in Obstetrics, Pregnancy, and Gynecology, ed. R. L. Bick *et al.* Published by Cambridge University Press.

Mechanism of hemostasis with menstruation

Intuitively, women with coagulation defects would be expected to have menorrhagia. The mechanism of hemostasis with menstruation is complex. Initially, the hemostatic response begins with constriction of endometrial arterioles and myometrial arteries.[7,8] Specific platelet membrane receptors at the site of vessel injury cause platelet adherence. Von Willebrand factor (VWF) anchors the platelet to a thrombogenic constituent of the vessel wall.[9] This activates further platelet aggregation by binding fibrinogen to glycoprotein forming a platelet plug. These plugs have been demonstrated in the first 20 hours of menstruation.[10]

Hemostasis is further maintained by fibrin deposition at the platelet plug, forming a stable clot. Involved in the fibrin deposition is the recruitment of circulating clotting factors. After the fibrin clot has been formed, the fibrinolytic system causes degradation of the clot. Balance between formation and lysis of the clot ultimately determines if hemostasis will be further maintained.

Determining menorrhagia

The perception of heavy menstrual bleeding by the patient can be very subjective. Unless specifically asked, patients may not realize that they are losing more than 80 ml of blood each cycle. Conversely, some patients complain of heavy bleeding when their total blood loss is less than 80 ml. The patient's bleeding perception is biased by upbringing and misconceptions.[11] Objective analysis of bleeding can be done with quantitative analysis of blood collected on sanitary napkins, but in practical clinical situations this is not feasible. An alternative method of determining if a patient is experiencing excessive bleeding is with a pictorial blood measurement chart (PBMC). This easy method identified patients who have menorrhagia with specificity and sensitivities of greater than 80%.[12] The validity of this method has recently come under question when a validation study using the PBMC failed to show its ability to objectively make the diagnosis of menorrhagia.[13] In a recent prospective study, the PBMC was modified to be more accurate and renamed the menstrual pictogram (Figure 19.1). This study found a high level of correlation between blood loss estimated by the menstrual pictogram as compared to the quantitative alkaline hematin method. The menstrual pictogram had a sensitivity of 86% and specificity of 88% in diagnosing menorrhagia.[14] Thus, using the menstrual pictogram will allow objective assessment of blood loss and should be used to determine if menorrhagia is present prior to beginning the diagnostic work up.

Gynecologist under-appreciation of coagulation defects

Studies have shown a high prevalence of von Willebrand disease (VWD) and other bleeding disorders among women with menorrhagia. Gynecologists tend to be the first health practitioners who evaluate women with menorrhagia and do not

NAPKIN	TYPE	Score (ml of blood)
	BRAND	Kotex
	Day time	1
	Night time	1
	Day time	2
	Night time	3
	Day time	3
	Night time	6
	Day time	4
	Night time	10
	Day time	5
	Night time	15

TAMPON	TYPE	Score (ml of blood)
	BRAND	Tampax
	Regular	0.5
	Super	1
	Super Plus	1
	Regular	1
	Super	1.5
	Super Plus	2
	Regular	1.5
	Super	3
	Super Plus	6
	Regular	4
	Super	8
	Super Plus	12

Figure 19.1 Assessment of menstrual blood loss using the menstrual pictogram.
The scores (in milliliters) associated with each icon are given. Left: sanitary napkins. Right: tampons.

Data from *Wyatt, K. M. Determination of total menstrual blood loss. Fertil. Steril., 2001.*[14]

routinely consider coagulation defects as a cause for this condition. In a survey of Georgian obstetricians and gynecologists, only 4% considered VWD as a cause for menorrhagia in reproductive aged women. Among girls near menarche, physicians overwhelmingly felt that the likely diagnoses in those with menorrhagia was either anovulatory bleeding or within normal limits. Only 16% would entertain a possible diagnosis of VWD in this age group. In general, most respondents believed that most menorrhagia is caused by anovulation or is within normal limits. On average, these physicians believed that less than 1% of menorrhagia patients had an underlying inherited bleeding disorder. Multiple studies have shown that the prevalence of coagulation defects in women with menorrhagia is significantly higher than 1%. This discordance, between the physician practice and the role of bleeding disorders in menorrhagia, may be related to the gynecologist's under-appreciation of the importance of the role of bleeding disorders in menorrhagia, the complexity of these disorders, and the diagnostic criteria necessary to make a specific clinical diagnosis.[15]

Table 19.1 Initial tests for the investigation of coagulation defects.

Test	Abnormal results	Diagnosis
Platelet count	Decreased (<150K)	Thrombocytopenia – various causes
Prothrombin time	Prolonged (>17 s)	Clotting factor deficiency: Factor VII, X, II, fibrinogen
Partial thromboplastin time	Prolonged (>34 s)	Clotting factor deficiency: Factor XI, X, IX, VIII, V, II, fibrinogen, von Willebrand factor
Bleeding time	Prolonged (>9 min)	Vessel wall abnormalities: Platelet dysfunction (i.e. Glanzmann's thrombesthenia, von Willebrand disease)
If all above are normal: Platelet aggregation studies – induction with epinephrine and ristocetin	Decreased aggregation	Platelet function defect disorders

Partially adapted from Ellis, M. H., Beyth, Y.[17]

Work up of menorrhagia in the coagulation-defect patient

The possibility of a coagulation defect should be considered after a thorough history and physical examination. The patient should be asked about a family history of bleeding disorders and personal history of excessive bruising or bleeding. Bleeding after tooth extraction, postoperative bleeding, and postpartum bleeding are significantly associated with inherited bleeding disorders.[16] The clinical expression of inherited coagulopathy is variable, yet many inherited coagulation disorders present at menarche and in adolescence.[17] A menstrual history, asking specifically how often and how much sanitary protection is required with each cycle, will alert the physician to possible patients with coagulopathy. Using the menstrual pictogram (Figure 19.1) can substantiate menorrhagia. Pelvic ultrasound will identify those patients with gynecologic disorders that can present with menorrhagia. If all examinations are within normal limits, preliminary blood studies looking for coagulation defects are indicated. As outlined in Table 19.1, the initial studies should include a complete blood count with platelets, prothrombin time (PT), partial thromboplastin time (PTT), and bleeding time (BT). The phase of the menstrual cycle when these laboratory studies are obtained is critical because VWF is variable during the menstrual cycle. Von Willebrand factor has its lowest levels during the first 7 days of the menstrual cycle. Blood drawn during this phase will improve the sensitivity of detecting VWD. If all initial studies are

Table 19.2 Confirmatory tests for selected bleeding disorders.

Disease	Test	Result
Von Willebrand disease	Von Willebrand antigen level	Decreased
	Ristocetin cofactor activity	Decreased
	Factor VIII activity/ von Willebrand factor	Decreased
	von Willebrand factor multimeric analysis	von Willebrand multimeric pattern
Factor XI deficiency	Factor XI activity assay	Decreased
Glanzmann's thrombasthenia	Platelet aggregometry	Decreased aggregation with collagen, thrombin, ADP, epinephrine; normal with ristocetin

Partially adapted from Ellis, M. H., Beyth, Y.[17]

normal, evaluation for platelet aggregation disorders is in order. These specific tests are discussed under platelet function disorders. If any of the initial laboratory evaluations are abnormal, Table 19.2 outlines specific additional laboratory studies that can help in making a clinical hematological diagnosis.

Typically, the initial presentation of a coagulation disorder is at menarche and in adolescence. In women who had menorrhagia at menarche, 20% were found to have some coagulation defect. Von Willebrand disease was most often seen. Thrombocytopenia and other less common disorders were also found.[7] Menorrhagia seen later in the reproductive years, after having had normal menstrual flows, are less likely due to coagulation defects. Yet, consideration for acquired VWD, thrombocytopenia, and platelet aggregation disorders is reasonable after other more likely causes for menorrhagia are not found.

Specific coagulation defects and menstrual abnormalities

Von Willebrand disease

Pathophysiology and prevalence

Von Willebrand disease is the most commonly inherited hematological disorder. Approximately 0.8% to 1.3% of the population has the disorder.[18,19] With VWD, VWF is diminished and hemostasis is affected. Von Willebrand factor binds platelets to the subendothelial matrix and plays an essential role in facilitating platelet adhesion and aggregation.[20] Von Willebrand factor additionally localizes FVIII to

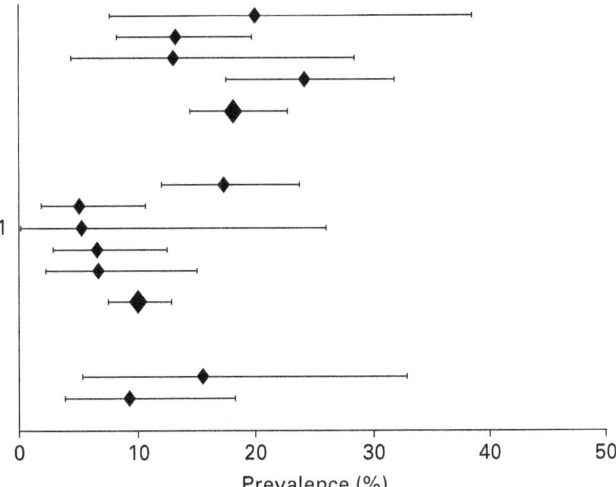

Figure 19.2 Prevalence rates of von Willebrand disease with confidence intervals.
Shankar, M., *et al.* Copyright permission obtained from *BJOG*.[23]

the vessel injury site. Seventy-four percent of patients with VWD have menorrhagia.[21] In type 2 and 3 VWD, menorrhagia occurs in 80% of women.[3] Von Willebrand disease, especially type 1, is often found at menarche. Patients with VWD type 2 and 3 have frequently evidence of a bleeding diathesis prior to menarche, necessitating an earlier evaluation and diagnosis.

Bleeding patterns of women with VWD are not always regular. Forty-four percent of women reported irregular bleeding lasting on average 11.5 days. Blood transfusion was required in 20% and the majority had been treated in the past for heavy bleeding. As previously noted, almost all women remember the start of menorrhagia at menarche.[22]

Figure 19.2 summarizes a review of studies that assessed the prevalence of VWD in women who were identified with menorrhagia and evaluated for coagulation defects. When the data from these individual studies was combined, the overall prevalence of VWD in women with menorrhagia was 13%.[23] There is a discrepancy between the approximately 1% prevalence of VWD in the general population and the prevalence of women having symptoms. This may be linked to many different factors, including how study populations were recruited and how the diagnosis of menorrhagia was made and objectively determined. Also, genetic factors, including race and blood type, will cause variability in the prevalence of VWD. In those studies that recruited women from the general population, VWD prevalence was the lowest. To definitively determine why this discrepancy is seen, a multi-center trial using similar inclusion criteria, objective analysis of blood loss, diagnostic testing, and inclusion for diagnosis will need to be performed. Regardless of the reasons for this difference, prevalence of VWD is increased in women with menorrhagia and should be considered when no obvious etiology for heavy bleeding is found.

Diagnostic requirements for VWD

When in its mild form, establishing the diagnosis of VWD is difficult and complex.[24] The levels of VWF and factor VIII c change within the individual's menstrual cycle.[25] The least amount of variability among patients is during menstrual bleeding. Testing for the diagnosis of VWD during the menses affords the best opportunity to identify those with the condition.[26] Most studies have shown variations within the menstrual cycle with VWF, yet one study did not appreciate cyclic changes.[27] Abnormal laboratory assessment of von Willebrand factor antigen, von Willebrand factor functional activity assay (VWF:Ac) or plasma factor VIII will aid in the diagnosis and classification of VWD. VWF:Ac is the single most sensitive test for most forms of VWD.[28] Additional tests for hypothyroidism when determining VWF levels will identify a subgroup of patients whose low VWF levels are due to hypothyroidism and not VWD.[29,30]

Treatment of menorrhagia and VWD

Desmopressin

Type 1 VWD responds to desmopressin (DDAVP).[31] This occurs by increasing the VWF synthesis and its release from its storage site in the endothelial cells. Desmopressin is available as a nasal spray and can be given intravenously or subcutaneously. Subcutaneous DDAVP was given to 14 women who had menorrhagia and VWD. Eighty-six percent of the women noted that the DDAVP was either very effective or effective in improving menstrual flow.[32]

The dosage of DDAVP is dependent on the weight of the patient. In those over 50 kg, two intranasal sprays, each 150 μg, one in each nostril is recommended. Those under 50 kg, only one intranasal dose of 150 μg is required. A decrease in bleeding with a single dose is considered an excellent response. Treatment should be limited to a maximum of 2 days during menstruation.[33]

Desmopressin is not generally recommended in type 2 and 3 VWD. In type 2 the VWF is dysfunctional, hence additional release of the defective VWF will not improve hemostasis. In type 3 VWD, there are inadequate stores of VWF so that DDAVP does not improve VWF levels. There are rare exceptions when DDAVP has efficacy in patients with type 2 and 3 VWD.[34,35]

Adverse reactions to DDAVP are common but mild. Tachycardia, headache, and facial flushing are most frequently seen. Because of the antidiuretic effect of

DDAVP, water intoxication and hyponatremia can rarely occur. There are insufficient studies looking at specifically menorrhagia and treatment with desmopressin, yet initial treatment reports appear promising.

Oral contraceptives

In oral estrogen-progestin preparations (OCPs) with estrogen greater than 50 μg of ethynyl estradiol, VWF increases and may of itself improve bleeding in women with VWD.[36] An increase in factor VIII activity, VWF-ristocetin cofactor activity has been reported with estrogens.[37] The increase in clotting factors due to estrogen is dose dependent, with smaller amounts of estrogen showing little or no increase in clotting factors.[38]

If the mechanism of improved hemostasis with OCPs is due to increased VWF, then menorrhagia should improve from its use. However, there is conflicting data on efficacy of OCPs in treatment of menorrhagia and VWD. In women with type 2 and 3 VWD, who were unresponsive to DDAVP, 88% showed clinical improvement with OCPs.[39] However, a survey of women with type 1 VWD treated with standard OCPs found OCPs to be only 24% effective at reducing blood loss. The authors concede that this low efficacy rate was determined by a questionnaire and not with objective analysis.[6] This lack of response by OCPs is intuitively contradictory, for patients with type 2 and 3 VWD have less circulating VWF and presumably the increases in the VWF from the estrogen should have affected bleeding in type 1 VWD patients also. The most likely mechanism of improved hemostasis with OCPs is due to a combination of the change in VWF and OCPs direct effect on menstrual blood flow by reducing the proliferation of endometrium. Irrespective of its action on clotting factors, use of OCPs is the most recommended treatment for women with VWD who have menorrhagia. Further investigations of the mechanisms by which OCPs have their effect on reducing menstrual flow need to be completed to fully understand the mechanism of action.

Antifibrinolytics: Tranexamic acid and Epsilon-aminocaproic acid

Tranexamic acid (TA) is a synthetic derivative of the amino acid lysine that exerts its antifibrinolytic effect through competing for lysine binding sites on plasminogen molecules, resulting in the inhibition of plasminogen activation to plasmin and binding to fibrin. Fibrinolysis is increased during menstruation.[40]

Menorrhagia in VWD has been successfully treated with TA.[41,42] There have been reductions of 34 to 57.9% in mean menstrual blood loss with treatment with TA therapy in women with menorrhagia.[43] The optimal dosing regimen and duration of treatment have not yet been determined. The medication has been given as a single 3 g dose,[44] 1 g every 6 hours,[45] 1–1.5 g three times a day,[46] and 4 g daily for 3–5 days.[47] While the medication is generally well tolerated with only mild gastrointestinal side effects, thromboembolic potential can cause serious complications.

Epsilon-aminocaproic acid (EACA), another antifibrinolytic amino acid that functions by binding to plasminogen, has been used in patients with menorrhagia. Five grams three times a day for 4 days resulted in a significant reduction in menstrual flow. Serious side effects were not seen and only nausea, vomiting, and giddiness were reported.[48] EACA and TA are often sufficient to control bleeding or can be used as an adjunct treatment with DDAVP.

Acquired von Willebrand syndrome

Acquired von Willebrand syndrome (aVWS) is a rare bleeding disorder with laboratory findings similar to VWD. AVWS arises out of persons who previously had no coagulation problems. Similar to VWD, patients will have a prolonged bleeding time, decreased factor VIII procoagulant activity, low VWF ristocetin cofactor activity, and low VWF antigen. Most present with bleeding from mucocutaneous sites, including menorrhagia.[49] Acquired von Willebrand syndrome is caused by a variety of systemic conditions, including lymphoproliferative (48%) and myeloproliferative (15%) disorders. Other conditions that produce the syndrome include malignancy, autoimmune disorders, and hypothyroidism.[50] Primary treatment is directed at the underlying disorder. With acute bleeding, the treatment for aVWS is the same as required for VWD.

Platelet dysfunction disorders

Pathophysiology and prevalence

Platelet function disorders is a general term for a variety of defects in which there is an alteration in platelet adhesion, aggregation, secretion, or elaboration to procoagulant activity. These disorders can be inherited or acquired. Acquired platelet function disorders can occur from drugs, systemic disease, or hematological disease. There is a broad range of clinical presentation, and mild conditions may be easily unrecognized.[51]

Previously, studies of women with menorrhagia without an obvious etiology, have determined that a significant percentage of these women have VWD. However, a substantial number have heavy bleeding without explanation. Until recently, the prevalence of platelet defects in women with menorrhagia has not been fully investigated. Recent studies have carefully evaluated for platelet aggregation and platelet ATP release defects and have found that this category of bleeding disorders may indeed be a more frequent cause for menorrhagia than VWD.

In a recent study, the frequency of qualitative platelet function defects was substantial among women with menorrhagia and was seen more often than coagulation defects. Of 337 women with menorrhagia determined to have a bleeding disorder, 16% had inherited defects and 84% had platelet function defects. Among those with platelet function defects, 48% had isolated PF3 availability defects, 9% Glanzmann's thrombasthenia, and 25% had an unclassified platelet disorder.[52] In another recent study evaluating platelet function, 47% of women had decreased platelet aggregation with one or more agonist. The prevalence odds of platelet aggregation abnormalities were 4.2 fold higher among women with menorrhagia than among control women.[53]

Glanzmann's thrombasthenia is a condition characterized by abnormal platelet aggregation because of a deficiency of platelet glycoprotein IIb/IIIa. The clinical presentation is usually with mucocutaneous bleeding, and severe bleeding at menorrhagia has been reported.[54]

Diagnostic studies to determine platelet dysfunction

Bleeding time, which has been used as a screening test for platelet function, did not identify 57% of women with abnormal platelet aggregation studies. Therefore, platelet aggregation studies are required to make the diagnosis. Platelet aggregation, induced by epinephrine and ristocetin agonists, show a reduced aggregation response when a defect is present. Black women with menorrhagia had a greater reduction with ristocetin-induced aggregation and epinephrine-induced aggregation than white women.[53] Flow cytometry for identification of the genetic defect is usually available in research facilities.[51]

Treatment

Desmopressin can be used for the treatment of platelet aggregation disorders. Seventy-three percent of patients, with inherited disorders of platelets, showed improvement in bleeding times, when given DDAVP.[55] Plasmapheresis, dialysis, transfusion of normal platelets, administration of cryoprecipitate, and administration of corticosteroids are all acceptable alternative treatments, depending on specific clinical situations.[56]

Thrombocytopenia

Hematological disorders causing thrombocytopenia are immune thrombocytopenia purpura, aplastic anemia, acute leukemia and hypersplenism. Often these conditions will initially present with other manifestations of bleeding, yet menorrhagia can be the predominant symptom. In adolescents, who presented with menorrhagia, 13% had thrombocytopenia. The most common cause was immune thrombocytopenia purpura, followed by myelosuppression caused by chemotherapy.[57] Another study looking at adolescents, with menorrhagia requiring hospitalization, found that 43% had thrombocytopenia due to primary hematological disease or platelet suppression from chemotherapy.[58] Determination of the cause of the thrombocytopenia will dictate the appropriate therapy.

Menstrual cyclic thrombocytopenia is a rare condition in which platelet counts reached their nadir at the onset of menses followed 5–14 days later with normal or elevated platelet counts. This condition was associated with bruising, epistaxis and menorrhagia. The authors propose that the mechanism for this condition is based on estrogen changes during the menstrual cycle that alter receptor mediated clearance of antibody coated platelets by macrophages, modulating platelet survival and causing thrombocytopenia.[59]

Hemophilia carriers

Women who are carriers for hemophilia A and B can have menorrhagia. There is wide variation in clinical presentation and menorrhagia. In women with low levels of factor VII, DDAVP will likely improve symptoms. In women with low levels for factor IX, DDAVP will not likely help.

Factor XI deficiency

Factor XI is an autosomal disorder, with homozygous patients having very low factor XI concentrations. This disorder occurs most commonly in Ashkenazi Jews, with a gene frequency of 4.3%.[58] The frequency of factor XI deficiency in women with menorrhagia was 4%, with the estimated prevalence of 0.001% in the general population.[25] Women with either homozygous or heterozygous factor XI deficiency are more likely to have menorrhagia than their unaffected relatives.[60] The PTT may be normal in heterozygous factor XI deficiency patients, and determining factor XI levels will be required to make the diagnosis.

TA has been recommended as treatment for menorrhagia in women with factor XI deficiency.[61] The only specific therapy is infusion of fresh frozen plasma (FFP) that contains factor XI. FFP is impractical for recurring treatment, since administration is costly and places the patient at risk of infection of enveloped viruses. Treatment with TA and oral contraceptives is more practical and generally effective.

Other coagulation deficiencies

Rare clotting disorders, like factor V and factor VII deficiency, will usually present in childhood, prior to menarche, with other bleeding tendencies. These include epistaxis, gastrointestinal bleeding, hemarthrosis, or hematuria. Because of their rarity, optimum management of menorrhagia with factor V deficiency and factor VII deficiency is not known. Factor V deficiency has been reported with menorrhagia.[62] Treatment with GnRH agonists has been successfully utilized.[63] Factor VII deficiency has been treated with recombinant VIIa, endometrial ablation,[64] and thermal balloon endometrial ablation.[65]

Warfarin

Clearly, iatrogenic coagulation defects secondary to heparin and oral anticoagulants, have their own special ramifications, when they are associated with menorrhagia. In a limited study of 11 women on warfarin, 5 were noted to have greater than 80 ml menstrual flow. This data suggests that oral anticoagulants may increase menstrual blood loss. The authors propose that definite clarification of the relationship between oral anticoagulants and menstrual blood loss should come from studies comparing flow prior to and after the instituting drug therapy.[66]

Alternative and surgical management of menorrhagia

Alternative treatments for menorrhagia

Alternative modalities can be used in the treatment of menorrhagia. These treatments are designed to reduce endometrial proliferation and subsequently menstrual flow. Danazol, an androgenic hormone, causes a hypoestrogenic environment by suppression of luteinizing hormone (LH) and follicular stimulating hormone (FSH). This leads to hypomenorrhea or amenorrhea. Many patients will experience side effects related to prolonged excessive androgen therapy, making long-term treatment unrealistic in patients with coagulation defects. Similarly, gonadotropin releasing hormone (GnRH) agonists, suppress FSH and LH by the reduction of GnRH secretion, causing hypoestrogenization and atrophy of the endometrium. The medication should not be given for long-term treatment, owing to osteoporosis that develops with its use. GnRH agonists are therefore impractical for long-term use in patients with coagulation defects.

The hormone releasing intrauterine device (IUD) has been used in patients with menorrhagia. IUDs containing progesterone and progestin are used for contraception and will reduce bleeding. This occurs from decidualization and atrophy of the endometrial glands. Blood loss is reduced by 40–50%. The literature has no reports of its specific use in women with coagulation defects and menorrhagia. On a theoretical basis, the progestin IUD should be efficacious.

Surgical treatment for menorrhagia

A surgical approach for control of menorrhagia in a patient with coagulopathy should be the last option. Surgery is indicated when medical and alternative management will not control menstrual bleeding and especially when excessive bleeding produces anemia. The definitive surgical treatment in women with menorrhagia is hysterectomy. Because hysterectomy will render the patient sterile, temporizing measures should always be attempted until the patient has finished her reproductive life. Hysterectomy was performed in 44% of type 2 and 3 VWD patients.[39] In type 1 VWD patients, 16% underwent hysterectomy, some for indications other than menorrhagia and others prior to diagnosis of VWD.[6] Often, hysterectomy is performed when patients have completed their childbearing and have either failed medical management or no longer want to continue medical therapy. With superior surgical management and a good working knowledge of the patient's coagulation defect, surgical treatment with hysterectomy is not an unreasonable choice for some patients.

With the advent of endometrial ablation, less invasive surgery is now available to the gynecologist for patients whose bleeding is not controlled with medical therapy and who are either not stable to undergo a hysterectomy or for those who prefer not to have a major surgery. Endometrial ablation can be accomplished with endometrial resection using both the laser and electrocautery. Endometrial ablation is also accomplished with cryoablation and thermal ablation. Depending on the technique and indications, successful reduction of flow or amenorrhea is seen in the majority of patients. Severe menorrhagia caused by factor VII deficiency has successfully been treated by thermal balloon ablation.[65] Emergency endometrial ablation was successfully performed in 3 patients with life-threatening uterine bleeding due to a variety of coagulopathies.[67]

Surgical considerations when operating on patients with a coagulation defect

In patients with coagulopathy undergoing any gynecological operations, hemorrhage during surgery can be a major complication. Minor operations, including dilatation and curettage, have also been associated with significant hemorrhage.[21] A collaborative team approach to management with the hematologist and anesthesiologist is essential. A clear understanding of the patient's coagulopathy is critical for preoperative planning and intraoperative and postoperative management. Levels of the appropriate clotting factors should be checked preoperatively. Depending on the type of coagulation defect, the surgical team must assemble the effective treatment modalities that will maintain hemostasis during and after surgery.

The most senior and experienced surgeon should perform surgery. Good surgical technique must be strictly adhered to, including suture ligation of significant bleeding vessels instead of electrocautery and the placement of surgical drains in operative fields for postoperative bleeding surveillance. If all clotting factors are maintained and excessive postoperative bleeding is encountered, the surgeon should also always consider that the bleeding is due to a surgical complication and not inadequate hemostasis.[68]

When operating on a VWD patient, the surgeon should make an assessment of the patient's response to DDAVP prior to surgery. In VWD patients undergoing elective surgery, the hemostatic response to DDAVP was 91% in patients treated.[69] Preoperative treatment with intravenous DDAVP is recommended. Postoperatively, continued intravenous DDAVP is appropriate for major surgical cases and intranasal DDAVP for minor surgery. Treatment should continue for at least 2 days in the postoperative period or longer until complete healing has occurred. Postoperative serum sodium levels should be followed so the physician can be alert to the development of hyponatremia that is occasionally associated with DDAVP.[70]

Approximately 10% of VWD patients fail to achieve minimal therapeutic response to DDAVP.[70] Replacement of deficient clotting factors during surgery is the mainstay of management of patients with VWD who do not respond to DDAVP. Fresh frozen plasma contains both factor VIII and VWF, but in small concentrations. Large amounts of FFP are needed to maintain hemostasis. When necessary, cryoprecipitate can be given because it contains higher concentrations of factor VIII and VWF, but is not preferable owing to the risk of occult virus transmission. In a study of VWD patients who were unresponsive to DDAVP, factor VIII concentrates and cryoprecipitate were given prophylactically to those undergoing surgery. Surgical hemostasis was satisfactory to excellent in 75 of 76 cases. In this report, factor VIII concentrates were subjectively as efficacious as cryoprecipitate.[71] The introduction of virucidal methods used in factor VIII concentrates make this treatment preferable to cryoprecipitate.[72] Replacement therapy with highly purified, virus inactivated factor VIII/VWF concentrate was effective in 93% of VWD patients undergoing surgery.[73] Humate-P and Alphanate are two commercial concentrates that contain VWF and factor VIII. These concentrates provided adequate hemostasis for invasive and surgical procedures.[74] Dosing recommendations are dependent on the procedure performed. Intraoperatively and postoperatively, factor VIII activity should be monitored daily. Factor VIII is a good predictor of surgical hemostasis.[75] For major surgery, trough factor VIII target levels should be >50% of normal levels. These should be maintained for 5–10 days, until healing is complete. For minor surgery, trough target levels should remain at >30% of normal until healing is complete in 2–4 days. Very high factor VIII levels should be avoided to prevent thromboembolic complications.[76]

Patients with platelet function disorders should be treated with DDAVP in the immediate preoperative and postoperative period. If bleeding is encountered, transfusion with normal platelets, cryoprecipitate and administration of corticosteroids are all acceptable treatment protocols in specific situations.[56]

To achieve acceptable surgical outcomes in patients with coagulation defects, the surgeon and collaborating physicians must have a superior working knowledge of the patient's condition, a preoperative treatment plan for dealing with intraoperative bleeding complications, and careful postoperative assessment of hemostasis and observation for bleeding.

REFERENCES

1 Hallberg, L., Hogdahl, A. M., Nilsson, L., *et al.* Menstrual blood loss – a population study. Variation at different ages and attempts to define normality. *Acta Obstet. Gynecol. Scand.*, 1966; **45**: 320–51.

2 Oehler, M. K., Rees, M. C. Menorrhagia: an update. *Acta Obstet. Gynecol. Scand.*, 2003; **82**: 405–22.

3 van Eijkeren, M. A., Christianens, G. C., Sixma, J. J., *et al.* Menorrhagia: A review. *Obstet. Gynecol. Surv.*, 1989; **44**: 421.

4 Edlund, M., Bolmback, M., von Schoultz, B., *et al.* On the value of menorrhagia as a predictor for coagulation disorders. *Am. J. Hematol.*, 1996; **53**: 234–8.

5 Kadir, R. A., Sabin, C. A., Pollard, D., *et al.* Quality of life during menstruation in patients with inherited bleeding disorders. *Haemophilia*, 1998; **4**: 836–41.

6 Kouides, P. A., Phatak, P. D., Burkart, P., *et al.* Gynaecological and obstetrical morbidity in women with type I von Willebrand disease: results of a patient survey. *Haemophilia*, 2000; **6**: 643–8.

7 Markee, J. E. Menstruation in intraocular endometrial transplants in the Rhesus monkey. *Contrib. Embryol.*, 1940; **28**: 221–308.

8 Bartelmez, G. W. Histological studies on the menstruating mucous membrane of the human uterus. *Contrib. Embryol.*, 1933; **24**: 141–86.

9 Fauvel, F., Grant, M. E., Legrand, Y. J., *et al.* Interaction of blood platelets with a microfibrillar extract from adult bovine aorta: requirement for von Willebrand factor. *Proc. Natl. Acad. Sci. USA*, 1983; **80**: 551–4.

10 Christianes, G. C., Sixma, J. J., Haspels, A. A. Morphology of haemostasis in menstrual endometrium. *Br. J. Obstet. Gynaecol.*, 1980; **87**: 425–39.

11 Fraser, I. S., McCarron, G., Markham, R. A preliminary study of factors influencing perception of menstrual blood loss volume. *Am. J. Obstet. Gynecol.*, 1984; **149**: 788–93.

12 Higham, J. M., O'Brien, P. M., Shaw, R. W. Assessment of menstrual blood loss using a pictorial chart. *Br. J. Obstet. Gynaecol.*, 1990; **97**: 734–9.

13 Reid, P. C., Coker, A., Coltart, R. Assessment of menstrual blood loss using a pictorial chart: a validation study. *Br. J. Obstet. Gynaecol.*, 2000; **107**: 320–2.

14 Wyatt, K. M., Dimmock, P. W., Walker, T. J., *et al.* Determination of total menstrual blood loss. *Fertil. Steril.*, 2001; **76**: 125–31.

15 Dilley, A., Drews, C., Lally, C., *et al.* A survey of gynecologists concerning menorrhagia: perceptions of bleeding disorders as a possible cause. *J. Womens Health Gend. Based Med.*, 2002; **11**: 39–44.

16 Kadir, R. A., Aledort, L. M. Obstetrical and gynaecological bleeding: a common presenting symptom. *Clin. Lab. Haematol.*, 2000; **22** (Suppl. 1): 12–6; discussion, 30–2.

17 Ellis, M. H., Beyth, Y. Abnormal vaginal bleeding in adolescence as the presenting symptom of a bleeding diathesis. *J. Pediatr. Adolesc. Gynecol.*, 1999; **12**: 127–31.

18 Werner, E. J., Broxson, E. H., Tucker, E. L., *et al.* Prevalence of von Willebrand disease in children: a multiethnic study. *J. Pediatr.*, 1993; **123**: 893–8.

19 Rodeghiero, F., Castaman, G., Dini, E. Epidemiological investigation of the prevalence of von Willebrand's disease. *Blood*, 1987; **69**: 454–9.

20 Ruggeri, Z. M. Mechanisms initiating platelet thrombus formation. *Thromb. Haemost.*, 1997; **78**: 611–16. Erratum in: *Thromb. Haemost.*, 1997; **78**: 1304.

21 Kadir, R. A., Economides, D. L., Sabin, C. A., *et al.* Assessment of menstrual blood loss and gynaecological problems in patients with inherited bleeding disorders. *Haemophilia*, 1999; **5**: 40–8.

22 Goodman-Gruen, D., Hollenbach, K. The prevalence of von Willebrand disease in women with abnormal uterine bleeding. *J. Womens Health Gend. Based Med.*, 2001; **10**: 677–80.

23 Shankar, M., Lee, C. A., Sabin, C. A., *et al.* Von Willebrand disease in women with menorrhagia: a systematic review. *Br. J. Obstet. Gynaecol.*, 2004; **111**: 734–40.

24 Federici, A. B., Mannucci, P. M. Advances in the genetics and treatment of von Willebrand disease. *Curr. Opin. Pediatr.*, 2002; **14**: 23–33.

25 Kadir, R. A., Economides, D. L., Sabin, C. A., *et al.* Variations in coagulation factors in women: effects of age, ethnicity, menstrual cycle and combined oral contraceptive. *Thromb. Haemost.*, 1999; **82**: 1456–61.

26 Edlund, M., Blomback, M., von Schoultz, B., *et al.* On the value of menorrhagia as a predictor for coagulation disorders. *Am. J. Hematol.*, 1996; **53**: 234–8.

27 Onundarson, P. T., Gudmundsdottir, B. R., Arnfinnsdottir, A. V., *et al.* Von Willebrand factor does not vary during normal menstrual cycle. *Thromb. Haemost.*, 2001; **85**(1): 183–4.

28 Werner, E. J., Abshire, T. C., Giroux, D. S., *et al.* Relative value of diagnostic studies for von Willebrand disease. *J. Pediatr.*, 1992; **121**: 34–8.

29 Coccia, M. R., Barnes, H. V. Hypothyroidism and acquired von Willebrand disease. *J. Adolesc. Health*, 1991; **12**: 152–4.

30 Blesing, N. E., Hambley, H., McDonald, G. A. Acquired von Willebrand's disease and hypothyroidism: report of a case presenting with menorrhagia. *Postgrad. Med. J.*, 1990; **66**: 474–6.

31 Mannucci, P. M. Desmopressin (DDAVP) in the treatment of bleeding disorders: the first 20 years. *Blood*, 1997; **90**: 2515–21.

32 Rodeghiero, F., Castaman, G., Mannucci, P. M. Prospective multicenter study on subcutaneous concentrated desmopressin for home treatment of patients with von Willebrand disease and mild or moderate hemophilia A. *Thromb. Haemost.*, 1996; **76**(5): 692–6.

33 Siegel, J. E., Kouides, P. A. Menorrhagia from a haematologist's point of view. Part II: management. *Haemophilia*, 2002: **8**: 339–47.

34 Federici, A. B., Mazurier, C., Berntorp, E., *et al.* Biologic response to desmopressin in patients with severe type 1 and type 2 von Willebrand disease: results of a multicenter European study. *Blood*, 2004; **103**: 2032–8.

35 Castaman, G., Lattuada, A., Mannucci, P. M., *et al.* Factor VIII: C increases after desmopressin in a subgroup of patients with autosomal recessive severe von Willebrand disease. *Br. J. Haematol.*, 1995; **89**: 147–51.

36 Alperin, J. B. Estrogens and surgery in women with von Willebrand's disease. *Am. J. Med.*, 1982; **73**: 367–71.

37 David, J. L., Gaspard, U. J., Gillain, D., *et al.* Hemostasis profile in women taking low-dose oral contraceptives. *Am. J. Obstet. Gynecol.*, 1990; **163**: 420–3.

38 Beller, F. K., Ebert, C. Effects of oral contraceptives on blood coagulation. A review. *Obstet. Gynecol. Surv.*, 1985; **40**(7): 425–36.

39 Foster, P. A. The reproductive health of women with von Willebrand disease unresponsive to DDAVP: results of an international survey. On behalf of the Subcommittee on von Willebrand Factor of the Scientific and Standardization Committee of the ISTH. *Thromb. Haemost.*, 1995; **74**: 784–90.

40 Cederblad, G., Hahn, L., Korsan-Bengtsen, K., *et al.* Variations in blood coagulation, fibrinolysis, platelet function and various plasma proteins during the menstrual cycle. *Haemostasis*, 1977; **6**: 294–302.

41 Ong, Y. L., Hull, D. R., Mayne, E. E. Menorrhagia in von Willebrand disease successfully treated with single daily dose tranexamic acid. *Haemophilia*, 1998; **4**: 63–5.

42 Mohri, H. High dose of tranexamic acid for treatment of severe menorrhagia in patients with von Willebrand disease. *J. Thromb. Thrombolysis*, 2002; **14**: 255–7.

43 Dunn, C. J., Goa, K. L. Tranexamic acid: a review of its use in surgery and other indications. *Drugs*, 1999; **57**: 1005–32.

44 Vermylen, J., Verhaegen-Declercq, M. L., Verstraete, M., *et al.* A double blind study of the effect of tranexamic acid in essential menorrhagia. *Thromb. Diath. Haemorrh.*, 1968; **20**: 583–7.

45 Bonnar, J., Sheppard, B. L. Treatment of menorrhagia during menstruation: randomised controlled trial of ethamsylate, mefenamic acid, and tranexamic acid. *BMJ*, 1996; **313**: 579–82.

46 van Eijkeren, M. A., Christiaens, G. C., Scholten, P. C., *et al.* Menorrhagia. Current drug treatment concepts. *Drugs*, 1992; **43**: 201–9.

47 Ong, Y. L., Hull, D. R., Mayne, E. E. Menorrhagia in von Willebrand disease successfully treated with single daily dose tranexamic acid. *Haemophilia*, 1998; **4**: 63–5.

48 Mehta, B. C., Parekh, D. S. Epsilon-amino-caproic acid in the treatment of menorrhagia. *J. Postgrad. Med.*, 1977; **23**: 121–3.

49 Nitu-Whalley, I. C., Lee, C. A. Acquired von Willebrand syndrome – report of 10 cases and review of the literature. *Haemophilia*, 1999; **5**: 318–26.

50 Federici, A. B., Rand, J. H., Bucciarelli, P., *et al.* Acquired von Willebrand syndrome: data from an international registry. *Thromb. Haemost.*, 2000; **84**: 345–9.

51 Garewal, G., Ahluwalia, J. Platelet function disorders. *Indian J. Pediatr.*, 2003; **70**: 983–7.

52 Saxena, R., Gupta, M., Gupta, P. K., *et al.* Inherited bleeding disorders in Indian women with menorrhagia. *Haemophilia*, 2003; **9**: 193–6.

53 Philipp, C. S., Dilley, A., Miller, C. H., *et al.* Platelet functional defects in women with unexplained menorrhagia. *J. Thromb. Haemost.*, 2003; **1**: 477–84.

54 Markovitch, O., Ellis, M., Holzinger, M., *et al.* Severe juvenile vaginal bleeding due to Glanzmann's thrombasthenia: case report and review of the literature. *Am. J. Hematol.*, 1998; **57**: 225–7.

55 DiMichele, D. M., Hathaway, W. E. Use of DDAVP in inherited and acquired platelet dysfunction. *Am. J. Hematol.*, 1990; **33**: 39–45.

56 Bennett, J. S. Disorders of platelet function: evaluation and treatment. *Cleve. Clin. J. Med.*, 1991; **58**: 413–17.

57 Bevan, J. A., Maloney, K. W., Hillery, C. A., *et al.* Bleeding disorders: A common cause of menorrhagia in adolescents. *J. Pediatr.*, 2001; **138**: 856–61.

58 Smith, Y. R., Quint, E. H., Hertzberg, R. B. Menorrhagia in adolescents requiring hospitalization. *J. Pediatr. Adolesc. Gynecol.*, 1998; **11**: 13–15.

59 Tomer, A., Schreiber, A. D., McMillan, R., *et al.* Menstrual cyclic thrombocytopenia. *Br. J. Haematol.*, 1989; **71**: 519–24.

60 Bolton-Maggs, P. H., Patterson, D. A., Wensley, R. T., *et al.* Definition of the bleeding tendency in factor XI-deficient kindreds – a clinical and laboratory study. *Thromb. Haemost.*, 1995; **73**: 194–202.

61 Kadir, R. A., Economides, D. L., Lee, C. A. Factor XI deficiency in women. *Am. J. Hematol.*, 1999; **60**: 48–54.

62 Sapuri, M., Amoa, A. B., Kariwiga, G., *et al.* A case of factor V deficiency presenting as menorrhagia. *P. N. G. Med. J.*, 1997; **40**: 92–5.

63 Bennett, K., Daley, M. L., Pike, C. Factor V deficiency and menstruation: a gynecologic challenge. *Obstet. Gynecol.*, 1997; **89**: 839–40.

64 White, B., O'Connor, H., Smith, O. P. Successful use of recombinant VIIa (Novoseven) and endometrial ablation in a patient with intractable menorrhagia secondary to FVII deficiency. *Blood Coagul. Fibrinolysis* 2000; **11**: 155–7.

65 Fasouliotis, S. J., Shushan, A. Severe menorrhagia due to factor VII deficiency successfully treated by thermal balloon endometrial ablation. *J. Am. Assoc. Gynecol. Laparosc.*, 2003; **10**: 116–18.

66 van Eijkeren, M. A., Christiaens, G. C., Haspels, A. A., *et al.* Measured menstrual blood loss in women with a bleeding disorder or using oral anticoagulant therapy. *Am. J. Obstet. Gynecol.*, 1990; **162**: 1261–3.

67 Milad, M. P., Valle, R. F. Emergency endometrial ablation for life-threatening uterine bleeding as a result of a coagulopathy. *J. Am. Assoc. Gynecol. Laparosc.*, 1998; **5**: 301–3.

68 Lee, C. A. Women and inherited bleeding disorders: menstrual issues. *Semin. Hematol.*, 1999; **36**: 21–7.

69 Nitu-Whalley, I. C., Griffioen, A., Harrington, C., *et al.* Retrospective review of the management of elective surgery with desmopressin and clotting factor concentrates in patients with von Willebrand disease. *Am. J. Hematol.*, 2001; **66**: 280–4.

70 Kouides, P. A. Obstetric and gynaecological aspects of von Willebrand disease. *Best Pract. Res. Clin. Haematol.*, 2001; **14**: 381–99.

71 Foster, P. A. A perspective on the use of FVIII concentrates and cryoprecipitate prophylactically in surgery or therapeutically in severe bleeds in patients with von Willebrand disease unresponsive to DDAVP: results of an international survey. On behalf of the Subcommittee on von Willebrand Factor of the Scientific and Standardization Committee of the ISTH. *Thromb. Haemost.*, 1995; **74**: 1370–8.

72 Federici, A. B., Mannucci, P. M. Optimizing therapy with factor VIII/von Willebrand factor concentrates in von Willebrand disease. *Haemophilia.*, 1998; **4** (Suppl. 3): 7–10.

73 Mannucci, P. M. Treatment of von Willebrand's Disease. *N. Engl. J. Med.*, 2004; **351**: 683–94.

74 Mannucci, P. M., Chediak, J., Hanna, W., *et al.* Treatment of von Willebrand disease with a high-purity factor VIII/von Willebrand factor concentrate: a prospective, multicenter study. *Blood*, 2002; **99**: 450–6.

75 Biggs, R., Matthews, J. M. The treatment of haemorrhage in von Willebrand's disease and the blood level of factor VIII (AHG). *Br. J. Haematol.*, 1963; **9**: 203–14.

76 Federici, A. B., Baudo, F., Caracciolo, C., *et al.* Clinical efficacy of highly purified, doubly virus-inactivated factor VIII/von Willebrand factor concentrate (Fanhdi) in the treatment of von Willebrand disease: a retrospective clinical study. *Haemophilia*, 2002; **8**: 761–7.

Index